THE CALORIEKING®
Calorie, Fat & Carbohy[illegible]

Contents

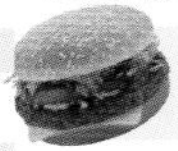

BONUS DIET GUIDES & COUNTERS

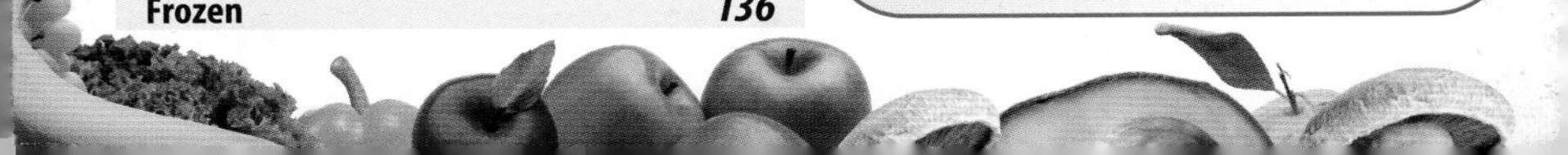

Weight Control Tips

✓ Eat & Drink Sensibly

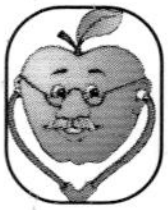

- **Eat 2-3 sensible meals daily,** ideally within an 8-10 hour window. Fast for the remaining 14-16 hours (except for water, coffee/tea without milk or sugar).
- **Eat mainly wholefoods** with adequate protein, healthy fats, and ample lower starch vegetables, beans, lentils and nuts.
- **Avoid highly processed foods** with seed oils, refined grains/flour and added sugar (particularly soda and candy).
- **Quench your thirst with water.**

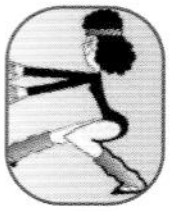

✓ Exercise Daily

- Aim for at least 30 minutes daily – even in 5-10 minute lots. For motivation, find an exercise buddy, personal trainer or join a gym. *(Extra Notes ~ Page 12)*

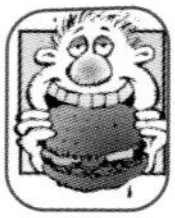

✓ Reshape Eating Behaviors

- **Keep a Food & Exercise Journal.** A journal helps you see exactly what you eat and drink, and how much you exercise. An excellent motivator and proven weight loss aid.

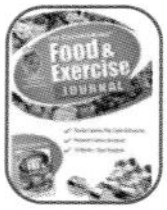

- **Also focus on social and emotional situations** that may trigger compulsive eating. *(Extra Notes ~ Page 14)*

✓ Arrange Moral Support

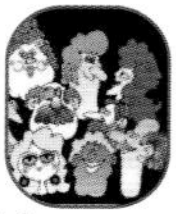

- Gain the support of workmates, family and friends.
- Get extra professional help and coaching, from your doctor, dietitian/nutritionist, psychologist, personal trainer, or slimming group.

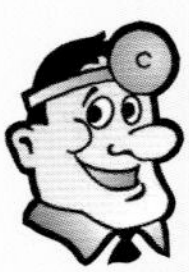

DOCTOR CHECK-UP

Ask your doctor to check your blood pressure, blood sugar and fats levels – even your insulin levels.

Dont wait to develop insulin resistance, prediabetes, or a fatty liver!

HEALTHY WEIGHTS ~ MEN & WOMEN ~ (Over 18 Years)

Based on weights with least risk of disease or death from heart disease, diabetes, stroke and cancer.

Based on Body Mass Index of 20-25

BMI calculated as: $\frac{\text{Weight (kg)}}{\text{Height (m)}^2}$

Height (No Shoes) Ft Ins		Healthy Weight Range (Pounds)
4'7"	~	86-108
4'8"	~	88-110
4'9"	~	92-114
4'10"	~	97-121
4'11"	~	99-123
5'0"	~	101-127
5'1"	~	105-132
5'2"	~	110-136
5'3"	~	112-140
5'4"	~	114-145
5'5"	~	119-149
5'6"	~	123-156
5'7"	~	127-158
5'8"	~	129-162
5'9"	~	134-167
5'10"	~	138-173
5'11"	~	143-178
6'0"	~	145-182
6'1"	~	149-187
6'2"	~	156-193
6'3"	~	158-198
6'4"	~	162-202
6'5"	~	170-211
6'6"	~	172-215
6'7"	~	175-220

Body Fat Distribution & Health

Moderate amounts of body fat do not compromise health. However, excess fat above the hips carries a far greater health risk than fat on or below the hips - better to be a 'pear-shape' than an 'apple-shape'.

Abdominal obesity greatly increases the risk of developing diabetes, heart disease, high blood fats, hypertension, stroke, sleep apnea, arthritis, fatty liver, and some cancers. So-called 'cellulite' carries no extra health risk.

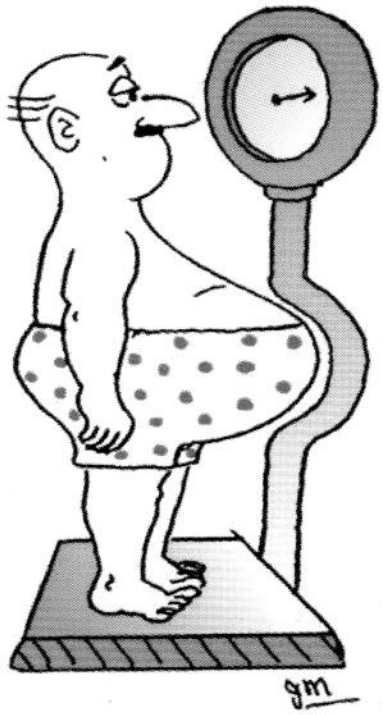

Abdominal obesity greatly increases the risk of ill-health and earlier death.

Waist Circumference directly reflects the increased health risk of abdominal obesity. Waist size associated with a higher health risk:

Men ~ Over 40 inches **Women** ~ Over 35 inches

Body Mass Index (BMI)

BMI is a general (but not specific) indicator of body fatness. Although BMI alone is not diagnostic, the higher the BMI, the greater the health risk of developing diabetes, high blood pressure and heart disease. BMI does not apply to heavily muscled persons. BMI is used in a different way for children.

Check Your BMI: **Find your height (no shoes) - look across the row to the weight nearest your own. Then track down to BMI.**

Ht	WEIGHT (LBS) ~ ADULTS													
5'1"	100	106	111	116	122	127	132	137	143	148	153	158	185	211
5'2"	104	109	115	120	126	131	136	142	147	153	158	164	191	218
5'3"	107	113	118	124	130	135	141	146	152	158	163	169	197	225
5'4"	110	116	122	128	134	140	145	151	157	163	169	174	204	232
5'5"	114	120	126	132	138	144	150	156	162	168	174	180	210	240
5'6"	118	124	130	136	142	148	155	161	167	173	179	186	216	247
5'7"	121	127	134	140	146	153	159	166	172	178	185	191	223	255
5'8"	125	131	138	144	151	158	164	171	177	184	190	197	230	262
5'9"	128	135	142	149	155	162	169	176	182	189	196	206	236	270
5'10"	132	139	146	153	160	167	174	181	188	195	202	207	243	278
5'11"	136	143	150	157	165	172	179	186	193	200	208	215	250	286
6'0"	140	147	154	162	169	177	184	191	199	206	213	221	258	294
6'1"	144	151	159	166	174	182	189	197	204	212	219	227	265	302
6'2"	148	155	163	171	179	186	194	202	210	218	225	233	272	311
6'3"	152	160	168	176	184	192	200	208	216	224	232	240	279	319
6'4"	156	164	172	180	189	197	205	213	221	230	238	246	287	328
BMI	19	20	21	22	23	24	25	26	27	28	29	30	35	40

BMI Classification:

BMI Below 19
Underweight

BMI 19-24.9
Healthy Weight (Low Health Risk)

BMI 25-29.9
Overweight (Moderate Health Risk)

BMI 30-40
Obese (High Health Risk)

BMI Over 40
Morbid Obesity (Very High Risk)

Interactive BMI Calculator www.calorieking.com

Calories & Weight Loss

Calories in Food

Calories in food are derived from protein, fat and carbohydrate. Alcohol also provides calories. Vitamins, minerals and water provide no calories.

Calorie Values Per Gram

Fat/Oil	~ 9 Calories
Carbohydrate	~ 4 Calories
Protein	~ 4 Calories
Alcohol	~ 7 Calories

Note that fats have over double the calories of protein and carbohydrate. The higher the fat content of food, the higher the calories.

Sample Calculation

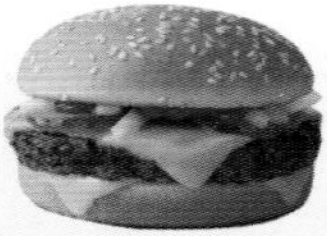

QUARTER POUNDER® WITH CHEESE has 520 calories derived from:

26g Fat (x 9 cals/gram)	= 234
42g Carbohyd.(x 4 cals/gram)	= 168
30g Protein (x 4 cals/gram)	= 120
Total Calories (rounded)	= 520

Calorie Levels for Weight Loss

Start with a calorie-controlled diet that allows a moderate weight loss of ½ - 1 pound per week. Weight loss is usually much greater in the first few weeks due to extra fluid losses.

Note: It is better to increase exercise rather than lessen food calories too drastically.

Suggested Calories for Weight Loss

Women:	Non-active	1000 - 1200
	Active	1200 - 1500
Men:	Non-active	1200 - 1500
	Active	1500 - 1800
Teenagers:		1200 - 1800

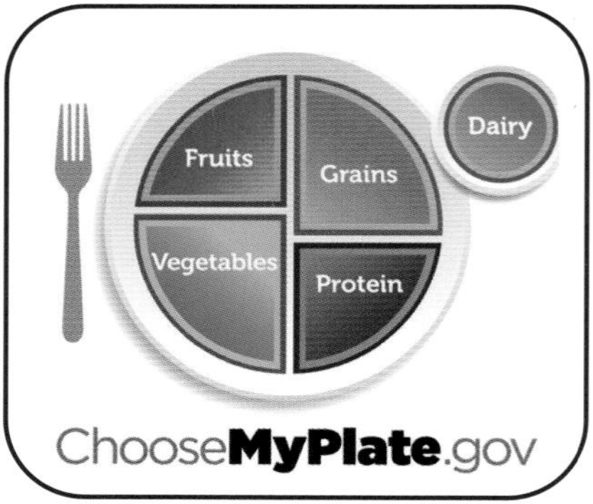

The MyPlate symbol represents the recommended proportion of foods from each food group. It focuses on the importance of making smart food choices in every food group, every day. Daily physical activity is also important. ***(More info: www.ChooseMyPlate.gov)***

Examples of Single Serving Sizes

Grains **(Eat 3-4 servings per day):**

- 1 slice wholegrain bread (1 oz)
- ½ bun, small bagel or English muffin
- 4 small crackers or 1 tortilla
- 1 oz ready-to-eat wholegrain cereal
- ½ cup cooked cereal, rice or pasta

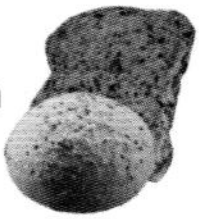

Vegetables **(Eat 3-5 servings per day):**

- 1 cup raw leafy vegetables
- 1½ cups raw chopped vegetables
- ½ cup cooked vegetables
- ½ - ¾ cup vegetable juice

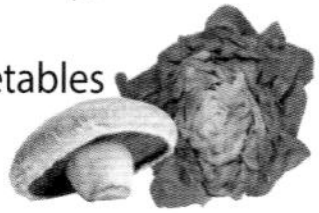

Fruit **(Eat 2-3 servings per day):**

- 1 medium apple, orange, banana
- ½ cup canned fruit (in own juice)
- ¼ cup dried fruit
- ½ cup fruit juice (unsweetened)
- ¼ medium avocado

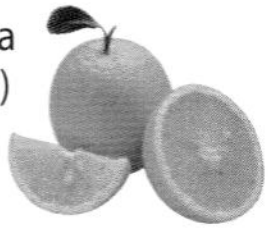

Protein **(2-3 servings per day):**

- 2-3 oz (cooked) meat/poultry/fish
- 2 eggs **or** 6 oz tofu **or** ¼ cup nuts
- 1 cup (cooked) dried beans **or** chickpeas

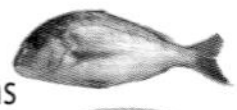

Dairy **(2-3 servings per day):**

- 1 cup (8 fl.oz) milk/soy (enriched)/yogurt
- 1½ oz cheese or ½ cup cottage cheese

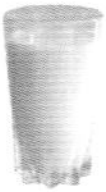

Portion Size Counts!

Food portion size is critical to controlling calorie intake for weight control.

Supersized food servings have become more common when eating out and in the home. This can mean a day's worth of calories being consumed in one meal; or a snack being equivalent to a full meal.

For example, some giant size bakery items such as muffins and sweet buns can have more calories, fat and carbs than a large burger – as shown below.

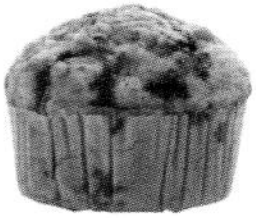

Hostess Double Choc Mega Muffin (5.5 oz):
580 calories, 33g fat, 71g carbs

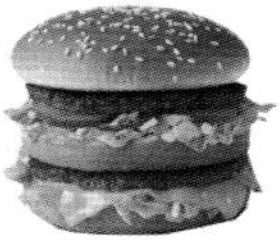

McDonald's Big Mac:
550 calories, 30g fat, 45g carbs

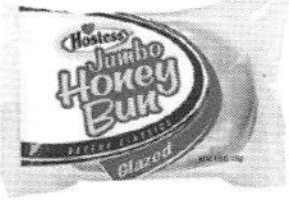

Hostess Jumbo Honey Bun (4.75 oz):
560 calories, 29g fat, 68g carbs

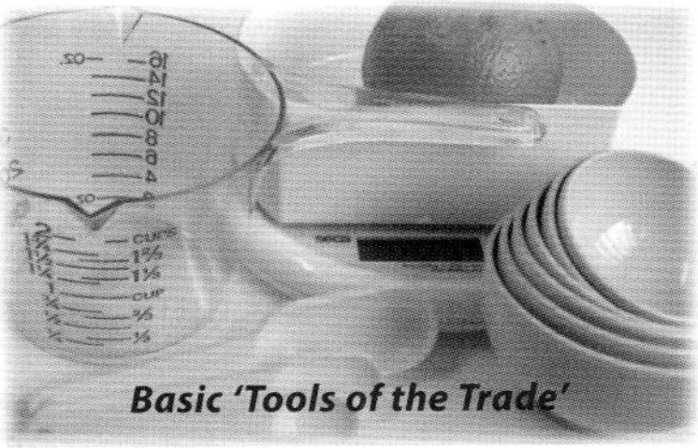

Basic 'Tools of the Trade'

CALORIEKING PORTION WATCH

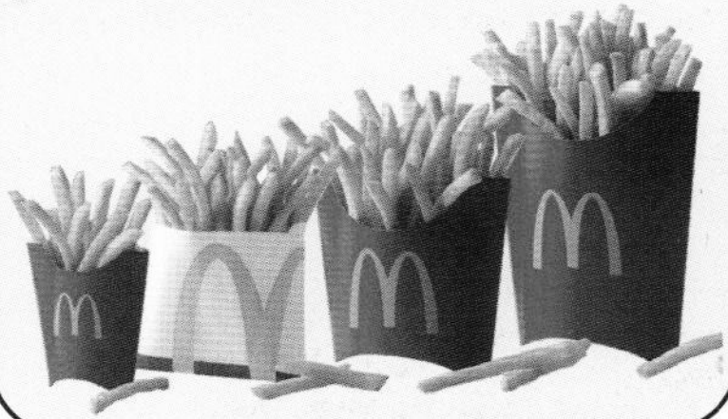

Fries	Cal	Fat	Carb
Kids	110	5	15
Small	220	10	29
Medium	320	15	43
Large	490	23	66

Weigh and Measure Your Portions

It is easy to underestimate portion size of foods and drinks, and unwittingly consume excess calories – even if the fat content is low or even zero!

To more accurately estimate portion size of different foods, weigh and measure your food with food scales, measuring spoons and cups. Better control of calories will result.

Allow for Extra Calories in Packaged Food

The actual weight of packaged foods is usually 5-10% more than the label net weight (the minimum legal weight) – and in some cases up to 50% more (particularly in-store bakery items such as muffins). However, manufacturers calculate the calories based on the net weight. For actual calories, weigh the product and calculate the extra calories.

CALORIEKING PORTION WATCH

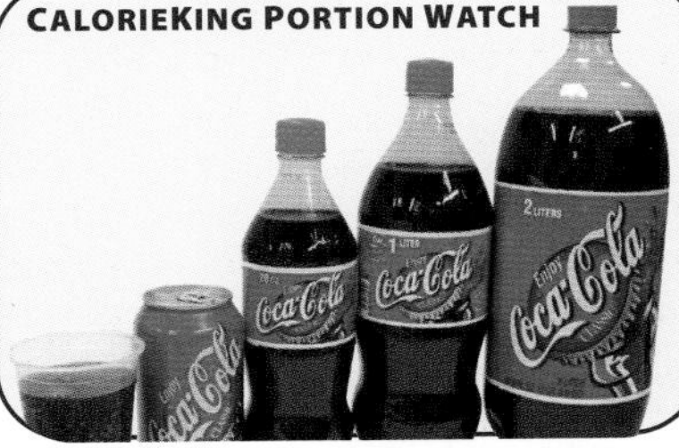

Cola	Cal	Fat	Carb
8 fl.oz Cup	100	0	25
12 fl.oz Can	150	0	37
20 fl.oz Bottle	250	0	63
1 Liter Bottle	400	0	100
2 Liter Bottle	800	0	200

► Fats in the diet are essential for good health.

Examples of fats' roles in the body include:

- important concentrated fuel source of energy for all cells
- major storage form of energy in the body
- provides structure and functionality to all body cell membranes
- important component of brain tissues
- helps the absorption of nutrients such as fat-soluble vitamins
- satisfies hunger more readily than fat-free foods
- produce important hormones
- protects your organs and keeps the body warm

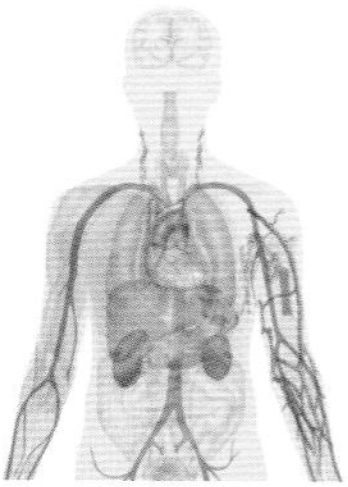

Healthy dietary fats are essential for good health.

Dietary fats and oils have over double the calories (9 calories per gram) of carbohydrates or proteins (4 calories per gram).

Low Fat vs Higher Fat Diets:

While low-fat diets have generally been recommended for weight control in past decades, they have not been successful in reducing the incidence of obesity, In fact, obesity rates have been steadily increasing. **Some problems with low-fat diets include:**

- **Carbohydrates take the place of fats,** so the diet becomes a 'low-fat, high-carbohydrate' diet. This can lead to greater difficulty in losing weight from adipose fatty tissue. When those extra carbohydrates are largely refined ones, this can also result in excessive fat triglycerides in the blood (a risk factor for heart disease), unstable blood sugar levels and a fatty liver leading to insulin resistance and Type 2 diabetes.
- **Low-fat diets do not generally satisfy the hunger** that often results from reduced calories.

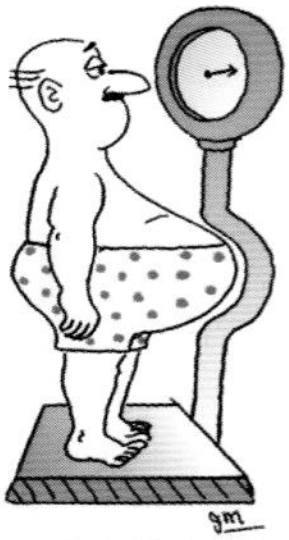

Low-fat diets have not been successful in reducing obesity.

Subsequently, research has shown **a diet lower in carbohydrate and higher in fat to be more effective for weight loss**. It is more sustainable and better satisfies hunger. Additionally, there are generally improvements in blood glucose levels, blood triglyceride fats and 'good' HDL-cholesterol levels – which in turn lowers the risk of heart disease and diabetes. This is in the context of sensible portion sizes, and incorporating healthy, high-quality foods.

The Mediterranean Diet is often used as a good example of healthy eating. It includes moderate amounts of meat, regular fish meals, generous lower starch vegetables, fruit, legumes, whole-grains, extra-virgin olive oil, nuts, seeds and herbs. Other important aspects include avoidance of highly processed foods as well as adequate physical activity, clean air, sunshine and sleep.

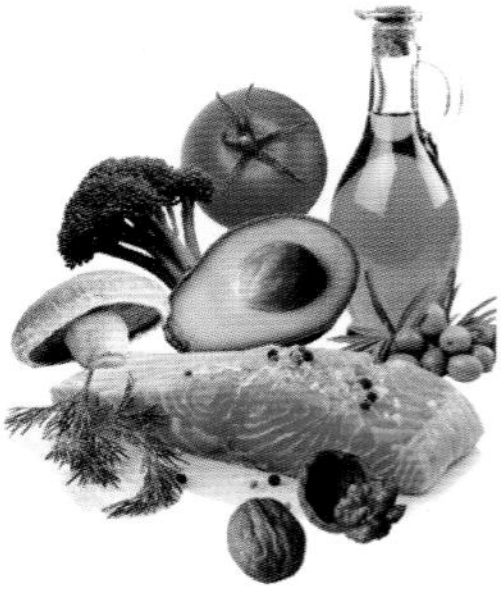

Mediterranean Diet food examples

Of course, there is no one perfect or 'one-size-fits-all' diet that suits all people. Rather, a personalized diet should also consider the person's food philosophy, food allergies / sensitivities, medical condition, medications and genetic predisposition.

Healthy Fats vs Unhealthy Fats

There are three main types of fat in food: saturated fats, monounsaturated fats, and polyunsaturated fats.

Different foods generally have a mixture of all three types with animal fats being rich in saturated fats, and plant foods generally higher in mono- and polyunsaturated fats. *(Extra notes on fats and heart health ~ See page 206)*

When consumed as part of wholefoods (unprocessed), these fats have important functions in maintaining our health. Examples of foods with healthy fats include avocados, olives, nuts, seeds, cheese, milk, fish, meats and eggs.

However, when fats and oils are isolated from their naturally occurring wholefood source, their physico-chemical properties can be altered; and there is the potential for them to affect our health. Ultraprocessing of foods can destroy the accompanying vitamins and antioxidants that would normally protect the fats or oils from oxidation.

Such is the case with so-called 'seed oils' or 'industrial vegetable oils' (such as corn, sunflower, safflower, soy bean and canola oils) which have a high omega-6 fatty acid content. Their polyunsaturated chemical structure is unstable and makes them more prone to oxidation – particularly when used in high-heat cooking

Oxidized fats can damage cellular components, cause inflammation and lead to metabolic dysfunction.

Oxidized fats can also adversely affect all body organs including the pancreas (insulin production), liver, brain, kidneys, eyes, lungs; and can even initiate inflammation of artery linings leading to atherosclerosis (by oxidation of lipoprotein carriers of cholesterol in the blood).

Researchers suggest that the 12-fold increase in consumption of these polyunsaturated seed oils over the last 100 years is largely responsible for the epidemics of obesity, insulin resistance, diabetes, heart disease, fatty liver and even many cancers.

Polyunsaturated omega-3 fats in oily fish, walnuts, hempseed, flaxseed and chia seed have an anti-inflammatory effect which can benefit many health conditions including heart health, insulin resistance, diabetes and brain health. Most Americans are deficient in omega-3 fats. *(Extra notes ~ page 263)*

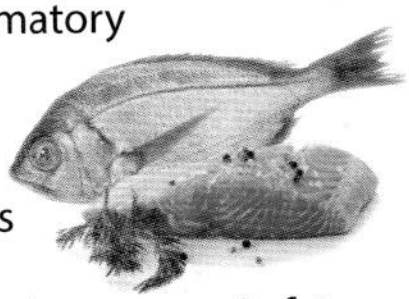

Monounsaturated oil such as extra-virgin olive oil is more stable and has protective antioxidants.

MCT oil (medium chain triglycerides) from coconut oil is also very stable and has some metabolic benefits.

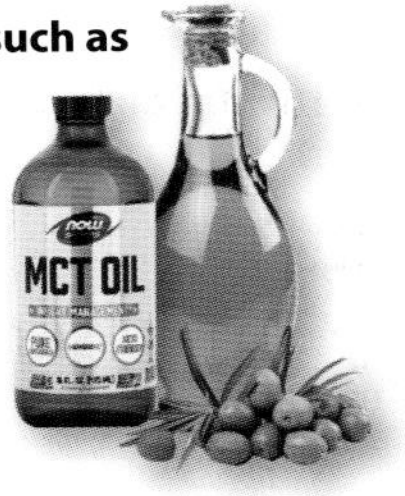

Vegetable seed oils are widely used in processed foods: Examples:

- spreads, dressings
- sauces, dips
- cakes, cookies, pastries
- fried snacks, snack bars
- vegetarian meat and milk alternatives
- fried foods
- cafe and restaurant foods.

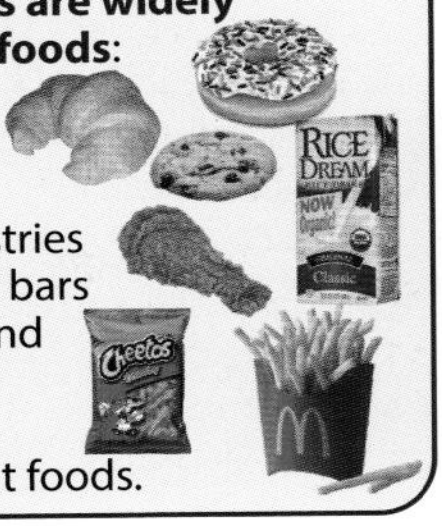

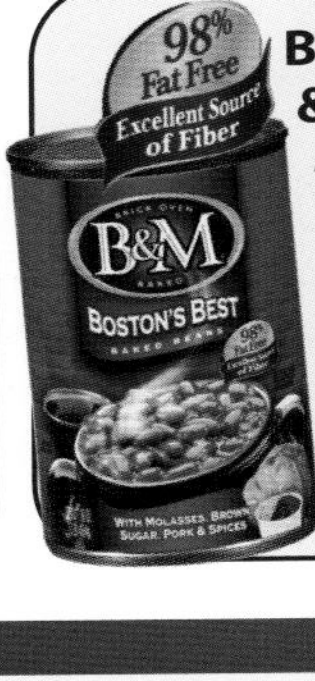

BEWARE OF LOW-FAT & FAT-FREE FOODS

They can be high in sugar!

This brand of baked beans hides 7 teaspoons of sugar (added) per 8 oz serving (½ of 16 oz can).

Carbohydrates ~ Friend or Foe?

Naturally-Friendly Carbs

Carbohydrate foods in their more natural wholefood forms (minimally processed) are essential to good health. They are the main source of fuel for the body, and also provide important vitamins, minerals, antioxidants and fiber.

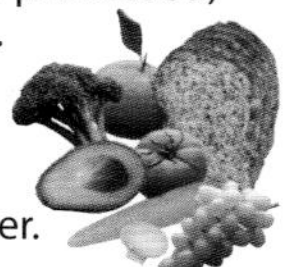

How Much Do We Need?

Most Americans consume excessive amounts of carbohydrate – particularly as refined white flour and sugar. This greatly increases the risk of obesity, high blood glucose levels, and insulin resistance – which can lead to Type 2 diabetes, fatty liver, heart disease and many other chronic diseases.

As such, many health authorities are now recommending a much lower carbohydrate intake – around 20-25% of total calories. *(See chart below)*

This lower carbohydrate intake still allows for adequate intake of fruit, vegetables and wholegrains in their wholefood forms.

The emphasis is on minimizing refined carbohydrates and sugar.

LOW CARBOHYDRATE DIET ~ DAILY AMOUNTS (Grams) ~

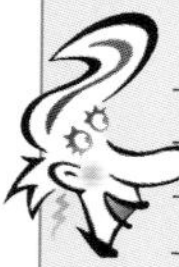

Calories		Carbohydrate
1200 Cals	~	60 - 75g
1600 Cals	~	80 - 100g
2000 Cals	~	100 - 125g
2400 Cals	~	120 - 150g

Note: The carbohydrate range for each calorie level corresponds to 20-25% of total calories.

Ketogenic diets generally contain 20-50 grams of carbohydrate (5-10% total calories). This diet is best planned and supervised by your doctor and dietitian – particularly if on medications to control blood glucose and/or thyroid hormone levels. (Dosage strength of medications may need to be adjusted.)

CARBOHYDRATE CONTENT OF SOME COMMON FOODS

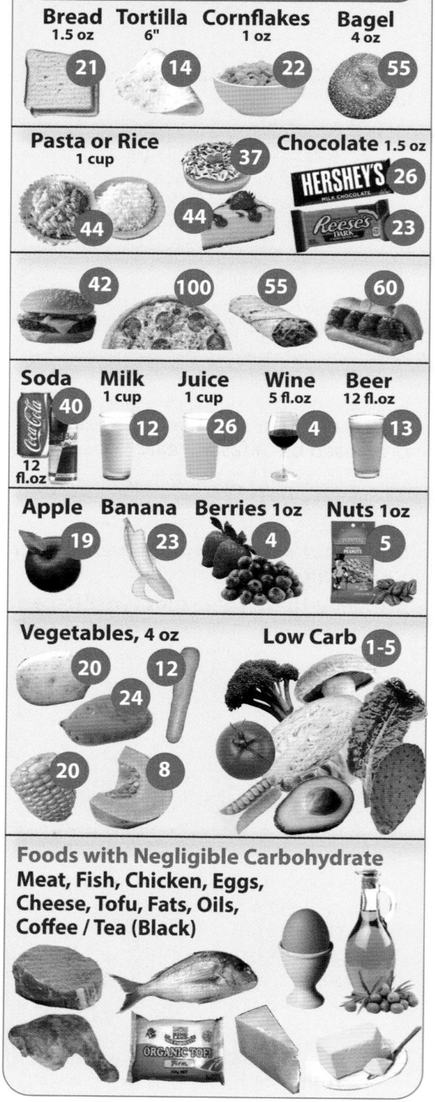
Bread 1.5 oz 21
Tortilla 6" 14
Cornflakes 1 oz 22
Bagel 4 oz 55
Pasta or Rice 1 cup 44
37
44
Chocolate 1.5 oz
HERSHEY'S 26
Reese's DARK 23
42
100
55
60
Soda 40
12 fl.oz
Milk 1 cup 12
Juice 1 cup 26
Wine 5 fl.oz 4
Beer 12 fl.oz 13
Apple 19
Banana 23
Berries 1oz 4
Nuts 1oz 5
Vegetables, 4 oz
20
12
24
20
8
Low Carb 1-5
Foods with Negligible Carbohydrate
Meat, Fish, Chicken, Eggs,
Cheese, Tofu, Fats, Oils,
Coffee / Tea (Black)
ORGANIC TOFU

- **Excess Sugar:**

  Many overweight, inactive people consume over 500 calories of refined sugars per day, either self-added or as part of food products. This is equivalent to over 30 level teaspoons. For context, just one 12-ounce can of soda contains 10 teaspoons of added sugar.

  Note: Naturally occurring sugars in fruits, vegetables and milk are fine when consumed in normal recommended amounts. These foods are also rich in other nutrients.

  Refined sugar is referred to as having **'empty calories'**. Sugar supplies calories but negligible nutrients and no fiber.

- **Most sugar in our diet is 'hidden'** in processed foods such as soft drinks, fruit drinks, candy, cookies, cake, jam, sauces, ice cream, desserts, canned foods, and processed breakfast cereals.

For serious weight control, as well as better control of blood glucose and blood fat levels, severely limit these foods and substitute healthier, higher fiber wholefoods.

- **Be aware that sugar comes in different forms** such as sucrose, glucose, fructose, malt, high-fructose corn syrup, molasses, honey and maple syrup. Check the label.
- **Sugar alcohols** such as sorbitol, mannitol and maltitol are carb-based and have ½ - ¾ the calories of regular sugar. While not counted as sugar on food labels, they do add to the carb count. Excess amounts can cause bloating, gas and diarrhea.
- **Sugar-free sweeteners** make it easy to reduce sugar in drinks and recipes. However, use minimally since research suggests possible ill-effects of some artificial sweeteners on friendly gut microbes. This may increase the risk of glucose intolerance and an increase in appetite.

  Plant-based sweeteners like stevia or monk fruit appear to be better choices.

SUGAR CONTENT OF SOME COMMON FOODS

	Teaspoons of Sugar
Coca Cola or *Pepsi,* 12 fl.oz	10
20 fl.oz size	17
Iced Tea, sweetened, 12 fl.oz	8
Energy Drink *(Red Bull),* 8.4 fl.oz	7
Chocolate Milk, 12 fl.oz	6
Frappuccino, 16 fl.oz	6
Fruit Drink, sweetened, 8 oz	6
Slurpee, 12 oz	6
Gatorade, 12 fl.oz	5
Shakes, medium, 16 fl.oz	12
Baked Beans *(B&M),* 8 oz	5
Honey Smacks Cereal, 1 cup, 1 oz	4.5
Popcorn, caramel, 1 cup	3.5
Chocolate Bar, 1.5 oz	5
M&M's, 1.7 oz pkg	7
Baby Ruth, King Size, 3.5 oz	8
Jelly Beans (10 medium), 1 oz	6
Life Saver, 1 roll, 1.2 oz	8
Lollipop, medium, 1 oz	6
Marshmallows, 4 pcs, 1 oz	5
Snickers Bar, 1.9 oz	6
Ice Pop/Popsicle	5
Ice Cream, ½ cup	4
Yogurt, sweetened, 6 oz	4
Muffin, large, 4 oz	6
Honey Bun, jumbo, 4.75 oz	6
Twinkies (2)	8
Choc Chip Cookie, 1 oz	2
Donut, iced	6
Apple Pie, 1 piece	7
Jell-O, snack cup, 3.5 oz	4
Jam, 1 Tbsp, ¾ oz	2.5
Nutella, 1 Tbsp	2.5
Syrup, maple, 1 Tbsp	3

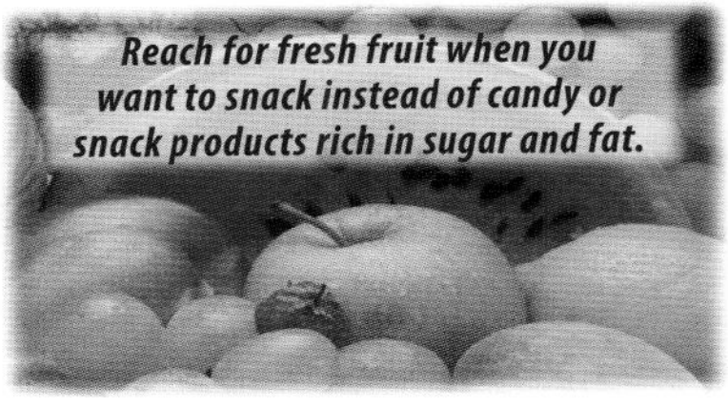
Reach for fresh fruit when you want to snack instead of candy or snack products rich in sugar and fat.

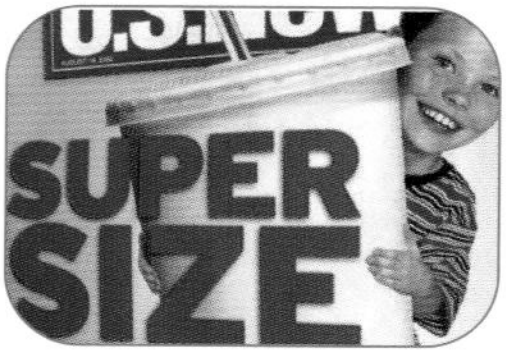

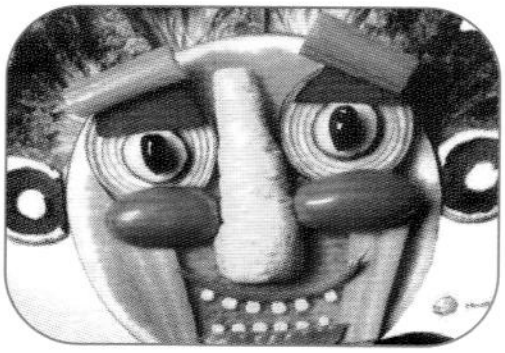

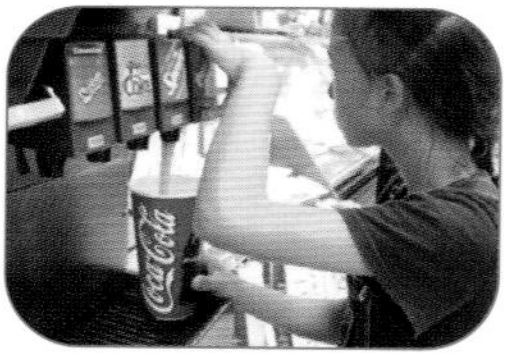

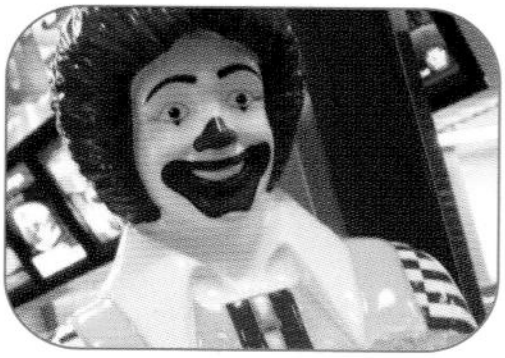

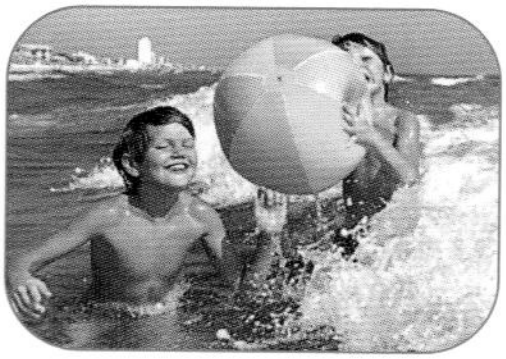

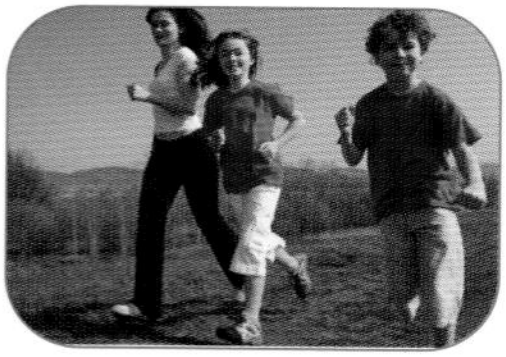

The XL Generation

Some 20% of American kids and adolescents are obese; and childhood obesity has doubled over the last 20 years. Diabetes, high blood pressure and high cholesterol are major problem areas for overweight children and adolescents, as are depression, low self-esteem, sleep apnea and bone joint problems.

To address this problem, cooperation is required between kids, parents, schools and government. Weight control is a family and community affair.

Five Simple Tips To Get Started:

❶ Watch Soda Intake

Limit soda and sugary drinks to one serving on the weekends. Soda should not be an everyday beverage – water should be. When at restaurants or using a soda fountain, choose small servings with ice or choose diet soda instead. Schools should provide water and restrict access to soda as should parents when eating out or in the home!

Also limit sports and energy drinks, fruit juice and flavored milks.

❷ Cut back on Fast-Foods and Eating Out

Many more calories are consumed when you eat out. Healthy meals prepared at home are best for the whole family.

❸ Say "No" to Super-Sizing

When meals are upsized, loads more calories are consumed. Choose sensible portion sizes when eating out and at home. Use smaller plates and choose smaller package sizes.

❹ Limit Between-Meal Snacking

Watch out for high-fat and high-calorie snacks – they can have more calories than a meal! Keep your eye on portion sizes and limit salty snack foods and candy to parties and special occasions. Choose fresh fruit, vegetables, nuts and milk instead.

❺ Get Moving ~ Watch Less TV

Kids need at least 60 minutes of physical activity every day. It's critical for their fitness, and greatly lessens the risk of obesity.

Encourage kids to be active out of school hours. Wearing a pedometer can be highly motivational for kids to move more – as can playing dance video games such as *Dance Dance Revolution. Dance Central* (XBox360) and *Wii Fit (Nintendo)* are also excellent fitness motivators.

Limit TV and non-active computer games to just one hour per day. Also limit the accompanying snacks! Include exercise in family activities.

Sample Meal Plan ~ 1400 Calories

For Healthy, Overweight Persons ~ Not for Persons With Any Medical Condition
~ Please Check With Your Doctor & Dietitian ~

Breakfast (approx. 300 cal)

	1 Small Fruit or ½ oz Dried Fruit
Plus	Cereal: 1½ oz Dry (high fiber) or 1 cup cooked Oatmeal/Quinoa or ½ Avocado
Plus	½ oz Almonds/Seeds
Plus	Milk (from daily allowance) or Yogurt (low-fat)

Daily Milk Allowance (approx.160 calories)
2 cups Non-Fat Milk or 1½ cups Low-fat (1%) Milk
or equivalent Soy Drink, Yogurt, Cheese, Tofu

Fat Allowance (140 calories; 15g Fat)
4 teasp. Butter/Spread or 3 teasp. Oil
or 1½ Tbsp Mayonnaise or ½ medium Avocado
or 1½ Tbsp Peanut Butter or 30g Nuts/Seeds

Lunch (approx. 440 calories)

	1 slice Wholegrain Bread (1 oz) or 2 Crispbreads/Crackers or 6" Pita
Plus	3 oz lean Meat, Chicken or Turkey or 3-4 oz Tuna (in water) or Salmon or 1½ oz Cheese or ¾ cup (6 oz) Cottage Cheese or ½ cup (4 oz) Ricotta Cheese or ¾ cup (6 oz) Fruit Yogurt (sugar-free) or ¾ cup (6 oz) Bean Salad
Plus	Large Salad (low-fat dressing)
Plus	1 small Fruit or ½ oz Dried Fruit

Dinner (approx. 360 calories)

	Soup (Vegetable), low-fat
Plus	3 oz lean Meat (cooked weight) or 4 oz Chicken Breast (no skin) or 3 oz Chicken Thigh/Leg (no skin) or 5 oz Fish (grilled) or ¾ cup (6 oz) Beans (Soy, Kidney, Pinto etc)/Lentils
Plus	1 small Potato or ½ cup Brown Rice/Pasta/Sweet Corn or 1 slice Wholegrain Bread
Plus	2-3 servings Vegetables (non-starchy) or large Salad
Plus	1 small fruit or ½ oz dark chocolate (over 70% cocoa)

Brealfast ~ Choice 2

	1 Small Fruit
Plus	2 Eggs (no added fat) or 2 oz Cheese (low-fat) or 4 oz Cottage Cheese (low-fat) or 2 oz Lean/Canadian Bacon
Plus	1 Tomato
Plus	1 Slice Wholegrain Toast

Between Meals

- Water, Coffee, Tea (sugar-free)
- Fruit from main meals; Raw Vegetables
- Milk from Daily Allowance

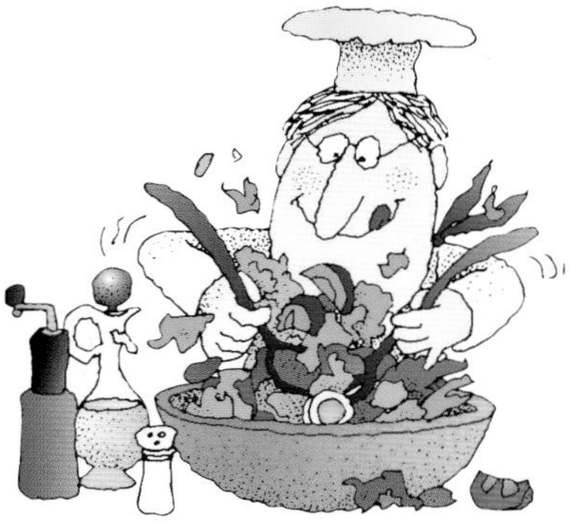

Exercise & Weight Control

- **Persons who exercise regularly lose more weight** and keep it off longer than non-exercisers. Blood glucose control also improves; as do beneficial gut microbes.
- **Exercise also improves general health and well-being.** Mood, confidence and self-esteem are also enhanced.
- **Exercise** is a good way to 'wake up' a sluggish metabolism and burn excess body fat.
- **Aerobic (huff and puff) exercise most days** is great for burning calories and for cardiovascular fitness. But, it is strength training that mainly builds the muscles that burn calories.
- **Strength training is the key to retaining or rebuilding muscles.** As we age, we lose some 6 pounds of muscle per decade. This results in a lower metabolism and fewer calories burnt.

  Muscles are the furnaces that burn calories. The more muscle you have, the more calories burnt – and as a bonus, the more food you can eat.
- **Regular strength training (2-3 times weekly)** can increase our metabolic rate for several days following exercise – with up to an extra 100 calories per day being burnt.

  While 2-3 pounds of muscle may be gained in the first 8-10 weeks, weight from exercised muscles is okay. It is excess fat (particularly abdominal fat) that is a potential health hazard.
- **Body reshaping** is enhanced by gaining muscle and losing fat - even if the scales don't show it.
- **Avoid injury** by beginning with walking, low impact aerobics, or weight-supported exercise (e.g. swimming, cycling). Avoid competitive sports. Allow 2-3 days of recovery between strength training sessions. Get professional advice.
- **How Much?** Start with 10-20 minutes per day and progress to 30-60 minutes per day. Also walk up stairs instead of using elevators. Take a brisk walk at lunch. Use an exercise bike, treadmill or stair machine while watching TV. Walk the dog.
- **How Often?** While aerobic fitness may require only 3-4 sessions weekly, **weight control is a daily event which requires daily exercise to burn calories.** Also add in strength training 2-3 times weekly.

Note: Persons on cholesterol-lowering statin drugs may experience muscle pains and weakness (as well as damage to muscle microfibrils). Supplementing with coenzyme Q10, magnesium, selenium, vitamins D and K2, may be beneficial. Check with your healthcare provider.

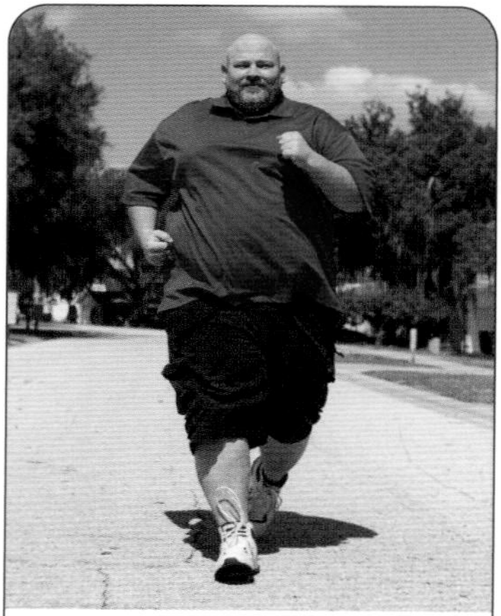

Brisk walking each day is a safe and effective way to burn calories and keep fit. Try it – you'll like it!

Be sure to wear sun-protective clothing.

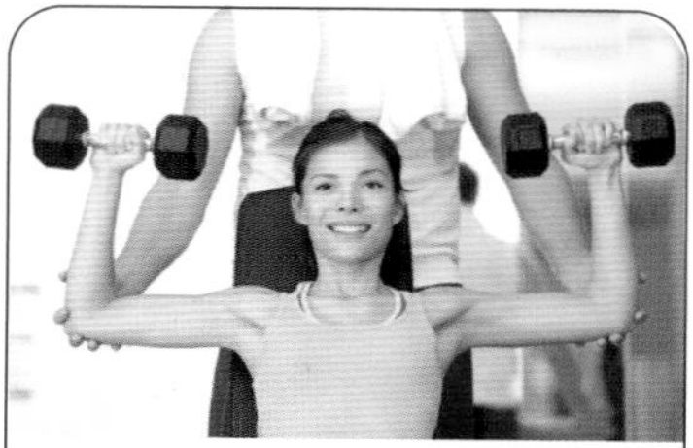

Strength training is the key to retain or rebuild muscles.

Exercized muscles burn extra calories even while you sleep.

For extra guidance and motivation, seek a qualified trainer or join a gym.

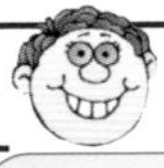

Calories Used in Exercise

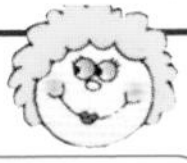

LIGHT

130 lbs ~ 3 Cals/Min

170 lbs ~ 4 Cals/Min

220 lbs ~ 5 Cals/Min

- Walking, slow
- Cycling, light
- Frisbee playing
- Gardening, light
- Golf, social
- Tennis, doubles
- Housework, cleaning
- Calisthenics, light
- Bowling
- Ping-pong, social
- Ice Skating, light
- Aquarobics, light
- Skate Boarding
- Line/Square Dancing
- Tai Chi, Yoga
- Volleyball

MODERATE

130 lbs ~ 5 Cals/Min

170 lbs ~ 6 Cals/Min

220 lbs ~ 7 Cals/Min

- Walking, brisk
- Cycling, moderate
- Swimming, crawl
- Weight-training, light
- Tennis, moderate
- Racquetball, beginners
- Aerobics, light
- Football, touch
- Basketball, Baseball
- Walking Downstairs
- Snow Skiing (downhill)
- Shovelling snow
- Dancing (ballroom)
- Rowing, moderate
- Volleyball, competitive

HEAVY

130 lbs ~ 8 Cals/Min

170 lbs ~ 10 Cals/Min

220 lbs ~ 12 Cals/Min

- Walking (power), Jogging
- Cycling (vigorous)
- Swimming, strenuous
- Weight-training, heavy
- Wrestling/Judo, advanced
- Racquetball, advanced
- Tae Bo, Kick Boxing
- Football, training
- Basketball (Pro)
- Climbing Stairs
- Skipping Rope
- Skiing (cross country)
- Aquarobics, advanced
- Dancing (strenuous), Zumba
- Rowing, vigorous
- Martial Arts

Note: Only those sports or activities that are sustained over a period of time (e.g running) qualify for heavy exercise. Stop-start sports such as tennis are considered 'moderate'.

WALKING PROGRAM

USE DISTANCE, STEPS OR TIME

Weeks	Distance	Steps (Pedometer)	Time
1-2	1 mile	2000	20 mins
3-5	1.5 miles	3000	28 mins
6-8	2 miles	3500	35 mins
9-10	2.5 miles	4500	45 mins
11+	3.5 miles	6000	60 mins

10,000 STEPS PER DAY

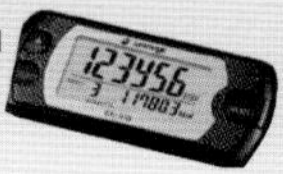

A pedometer can motivate you to be more active. It clips to your belt or waist band and registers each step.

Alternatively, use a *Fitbit*, *Garmin* or *Striiv* activity tracker, or your smartphone inbuilt accelerometer.

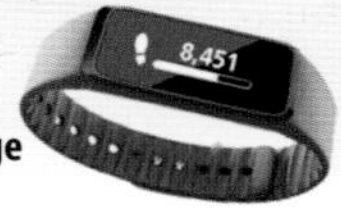

Aim for 8,000 - 10,000 steps per day, insead of an average of only 3,000 - 4,000 steps.

Reshaping Eating Behaviors

- Eating is a behavior that is largely controlled by people with whom we live or socialize, places in which we carry out our lives, and our emotions. Become aware of those situations that commonly lead to extra food being eaten.
- We may also be unaware of 'bad' eating habits that can lead to excess calorie intake; e.g. eating quickly, large mouthfuls, eating when tense or bored, finishing a large serving of food when not hungry.

Tips to help uncover and correct those 'bad' or problem eating habits:

- **Don't eat while engaged in other activities;** for example, watching TV, reading. Eat only at the table, not at the fridge or while standing.
- **Don't eat quickly.** Chewing slowly allows time to register a feeling of fullness. Don't use fingers, only utensils. Cut food into smaller pieces. Don't load your fork until the previous mouthful is finished.
- **Don't purchase problem high calorie foods.** Shop from a set list to prevent impulse buying. Avoid shopping with children.
- **Buy snack foods** in the smallest package. The larger the serving size or package, the more you are likely to eat or drink.
- **Plan meals in advance. Stick to a set menu.**
- **Plan a strategy to avoid uncontrolled eating** and drinking at social events, or when your emotions urge you to binge.

  Rehearse repeatedly in your mind exactly what you will do in such situations. Remind yourself several times each day that you are in charge of your actions and that you can be strong-willed. Seek counseling or coaching on various strategies.
- **Distract yourself** when you feel the urge to snack impulsively. Engage in some activity that will distract you from thinking about food. Examples: go for a walk, brush your teeth, phone a friend.

  If you eat out of boredom, find some new hobby or interest that gets you out of the house. Even enrol in an adult education class.

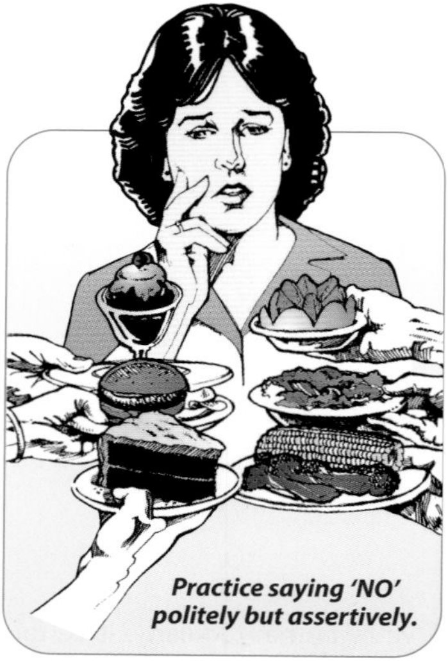

Practice saying 'NO' politely but assertively.

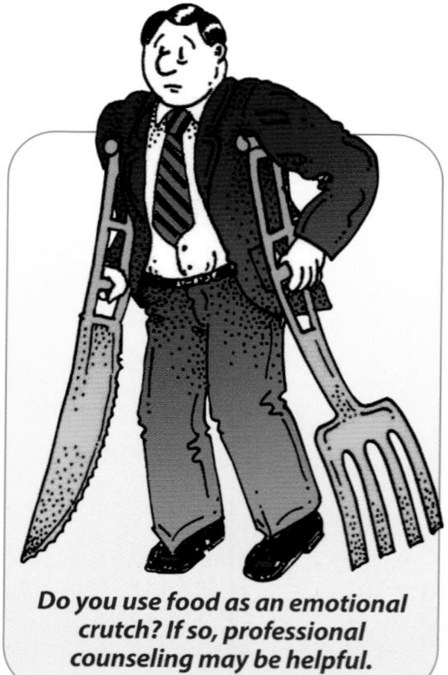

Do you use food as an emotional crutch? If so, professional counseling may be helpful.

The food journal is the most powerful proven aid for dieters. Persons who keep a food and exercise journal not only lose more weight, they also keep it off. Here are some of the reasons:

- **Recording your eating and exercise habits** jolts you into realizing just what you do eat and drink each day; and also whether you exercise sufficiently.
- **Helps you identify problem foods** and drinks with excessive calories and fat.
- **Helps identify moods**, situations and events that lead to excessive eating of unwanted calories. You can then plan to overcome or avoid them.
- **Prevents 'calorie amnesia'**, the forgetfulness that leads to rebound weight gain after successful weight loss. Recording puts you back on the right track.
- **Helps you develop greater self-discipline.** You will think twice about overindulging if you have to record it - especially if someone checks your journal regularly. It certainly keeps you honest!
- **Motivates you** to carefully plan your meals and to exercise each day.
- **Serves as a check system** for your doctor, dietitian or counselor to assess your progress and make recommendations.

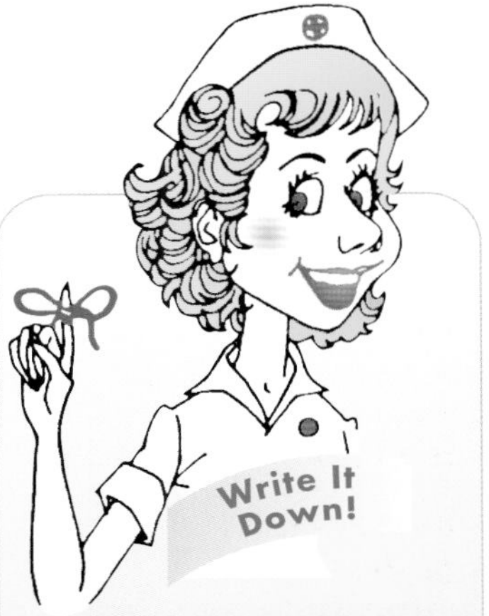

"Keeping a journal gives me feedback on exactly what I eat and drink each day.

It helps prevent 'calorie amnesia' and reminds me to exercise each day.

It's a 'must' for successful weight control!"

3 Easy Ways to Track Your Food & Exercise Calories!

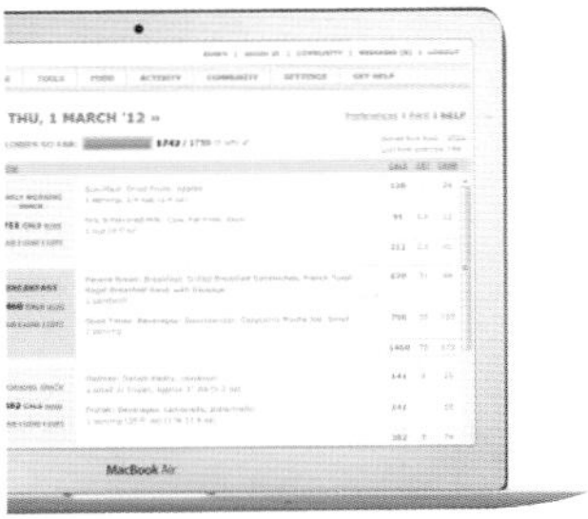

CalorieKing Online

Part of a comprehensive personalized program that includes tools, reports and a supportive community.

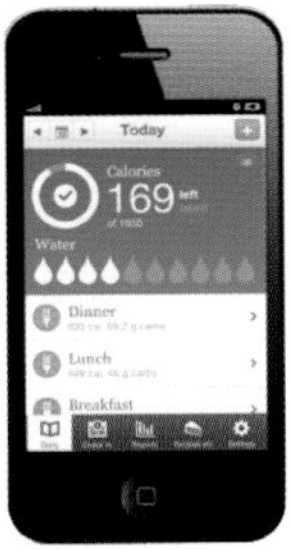

CalorieKing App

ControlMyWeight

Make smart food choices wherever you are! Easy to use.

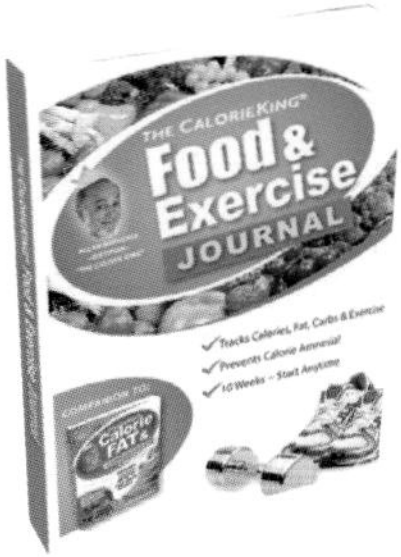

Book

A 10-week journal that fits in your pocket. Includes Weekly Summary page and Progress Checklist.

Extra Information ~ www.CalorieKing.com

Diabetes Guide

What is Diabetes?

Diabetes occurs when the body has difficulty processing glucose sugar in the blood.

- **After digestion**, sugar and starches are changed into **glucose** – the simplest form of sugar vital for body energy and growth.
- **Insulin** is the hormone which acts like a key that opens the door to body cells and allows glucose to enter.
- **Without enough insulin**, glucose builds up in the blood and passes into the urine. High blood glucose levels lead to frequent urination, extreme thirst, and tiredness.
- **Untreated diabetes increases the risk of damage to nerves and blood vessels.** This, in turn, increases the risk of heart disease, stroke, blindness, kidney damage, foot ulcers and gangrene (with amputation), impotence, Alzheimer's Disease and other problems.

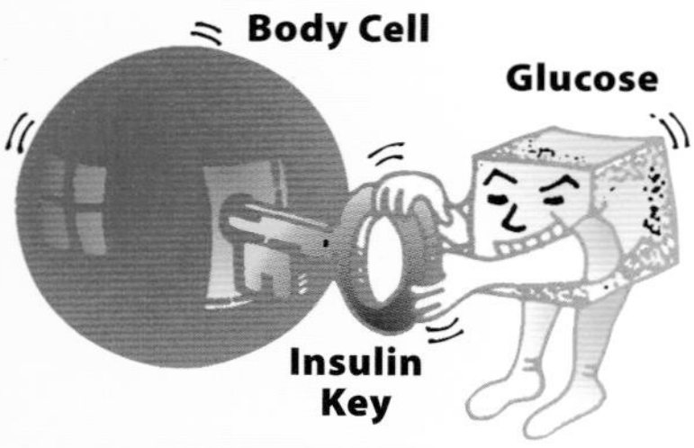

Insulin acts like a key. It opens the door to body cells and allows glucose to enter.

People with type 1 diabetes and some with type 2 have too few or no keys. They require insulin injections.

Others (primarily type 2) make enough insulin but the body doesn't use it as well as it should – particularly if obese and inactive.

SYMPTOMS OF DIABETES

- Frequent urination
- Extreme thirst
- Unusual hunger
- Rapid weight loss
- Extreme fatigue
- Blurred vision
- Skin infections that are slow to heal
- Tingling/numbness in feet

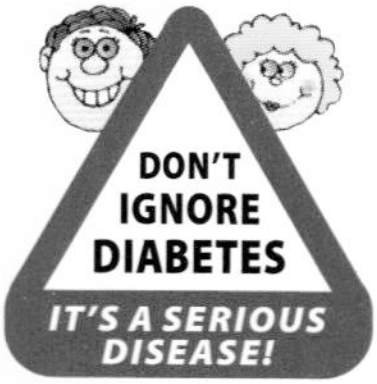

Note: Diabetes can be present even without symptoms.

TYPE 2 DIABETES

- Occurs in 90% of diabetes cases
- Occurs mainly in adults - particularly in overweight and inactive persons
- Insulin is produced but body cells resist its action and glucose cannot enter cells
- Usually treated with meal planning and physical activity. Sometimes requires medication (pills or insulin)

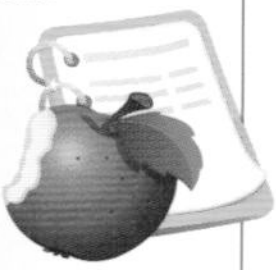

TYPE 1 DIABETES

- Occurs in 10% of diabetes cases
- Usually in children and young adults
- Pancreas produces little or no insulin. Daily insulin injections (or use of an insulin pump) are necessary, as well as:
  - matching pre-meal insulin to the amount of carbohydrate eaten
  - weight control and regular physical activity

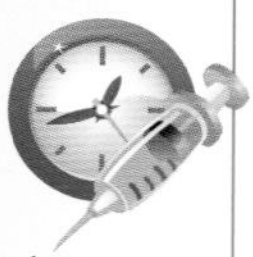

GESTATIONAL DIABETES

- Occurs in some women during pregnancy. It usually disappears after the baby's birth but still leaves mothers (1 in 3) at high risk of type 2 diabetes within 5-10 years.
- Check your blood glucose **before** and during pregnancy. High levels can harm the fetus, especially in the first 6 weeks.
- Requires weight control, a healthy lifestyle and regular medical checks.

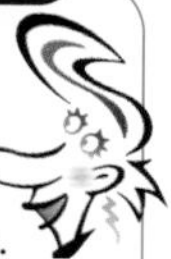

Are You At Risk for Diabetes?

Pre-Diabetes ~ An Early Warning!

Pre-diabetes means your blood glucose levels are higher than normal, but not high enough to be called diabetes.

If you have pre-diabetes, you have a higher risk for getting diabetes later on.

The good news is that you can start taking steps to prevent diabetes by making healthy lifestyle changes – such as losing weight if overweight, and being more physically active.

WHAT'S YOUR RISK?

Find out if you're at risk for diabetes by answering the following questions:

- ☐ I have been told I have pre-diabetes
- ☐ I have a family history of diabetes
- ☐ I am African American, Latino American, Asian American, Native American or a Pacific Islander
- ☐ I have had gestational diabetes (diabetes during pregnancy)
- ☐ I am over age 45
- ☐ I am overweight
- ☐ My waist is larger than: 35 inches (for a woman) or 40 inches (for a man)
- ☐ I get little or no physical activity
- ☐ My blood pressure is higher than 130 over 85
- ☐ My HDL (good cholesterol) is too low
- ☐ My triglycerides (blood fats) are too high

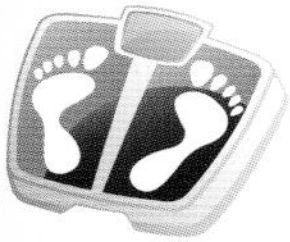

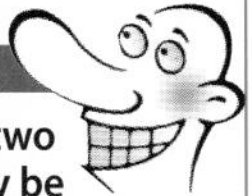

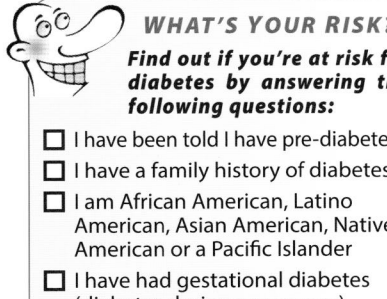

☑ CHECK YOUR RESULT

- **If you've put a check mark in two or more of the boxes, you may be more likely to develop type 2 diabetes.**
- **Talk with your healthcare provider to see if you should have a blood test for diabetes.**

BLOOD GLUCOSE CLASSIFICATION OF DIABETES

Normal:	**Below 100 mg/dl***
Pre-Diabetes:	**100-125 mg/dl***
Diabetes:	**Over 125 mg/dl***

(*Fasting Blood Glucose)

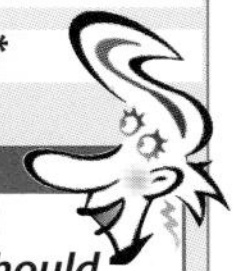

KNOW YOUR BGL

(Blood Glucose Level)

Everyone over the age of 45 should have a blood glucose test every three years.

Importance of Weight Control

- **Type 2 diabetes** is more common in people who are overweight.
- **Being overweight** means that your insulin doesn't work as well to control blood glucose levels.
- **Losing just 10 to 20 pounds** can help you better manage your diabetes and lower your risk for heart disease.

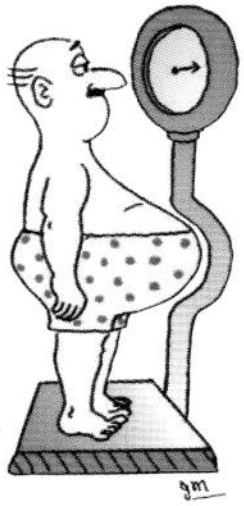

Keys to weight control include:

- Follow a healthy eating plan
- Control food portions.
- Be physically active every day. Track your daily activity.
- Keep food records ~ *See Page 15*
- Get the support of family and friends.
- **Work with a registered dietitian** who can help you reach a weight that's ideal for you.

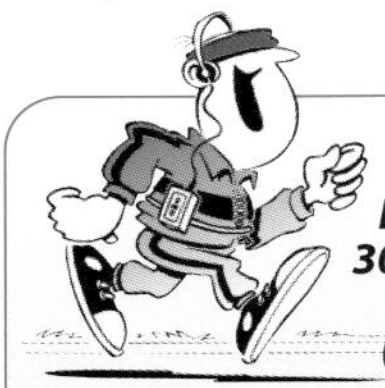

KEEP MOVING!

Every day, do at least 30 minutes of moderate intensity exercise. (even in 5-minute sets)

It's the key to improving insulin action. Add muscle strength training 3-4 times a week to double the benefits.

Managing Diabetes

Don't battle diabetes alone. Establish a partnership with your doctor, dietitian, certified diabetes educator, and pharmacist.

Extra Support:

- *American Association of Diabetes Educators*
- *American Diabetes Association*
- *BeyondType1.org* • *Joslin Diabetes Center*
- *Juvenile Diabetes Research Foundation*
- *National Diabetes Education Program*

Tips to keep blood glucose within safe limits:

- **Control your food intake.** Know what and when you will eat. Seek referral to a dietitian for expert advice.
- **Exercise daily.** It assists weight control and can improve sensitivity of body cells to insulin. Plan physical activity into your daily routine.
- **Take insulin or oral medication as prescribed.** If on insulin, know what action to take if hypoglycemia (low blood glucose) occurs. Also educate your family and friends.
- **Monitor your blood glucose** at home and work with a blood glucose meter or CGM system. It will help you become familiar with your blood glucose patterns, and the effects of food, activity and medication.
- **Continuous glucose monitoring (CGM) tracks** your glucose levels every few minutes by using a sensor (skin patch or insert) that measures glucose levels in the tissue just below the skin. This allows the user to see a graph of glucose levels – not just single measurements from fingerstick testing. Seeing trends and patterns can help to better manage diabetes. **This results in greater awareness of unnoticed highs and lows** (as illustrated below). CGM can also help to reduce A1C with less risk of hypoglycemia for people on insulin.

Blood glucose meter systems and insulin pumps can greatly improve control of diabetes

BLOOD GLUCOSE METERS (EXAMPLES)

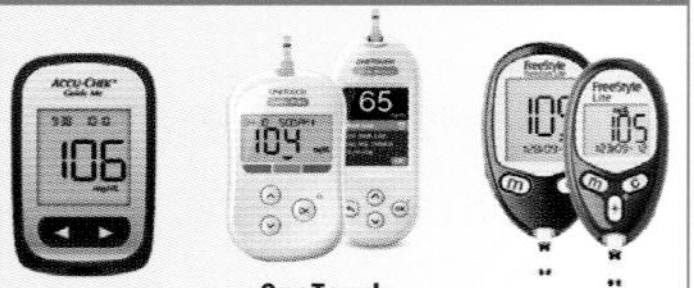

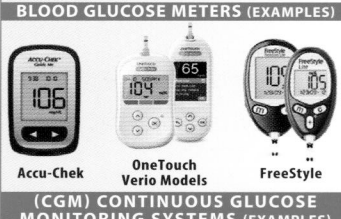

Accu-Chek | OneTouch Verio Models | FreeStyle

(CGM) CONTINUOUS GLUCOSE MONITORING SYSTEMS (EXAMPLES)

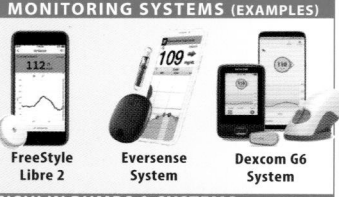

FreeStyle Libre 2 | Eversense System | Dexcom G6 System

INSULIN PUMPS & SYSTEMS (EXAMPLES)

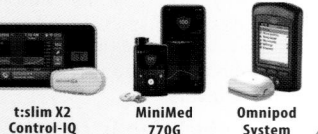

t:slim X2 Control-IQ | MiniMed 770G | Omnipod System

Hemoglobin A1C Target:
The hemoglobin A1C (A-one-C) test reflects your average blood glucose levels over the last 3 months. **Aim for less than 6.5%.**

Benefits of Continuous Glucose Monitoring

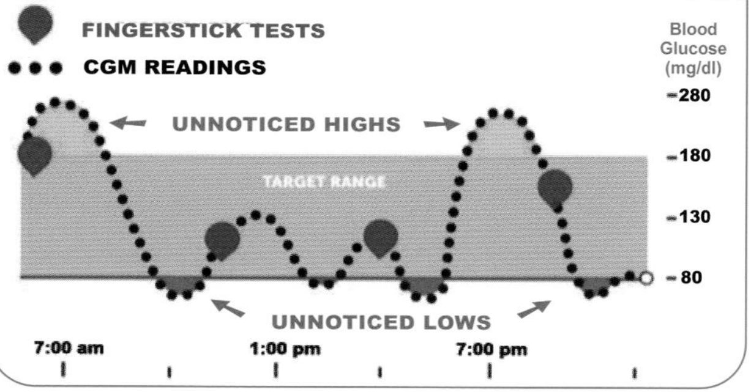

Target Blood Sugar Levels (ADA):

Before Meals:
Between 80 and 130 mg/dL

2 Hours After Meals:
Less than 180 mg/dL

Guidelines for choosing a healthy diet apply equally to people with or without diabetes.

Eat a wide variety of wholefoods that are minimally processed, low in refined grains/flour and added sugar, high in fiber, and moderate in protein.

However, actual food quantities, as well as when you eat, will also influence control of blood glucose. Your dietitian will individualize a meal plan to suit your food preferences, lifestyle and medical status.

Healthy Diet Tips:

- **Maintain a healthy weight.** If overweight, even a modest weight loss plus daily physical activity can help manage blood glucose in type 2 diabetes.

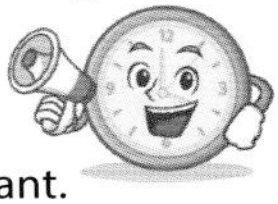

- **Don't skip meals.** If you take insulin or an oral hypoglycemic agent, regular meals are important.

  If on insulin, eat meals at the same time each day. Eat a similar amount of food at each meal. Eating about the same amount of carbohydrate over the day will make best use of insulin and prevent wide variations in blood glucose levels.

- **Know which foods contain carbohydrate;** and learn how to check the *Nutrition Facts Label* on foods. Check the serving size, total fat and total carbohydrate – not just the sugar content. All carbohydrate breaks down to sugars after digestion.

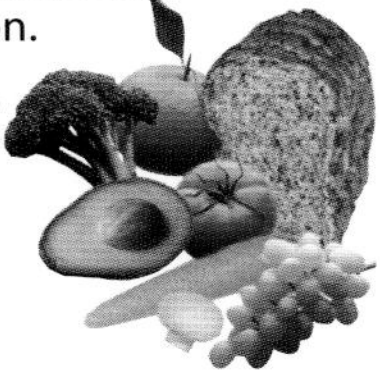

- **Choose wholegrain breads, cereals and pasta.** Eat fresh fruits, vegetables and legumes. These foods contain more fiber and slow the release of glucose into your blood after a meal.
- **Limit sugars and foods high in added sugar** particularly if overweight. *(Extra Notes: Page 9)*
- **Choose foods with healthy fats** such as fatty fish, avocados, olives and nuts, flaxseeds, chia seeds, hemp seeds.Avoid excess use of seed oils. Ideally, use extra virgin olive oil. Avoid fried foods. Frying can oxidize seed oils that can harm our health.

Eat a well-balanced diet with foods high in fiber and low in added sugars.

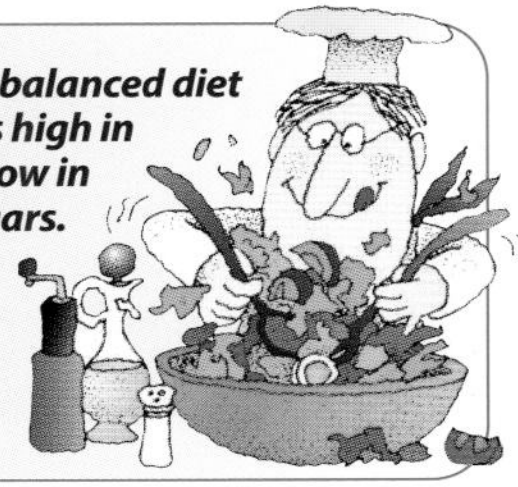

A fiber-rich diet assists the growth of friendly gut microbes that can benefit our metabolism, weight and blood glucose levels – as well as hunger, mood and our immune system.
(Also see Fiber Guide ~ Page 264)

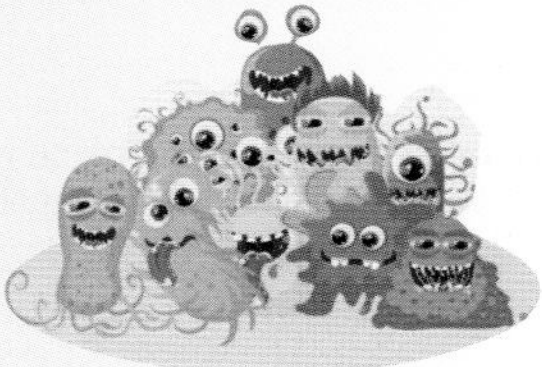

ALCOHOL TIPS

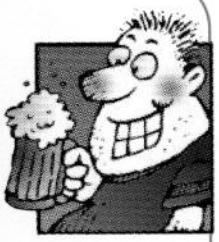

- **If you drink alcohol, have only moderate amounts:**
  Men ~ 1-2 drinks/day
  Women ~ 1 drink/day
  For some people, safe drinking will mean no alcoholic drinks at all.

(Also see Alcohol Guide ~ Page 23)

- **Drink along with your food –** especially if you use insulin or diabetes medication pills.
- **Do not omit any carb food** in exchange for an alcoholic drink. However, non-alcoholic beers (12 fl oz) count as one carb exchange.
- **Alcohol increases the risk of hypoglycemia** (low blood sugar) and drug interactions if you take insulin and certain types of diabetes pills.
- **Check with your doctor and dietitian.**

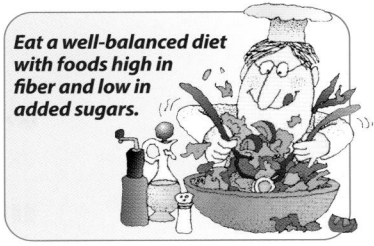

Notes for Pre-diabetes & Type 2 Diabetes
(Please discuss with your doctor)

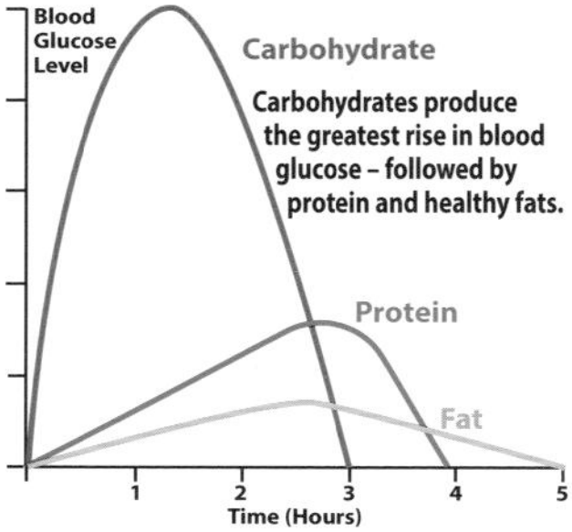

• **Benefits of Lower Carb Eating:**
Generally, following a lower carbohydrate pattern of eating is associated with more stable blood glucose levels (fewer highs and lows).

A reduction in blood glucose variation (high to low) can greatly reduce the need for diabetes medications (as assessed by your doctor) – as well as the risk of hypoglycemia and diabetic health complications.

Greater improvements are also usually seen with blood triglyceride fat levels and HDL-cholesterol.

• **Eat earlier in the day rather than at night.** The body's circadian rhythms allow for more efficient processing of foods in the first half of the day - with likely greater tissue sensitivity to insulin resulting in lower blood glucose levels. Eating late at night can lead to higher blood glucose levels and potential greater damage to body tissues – as well as reduced quality of sleep. Ideally make breakfast or lunch the main meal of the day.

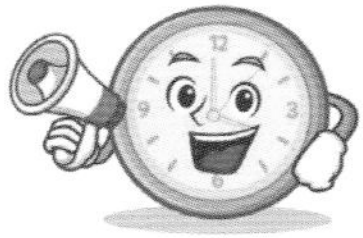

• **Consume fats and oils mainly as wholefoods in which they naturally occur** such as avocados, olives, cheese, milk, meats, fish, poultry and eggs.

Once vegetable seed oils (such as corn, sunflower, safflower, soy, canola) are isolated from their original food source, their unstable polyunsaturated chemical structure makes them more prone to oxidation particularly when used in high-heat cooking (broiling, frying, baking). The oxidative by-products can be toxic to body tissues and organs, including the pancreas which produces insulin *(Extra Notes ~ See page 6-7)*.

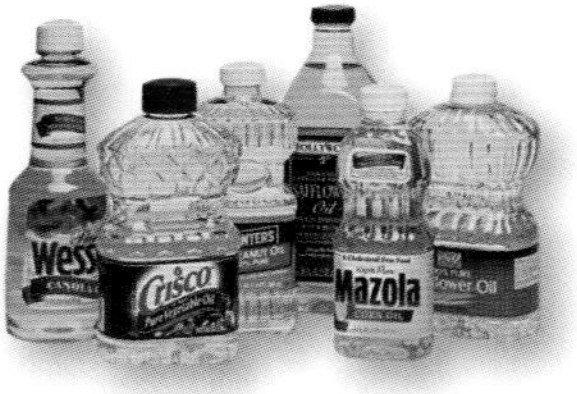

Avoid vegetable seed oils and processed foods that contain them.

• **Eat your protein and vegetables before carbohydrate-rich foods** such as fruit juice and bread. This greatly improves post-meal blood glucose balance (with fewer spikes), as well as insulin sensitivity. Post-meal insulin levels are also reduced.

• **Benefits of Nutrition Supplements:**
Persons with Type 2 diabetes are at greater risk of nutritional deficiencies due to the extra inflammatory stresses throughout the body. Further deficiencies can also result from prescribed drugs, such as statin cholesterol-lowering drugs, anti-inflammatory drugs for pain relief, stomach acid-suppressing drugs and antibiotics.

Check with your doctor about the potential benefits of supplements such as coenzyme Q10, multi-vitamins, vitamins D and K2, magnesium, omega-3 fish or algal oils, astaxanthin, berberine (if statin-intolerant), curcumin – all of which have clinical studies showing potential health benefits.

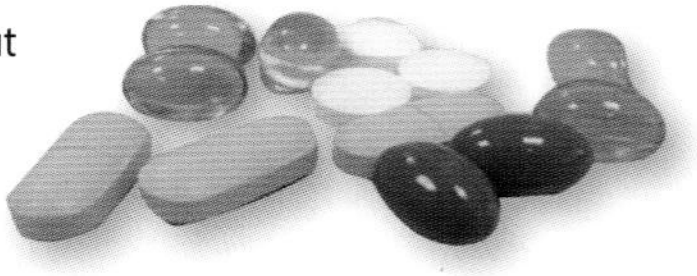

People with diabetes may benefit from nutrition supplements. Check with your doctor.

Carb Type Affects Blood Glucose

The various forms of carbohydrate affect blood glucose levels in different ways. It is difficult to predict the effect of particular foods, sugars, or meals, simply by their carbohydrate content.

Thus the same amount of carbohydrate from different foods may affect blood sugar levels very differently. **Many factors affect the rate of digestion and absorption such as:**

- the type of sugar, starch, and fiber
- the degree of processing and cooking (which increases digestion rate)
- the amount of protein and fat (which slow stomach emptying and digestion).

Additionally, the effect of particular foods on blood glucose can differ markedly between individuals.

Glycemic Index (GI)

The GI is a method of ranking carbohydrate foods on a scale (0-100) according to how they affect blood glucose levels. (See next column).

The higher the GI value, the greater the food's ability to rapidly raise blood glucose levels; and the more insulin that is needed by the body (not desirable).

Eating low-GI foods may lead to better control of blood glucose and insulin levels (which in turn lowers the risk of damage to blood vessels and nerves). The slower digestion of low-GI foods may also help to delay hunger pangs and benefit weight control.

Cautionary Notes on GI

Choosing low-GI foods is not a license to eat unlimited amounts. Calorie restriction and portion control for weight control is of prime importance.

Also remember, **low-GI foods are carbohydrate foods** and must still be counted as part of any dietetic carbohydrate plan.

GI is not meant to be used by itself without regard to portion size, and other dietary recommendations for healthy eating. Foods are not good or bad on the basis of their GI.

LOWER-GLYCEMIC FOODS

Slower-Acting Carbohydrates

These foods are more slowly digested and absorbed. They help maintain more even blood glucose levels, as long as excessive amounts are not eaten. Use these foods regularly but still limit portion size for weight control.

Examples:

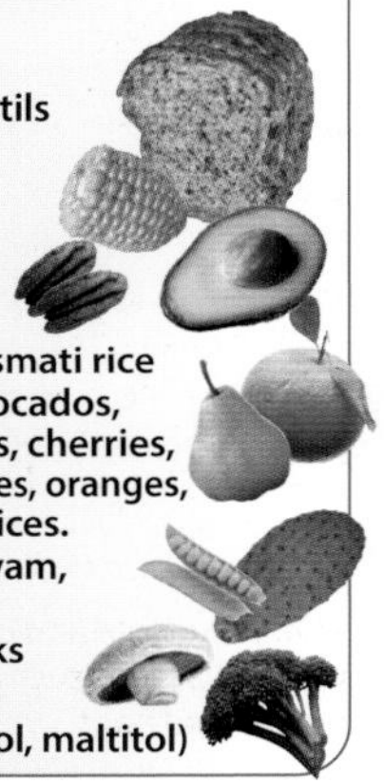

- **Dried beans, peas, lentils**
- **Nuts and seeds**
- **Wholegrain breads**
- **Bran cereals, oats**
- **Sweet corn, barley, quinoa buckwheat**
- **Wholegrain pasta, basmati rice**
- **Fresh fruit: apples, avocados, bananas (firm), berries, cherries, grapefruit, grapes, olives, oranges, pears, plums. Fresh juices.**
- **Vegetables: broccoli, yam, nopales, salad greens**
- **Milk, yogurt, soy drinks**
- **Dark chocolate, cacao**
- **Sugar alcohols (sorbitol, maltitol)**

HIGHER-GLYCEMIC FOODS

Quicker-Acting Carbohydrates

These foods more rapidly raise blood glucose levels. Eat only in moderation.

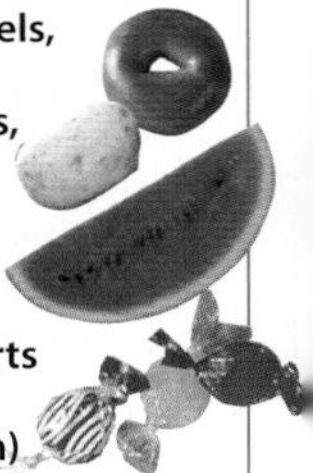

- **White bread, rice cakes, bagels, croissants, doughnuts**
- **Low-fiber cereals: Cornflakes, *Rice Krispies, Froot Loops***
- **White potatoes, white rice**
- **Watermelon, ripe bananas, cantaloupe, pineapple**
- **Soda, sugar-sweetened sports and energy drinks**
- **Sugar, candy, popcorn (plain)**
- **Ice cream (low-fat), frozen yogurt**

High-GI fruits and potatoes can be healthy choices when eaten in moderate amounts.

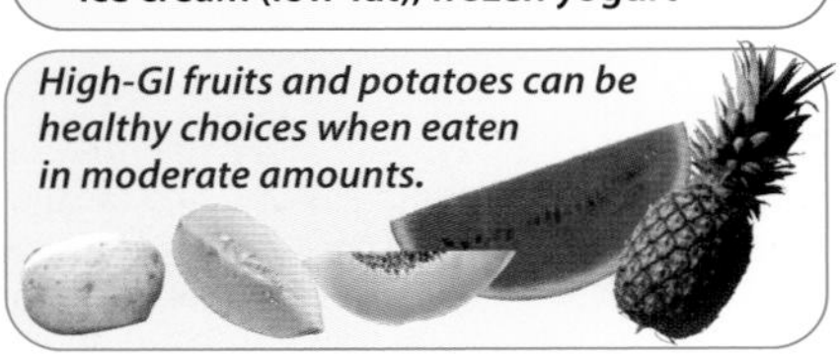

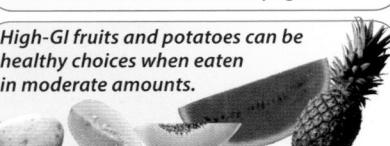

Notes ♦ Abbreviations ♦ Disclaimer

- **Calorie and fat values have been rounded off.** **Calories** ~ to the nearest 5 or 10 calories. **Fat** ~ to nearest half gram. **Note:** Trace amounts of fat (less than 0.3 grams) have been treated as zero.
- **Carbohydrate figures** in this book are for total carbohydrate, and not **Net Carbs** (which deducts fiber, polydextrose and sugar alcohols from total carbs).
- Because manufacturers' figures on labels are rounded off, figures in this book may differ slightly from the label. Serving sizes may also vary.

IMPORTANT DISCLAIMER

* The authors and publishers of this book are not physicians and are not licensed to give medical advice.This book is not a substitute for professional advice.Users should consult their medical professional before making any health, medical or other decisions based on the material contained herein.

* This book is a compilation of original material from other sources intended for educational purposes only. Because food manufacturers constantly change their products, only they are the authoritative source for food's most current nutritional information.

* Persons using the information herein for any medical purposes, such as matching insulin dosage to carbohydrate intake, should not rely solely on the accuracy of figures herein and should independently check food labels or contact the food manufacturer for the latest data.

Canadian Readers:

Please note that figures in this book are based on U.S. food products and restaurants. Equivalent Canadian foods may vary and should be checked independently.

* WARRANTY DISCLAIMER:

THE AUTHOR AND PUBLISHER DISCLAIM ANY LIABILITY ARISING DIRECTLY OR INDIRECTLY FROM THE USE OF THIS BOOK.THE INFORMATION HEREIN IS PROVIDED "AS IS" AND WITHOUT ANY WARRANTY EXPRESSED OR IMPLIED. ALL DIRECT, INDIRECT, SPECIAL, INCIDENTAL, CONSEQUENTIAL OR PUNITIVE DAMAGES ARISING FROM ANY USE OF THIS INFORMATION IS DISCLAIMED AND EXCLUDED.

This information is also provided subject to Family Health Publications' Terms and Conditions found at the website, www.calorieking.com/terms and incorporated herein.

C ~ Calories
F ~ Fat (grams)
Cb ~ Carbohydrate (grams)

Abbreviations

tsp = teaspoon
Tbsp or T = Tablespoon
oz = ounce(s)
c = cup
fl.oz = fluid ounce(s)
g = gram(s)
avg = average
pkg = package

Volume Measures

(All measures are level)
3 tsp = 1 Tbsp
2 Tbsp = 1 fl.oz
½ cup = 4 fl.oz
1 cup = 8 fl.oz
2 cups = 1 Pint
2 Pints = 1 Quart

Note: 8 oz weight is not the same as 8 fl oz volume (space occupied). Dense foods weigh more per set volume. Examples:
1 cup popcorn weighs ½ oz
1 cup milk weighs 8½ oz
1 cup pudding weighs 10 oz

Metric Conversion

½ oz = 14 grams
1 oz = 28.4 grams
2 oz = 57 grams
3½ oz = 100 grams
1 fl.oz = 30 mls
1 cup (8 fl.oz) = 240 mls
33 fl.oz = 1 liter (volume)

INFORMATION SOURCES

- U.S. Dept. of Agriculture
- U.S. Food Manufacturers
- Food Industry Boards & Councils
- Author extrapolations

FEEDBACK WELCOME!

Please contact the author with your queries and suggestions.
feedback@calorieking.com

- **Health Hazards: Excessive alcohol intake** contributes to obesity, high blood pressure, stroke, heart and liver disease, some cancers, and even impotence. **Concentration and short-term memory** are reduced as well as athletic performance.

  Other alcohol hazards include: Fetal Alcohol Syndrome, stomach upsets, gut dysbiosis, menstrual and menopausal problems, depression, snoring, sleep problems, work absenteeism, impaired judgement, risky behaviors and social/family problems.
- **Alcohol contributes to obesity** through its high calories and by lessening the body's ability to burn fat. Fat storage is promoted, particularly in the belly – a health danger zone. Alcohol can also stimulate the appetite; and weaken the dieter's resolve!
- **Alcohol is potentially more harmful while dieting:** Blood sugar levels may drop with resultant fatigue and further impairment of concentration, reflexes and driving skills.

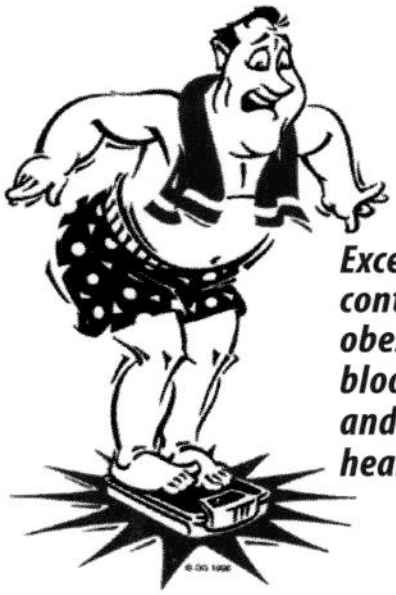

Excess alcohol contributes to obesity, high blood pressure and many other health problems

Lower Risk Alcohol Limits

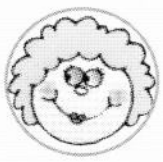

WOMEN:
No more than
1 drink per day

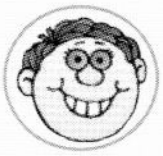

MEN:
No more than
2 drinks per day
(1 drink if over 65 y.o.)

(At least 2 days a week should be alcohol-free)

1 DRINK CONTAINS 14 GRAMS ALCOHOL
- **12 fl.oz Regular Beer** (5% Alc.)
- **OR 14 fl.oz Light Beer** (4.2% Alc.)
- **OR 5 fl.oz Wine** (12% Alc.)
- **OR 1½ fl.oz Spirits** (80 Proof)

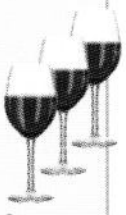

Note: You cannot save daily drinks for one occasion.
Binge drinking is particularly harmful:
4 drinks for males or 3 drinks for females (within 2 hours).

For some people, safe drinking means no alcohol at all. Even one drink may impair driving skills, particularly if tired. For women who drink frequently, breast cancer risk is increased by 9% for each drink after the first drink. In men, just 2 drinks a day doubles the risk of cancers of the mouth and throat.

It is advisable not to drink at all if you are:
- pregnant, trying to conceive or breastfeeding
- taking medication or have liver or heart disease (unless approved by your doctor or pharmacist)
- planning to drive, use machinery or play sports
- studying or needing to concentrate
- a child or adolescent

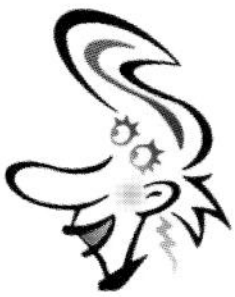

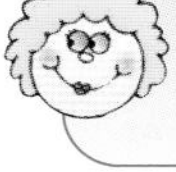

Women and adolescents are more prone to alcohol's ill-effects due to their lower body weight, smaller livers and lesser capacity to metabolize alcohol. As we age, our ability to handle alcohol decreases.

How To Calculate Alcohol Content

Percent alcohol on label refers to alcohol volume (ml alcohol/100ml).
Note: 100ml = 3½ fl.oz

To convert to grams (weight) of alcohol, multiply the alcohol volume by 0.8 – since 1 ml of alcohol weighs only 0.8 grams.

EXAMPLE:
12 fl.oz Can Beer
(5% alcohol)

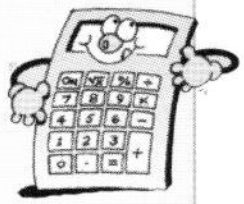

5% alc. volume
= 5% of 12 fl.oz = 0.6 fl.oz
= 18ml alcohol (Note: 1 fl.oz = 30ml)
Weight (18ml x 0.8) = 14.4g alcohol

Government Warnings!

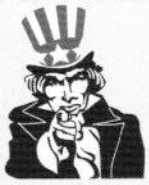

(1) According to the Surgeon General, women should not drink alcoholic beverages during pregnancy because of the risk of birth defects.

(2) Consumption of alcoholic beverages impairs your ability to drive a car or operate machinery, and may cause health problems.

Extra Information

Alcohol & Diabetes ~ See Page 19
Alcohol & The Heart ~ See Page 18
Tips to Avoid Harmful Drinking ~ Page 19

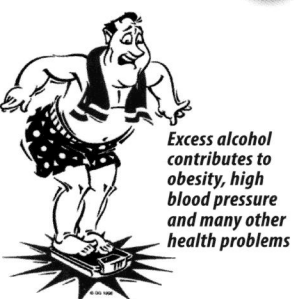

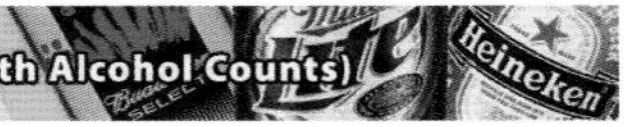

Quick Guide

Alc ~ Alcohol (Grams)

Beer:

Cb ~ Carbohydrate

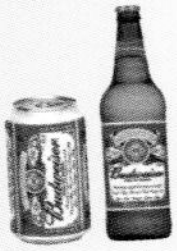
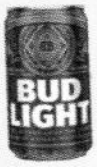

Beer Contains Zero Fat:	C	Alc	Cb
Regular Beer (5% Alc. Vol.):			
7 fl.oz Glass	80	8.5	4
12 fl.oz Bottle/Can/Glass	140	14	10
16 fl.oz/Pint	185	19	13
22 fl.oz Bottle	260	26	18
24 fl.oz Can	280	28	20
32 fl.oz/ ½ Yard	370	38	28
40 fl.oz Bottle	470	47	35
50 fl.oz Football	590	59	50
Light Beer (4.2% Alc. Vol.):			
7 fl.oz Glass	65	7	4
12 fl.oz Bottle/Can/Glass	110	12	7
16 fl.oz/Pint	145	16	9
22 fl.oz Bottle	200	22	13
24 fl.oz Can	220	24	14
Non-Alcoholic Brews:			
(Less than 0.5% alcohol by volume)			
Average all Brands, 12 fl.oz	70	1	14

Beer ~ Brands

Note: Figure shown are for the United States except for the states of Utah, Colorado, Kansas and Oklahoma who have certain restrictions limiting the alcohol content to not more than 4% by volume (3.2% by weight).

Percentage alcohol listed is by volume - not by weight.

Per 12 fl.oz Serving

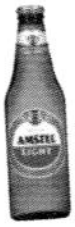
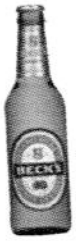
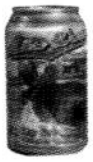
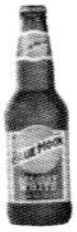

	C	Alc	Cb
Aguila (3.9%)	125	12	14
Amstel, Light (3.5%)	95	10	5
Anchor: Porter (5.6%)	210	16	23
Steam (4.9%)	160	14	14
Asahi: Kuronama (5.3%)	165	14	14
Select (4.7%)	140	13	11
Super Dry (4.9%)	150	14	11
Bass, Pale Ale (5.1%)	155	14	12
Beck's: Original (5%)	145	14	11
Premier Light (2.3%)	65	7	4
Sapphire (6%)	160	17	9
Big Sky: Original IPA (6.2%)	195	18	17
Moose Drool (5.3%)	175	15	16
Scape Goat (4.7%)	155	14	14
Trout Slayer Ale (4.7%)	145	14	12
Blatz: Original (4.6%)	145	13	13
Light (3.9%)	110	11	8
Blue Moon:			
Belgian White (5.4%)	170	15	14
Mango Wheat (5.4%)	175	15	16
Bohemia (4.73%)	140	14	12
Bud Ice (5.5%)	125	16	4

Brands (Cont)

Alc ~ Alcohol (Grams)

Per 12 fl.oz Serving

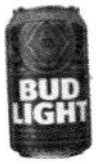
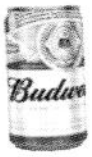
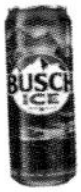
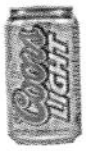
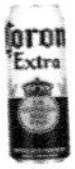
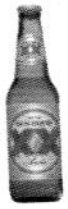
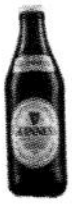
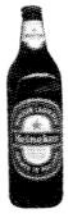
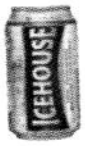

	C	Alc	Cb
Bud Light: Regular (4.2%)	110	12	7
Clamato Chelada: Orig. (4.2%)	150	12	16
Extra Lime; Mango (4.2%), av.	155	12	17
Lemonade (4.2%)	150	12	16
Lime (4%)	115	12	8
Orange (4.2%)	145	12	14
Platinum (6%)	140	17	5
Budweiser: Lager (5%)	145	14	11
Clamato Chelado (4.2%)	150	12	16
Discovery Reserve (5%)	155	14	13
Nitro Gold (5%)	170	14	15
Select (4.3%)	100	12	3
Select 55 (2.4%)	55	7	2
Zero (0%)	50	0	12
Busch: Original (4.3%)	115	12	7
Ice (5.9%)	135	17	4
Light (4.1%)	95	12	3
NA (0.4%)	60	1	13
Carlsberg, Pilsner (5%)	135	14	10
Carta Blanca (4.6%)	145	13	11
Cerveza, Aguila (4%)	125	11	11
Colorado Native, Amber (5.5%)	170	16	15
Colt 45, Malt Liquor (5.6%)	155	16	11
Coors: Banquet (5%)	145	14	12
Light (4.2%)	100	12	5
Non-Alcoholic	60	0	12
Corona: Extra (4.5%)	150	13	13
Light (4.1%)	100	12	5
Premier (4%)	90	11	11
Dos Equis XX: Ambar (4.7%)	145	14	12
Lager (4.5%)	140	13	11
Extra Gold (5%)	150	14	12
Fosters: Lager (5%)	145	14	11
Premium Ale (5.5%)	160	16	13
Genesee: Beer (4.5%)	145	13	13
Light (4%)	100	10	4
George Killian's, Irish Red (5.4%)	170	16	15
Goose Island, So-Lo (3%)	100	8	9
Grolsch, Premium (5%)	145	14	10
Guinness: Draught (4%)	125	12	10
Extra Stout (6%)	175	17	14
Blonde American (5%)	150	14	11
Nitro IPA (5.8%), 11.2oz	155	19	5
Hamm's: Original (4.7%)	145	13	12
Special Light (3.8%)	110	12	8
Heineken: Lager (5%)	140	14	10
Special Dark (5%)	165	14	15
Premium Light (3.5%)	100	10	7
0.0 (Alchohol-Free)	75	0	12
Hop Valley: Bubble Stash (6.2%)	195	17	16
Citrus Mistress (6.5%)	190	18	14
Hurricane: Malt Liquor (6%)	140	17	4
High Gravity (8.1%)	185	23	6
Icehouse, Original (5.5%)	150	16	10

Brands (Cont)

Alc ~ Alcohol (Grams) Cb ~ Carbohydrate

Beer Contains Zero Fat:
Per 12 fl.oz Serving

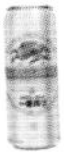
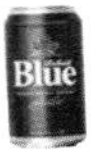
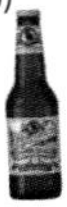
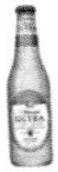
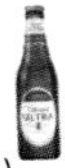
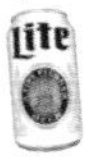
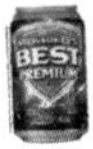
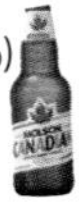
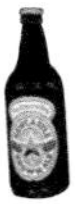
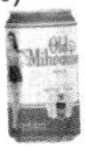
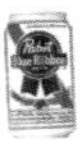

	C	Alc	Cb
Keystone: Ice (5.9%)	145	17	7
Light (4.1%)	100	12	5
King Cobra (6%)	135	17	4
Kirin: Ichiban (5%)	145	14	11
Light (3.2%)	95	9	8
Kokanee (5%)	145	14	11
Labatt: Blue (5%)	135	14	10
Blue Light (4%)	110	11	8
Laqunitas, Daytime (4%)	100	12	3
Landshark, Lager (4.6%)	150	13	13
Leinenkugel's: Original (4.7%)	150	13	15
Summer Shandy (4.2%)	135	12	13
Lone Star: Pale Lager (4.65%)	135	13	11
Light (3.85%)	110	11	8
Lowenbrau, Original (5%)	140	14	12
Magic Hat, #9 (5.1% alc)	165	15	15
Magnum, Malt Liquor (5.6%)	155	16	11
Michelob Ultra:			
Ultra Amber (4%)	100	11	5
Ultra Infusions, Lime (4%)	95	11	5
Ultra Light (4.2%)	95	12	3
Ultra Pure Gold (3.8%)	85	12	3
Mickey's, Malt Liquor (5.6%)	155	16	11
Miller:			
Genuine Draft/High Life (4.6%)	140	13	12
High Life Light (4.1%)	110	12	6
Lite (4.2%)	95	12	3
Miller64 (2.8%)	65	8	3
Milwaukee's Best:			
Ice (5.9%)	150	17	8
Light (4.1%)	95	12	4
Premium (4.8%)	145	14	12
Minnesota's Best, Original (4.9%)	140	14	10
Modelo, Especial (4.4%)	145	13	14
Molson Canadian: Ice (5.6%)	170	16	14
Lager (5%)	150	14	12
Canadian 67 (3%)	70	8	3
Moosehead, Lager (5%)	150	14	11
Natural: Ice (5.9%)	130	17	4
Light (4.2%)	95	12	3
Negra Modelo (5.4%)	175	15	16
Newcastle, Brown Ale (4.7%)	130	13	10
O'Douls: Amber (0.4%)	90	1	18
Original (0.4%)	65	1	13
Old Milwaukee: Lager (4.6%)	145	13	13
Light (3.8%)	110	11	8
Non-Alcoholic (0.4%)	60	1	12
Old Style: Lager (4.7%)	145	13	12
Light (4.2%)	115	12	7
Pabst: Blue Ribbon (4.8%)	145	13	12
Low Calorie (3.8%)	110	11	8
Pacifico, Clara (4.4%)	145	12	13

Per 12 fl.oz Serving Unless Indicated

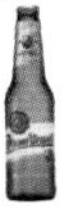
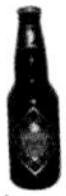
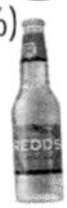
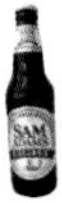
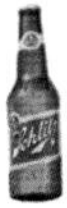
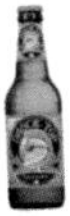
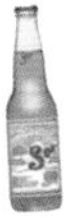
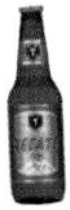
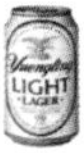

	C	Alc	Cb
Palmier, (4.2%), 11.2 fl.oz	90	11	3
Peroni, Nastro Azzurro (5.1%)	150	14	12
Piels, Lager (4.3%)	125	12	9
Pilsner Urquell, Lager (4.4%)	155	12	16
Point: Amber Classic (4.7%)	160	13	14
Special Lager (4.7%)	150	13	12
Presidente (5%)	175	14	5
Redbridge, Lager (4%)	135	10	14
Red Dog, Lager (4.8%)	145	14	12
Red Hook: ESB (5.8%)	185	16	16
India Pale Ale (4.7%)	190	13	19
Red Stripe, Jamaican Lager (7%)	150	13	14
Redd's: Apple Ale (5%), 12 fl.oz	165	14	17
Wicked Hard Ale (8%), av. 10 fl.oz	230	19	25
Saint Archer: Blonde (4.8%)	150	14	13
Pale Ale (5.5%)	170	16	13
Samuel Adams:			
Boston Lager (4.9%)	175	14	17
Sam Adams, Light Lager (4%)	120	13	8
Sapporo, Prem. Lager (4.9%)	135	14	9
Schaefer: Lager (4.6%)	145	13	12
Light (3.9%)	110	11	8
Schell's: Deer (4.7%)	145	14	13
Light (3.5%)	100	10	7
Schlitz: Pale Lager (4.6%)	145	13	12
Light (3.8%)	110	11	8
Schmidt's: Pale Lager (4.6%)	145	13	13
Light (3.8%)	110	11	8
Sharps, *(Miller)*, N.A., 12 fl.oz	60	0	12
Sheaf, Stout (5.7%)	190	16	19
Shock Top: Belgian White (5.2%)	165	15	15
Lemon Shandy (4.2%)	145	12	15
Sierra Nevada: Bigfoot (9.6%)	330	28	32
Draft Pale Ale (5%)	155	14	13
Pale Ale (5.6%)	175	16	14
Sol: Lager (4.5%)	140	13	12
Chelada (3.5%)	160	10	20
Sparks, Lager (6%)	250	17	34
Steel Reserve:			
High Gravity Malt Liquor (8.1%)	220	23	15
Steel 6.0 (6%)	165	17	11
Stella Artois, (5%), 11.2 fl.oz	140	14	11
Stroh's: Classic (4.5%)	145	13	12
Light (4.1%)	120	12	7
Tecate: Pale Lager (4.6%)	140	13	11
Light (4%)	110	11	8
Third Shift, Amber Lager (5.3%)	185	15	18
Trader Jose: Premium, 11.2 fl.oz	145	14	14
Light (3.8%), 11.2 fl.oz	105	14	8
Victoria Lager (4%)	135	11	14
Wild Blue, Lager (8%)	240	23	20
Yuengling: Light (3.2%)	99	9	9
Traditional Lager (4.5%)	140	13	12
ZeigenBock, Amber (4.9%)	145	14	11

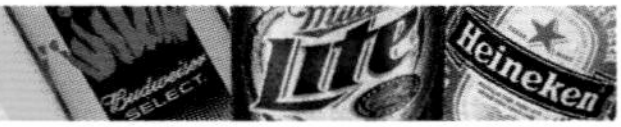

Alc ~ Alcohol (Grams) Cb ~ Carbohydrate

Ciders ~ Alcoholic/Hard

Per 12 fl.oz Unless Indicated

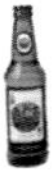
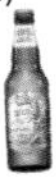
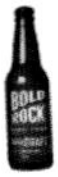
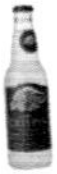
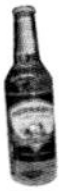
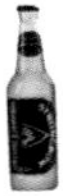
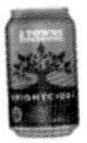
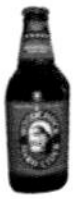
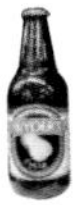

	C	Alc	Cb
Ace: Apple (5%), 12 fl.oz	**145**	14	12
Berry (5%), 12 fl.oz	**155**	14	14
Joker (6.9%), 12 fl.oz	**190**	19	13
Perry (5%), 12 fl.oz	**170**	14	18
Pineapple (5%), 12 fl.oz	**175**	14	19
Angry Orchard: Crisp Apple (5%)	**190**	14	25
Easy Apple (4.2%), 12 fl.oz	**150**	12	19
Green Apple (5.5%), 12 fl.oz	**210**	14	31
Pear (5%), 12 fl.oz	**160**	14	17
Rosé (5.5%), 12 fl.oz	**170**	16	17
Bold Rock: Apple, (4.7%), 12 fl.oz	**140**	13	12
Carolina Draft (4.7%), 12 fl.oz	**145**	13	13
IPA (4.7%), 12 fl.oz	**140**	13	12
Pear (4.7%), 12 fl.oz	**140**	13	12
Premium Dry (6%), 12 fl.oz	**140**	17	6
Crispin: Original (5%), 12 fl.oz	**160**	14	15
Blackberry Pear (5%), 12 fl.oz	**170**	14	16
Brut (5.5%), 12 fl.oz	**170**	16	13
Honey Crisp (6.5%), 12 fl.oz	**200**	18	16
Pacific Pear (4.5%), 12 fl.oz	**160**	13	17
Rosé (5%), 12 fl.oz	**160**	14	13
The Saint (6.9%), 12 fl.oz	**230**	19	20
Hornsby's: Amber (5.5%)	**180**	16	19
Crisp (5.5%), 12 fl.oz	**190**	16	26
Johnny Appleseed, (5.5%)	**210**	16	26
Magners, (4.5%)	**125**	13	9
Michelob, Ultra Light Cider (4%)	**120**	10	10
Saint Archer, Hard Cider (6.1%)	**170**	17	11
Smith & Forge, Hard Apple (6%)	**220**	17	26
Stella Artois Cidre, (4.5%)	**180**	13	22
Strongbow: *Per 11.2 fl oz*			
Cherry Blossom, (4.5%), av.	**155**	12	25
Original Dry (5%), 12 fl.oz	**145**	14	10
Rosé Apple (5%)	**140**	13	11
2 Towns Ciderhouse:			
Brightcider Apple (6%), 12 fl.oz	**145**	17	7
Ginger Ninja (6%), 12 fl.oz	**145**	17	7
Made Marion (6%), 12 fl.oz	**150**	17	8
Outcider (5%), 12 fl.oz	**155**	14	14
Pacific Pineapple (5%), 12 fl.oz	**150**	14	12
Woodchuck: Amber (5%)	**200**	14	21
Granny Smith (5%), 12 fl.oz	**160**	14	11
Pear (4%), 12 fl.oz	**150**	12	18
Raspberry (4%), 12 fl.oz	**170**	12	22
Semi-Dry (5.5%), 12 fl.oz	**160**	14	13
Wyder's: Pear (4%), 12 fl.oz	**140**	11	22
Prickly Pineapple (5%), 12 fl.oz	**180**	14	22
Raspberry (4%), 12 fl.oz	**120**	11	17
Reposado (6.9%), 12 fl.oz	**250**	19	30

Quick Guide ~ Table Wines

Average all Varieties (11.5% Alc.)
(Wine Contains Zero Fat)

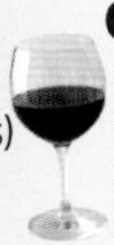
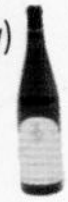

	C	Alc	Cb
4 fl.oz, 1 small wine glass OR ½ large wine glass	**100**	11	3
6 fl.oz, (¾ large wine glass)	**145**	16	5
8 fl.oz, (1 large wine glass)	**200**	21	7
½ Carafe/Bottle, 12 fl.oz	**300**	32	10
1 Bottle, 750ml, 25.4 fl.oz	**620**	68	21
Red Wines: *Per 4 fl.oz*			
Burgundy/Cabernet/Merlot, av.	**100**	11	4
White Wines: *Per 4 fl.oz*			
Dry (Chenin; Fume Blanc; Chardonnay)	**95**	11	4
Sparkling, 4 fl.oz	**95**	11	4
Zinfandel Sweet, (Moselle/Sauterne), 4 fl.oz	**85**	11	2

Other Wines

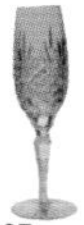

	C	Alc	Cb
Champagne: *Per 4 fl.oz*			
Average all types, 1 glass	**85**	11	2
with Orange Jce (3:1 orange)	**75**	8	4
with Orange Jce (1:1 orange)	**65**	5	7
Mulled Wine *(Gluhwein)*, 4 fl.oz	**180**	14	20
Non-Alcoholic Wine: *Less than 0.5% Alcohol*			
Ariel: White varieties, average, 4 fl.oz	**35**	0.5	8
Red varieties, average, 4 fl.oz	**25**	0.5	5
Flavored/Reduced Alcohol Wine:			
Average All Brands (6% alcohol):			
(Arbor Mist, Wild Vines, Boone's Farm):			
1 small wine glass, 4 fl.oz	**80**	6	10
1 large wine glass, 8 fl.oz	**160**	11	20
Skinnygirl, Red/White, (8.5%), 5 fl.oz	**100**	10	5
Sake *(Gekkeikan)*, (16%), 4 fl.oz	**120**	15	5
Sangria *(Skinnygirl)*, (4%), 5 fl.oz	**130**	5	23

Dessert Wines

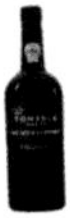

	C	Alc	Cb
Madeira (18%), 2 oz	**85**	9	5
Marsala (18%), 2 oz	**110**	9	11
Port, Muscatel (18%), 2 oz	**85**	9	5
Sherry (15%), 2 oz:			
Dry, 1 Sherry glass	**90**	7	7
Sweet/Cream, average	**90**	7	8
Vermouth *(Martini & Rossi)*:			
Extra Dry (18%), 2 oz	**65**	9	2
Martini Rosso (16%), 2 oz	**90**	8	8

Cooking Wines

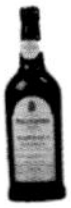

	C	Alc	Cb
Holland House:			
Marsala, (14%), 2 T., 1 fl.oz	**45**	4	4
Red/White, (10%): 2 T., 1 fl.oz	**20**	2	1
1 cup, 8 fl.oz	**160**	18	8
Sherry, (17%), 2 Tbsp, 1 fl.oz	**45**	5	2

Quick Guide

Alc ~ Alcohol (Grams)

Spirits/Liquors:
Includes Bourbon, Brandy, Gin, Rum, Scotch, Tequila, Vodka, Whiskey.
Note: All spirits with same alcohol proof have similar calories and zero fat.

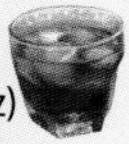

Average All Brands	C	Alc	Cb
80 Proof (40% Alcohol by Volume):			
1 fl.oz	65	9.5	0
1.5 fl.oz (1 shot)	100	14	0
3 fl.oz (Double shot)	195	28	0
½ Bottle, 350 ml (12 fl.oz)	770	113	0
1 Bottle, 700 ml (24 fl.oz)	1540	227	0
86 Proof (43% Alc), 1.5 fl.oz shot	105	15	0
100 Proof (50% Alc), 1.5 fl.oz	125	18	0
Shochu (Soju), av., (25% alc), 2 fl.oz	65	12	0

Flavored Spirits

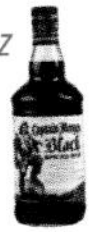

	C	Alc	Cb
Captain Morgan: *Per 1.5 fl.oz*			
Original (35%)	85	12	0.5
Black Spiced (47.3%)	115	14	1
Parrot Bay (21%), average	90	7.5	10
Silver Spiced (35%)	95	12	2
Malibu Rum, Orig,/Fruit (21%), 1.5 fl.oz	80	8	8
Southern Comfort (35%), 1.5 fl.oz	100	13	3

Hard Lemonade, Sodas, Seltzers & Tea

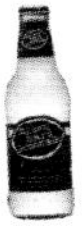

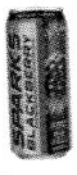

	C	Alc	Cb
Bud Light Seltzers, (5%), 12 fl.oz	100	14	2
Corona Seltzer, (4.5%), 12 fl.oz	90	12	0
Henry's Hard Soda:			
Grape (4.2%), 12 fl.oz	225	12	35
Lemon Lime/Orange (4.2%), 12 fl.oz	190	12	28
Labatt Blue Light Seltzer, (5%)	100	14	1
Margaritaville:			
Lime Margarita (8%), 12 fl.oz	310	23	30
Paradise Punch (8%), 12 fl.oz	340	23	46
Mike's Hard Lemonade:			
Black Cherry (5%), 11.2 fl.oz	220	13	33
Lite (5%), 11.2 fl.oz	150	13	15
Lemonade (5%), 11.2 fl.oz	220	13	33
Lite (5%), 11.2 fl.oz	100	13	4
Harder (8%), 16 fl.oz	395	31	44
Not Your Father's Root Beer, (5.9%), 12 fl.oz	195	17	20
Pabst Hard Coffee, (5%), 11 fl.oz	250	13	31
Platform Setzer, (5%), 11.2 fl.oz	110	13	4
Pura Still, (4.5%), 11.2 fl.oz	90	12	1
Redd's Wicked, (8%), av. 10 fl.oz	230	19	25
Social Club Seltzer, (7%), 12 fl.oz	150	20	2
Sparks, Original (6%), 16 fl.oz	335	23	45
Twisted Tea: Original (5%)	220	14	31
Half & Half (5%)	260	14	34
Zumbida Mango, (4.2%), 12 fl.oz	150	12	17

Coolers & Premix Cocktails

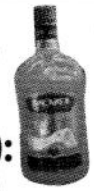

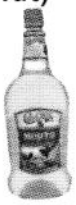

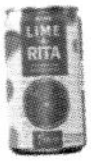

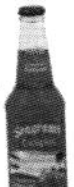

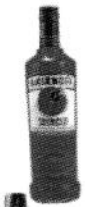

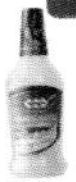

Ready-To-Drink: *Zero Fat Unless Indicated*	C	Alc	Cb
Bacardi: *Per 4 fl.oz*			
Party Drinks (Ready To Pour):			
Bahama Mama; Mai Tai (10%)	130	9	16
Mojito (15%)	160	14	16
Rum Island Ice Tea (12.5%)	150	12	16
Bacardi Silver: *Per 12 fl.oz*			
Lemonade/Sangria (6%), av.	270	17	41
Mojito/Raz/Strawberry (5%)	240	14	36
Bartles & Jaymes: *Per 11.2 fl.oz*			
Malt Based Coolers (3.2%):			
Exotic Berry	195	9	31
Fuzzy Navel	215	9	36
Margarita; Pina Colada, av.	245	9	44
Pomegranate Raspberry	205	9	35
Sangria	240	9	40
Strawberry Daiquiri	205	9	34
Cape Lime, Cocktails (4.5%), av. 12 fl.oz	120	13	9
Captain Morgan's,			
Parrot Bay (4.1%), all var. av., 11.2 fl.oz	210	10	35
Chi Chi's: Long Is. Iced Tea, 4 fl.oz	145	12	17
Mexican Mudslide, 4 fl.oz (8g fat)	240	2	42
Mojito, 4 fl.oz	160	11	21
Pina Colada, 4 fl.oz (6g fat)	240	4	42
White Russian, 4 fl.oz (7g fat)	245	2	43
Daily's, Frozen Pouches (5%), average all flavors, 10 fl.oz	285	12	47
Jack Daniels, Country Cocktails (4.8%), average all varieties, 10 fl.oz	200	9	30
Jose Cuervo:			
Margaritas: Classic Lime (10%), 6 fl.oz	210	14	29
Golden (12.7%), 4.7 fl.oz	170	14	19
Pabst, Hard Coffee (5%), 11 fl.oz	250	13	31
Ritas: Lime-A-Rita (8%), 8 fl.oz	220	15	29
Spritz (6%), av., 12 fl.oz	200	17	21
Seagram's:			
Escapes Coolers (3.2%):			
Bahama Mama, 11.2 fl.oz	200	9	36
Strawb. Daiquiri, 11.2 fl.oz	225	9	41
Skinnygirl:			
Vodka with flavors (30%), 1.5 fl.oz	75	11	0
Cocktails (10%), av., 3 fl.oz	70	8	4
Smirnoff:			
Ice (4.5%): Original, 11.2 fl.oz	220	13	33
Mango; Pineapple, av., 11.2 fl.oz	230	13	35
Sourced, Fruit Flavors, (4.5%), 11.2 fl.oz	160	12	20
Spiked Sparkling Seltzer, (4.5%), all flav., 12 fl.oz can	90	13	1
TGI Friday's:			
On The Rocks: *Per 6 fl.oz*			
Long Island Ice Tea (15%)	250	21	28
Margarita (7.5%)	185	11	29
Mudslide (10%)	365	14	31
Blenders (12.5%), Mudslide, 6 fl.oz	365	18	31

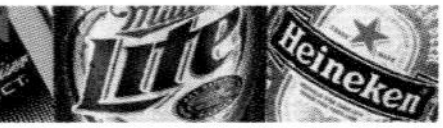

Coolers & Premix Cocktails (Cont)

Ready-To-Drink:

The Club Premix Cocktails: *Per 3.4 oz Serving (½ can)*	C	Alc	Cb
Censored on Beach; Margarita (7.5%)	**105**	6	17
Gin/Vodka Martini (21%), av.	**155**	17	0.2
Ice Tea (15%)	**145**	12	17
Manhattan (17%)	**115**	13	5
Mudslide/Pina Colada (10%), av.	**200**	8	16
Screwdriver (7.5%)	**95**	6	14
Whiskey Sour (10%)	**95**	8	11

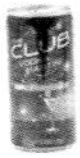

Shooters

Alc ~ Alcohol (Grams)

	C	Alc	Cb
Alabama Slammer	**110**	14	2
Amaretto Sour	**120**	6	19
B52	**145**	14	11
Beam Me Up Scotty	**145**	13	13
Blue Tequila	**160**	18	6
Jager Bomb	**205**	8	30
Jager Bomb, w/ Sugar-Free Red Bull	**155**	8	18
Jell-O Shot: 3 oz, with 1.5 oz Vodka	**180**	14	19
with Diet Jell-O	**110**	14	0
Kamikaze	**75**	8	3
Kool-Aid	**160**	15	14
Orgasm	**100**	12	6
Peppermint Patty	**195**	8	11
Stinger	**170**	18	12
Surfer on Acid	**90**	7	11

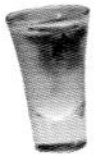

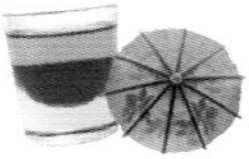

Cocktail Mixers ~ Non-Alcoholic

	C	Alc	Cb
Bacardi: *Per 8 fl.oz, Prepared from 2 fl.oz Concentrate*			
Daiquiris; Rum Runner	**120**	0	32
Margarita	**90**	0	25
Mojito	**110**	0	30
Pina Colada	**170**	0	36
Baja Bob's: *Per 4 fl.oz*			
Cranberry Cosmo Martini	**10**	0	2
Pina Colada	**30**	0	4
Jose Cuervo:			
Margaritas: Av. all flav., 4 fl.oz	**85**	0	21
Light (Sugar Free), Lime, 4 fl.oz	**5**	0	1
Mr & Mrs T:			
Bloody Mary: Original, 5 oz	**30**	0	7
Bold & Spicy, 4 oz	**35**	0	7
Mai Tai	**130**	0	32
Margarita	**100**	0	26
Pina Colada	**170**	0	44
Strawberry Daiquiri	**180**	0	46
TGI Friday's:			
Mudslide, 2.3 fl.oz	**110**	0	23
Cosmo; Berrytini, 2 fl.oz	**80**	0	20
Strawb. Daiquiri; Marg., 4 fl.oz	**190**	0	46

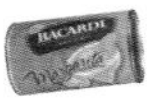

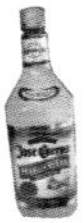

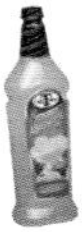

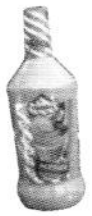

Cocktails

Alc ~ Alcohol (Grams)

Made to Standard Recipes (Standard Size):
(Main Reference: The New American Bartender's Guide)

Zero Fat Unless Indicated	C	Alc	Cb
Adios Mother F.	**260**	23	23
Bacardi & Coke (with 1.5 oz Bacardi)	**160**	14	17
Bellini, 4.5 fl.oz	**95**	11	7
Bloody Mary (with 1.5 oz Vodka)	**125**	10	7
Blushin' Russian (20g fat)	**405**	14	23
Bourbon & Soda (with 2 oz Bourbon)	**130**	19	0
Brandy Alexander (10g fat)	**300**	20	15
Chupa Naranjas (with 1.5 oz Tequila)	**150**	16	8
Cosmopolitan	**215**	24	12
Daiquiri (w/ 2 oz Rum), av. all types	**140**	19	4
Frozen Daiquiri (with 2 oz Rum):			
without fruit	**155**	19	6
with fruit (with 1.5 oz Rum)	**145**	14	11
Grasshopper	**260**	17	28
Harvey Wallbanger (2 oz)	**200**	19	17
Highball (1.5 oz Whiskey)	**100**	14	0
Irish Coffee (10g fat)	**205**	14	2
Kahlua Mudslide: with milk (3g fat)	**145**	11	12
with cream (12g fat)	**230**	11	10
Lemon Drop, 4 fl.oz	**130**	14	10
Long Island Iced Tea (with 3 oz Cola)	**270**	19	32
with 3 oz Diet Cola	**235**	19	22
Mai Tai (with 2 oz Rum)	**290**	24	33
Manhattan	**130**	17	5
Margarita	**160**	18	7
Martini: Dry, with 1.5 oz gin	**100**	14	0
Sour Apple, w/ 2 oz Vodka/1 oz Schnapps	**250**	31	10
Mint Julep (with 2½ oz Bourbon)	**180**	24	4
Mojito (with 2 oz rum)	**170**	19	9
Moscow Mule (with 1.5 oz Vodka)	**180**	14	20
Pina Colada (10g fat), 6 oz	**250**	15	18
Red Bull & Vodka (with 1.5 oz vodka)	**210**	14	28
with Sugar Free Red Bull	**105**	14	3
Rum & Coke (with 1.5 oz Rum)	**160**	14	17
Sake Bomb (1.5 oz Sake & 5 oz Beer)	**105**	12	7
Sangria: with 1 oz Fruit Juice, 5 oz	**120**	12	9
with 0.5 oz Brandy, 5.5 oz	**150**	17	9
Screwdriver	**160**	14	15
Sex On The Beach	**235**	19	25
Spritzer (with 3 oz Wine)	**65**	8	2
Tequila Sunrise	**200**	14	25
Tom Collins (with 2 oz Gin)	**210**	19	18
Vodka Soda (with 1.5 oz Vodka)	**100**	14	0
Vodka Tonic (with 1.5 oz Vodka)	**165**	14	18
Whiskey Sour (w/ 2 oz Whiskey)	**155**	19	7
White Russian (10g fat)	**240**	19	7
Non-Alcoholic:			
Cinderella	**45**	0	11
Shirley Temple (with 6 oz Ginger Ale)	**140**	0	34

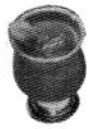

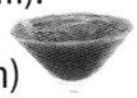

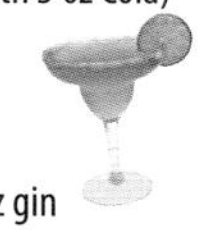

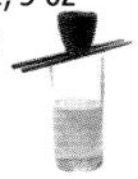

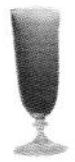

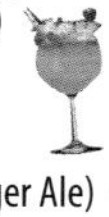

Liqueurs/Cordials

Per 1 fl.oz

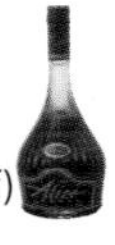
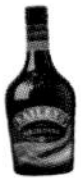
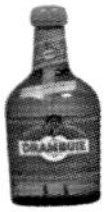
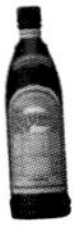
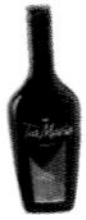

	C	Alc	Cb
Advocaat (36 Proof; 2g fat)	**85**	4	9
Alizé: Cognac (80 Proof)	**70**	9	2
Gold/Red Passion (32 Proof)	**105**	4	11
Amaretto (56 Proof)	**110**	7	17
Baileys Irish Cream (34 Proof; 4g fat)	**100**	4	8
Benedictine (80 Proof)	**90**	9	5
Chambord (33 Proof)	**105**	4	11
Chartreuse (80 Proof)	**100**	9	9
Cherry Brandy (48 Proof)	**80**	6	9
Coffee Liqueur (53 Proof)	**115**	7	16
Cointreau (80 Proof)	**95**	9	7
Creme de Cacao (54 Proof)	**100**	6	15
Creme de Menthe (72 Proof)	**125**	9	14
Curacao (70 Proof)	**95**	8	6
Drambuie (80 Proof)	**105**	9	9
Frangelico (40 Proof)	**65**	5	12
Galliano (86 Proof)	**100**	10	8
Grand Marnier (80 Proof)	**100**	9	7
(40 Proof)	**85**	5	14
Kirsch (68 Proof)	**80**	8	6
Midori (42 Proof)	**80**	5	11
Ouzo (80 Proof)	**105**	9	11
Pernod (80 Proof)	**75**	9	11
Sambuca (84 Proof)	**100**	10	11
Schnapps (100 Proof)	**115**	12	9
Southern Comfort (70 Proof)	**65**	8	3
Tia Maria (40% Proof)	**90**	7	10

Liqueur Coffee & Hot Drinks

Per Standard Drink

	C	Alc	Cb
Liqueur Coffee: Av. all types	**200**	10	10
Irish, 1.5 oz Whiskey & 1 oz whip	**205**	9	4
Hot Toddy, with 1½ oz liquor, av. all	**170**	9	19
Mulled Wine *(Glühwein)*, 4 fl.oz, av	**195**	14	25

"The doctor told him to cut down to just one glass a day."

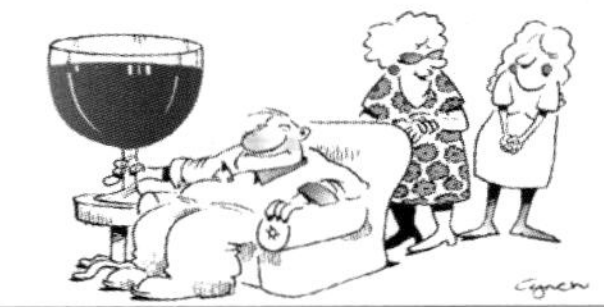

TEN TIPS TO AVOID HARMFUL DRINKING

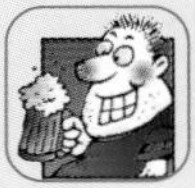

1. **Add up the alcohol** you typically drink each day and on social occasions. How does this compare with 'low risk' amounts? *(See page 23)*
2. **Compare the alcohol content** of different drinks and select the lowest. Request half shots of alcohol in cocktails and mixed drinks. Dilute them and keep topping off with non-alcoholic drinks.
3. **Go easy on 'Light' beers.** At 4% alcohol, on average, they are still high in alcohol compared to regular beer (5% alcohol).
4. **Try low alcohol or non-alcohol** alternatives such as fruit juices and mineral water. Take your own to parties.
5. **Before drinking alcohol,** quench your thirst with water and non-alcoholic drinks – particularly after vigorous exercise or sports.
6. **Slow the rate of drinking.** Chugging or drinking fast is the major cause of illness and death from alcohol poisoning.
7. **Avoid drinking in 'rounds'.**
8. **Have a non-alcoholic 'spacer'** between drinks (e.g. mineral water, orange juice).
9. **Don't drink on an empty stomach.** Food slows the rate of alcohol absorption.
10. **Keep track of the number of drinks** and know when to stop. Stick to a set limit.

Note: Alcohol can be very dangerous when taken with prescription or street drugs, or when you are very tired.

Extra Info: www.CalorieKing.com

Cocktail Mixers & Extracts

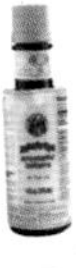
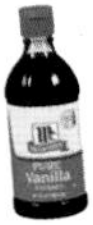

	C	Alc	Cb
Angostura Bitters, ¼ tsp	**2**	0	0.5
Grenadine, ½ tsp	**6**	0	2
Lime/Lemon Juice, 2 Tbsp, 1 oz	**10**	0	2
Maraschino Cherry, 1 small	**8**	0	2
Simple Syrup, 1 Tbsp, av.	**50**	0	14
Sweet & Sour Mix, 2 Tbsp, 1 oz	**30**	0	7
Tonic Water, 8 fl.oz	**80**	0	22
Flavor Extracts *(McCormick)*:			
Pure Lemon (83%), 1 tsp	**0**	3.5	0
Pure Vanilla (35%), 1tsp	**0**	1.5	0

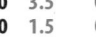

B Baking Ingredients

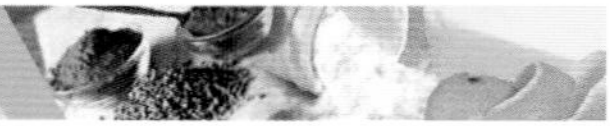

Baking Ingredients

Baking Ingredients	C	F	Cb
Almond Flour, ¼ cup, 1 oz	160	10	10
Almond Paste, (Marzipan), 2 Tbsp	170	7	24
Apple Pie Filling, Sweetened, 9.4 oz	290	0	69
(Bean Water), ¼ c., 2 oz	10	0	2
Amaranth Flour *(Bob's Red Mill)*, ¼ cup, 1 oz	110	2	20
Baking Powder: Regular, 1 tsp	5	0	1
Cream of Tartar, 1 tsp	10	0	2
Baking Mix *(Bisquick)*: Original, ⅓ cup, 1.5 oz	160	5	26
Batter Mix *(Golden Dipt)*, All Purpose, ¼ cup	100	0	20
Butter/Margarine, ½ cup, 4 oz	800	88	1
Stick *(Land O' Lakes)*, 0.5 oz	100	11	0
Cacao Butter, 2 Tbsp, 1 oz	240	28	0
Cacao Powder, raw: 1 Tbsp, 0.3 oz	35	2	3
¼ cup, 1 oz	150	9	11
Carob Flour, ½ cup	115	0.5	46
Cassava Flour, ½ cup, 70g	260	0	62
Chia Seed Protein Powder, 2 T., 0.5 oz	25	0	8
Chocolate Baking Bars: *Average all Brands*			
Sweet *(Baker's)*: 1 oz portion	120	7	16
4 oz bar	470	28	64
Semi-sweet, 1 oz	140	9	16
White Baking, 1 oz	160	9	16
Unsweetened: 1 oz	140	14	8
Grated, 1 cup, 4.5 oz	660	69	39
Chocolate Baking Chips: *Average all Brands*			
Milk Choc./Semi Sweet, 1 oz	140	8	18
½ cup, 3 oz	420	24	54
1 cup, 6 oz	840	48	108
Dark, 1 Tbsp, 0.5 oz	70	5	3
Mini Kisses *(Hershey)*, 1 piece	5	0.5	1
Cocoa Powder, unsweetened:			
1 Tbsp, 0.2 oz	15	0.5	3
⅓ cup, 1 oz	60	4	17
Coconut, dried:			
Sweetened/Flaked: 1 oz	130	8	15
½ cup, 1.3 oz	195	12	22
Tsd *(Baker's)*, 1 oz	170	13	13
Unsweetened, 1 oz	190	18	7
Coconut Cream/Milk ~ *See Page 89*			
Coconut Flour, 2 Tbsp, 0.5 oz	60	2	8
Coconut Manna *(Nutiva)*, 1 Tbsp	100	9	3
Cornstarch, 1 Tbsp	30	0	7
Eggs: Large (1)	75	5	0
Jumbo (1)	90	6	0.5
Egg White: 1 Egg White	15	0	0
½ cup (4 egg whites), 4 oz	60	0	1

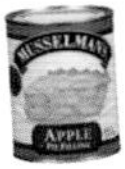

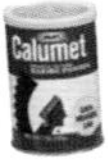

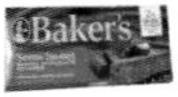

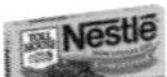

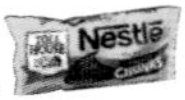

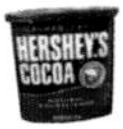

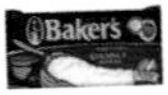

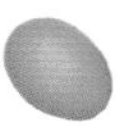

Flour:	C	F	Cb
Whole Wheat, 1 cup, 4.2 oz	400	2	84
White: 1 Tbsp, 0.3 oz	25	0	5.5
1 cup, 4.2 oz	400	1	88
Flavor Extracts: *Av. all Brands*			
Imitation, 1 tsp	10	0	2
Pure Extract, 1 tsp	10	0	0.5
Almond; Vanilla, 1 tsp	10	0	0.5
Fruit Pectin: Swtnd, ¼ tsp	5	0	1
Unsweetened, ¼ tsp	0	0	0
Gelatin, dry, unsweetened, 0.3 oz	20	0	0
Glaze *(Duncan Hines)*: Choc., 2 T.	150	7	21
Vanilla, 2 Tbsp	140	6	22
Hazelnut Meal/Flour, ¼ cup, 1 oz	160	12	8
Hemp Protein Powder, ¼ cup, 1.1 oz	120	3	10
Honey, ½ cup, 6 oz	515	0	145
Lemon/Orange Peel, ¼ cup	25	0	6
Lighter Bake *(Sunsweet)*: (Butter & Oil replacement)			
1 Tbsp, ½ oz	35	0	9
¼ Cup, 2.7 oz	140	0	36
Masa Harina *(Bob's Red Mill)*, ½ cup, 2 oz	220	2	47
Milk: Whole, 1 cup, 8 fl.oz	150	8	12
2%, 1 cup, 8 fl.oz	120	5	12
1%, 1 cup, 8 fl.oz	100	2.5	12
Fat-Free, 1 cup, 8 fl.oz	90	0.5	13
Oat Flour *(Bob's Red Mill)*, ⅓ cup, 1.5 oz	120	3	26
Pastry ~ *See Page 134*			
Pie Crusts ~ *See Page 134*			
Pie Fillings, Fruits ~ *See Page 134*			
Lemon Creme, ⅓ cup	130	1.5	28
Mincemeat, 3.5 oz	190	5	45
Pumpkin, 1 cup, 9.3 oz	270	1.5	60
Prune Puree, ¼ cup, 3 oz	220	0	55
Quinoa Flour, ¼ cup, 1 oz	110	1.5	18
Raisins, ½ cup, 2.8 oz	240	0.5	63
Rennin, 0.4 oz pkt	10	0	2
Rice Flour, ½ cup, 2.8 oz	290	1	63
Soy Milk ~ *See Pages 49-50*			
Soy Flour, *(Bob's Red Mill)*, 100% Whole Ground, ¼ cup, 1 oz	120	6	8
Sprinkles, all types, 1 tsp	20	1	3
Sugar: 1 Tbsp, 0.5 oz	55	0	14
1 oz	110	0	28
1 cup, 7 oz	775	0	195
16 oz (1 lb)	1760	0	454
Sweeteners & Sugar Substitutes ~ *See Page 156*			
Vinegar, average all types, 1 oz	5	0	1
Whey, sweet, dry, 1 oz	100	0.5	21
Yeast:			
Active, dry, 0.3 oz pkg	25	0.5	3
Bakers, compressed, 1 oz	30	0.5	5
Fleischmann's, 0.6 oz pkg	0	0	0

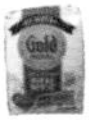

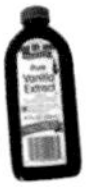
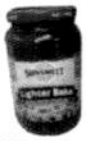
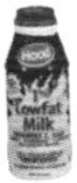

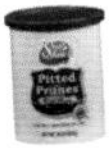
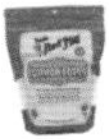
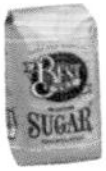

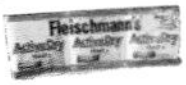

Note: Actual weight of bars is usually 5-10% more than label Net Weight. Weigh bar and allow extra calories.

Bars ~ Brands

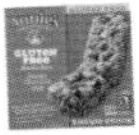
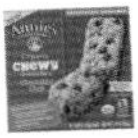
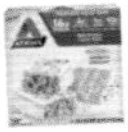
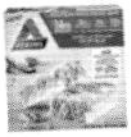
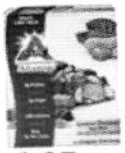
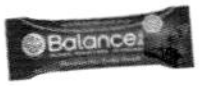

Per Bar	C	F	Cb
AdvantEdge ~ *See EAS*			
Annie's Homegrown:			
Gluten Free, all varieties, 1 oz	110	3	20
Organic Chewy Granola Bars: *Per 0.9 oz Bar*			
Chocolate Chip	100	2.5	18
Oatmeal Raisin	90	1.5	19
PB Chocolate Chip	110	3.5	17
Organic Crispy, P'nut Butter, 0.9 oz	80	2	15
Protein, Choc. P'nut Butter, 1.2 oz	140	7	16
Atkins:			
Meal Bars: *Per 1.7 oz Unless Indicated*			
Birthday Cake	190	10	17
Blueberry Greek Yogurt	190	9	21
Choc. Almond Caramel	180	9	17
Chocolate Chip Granola	200	9	18
Chocolate Peanut Butter, 2 oz	240	15	23
Cookies 'n Crème, 1.76 oz	190	11	22
Peanut Fudge Granola	200	11	17
Vanilla Pecan Crisp	190	10	17
Note: Carb figures include 12-15g Fiber & Glycerin			
Snack Bars: *Per 1.55 oz Bar Unless Indicated*			
Caramel Chocolate Nut Roll	180	12	20
Caramel Chocolate Peanut Nougat	170	11	19
Caramel Double Chocolate Crunch	150	9	20
Choc. Chip Crisp, 1.23 oz	140	6	16
Cranberry Almond, 1.27 oz	140	6	16
Lemon Bar, 1.4 oz	150	7	15
Peanut Butter Fudge Crisp, 1.27 oz	140	8	13
Triple Chocolate, 1.4 oz	160	8	15
White Chocolate Macadamia, 1.4 oz	160	8	15
Note: Snack Bars Carb figures includes 14-16g Sugar Alcohol			
Protein Wafer Crisps, average	190	14	9
Balance:			
Original Bars:			
Average, 1.8 oz	205	7	21
Dark Chocolate var., av., 1.6 oz	180	7	22
Duo-licious: *Per 2 Pieces*			
Choc. Pepeprmint Patty, 1.4 oz	160	4	27
Dark Chocolate Turtle, 1.55 oz	190	8	24
Dulce De Leche & C'rml, 1.4 oz	150	5	24
Bounce: Caramel Sea Salt Ball, 1.4 oz	170	7	17
Peanut Chocolate Chip Ball, 1.4 oz	180	9	16

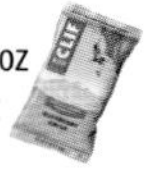
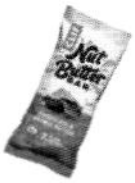
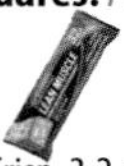
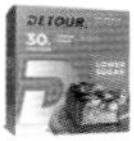
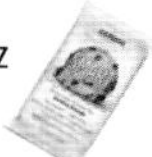
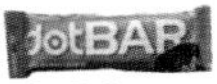

Per Bar	C	F	Cb
Cascadian Farms *(General Mills):*			
Chewy Granola:			
Dark Choc Chip, 1.2 oz	140	3.5	25
Harvest Berry, 1.2 oz	130	2	27
Crunchy Granola, av., 2 bars, 1.4 oz	190	7	27
Fruit Infused, av., 1.23 oz	140	3	25
Protein Granola Bars, av., 1.76 oz	250	15	20
Soft Baked Squares, av., 1.23 oz	150	5.5	23
Sweet & Salty, av. 1.2 oz	170	9	20
Clif:			
Original: Blueb. Crisp, 2.4 oz	250	5	44
Dark Choc. Mocha, 2.4 oz	250	5	44
Av. other flavors, 2.4 oz	255	7	42
Mini Bar, Chocolate Brownie, 1 oz	100	2	18
Bloks, av. all flavors, 3 pieces	100	0	24
Builder's, average, 2.4 oz	285	10	30
Fruit Smoothie, 1.76 oz	230	11	29
Kid Z-Bar, av., 1.27 oz	150	5	24
Nut Butter, av, 1.76 oz	230	11	27
Sweet & Salty, average, 2.4 oz	255	6.5	43
Whey, P'B & Chocolate, 2 oz	260	13	23
Corazonas:			
Heartbar Oatmeal Squares: *Per 1.8 oz Bar*			
Average all varieties	190	6	30
Detour:			
Lean Muscle:			
Cookie Dough Caramel Crisp, 3.2 oz	370	12	33
M&M's: Choc. Candy Crunch, 1.9 oz	210	2	27
PB Candy Crunch, 1.9 oz	250	3	25
P'nut Butter Choc. Crunch, 3.2 oz	420	18	33
Lower Sugar: *Average all flavors*			
Full Size, 3 oz	350	11	32
Snack Size, 1.5 oz	170	5	17
Protein Boost:			
Full size, 20g Protein, av., 2 oz	225	7	24
Snack size, 10g Protein, av., 1 oz	115	3	12
Smart:			
Coconut Almond, 1.3 oz	150	5	16
Cookie Dough, 1.3 oz	150	4	18
Fruit varieties, 1.3 oz	130	2.5	18
dotFIT:			
dotBAR:			
Double Choc. Brownie, 3.3 oz	370	13	38
Peanut Butter Crisp, 1.4oz	150	5	16
Vegan Chocolate Choc. Chip, 1.9 oz	260	9	24
Note: dotBARS Carb figures includes 7-21g Sugar Alcohol			
Extend Bar: Yogurt, av., 1.4 oz	150	5.5	23
Average Other Flavors	150	3	21
Note: Extend Bars Carb figure includes 3-8g Sugar Alcohol			

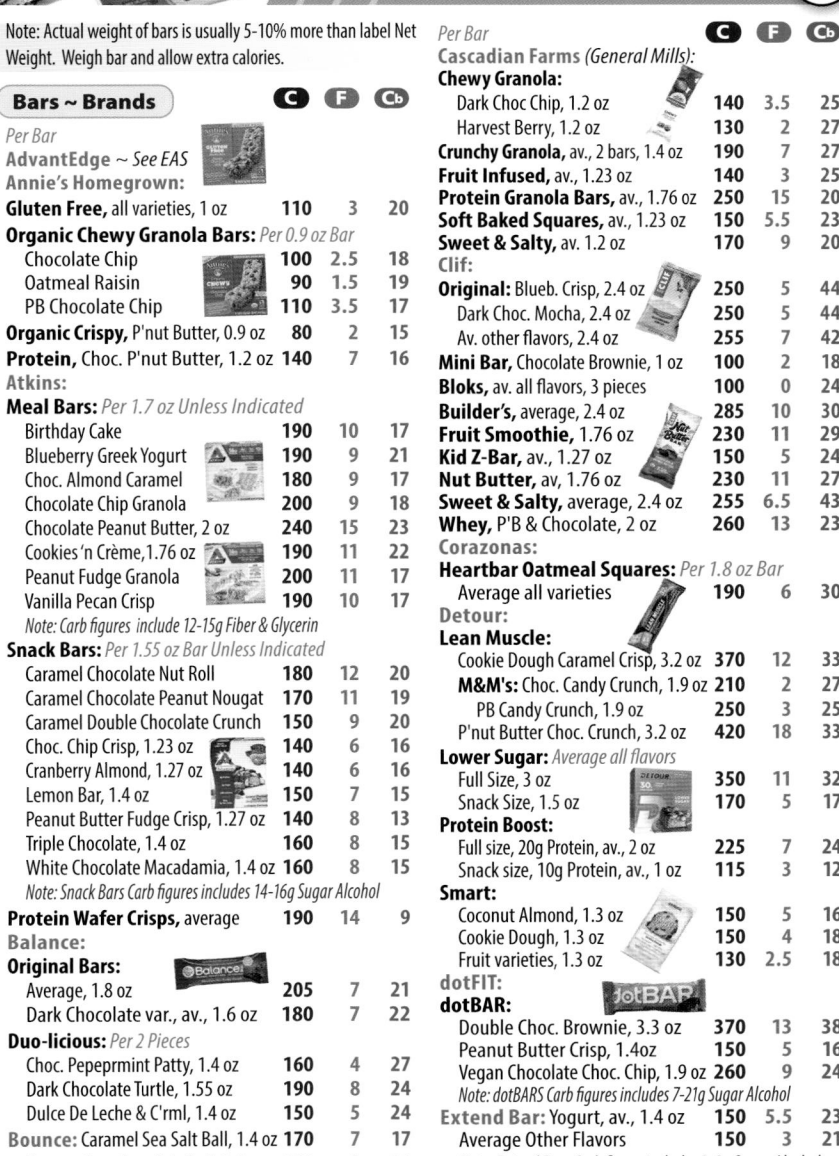

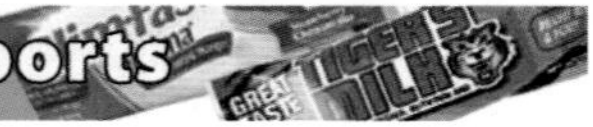

Bars ~ Brands (Cont)

Per Bar	C	F	Cb
Fiber One: *Per 0.8 oz Bar*			
Chewy: Choc.; Choc. Caramel & Pretzel	70	2	14
Chocolate Peanut Butter	70	2.5	13
Note: Carbohydrate figure includes 3g Sugar Alcohol			
General Mills: *Per 1.6 oz Bar*			
Milk 'n Cereal Bar, Honey Nut Cheerios 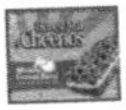	160	7	17
Glucerna: 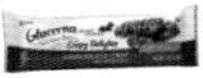			
Snack Bars, Peanut/Choc. Chip, av., 1.4 oz	155	5.5	20
Note: Carbohydrate figure includes 7g Sugar Alcohol			
Mini Snack Bar, average, 0.7 oz	80	3.5	11
Note: Carbohydrate figure includes 2g-4g Sugar Alcohol			
Great Value *(Walmart):*			
Cereal Bars, Fruit & Grain, 1.3 oz	130	3	24
Chewy Granola: 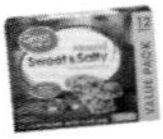			
Protein, average, 1.4 oz	190	12	14
Snack Size Variety Pack, average. 0.84 oz bar	100	2.5	19
Sweet & Salty, Almond, 1.23 oz	170	8	20
Crunchy Granola, Oats & Honey, 2 bars, 1.48 oz	190	7	29
Grenade:			
Carb Killa: Choc Chip Cookie Dough, 2 oz	220	9	24
Dark Chocolate Raspberry, 2 oz	220	10	21
Go Nuts Vegan Nut Bar, Spicy Chili, 1.4 oz 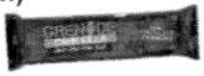	170	9	16
Peanut Butter, 2 oz	220	9	22
Health Valley,			
Multigrain, Cobbler Cereal Bars, all flavors, 3 oz	130	2	25
HMR, Benefit Bars, av. all, 1.4 oz	160	5	22
Init: *Per 1.4 oz Bar* 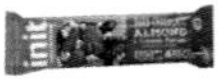			
Dark Choc., average	180	10	23
Mixed Nut & Sweet Berries	180	9	24
Roasted Nuts & Honey Chipotle	190	13	18
Jenny Craig, all var., 1.2 oz	125	6	11
Kashi:			
Breakfast, Soft Baked, 1.26 oz	120	2.5	25
Go, Protein Bars, average, 1.76 oz	223	13	19
Granola Bars:			
Chewy, average all varieties, 1.3 oz	135	5	23
Chewy Nut Butter, av., 1.23 oz	150	7	21
Crunchy, all varieties, 2 bars, 1.4 oz 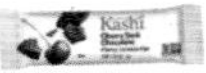	175	6	26
Layered, Dark Choc. Coconut	120	3.5	21
Kellogg's:			
Nutrigrain ~ *See page 33*			
Special K ~ *See page 34*			

Per Bar	C	F	Cb
Kind Bars: *Per 1.4 oz Bar* 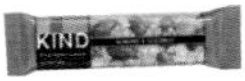			
Almond & Apricot	170	11	21
Almond & Coconut	180	12	21
Blueberry Vanilla Cashew	160	12	19
Cranberry Almonds with Macadamia	170	13	18
Dark Choc. Almond Coconut	180	12	21
Dark Chocolate Cherry Cashew	160	10	22
Honey Roasted Nuts & Sea Salt	180	15	15
Maple Glazed Pecan & Sea Salt	200	17	14
Milk Chocolate Almond 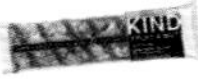	180	14	17
Peanut Butter Dark Choc	200	13	16
Raspberry Cashew Chia	170	11	21
Salted Caramel Dark Chocolate Nut	190	15	16
Breakfast Probiotics: *Per 2 Bars, 1.76 oz*			
Apple Cinn.; Or. Cranberry, av.	210	7	33
Peanut Buter Dark Chocolate	230	12	28
Kids, average all varieties,	95	3	16
Minis, Chewy, av all varieties, 0.8 oz	100	4	15
Kudos, av. all varieties, 0.9 oz	100	3	17
Kuli Kuli:			
Moringa Energy Bars: *Per 1.6 oz Bar* 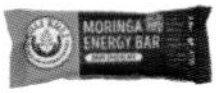			
Black Cherry	170	4	29
Dark Chocolate	210	11	22
Labrada:			
Lean Body Protein Bar: *Per 2.54 oz*			
Cookie Dough; Fudge Brownie	290	9	32
PB Chocolate Chip 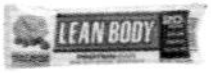	310	11	32
Larabar:			
Original Fruit & Nut, av.	205	10	26
Fruits & Greens, av. 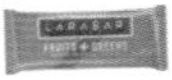	130	3	23
Protein, av., 1.83oz	220	8	25
Lindora Bars:			
Protein Bars: 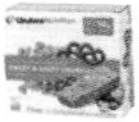			
Caramel Cocoa,1.6 oz	160	5	18
Chocolate Mint, 1.45 oz	150	4.5	21
Dark Chocolate S'mores, 1.6 oz	160	5	18
Oatmeal Cinnamon Raisin, 1.5 oz	150	4.5	19
Sweet & Salty Crunch. 1.4 oz	160	5	21
Zesty Lemon Crunch, 1.5 oz	160	7	16
Note: Carbohydrate figure includes 0.5g-4g Sugar Alcohol			
Luna Bars: 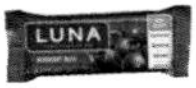			
Regular, av., 1.7 oz	185	7	20
Protein: Av. all varieties, 1.6 oz	175	5	21
Mini, Choc. Chip Cookie Dough, 1.1 oz	120	3.5	14
Mars, Protein Bar, 2 oz	200	4.5	22

Bars ~ Brands (Cont)

Per Bar	C	F	Cb
Medifast:			
Chewy, all varieties, 1.3 oz	110	3	15
Crunch, av. all varieties, 1.2 oz	105	3	13
Note: Crunch Bars Carb figure includes 2-3g Sugar Alcohol			
Maintenance, Cararmel Nut, 1.5 oz	160	5	20
Met-Rx:			
Big 100: *Per 3.52 oz*			
Crispy Apple Pie	400	10	48
Chocolate Toasted Almond	410	13	46
Peanut Butter Caramel Crunch	400	13	44
Peanut Butter Pretzel	410	12	47
Super Cookie Crunch	410	14	42
Protein Plus: Choc. Choc. Chunk, 3 oz	310	10	29
Choc. Roasted Peanut w/ Crml, 3oz	320	10	33
Peanut Butter Cup, 3 oz	300	10	34
Mojo Bars ~ *See Clif*			
Muscle Milk *(Cytosport):*			
15G Protein Bars: Cookies & Cream	180	5	23
Peanut Butter Cookie	190	6	22
20G Protein Bar, Choc P'nut Butter	250	9	27
Note: Protein Bars Carb figures include 6-14g Sugar Alcohol			
Nature's Path:			
Love Crunch, av., 1.1 oz	150	7	19
Nut Butter, av., 1.2 oz	170	10	17
Sunrise Chewy B'fast, av., 1.2 oz	140	4	25
Nature Valley:			
Chewy, XL Protein, average, 2 oz	290	19	21
Crunchy, 2 bars, average, 1.5 oz	190	8	29
Layered Granola Nut, average	190	11	20
Nut Crunch, Almond, 1.23 oz	190	14	14
Protein, all var., 1.4 oz	190	12	14
Sustained Energy, av., 1.7 oz	240	13	24
Sweet & Salty, average, 1.3 oz	160	7	22
Wafer, av., 1.3 oz	200	12	17
NuGo:			
Dark, average all varieties, 1.76 oz	200	6	25
Fiber d'Lish: Orange Cranb., 1.6 oz	150	3	31
Coc. Macaroon; P'nut Choc. Chip, 1.6 oz	160	6	28
Gluten Free, av. all varieties, 1.6 oz	180	4	27
Organic, all varieties, 1.6 oz	190	5	26
Slim: Espresso, 1.6 oz	170	5	20
Av.e other varieties	185	5	19

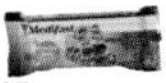
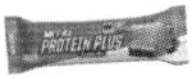
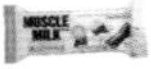
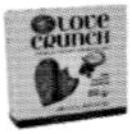
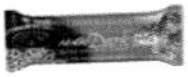
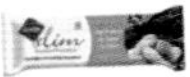

Per Bar	C	F	Cb
NuGo (Cont):			
Smarte Carb: Choc. Black Berry, 1.76 oz	150	3	22
Peanut Butter Crunch, 1.76 oz	160	5	19
Note: Carbohyrate figures include 12-14 g Sugar Alcohol			
Stronger: Peanut Cluster, 2.8 oz	330	14	36
Average other varieties, 2.8 oz	300	9	37
Nutri-Grain *(Kellogg's):*			
Kids, all varieties, 1.3 oz	140	3.5	27
Soft Baked B'fast Cereal Bars, all varieties, 1.3 oz	130	3.5	25
NutriSystem:			
Breakfast, Apple Streudel Bar	160	3	28
Lunch: Choc. P'nut Butter Bar	200	8	25
Double Chocolate Caramel	180	6	28
Snack, Dark Chocolate & Sea Salt Nut	190	14	16
Oh Yeah! (ISS):			
Original: *Per 3 oz Bar*			
Almond Fudge Brownie	350	13	27
Choc. Caramel Candies	340	13	32
Cookie Caramel Crunch	340	13	32
Peanut Butter & Caramel	380	19	30
Note: Carbohydrate figure includes 13g-14g Sugar Alcohol			
Good Grab, PB Crunch Bar	190	10	19
Note: Carbohydrate figure includes 4g Sugar Alcohol			
Optifast:			
800 Bars:			
Apple Cinnamon, 1.52 oz	160	4	18
Chocolate, 1.65 oz	160	4.5	18
Peanut Butter Chocolate, 1.52 oz	160	5	18
Note: 800 Bars Carb figures include 1-4g Sugar Alcohol			
PowerBar:			
Protein Plus, average, 1.4 oz	220	14	11
Note: Carbohydrate figures include 16-18g Sugar Alcohol			
Snack Bar, average	230	13	23
Power Crunch *(BNRG):*			
Orig. Protein Bar, av. all var., 1.4 oz	215	12	11
Power Crunch, Choklat, av., 1.5 oz	215	12	18
PR:			
Protein: Chocolate Mint, 2.1 oz	200	6	22
Chocolate Peanut, 1.8 oz	200	7	22
Oatmeal Raisin Granola, 1.8 oz	210	7	22
Premier Protein *(Premier Nutrition): 12G Protein*			
Chocolate Peanut Butter, 1.5 oz	180	10	17
Salted Caramel Cashew, 1.65 oz	190	10	19
Vanilla Almond Coconut, 1.65 oz	190	11	18

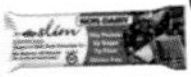
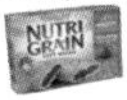
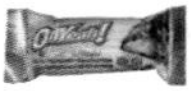
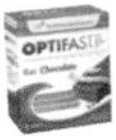

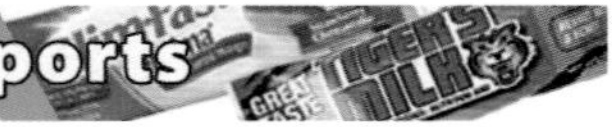

Note: Actual weight of bars is usually 5-10% more than label Net Weight. Weigh bar and allow extra calories.

Bars ~ Brands (Cont)

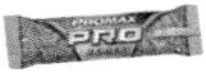

Per Bar	C	F	Cb
Promax:			
Original, av. all varieties, 2.6 oz	**290**	7.5	39
Lower Sugar, av. all varieties, 2.4 oz	**215**	7	32
Note: Lower Sugar Carbohydrate figures include 5-6g Sugar Alcohol			
Proti Bars *(Bariatrix)*:			
Almond Coconut, 1.76 oz	**190**	9	17
Chocolate/Vanilla Wafers (2), 1.4 oz	**205**	10	14
Note: Carbohydrate figures include 2g -5g Sugar Alcohol			
Salted Toffee Pretzel Bar, 1.75 oz	**160**	6	18
PureFit, Protein av. all varieties, 2 oz	**225**	7	25
Pure Protein:			
Hi Protein, av. all varieties, 1.76 oz	**195**	5	18
Note: Carbohydrate figures include 2-13g Sugar Alcohol			
Quaker:			
B'fast Flats: Banana Honey Nut (3)	**170**	7	28
Av. other varieties (3)	**175**	6.5	28
B'fast Squares: P'nut Butter, 2.1 oz	**250**	10	35
Other flavors, 2.1 oz	**210**	4.5	42
Granola Bars:			
Chewy: 25% Less Sugar, average, 0.8 oz	**95**	3	17
Big, average all varieties, 1.9 oz	**175**	6	30
Note: Big Bar Carbohydrate figure include 2g Sugar Alcohol			
Bites, average, 8 pieces	**135**	5	21
Dipps, average, 1.2 oz	**140**	6	22
Yogurt, Srawb., 1.2 oz	**140**	4.5	25
Quest Bar:			
Hero: Choc.Pnut Butter, 1.9 oz	**200**	12	18
Average other varieties, 2.1 oz	**175**	8	30
Note: Carbohydrate figure include 4g Sugar Alcohol			
Protein,, av., 2.1 oz	**185**	6	23
Note: Carbohydrate figures includs 1-6g Sugar Alcohol			
RX Bar:			
Protein: Average, 1.83 oz	**215**	9	24
Kids, average, 1.2 oz	**135**	5	16
Skratch Bars:			
Anytime Energy: *Per 1.76 oz Bar*			
Cherries & Pistachios; Savory Miso, av.	**220**	9	30
Choc. Chips & Almonds;PB & Strawb.	**220**	8	33
Slim-Fast:			
Bake Shop Bars, average all, 1.6 oz	**180**	6.5	17
Note: Carb includes 12g Sugar Alcohol + 5g Fibre			
Keto: Bars, av., 1.48 oz	**190**	14	15
Note: Carb includes 12g Sugar Alcohol + 9g Fibre			
Fat Bomb, P'But Butter, 1 cup	**90**	9	6
Snickers, Protein Bar, 1.8 oz	**200**	7	18
Solo, Gi, average all varieties 1.76 oz	**195**	7	26

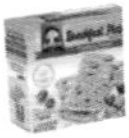

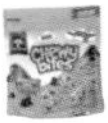

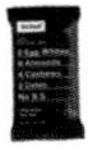

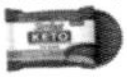

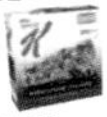

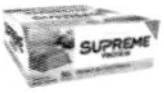

Per Bar	C	F	Cb
Special K:			
Chewy Nut Bars, av., 1.16 oz	**165**	8	18
Chewy Snack Bars, av. all varieties, 0.88 oz	**100**	2	19
Protein Snack, av. all var., 1.23 oz	**155**	7	17
Supreme Protein:			
High Protein:			
Caramel Nut Chocolate, 3.4 oz	**390**	15	36
PB Crunch, 3.38 oz	**390**	18	26
Note: Carbohydrate figures include 14-27g Sugar alcohol			
thinkThin: *Per Bar*			
High Protein, av. all flavors, 1.94 oz	**235**	9	25
Note: Carbohydrate figure includes 5-22g Sugar Alcohol			
Keto, Choc. Peanut Butter Pie, 1.4 oz	**180**	14	14
Note: Carbohydrate figure includes 4-5g Sugar Alcohol			
Protein + 150 Calorie, av., 1.4 oz	**150**	5	20
Vegan High Protein:			
Choc. Mint; Sea Salt Alm. Choc., 1.95 oz	**230**	8	28
PB Chocolate Chip, 1.76 oz	**190**	6	24
Note: Carbohydrate figure includes 9g Sugar Alcohol			
Tiger's Milk:			
Protein Rich, 1.2 oz	**140**	5	19
Peanut Butter Crunch, 1.2 oz	**150**	6	18
King Size, average all varieties, 2 oz	**225**	9	28
Trader Joe's:			
Hemp Seed Bar, 0.9 oz	**120**	7	11
Organic Granola Bar, Chocolate Chip, 0.85 oz	**100**	2.5	18
PB & J Bar, 1.2 oz	**150**	4	23
Simply Nutty Bars, av. , 1.4 oz	**200**	15	15
Vega:			
Protein Bars: 20G, 2.47 oz	**290**	10	26
Snack Bar, Choc. Caramel, 1.6 oz	**190**	8	20
Sports Bar, 2.47 oz	**300**	11	27
Wickedly Prime: *Per 1.4 oz Bar*			
Banana Nut	**180**	11	21
Cashews & Cranberry	**170**	9	24
Cherry Nut Crunch	**190**	14	15
Nuts & Sea Salt; Peanut Almond	**200**	16	14
Zone Perfect:			
High Protein Bars, average, 2 oz	**235**	9	22
Nutrition Bars:			
Chocolate Peanut Butter, 1.76 oz	**220**	8	24
Dark Choc. Almond, 1.58 oz	**190**	7	20
Salted Caramel Brownie, 1.58 oz	**200**	9	20

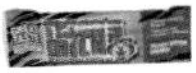

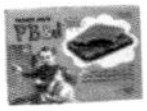

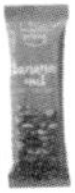

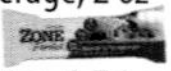

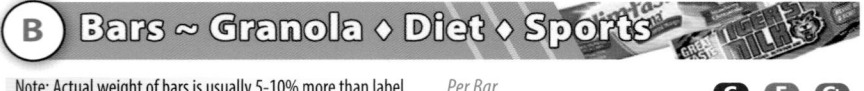

Cocoa & Hot Chocolate

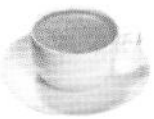

	C	F	Cb
Cocoa:			
Small (8 fl.oz):			
with Whole Milk	**205**	8.5	22
with Nonfat Milk	**145**	1	23
Tall (12 fl.oz): with Whole Milk	**280**	12	26
with Nonfat Milk	**185**	1	28
Hot Chocolate:			
Small (8 fl.oz): with Whole Milk	**180**	7	26
with Nonfat Milk	**140**	2	27
Tall (12 fl.oz): with Whole Milk	**260**	10	36
with Nonfat Milk	**190**	2	37
Cinnabon, Mochalatta Chill, 16 oz	**420**	17	63

Cocoa - Chocolate Mixes

Add extra cals/fat/carbohydrate for milk

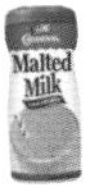

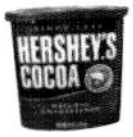

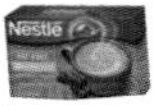

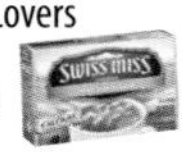

	C	F	Cb
Caffé D'Vita: *Per Singe Serve Envelope*			
Hot Cocoa, 1 oz	**110**	1.5	24
Hot Cocoa, Sugar Free	**70**	4.5	7
Carnation Breakfast Drinks ~ *See Page 38*			
Carnation: *Per 3 Tbsp*			
Malted Milk: Original	**90**	2	15
Chocolate	**90**	1	18
Ghirardelli:			
Premium Hot Cocoa:			
with Chocolate Chips, 1 oz	**110**	2	23
Double Chocolate, 2 Tbsp	**90**	1	20
Hershey's, Cocoa,			
Natural, unsweetened,			
1 Tbsp, 0.2 oz	**10**	0.5	3
Land O Lakes:			
Arctic White Coccoa, 1.3 oz	**160**	6	26
Other varieties, 1.3 oz	**140**	3.5	26
Nestle: *Per Per Single Serve Envelope*			
Rich Milk Chocolate:			
Regular	**80**	2	15
Fat Free	**25**	0	4
with Mini Marshmallows	**80**	1.5	15
Nesquik Powder: *Per 2 Tbsp*			
Chocolate	**50**	0	12
No Added Sugar	**40**	0.5	8
Strawberry	**45**	0	12
Ovaltine, average all flav., 2 Tbsp	**40**	0	10
Swiss Miss: *Per Single Serve Envelope*			
Cafe Blends, Mocha	**150**	2.5	28
Classics: Marshmallow Lovers	**190**	2.5	39
Milk Chocolate	**160**	2.5	34
Indulgent Collection:			
Caramel Delight	**160**	2.5	34
Dark Chocolate Sensation	**150**	3.5	28
Sensibly Sweet,			
Milk Choc. Flavor, No Sugar Added	**80**	1.5	14
Simply Cocoa, Milk Chocolate	**100**	0	22

Instant Coffee

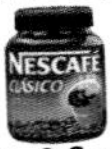

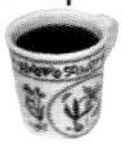

	C	F	Cb
Powder/Granules: *Regular or Decaffeinated,*			
1 level tsp	**2**	0	0.5
1 rounded tsp	**4**	0	1
Ground, 3 tsp	**7**	0	2
Brewed/Percolated, 1 cup, 8 fl.oz	**4**	0	1
Coffee with Milk/Cream/Creamers: *Per 8 oz Cup*			
Black:	**4**	0	1
with Whole Milk: Dash, 1 Tbsp	**15**	0.5	2
2 Tbsp, 1 fl.oz	**25**	1	2.5
with 2% Milk, 2 Tbsp	**20**	0.5	2.5
with 1% Milk, 2 Tbsp	**20**	0.5	2.5
with Fat Free Milk, 2 Tbsp	**15**	0	2.5
with Soy Milk: 1 Tbsp	**10**	0	1.5
2 Tbsp, 1 oz	**15**	0.5	2
with Half & Half: 2 Tbsp	**50**	3	3
¼ cup, 2 fl.oz	**90**	6	4
with Cream (light coffee), 2 Tbsp	**65**	6	2
with Coffee Mate: Liquid, reg., 1 T.	**20**	1	3
Liquid Fat Free, 1 Tbsp	**25**	0	2
Powder, 1 heaping tsp	**15**	1	2
Sugar ~ Add Extra: 1 heaping tsp	**25**	0	6
Single portion, 1 package	**25**	0	6
Sweeteners, *(Equal/Splenda/Sweet N Low),*			
Powder, 1 package	**0**	0	0

Flavored Coffee Mixes

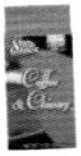

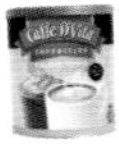

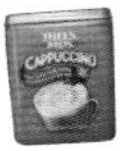

	C	F	Cb
Chicory:			
Instant Coffee, 1 tsp	**5**	0	1
Coffee Essence, 1 tsp	**15**	0	4
Caffé D'Vita:			
Cappuccino: Caramel, 3 tsp	**60**	2	10
English Toffee, 3 tsp	**70**	2.5	11
French Vanilla, 3 tsp	**70**	3	10
Mocha; Peppermint Mocha, av., 3 tsp	**60**	2.5	11
Iced, Caramel Latte, 3 tbsp	**180**	6	32
Sugar Free Cappuccino, Mocha, 2 tsp	**40**	2.5	4
General Foods International:			
Cappuccino: Hazelnut Belgian, 1.3 oz	**160**	4	29
Suisse Mocha, 1.3 oz	**150**	5	28
White Chocolate Caramel, 1.3 oz	**150**	3	30
Hills Bros: *Per 3 Tbsp, 1 oz*			
Cappuccino: French Vanilla	**110**	3.5	19
Sugar Free	**50**	2	8
Double Mocha, Sugar Free	**50**	2	8
English Toffee	**110**	3	19
White Chocolate Caramel	**120**	4.5	19
Nescafe, Memento, 1 stick,			
average all varieties	**100**	2.5	19

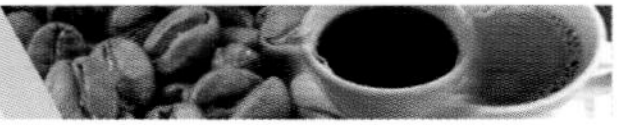

Coffee Shops/Restaurants

Per 8 fl.oz Cup (Unless Indicated)	C	F	Cb
Coffee, Regular/Percolated/Filtered	5	0	0
Americano Drip Coffee, 1 cup	7.5	0	1
Cafe Au Lait: 1 cup, 8 fl.oz	60	3.5	5
Nonfat Milk, 1 cup, 8 fl.oz	35	0	5
Caffe Latté:			
8 fl.oz cup: with Whole Milk	110	6	9
with 2% Milk	100	3.5	9
with Nonfat Milk	70	0	10
12 fl.oz: with Whole Milk	180	9	14
with Nonfat Milk	100	0	15
16 fl.oz: with Whole Milk	220	11	18
with Nonfat Milk	130	0	19
Cafe Mocha (Mochaccino): 8 fl.oz	150	6	20
12 fl.oz	230	9	31
16 fl.oz	290	12	41
Cappuccino:			
8 fl.oz cup: with Whole Milk	90	3.5	7
with 2% Milk	80	3	8
with Nonfat Milk	50	0	8
12 fl.oz: with Whole Milk	110	6	9
with 2% Milk	90	3.5	9
with Nonfat Milk	60	0	9
16 fl.oz: with Whole Milk	140	7	11
with 2% Milk	120	3.5	11
with Nonfat Milk	80	0	12
Mocha: *With Cream*			
8 fl.oz: with Whole Milk	200	11	22
with Nonfat Milk	160	6	22
12 fl.oz: Whole Milk	290	15	33
with Nonfat Milk	230	8	34
Iced Mocha: *Without Cream*			
12 fl.oz: with Whole Milk	170	6	26
with Nonfat Milk	130	2	27
Espresso: Single (Solo), 1 fl.oz	5	0	1
Double (Doppio), 2 fl.oz	10	0	2
Espresso con Panna,			
(w/ dollop wh. cream), solo, 1 fl.oz	30	2.5	2
Espresso Macchiato, solo, 1 fl.oz	5	0	1
Frappuccino: Tall, 12 fl.oz	180	2.5	37
Grande, 16 fl.oz	240	3	48
Frappuccino Mocha:			
(with Cream): Tall, 12 fl.oz	280	11	43
Grande, 16 fl.oz	380	15	57
Iced Latte, Similar to Caffe Latte			

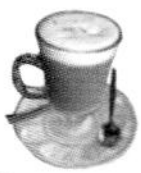
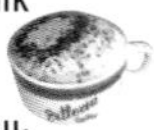
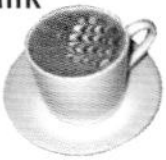
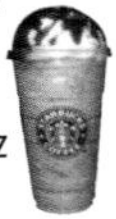

McCafe (McDonald's) ~ *See Fast Food, Page 216*
Starbucks ~ *See Fast-Foods Section, Page 243*

Coffee Substitute Mixes

	C	F	Cb
Roasted Cereal Beverages ~ *(No Caffeine)*			
Cafix, Instant Beverage, 1 tsp	5	0	1
Kaffree Roma, Instant Beverage, 1 tsp	10	0	2
Teeccino, Herbal Coffees, 1 tsp	10	0	2

Irish & Liqueur Coffees

	C	F	Cb
Irish Coffee, without sugar	175	10	0
Liqueur Coffee, with cream,			
all varieties, av., 1 fl.oz	100	5	7

Coffee Extras

	C	F	Cb
Chocolate (Cocoa) Topping, ½ tsp	5	0	1
Flavored Syrups: Regular, 2 Tbsp	80	0	20
Sugar-free, 2 Tbsp	0	0	0
Half & Half Cream: 2 Tbsp	40	3.5	1
Single serve pkg, ⅜ fl.oz	15	1.5	0.5
Light whipped cream, 2 Tbsp	15	1.5	1
Marshmallows, miniature (2)	5	0	1
Sugar:			
1 single portion package	20	0	5
1 level tsp	15	0	4
1 heaping tsp	25	0	6
Equal/Splenda/Sweet 'N Low	0	0	0

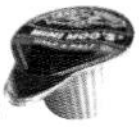
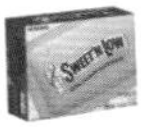

Coffee Shop ~ Cakes, Cookies

	C	F	Cb
Cookies:			
Biscotti, 1 oz	140	6.5	18
Chocolate Chip, 3 oz	350	15	54
Oatmeal Raisin, 3 oz	350	12	56
Peanut Butter, 3 oz	410	25	39
White Choc. Macadamia, 3.33 oz	420	20	55
Cakes/Pastries:			
Almond Croissant, 5 oz	620	35	67
Apple Danish, 5 oz	450	18	67
Banana Walnut, 4.5 oz	410	17	60
Brownie, 3 oz	390	24	42
Bundt, Chocolate, 4 oz	440	21	61
Carrot Cake, 4 oz	400	22	45
Chocolate Cake, 5 oz	530	28	65
Crumble Coffee Cake, 4.5 oz	500	25	65
Cupcake, 3 oz	330	16	43
Pound Cake, av., 3 oz	330	17	40
Cinnamon Roll, 6 oz	500	15	83
Donuts:			
Sugared, 1.8 oz	220	11	27
Glazed, 2 oz	250	12	34
Pretzel, large, 4 oz	290	5	52

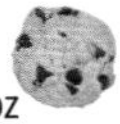
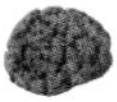
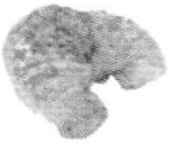

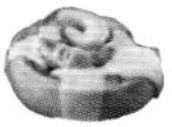
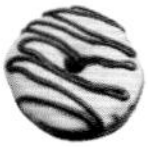

Starbucks Bakery Items ~ *See Page 244*

Ready To Drink Coffee

	C	F	Cb
Bottled & Chilled:			
Califia Farms: *With Almond Milk*			
Cold Brew Coffee: Cafe Latte, 12 fl.oz	100	4	15
Mocha, 12 fl.oz	130	4.5	21
Dunkin Donuts, Mocha, 13.7 fl.oz	280	9	44
International Delight:			
Iced, all flavors, 8 fl.oz	120	2.5	21
Light varieties, 8 fl.oz	80	2.5	13
Kahlua, Cappuccino Shake, 10.5 fl.oz	130	2	24
Starbucks:			
Cold Brew: *Per 11 fl.oz*			
Black, sweet	50	0	12
Black, unsweetened	15	0	2
Cocoa & Honey, with Cream	150	4	23
Vanilla & Fig, with Cream	150	4	24
Doubleshot Energy: *Per 15 fl.oz Can*			
Coffee Drink	220	3	35
Hazelnut Drink	210	3	34
Mocha/Vanilla Drink, av.	210	3	34
White Chocolate Drink	210	3	34
Doubleshot Espresso: *Per 6.5 fl.oz Can*			
Espresso/Salted Caramel & Cream	140	6	18
Espresso & Light Cream	70	4	5
Frappuccino Coffee Drink: *Per 9.5 fl.oz Bottle*			
Regular; Caramel; Vanilla, av.	205	3.5	37
AlmondMilk Mocha	120	3.5	21
Mocha	190	3.5	33
Light Mocha	100	3	12
Iced Espresso Classics (Chilled): *Per 12 fl.oz serving*			
Caffe Mocha	200	4	35
Caramel Macchiato; Van. Latte	190	4	32
Skinny, Caramel Macchiato, Van. Latte	100	0	15
Iced Latte: *Per 14 fl.oz Bottle*			
Regular, reduced fat milk	220	4.5	37
Vanilla, reduced fat milk	220	4.5	36
White Choc. Mocha, red. fat milk	260	4.5	44

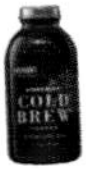
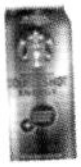
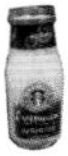

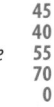

Starbucks Refreshers ~ *See Page 40*

Tips to Reduce the Calories in Your Coffee Drinks:

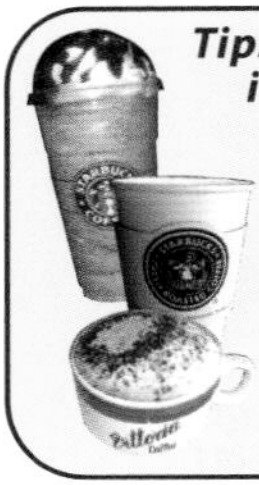

- Request non-fat milk in place of whole or 2% milk
- Downsize to 8 fl.oz or 12 fl.oz
- Avoid cream on frappuccinos
- Replace sugar with *Equal, Splenda, Stevia* or *Sweet 'N Low*
- Avoid syrup add-ons

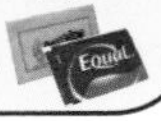

Caffeine Counter

Moderate caffeine intake is not harmful to healthy adults. However, frequent large amounts (over 400 mg/day) may cause dependency ('caffeinism') and adversely affect health. **To be safe, limit caffeine to 200mg/day.** Avoid if pregnant, breastfeeding, a child under 8, have sleep problems, an overactive bladder or heart arrhythmia.

	Caffeine (mg)
Coffee: Instant: Weak, 1 level teaspoon	30
Medium, 1 rounded teaspoon	60
Strong, 1 heaping teaspoon	100
Decaffeinated, 1 rounded teaspoon	2
Bags (Folgers), 1 bag (6-8 fl.oz)	115
Ground, 1 Tbsp, 0.2 oz	60
Bottled (Ready-To-Drink), 9.5 fl.oz	70
Coffee Shop: Brewed, 8 fl.oz	110 -150
Cappuccino/Latte: 1 cup, 8 fl.oz	75
Tall, 12 fl.oz	110
Large, 16 fl.oz	150
Decappuccino, decaffeinated	5
Espresso: Regular/Single/Solo	75
Double/Doppio	150
Iced Coffee w/o Milk, 12 fl.oz	140
Latte, 1 cup, 8 fl.oz	75
Mocha, 1 cup, 8 fl.oz	90
Hot Chocolate, 8 fl.oz	15
Black Tea: Weak, 1 cup	20
Medium Strength, 1 cup	40
Strong, 1 cup	70
Decaffeinated Tea, 1 cup	0-5
Herbal Tea, 1 cup	0
Green Tea, 1 cup	20
Iced Tea, tall glass/can, 12 fl.oz	20-30
Soft Drinks: *Per 12 fl.oz Can*	
Coca-Cola; Pepsi (Regular/Diet)	35
Diet Coke; TAB; RC Cola (Regular)	45
Dr. Pepper; Sunkist Orange	40
Pepsi One; Mountain Dew; Mellow Yellow; Surge	55
Pepsi Max (Regular/Diet) Sun Drop (Reg/Diet)	70
7-Up, Fanta, Sprite, Fresca, Diet Rite Cola	0
Energy Drinks (with added caffeine): *(AMP, Adrenaline Rush, Full Throttle Monster, No Fear, Red Bull, Rockstar)*	
Average all brands: 8 fl.oz	80
16 fl.oz	160
NOS Energy, 16 fl.oz	260
Chocolate Bars: Milk Chocolate, 2 oz	20
Dark Chocolate, 2 oz	30
Choc Chip Cookies, 2 medium, 2 oz	6
Chocolate Syrup, 2 Tbsp, 1.4 oz	5
Guarana, *GNC*, 1 tablet	90
Medicinals: *Excedrin Extra*/Migraine, 1 tab.	65
Jet Alert/NoDoz, 1 tablet	200
Stay Awake (Walgreens), *Vivarin*, 1 tab.	200

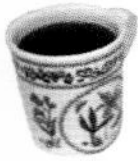
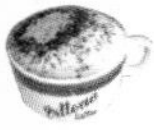
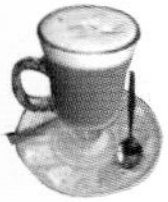
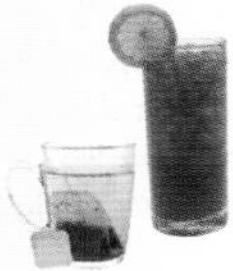 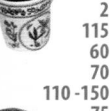
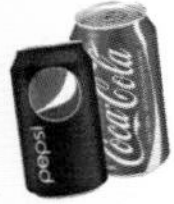

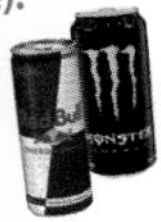
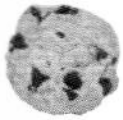
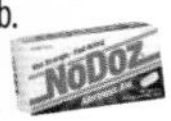

Energy/Protein Drinks

	C	F	Cb
5-hour Energy, 2 fl.oz 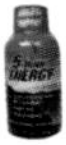	4	0	1
A.B.B:			
Post Workout Pure-Pro:			
Pure Pro 50, all flavors, 14.5 fl.oz	260	4.5	7
Maxx Recovery, all flavors, 18 fl.oz	390	0.5	60
Pre Workout, Speed Stack Pumped, 22 fl.oz	30	0	8
AllSport Hydration:			
Regular, all flavors, 20 fl.oz	150	0	40
Zero, 20 fl.oz	0	0	0
AMP Energy: *Per 16 fl.oz Can* 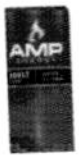			
Original; Strawberry Limeade	220	0	58
Cherry Blast	120	0	31
Tropical Punch	100	0	26
Arbonne,			
Protein Shakes, av., 2 sc., 1.4 oz	165	3	13
Arizona:			
Green Tea Energy Shot, Extra Str., 2 fl.oz	5	0	1
Natural Energy, average, 8 fl.oz	70	0	19
Rx Energy, Herbal Tonic, 8 fl.oz	100	0	26
Atkins: *Per 11 fl.oz*			
Plus 30G Prot. Shakes, Choc./Van., av.	190	5	9
Shakes, average, 11 fl.oz	165	9	7
Bariatrix, Proti-Max, Ready to Drink			
Chocolate/Vanilla, av., 8.45 fl.oz	105	4	3
Bawls Guarana: *Per 10 fl.oz Bottle*			
Original; Cherry; Ginger	130	0	33
Orange; Root Beer, average	140	0	35
Beet It: 			
Organic Beet Juice: 8.5 fl.oz	80	0	17
25.4 fl.oz Bottle	240	0	51
Shot, 2.4 fl.oz	95	0.2	20
BodyArmor, SuperDrinks, 16 fl.oz	120	0	28
Bolthouse: *Per 15.2 fl.oz*			
Bolts Energy, 2 fl.oz	25	0	6
Protein Keto, average all flavors	280	22	14
Protein Plus: Chocolate	390	6	55
Dutch Choc.; Banana;Van. Bean. av	345	6	46
Mango	375	1	62
Boost *(Nestle):* 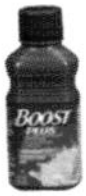			
Original, all flavors, 8 fl.oz	240	4	41
High Protein, all flav, 8 fl.oz	240	6	28
Glucose Control, 8 fl.oz	190	7	16
Max 30g Protein, 11 fl.oz	160	2	7
Men, 8 fl.oz 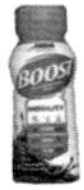	220	6	24
Mobility, 8 fl.oz	180	4	16
Plus, all flavors, 8 fl.oz	360	14	45
Women, 8 fl.oz	180	7	14

	C	F	Cb
Carnation:			
B'Fast Essentials, Powder:			
Original,av. all flav., 1.3 oz envelope	135	0	27
Light Start, av. , 0.7 oz	60	0.5	11
Probiotic, 1.3 oz envelope	140	1	27
Ready To Drink: Reg., all flav., 8 fl.oz	240	4	41
High Protein, average, 8 fl.oz	220	6	26
CeraSport:			
Powders: Endurance, Vanilla, 1 pkt	150	0	30
Plus Hydration, Strawb., 1 pkt	120	0	30
Ready To Drink, Citrus Drink, 8.5 fl.oz	40	0	10
Champion Performance: 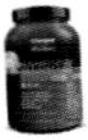			
Heavyweight Gainer 900,			
av. all flavors, 4 scps, 5.4 oz	600	7	102
Metabolol II, 2 scoops, 2.3 oz	260	3	40
Pure Whey Plus, av., 1 scoop, 1.2 oz	130	2	5
UltraMet, 2.7 oz pkt	280	4	20
Clif: Hydration Mix, 0.4 oz pkt	40	0	10
Recovery Powder, Choc., 1.6 oz	160	0	31
Cocaine, Energy, 12fl.oz can	90	0	23
Core Power *(fairlife):* 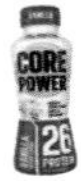			
26g, av. all flavors, 11.5 fl.oz	240	3.5	27
Elite, 42g, av. all flav., 14 fl.oz	240	3.5	12
Curves, Protein Drink,			
Choc.; Vanilla, 2 scoops, 1 oz	120	1	12
Ensure: *Per Bottle* 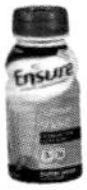			
Original, all flavors, 8 fl.oz	220	6	33
Clear, all flavors, 10 fl.oz	180	0	37
Enlive, av. all flavors, 8 fl.oz	350	11	44
High Protein , all flav., 8 fl.oz	160	2	19
Plus, all flavors, 8 fl.oz	350	11	50
Enterex, Diabetic, all flavors, 8 fl.oz	220	8	25
Enu, Nutritional Shakes, av., 8.5 fl.oz	340	13	39
FRS, Energy Concentrate, 2 fl.oz	10	0	3
Fruit$_2$O *(Veryfine)*: Classic 20 fl.oz	0	0	0
Sparkling, 20 fl.oz	0	0	1
Full Throttle: *Per 16 fl.oz*			
Energy, Citrus; Blue Agave	220	0	58
Gatorade G Series: 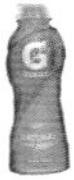			
Endurance: Powder, 1½ Tbsp	90	0	22
Thirst Quencher, 12 fl oz	90	0	22
Lower Sugar, 12 fl.oz	30	0	8
Protein: Chocolate Shake, 11.16 fl.oz	280	1	47
Super Shake, Chocolate, 11.16 fl.oz	190	1	12
Whey Protein Powder, ⅓ cup 1.1 oz	120	2	6
Sports Fuel Drink, 4 fl.oz	100	0	25
Glaceau:			
Smartwater, 8 fl.oz	0	0	0
Vitaminwater: Revive Punch, 20 fl.oz	120	0	32
Average other flavors, 20 fl.oz	100	0	27

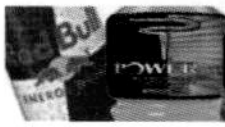

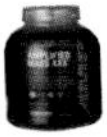

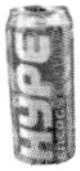

	C	F	Cb
Glucerna:			
Shakes, all flavors, 8 fl.oz	180	9	16
Advance Shakes, average., 8 fl.oz	200	7	27
Hunger Shakes, average, 8 fl.oz	180	8	15
GNC:			
Pro Performance:			
Amplified: Mass XXX,			
av. all flavors, 4 scoops	745	6	123
RTD, Wheybolic, all flavors, 14 fl.oz	190	1.5	6
Total Lean:			
Powders: All flavors, 1 pkt	200	3	18
Classics, Swiss Choc., 1 Heaping Scoop	180	2	31
RTD Shakes: 25, all flavors, 14 fl.oz	170	6	6
Burn, all flavors, 14.fl.oz	170	6	8
Guru:			
Org. Energy Drink: Regular, 8 oz can	80	0	21
Lite,12 oz can	10	0	3
Herbalife: Nutr. Shake, 1 scoop, 0.9 oz	90	1	13
Protein Drink Mix, 2 scoops, 1 oz	110	3	5
Hormel:			
Plus-2 Protein Shakes, all flav., 8 fl.oz	480	23	49
Vital Quisine 500, av. all flav., 8.5 fl.oz	520	21	60
Hype: *Per 8 fl.oz Can*			
Enlite	25	0	4
Energy: After Dark, Hype	130	0	30
MFP	110	0	25
Up, Ice Berry Max	120	0	28
Twisted, average all flavors	110	0	26
Jarrow:			
Optimal Plant Proteins, 2 scoops, 1.2 oz	140	3	8
Organic Plant Protein, Van., 1 oz	120	3	6
Rice Protein, Vanilla, Tbsp, 0.6 oz	60	0	3
Whey Protein: Unflavored, 0.8 oz sc.	90	2	1
Chocolate; Vanilla, 0..9 oz scoop	100	1.5	3
Knudsen: Recharge, average, 8 fl.oz	75	0	18
Simply Nutritious, av. all, 8 fl.oz	115	0	28
Kroger: *Per 8 fl.oz Bottle*			
Nutrutional Shake, all flavors	190	7	23
Nutrition Shake, Fortify Plus, av.,	350	11	50
La Brada:			
Lean Body, Meal Repl., 2.47 oz sc.	285	7	19
RTD, Lean Body, 17 fl.oz	280	9	9
Lindora:			
Powder: Berry Cream Smoothie	100	1	7
Creamy Chocolate; Vanilla	90	1	7
Ready To Drink Shakes, 8 fl oz	110	4.5	4

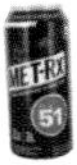

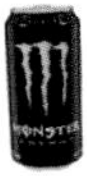

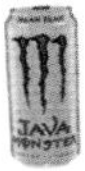

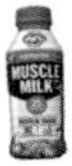

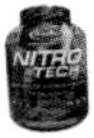

	C	F	Cb
Liquid Ice:			
Black, 8.3 fl.oz	110	0	26
Other Flavors, 8.3 fl oz	120	0	28
Met-Rx, 51 Shake,			
Chocolate, 15 fl.oz	250	2	6
Monster:			
Energy: 16 fl.oz can	210	0	54
Lo-Carb, 16 fl.oz	25	0	7
M-80, 16 fl.oz	180	0	46
Mixxd (with Juice), 16 fl.oz	220	0	54
Java Monster: All flav., 15 fl.oz	190	3	33
Light, Vanilla, 15 fl.oz	95	3	13
Shakes, 16 fl.oz can	220	4	20
MRM:			
Veggie Meal Replacement, 1.7 oz	190	5	14
Whey Protein, 1 scoop, 0.9 oz	100	1.5	4
Muscle Milk *(Cytosport)*:			
Gainer, 4 scoops, 5.71 oz	650	9	109
Genuine Protein Powder:			
Real Chocolate; Vanilla, 2 sc., 2.47 oz	310	11	20
Other Flavors, 2 scoops, 2.47 oz	280	9	21
Non Dairy Ready To Drink:			
100 Calorie, Vanilla Creme, 11 fl.oz	100	1.5	5
Genuine, average all flavors, 11 fl.oz	160	4.5	6
Original, all flavors, 17 fl.oz	320	15	13
Pro Series, Go Bananas, 14 fl.oz	200	2.5	8
Yogurt Smoothies, 11 fl.oz	180	3	18
Muscle Tech:			
Mass-Tech Powder,			
Milk Choc., 5 scoops, 9 oz	1000	9	168
Nitro Tech Ripped Powder, 1.5 oz	170	4	4
Nature's Best:			
Isopure: 20G Protein, 16 fl.oz	80	0	0
Mass, all flavors, 20 fl.oz	350	0	53
Zero Carb, all flavors, 20 fl.oz	160	0	0
JavaPro Ready To Drink + Coffee,			
average all flavors, 8 fl.oz	110	2	3
Nestle Health Science,			
Diabetishield, Mixed Berry, 8 fl.oz	150	0	30
NOS, High Performance Energy,			
Grape, 16 fl.oz can	210	0	54
Av. other flavors, 16 fl.oz	215	0	53
Turbo, 16 fl.oz	10	0	3
Nutrament *(Nestle)*, 12 fl.oz can	360	10	52
Nutrilite *(Amway)*:			
BodyKey Meal Replacement Shakes,			
Powder, av. all flavors, 2 oz scoop	230	5	25

Energy/Protein Drinks (Cont)

	C	F	Cb
Optifast: *(Nestle):*			
HP Shake Mix, 1 pkg	200	6	10
Ready To Drink Shakes, 8 fl.oz	160	3.5	18
Shake Mix, 1 pkg	160	3.5	18
Optimum Nutrition: *Powder*			
Gold Standard:			
100% Whey, av. all flavors, 1 oz scp	120	1	4
100% Plant, 1 scoop, 1.3 oz	145	2.5	6
Optisource *(Nestle)*,			
Very High Prot. Drink, Strawb., 8 fl.oz	200	6	12
OrGain:			
Organic Ready To Drink: 11 fl.oz	250	7	32
Van. Almond Milk Shake, Unsw., 8 fl.oz	80	3.5	4
Organic Plant Based Powders,			
Average all flavors, 2 scps, 1.62 oz	150	4	15
Powerade, av. all flavors, 12 fl.oz	80	0	21
PowerBar:			
Protein Plus 50G, Choc., 17 fl.oz	315	2	24
Power Gel Smoothie, av., 1.5 oz pkg	110	0	27
Premier Protein *(Premier Nutrition):*			
Clear, Tropical Punch, 16.9 fl.oz	60	0	1
Shakes, average, 11 fl.oz bottle	160	3	5
Propel: Purified Water, 12 fl.oz	0	0	0
Vitamin Boost, all flavors, 20 fl.oz	10	0	2
Protein2O: Tropical Coconut, 16.9 fl.oz	60	0	1
Aveage other flavors, 16.9 fl oz	55	0	7
Pure Protein: *Per 11 fl.oz Bottle or Can*			
30 Gram Shakes, average	140	2	6
35 Gram Shakes: Banana	150	1	1
Average other flavors	165	1	3
Powder, Plant Based, Van. Bean, 1.3 oz	140	3.5	8
Red Bull:			
Energy Drink: Average, 8.4 fl.oz	110	0	29
12 fl.oz can	160	0	40
Sugar-Free, 8.4 fl.oz	10	0	3
Zero Calories, 8.4 fl.oz	0	0	0
Revival:			
Soy Mix, unsweetened:			
Plain, 2 scoops, 0.95 oz	105	1	4
Average all flavors, 2 scoops	115	2.5	5
Rhino, Rush Drink, all flav., 2 fl.oz	6	0	2
Rip It, Energy Fuel, Citrus X, 16 fl.oz	200	0	52
Rockstar: *Per 16 fl.oz Can*			
Energy Drink: Original	130	0	32
Sugar Free	0	0	0
Rumble, Supershake, 12 fl.oz	250	8	26
Rush: *Per 8.4 fl.oz*			
Energy Drink: Regular	120	0	32
with Maca, 8 fl.oz	130	0	30

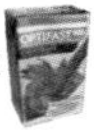
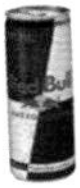
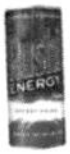

	C	F	Cb
Skratch Labs:			
Hydration Drink Mix: *Per Packet*			
Hyper, Passion Fruit, 0.9 oz	80	0	17
Sport Mix, average, 1 scoop, 0.78 oz	80	0	20
Wellness, Lemon & Limes, 0.6 oz	70	0	18
Sport Recov. Mix, average, 1.76 oz	200	3.5	35
Super Fuel, Lemon & Lime, 3.7 oz	400	0	100
Slim-Fast:			
Original: Protein Shakes, av., 11 fl.oz	180	5	24
Powder, average, 0.9 oz scoop	110	3.5	18
Advanced, High Protein, 11 fl.oz	180	9	7
Smoothie Mix, 1 scoop, 0.9 oz	100	3	7
Diabetic Wt. Loss, av., 1 sc., 26g	100	7	11
Keto Meal Shake, 2 sc, 38g	180	14	7
SoBe: *Per 20 fl.oz Can/Bottle*			
Citrus Energy Fruit Drink	250	0	64
Water, average all flavors	0	0	0
Solixir, Energy Drink, av. all, 12 fl.oz	55	0	13
Special K,			
Protein Shakes, av. all flav.	185	5	23
Spiru-Tein:			
Energy Meal Shake Powder:			
Banana, 1.3 oz	110	0	15
Cappuccino, 1.1 oz	100	0	13
Gold: Chocolate, 1.3 oz	90	0	21
Strawberry,1.3 oz scoop	125	0	20
Note: Gold Products Contains 12 G Xylitol			
Sport, Vanilla, 2.25 oz scoop	260	7	27
Whey, Cookies & Cream, 1.2 oz sc.	125	2	15
Starbucks: Refreshers, av.,12 fl.oz	90	0	22
Doubleshot Energy ~ *See page 37*			
Steaz: Energy, all flav., 12 fl.oz	140	0	35
Zero Berry, 12 fl.oz	0	0	0
Shakeology:			
Beachbody Whey Prot. Powder,			
Chocolate, 1.45 oz	160	2.5	17
Twin Lab, MVP Fuel, all flav.,1 sc., 0.5 oz	25	0	6
Vega, Protein Shake, 11 fl.oz	170	5	14
Venom, av all flavors, 16 fl.oz	235	0	57
Vital: Organic Greens, 0,17 oz	20	0.2	2.3
Pea Protein, 0.9 oz	90	0.3	0.7
Weider:			
Mega Mass: 2000, 2 scoops, 3.5 oz	400	7	61
4000, 2 scoops, 3.5 oz	400	6	59
4000, Extreme Gainer, 7 sc., 11.8 oz	1275	19	247
XS *(Amway)*: Energy & Burn, 8 fl.oz	10	0	1
Energy, Summit 8.45 fl.oz	10	0	0
Zola: Energy Drinks, av., 12 fl.oz	115	0	27
Flavored Coconut Water, av., 8 fl.oz	60	0	15

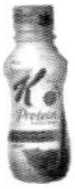
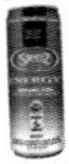
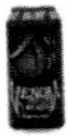

Quick Guide

Orange Juice

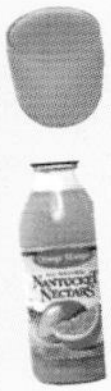

Average ~ Fresh	C	F	Cb
½ Cup, 4 fl.oz	**55**	0	13
Small Glass, 6 fl.oz	**85**	0	19
Regular Cup 8 fl.oz	**110**	0.5	26
Regular Glass, 12 fl.oz	**160**	0.5	39
10 fl.oz Bottle	**140**	0.5	32
11.5 fl.oz Can	**160**	0.5	37
16 fl.oz Bottle	**225**	1	52
20 fl.oz Bottle	**280**	1	64

Juices ~ Generic

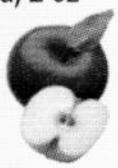
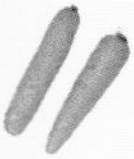
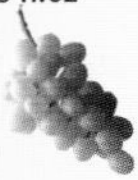
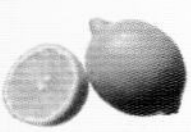
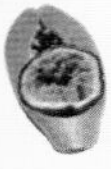
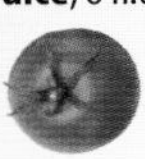
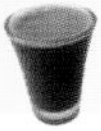

Average All Brands:	C	F	Cb
Aloe Vera Juice, unsweetened, 2 oz	**10**	0	0
Apple Juice: 8 fl.oz	**120**	0	29
10 fl.oz Bottle	**145**	0.5	36
16 fl.oz	**235**	0.5	58
Cactus Water, 1 Cup, 8 oz	**25**	0	6
Carrot Juice: Fresh, 6 fl.oz	**35**	0	8
Sweetened, 6 fl.oz	**75**	0	17
Coconut Water, 8 fl.oz	**50**	0.5	9
Cranberry Juice, Cocktail/Blend	**140**	0	34
Fruit Blends, average all, 8 fl.oz	**110**	0	27
Fruit Nectars, average all, 8 fl.oz	**140**	0	36
Grape Juice, 8 fl.oz	**155**	0	38
Grapefruit Juice, 8 fl.oz	**95**	0	22
Lemon/Lime Juice: 1 Tbsp	**5**	0	1
1 cup, 8 fl.oz	**50**	0.5	16
Concentrate, 1 tsp	**0**	0	0
Noni Juice:			
Tahitian, 2 Tbsp, 1 fl.oz	**15**	0	3
Tahiti Traders, 1 fl.oz	**20**	0	5
Papaya/Peach Nectar, av., 8 fl.oz	**140**	0	36
Passion Fruit Juice, Fresh:			
Purple, 1 cup, 8 fl.oz	**125**	0	34
Yellow, 1 cup, 8 fl.oz	**80**	1.5	14
Pear Nectar, 8 fl.oz	**150**	0	40
Pineapple Juice, 8 fl.oz	**130**	0	32
Pomegranate Juice, 8 fl.oz	**160**	0	40
Prune Juice, 8 fl.oz	**180**	0	45
Strawberry/Raspberry Juice, 8 fl.oz	**100**	0	23
Tangerine Juice, 8 fl.oz	**105**	0.5	25
Tomato Juice, 8 fl.oz	**40**	0	10
Vegetable Juice, 8 fl.oz	**45**	0	11
Wheat Grass Juice:			
1 fl.oz 'Shot'	**10**	0	1.5
2 fl.oz 'Shot'	**20**	0	3

Quick Guide

Fruit Smoothies (Jamba Juice; Smoothie King)

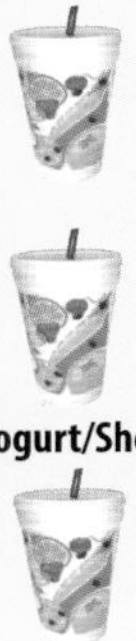

Average All Brands	C	F	Cb
Fruit Only: 8 fl.oz	**115**	0.5	29
12 fl.oz	**175**	1	43
16 fl.oz	**230**	1	58
24 fl.oz	**350**	1	78
Fruit + Non-Fat Milk/Soy:			
12 fl.oz	**135**	0	29
16 fl.oz	**155**	0	37
24 fl.oz	**265**	1	59
Fruit + Non-Fat Frozen Yogurt/Sherbet:			
12 fl.oz	**200**	0.5	47
16 fl.oz	**265**	1	63
24 fl.oz	**395**	1.5	95

Juice ~ Brands

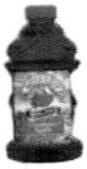

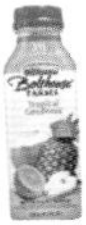

Per 8 fl.oz Unless Indicated	C	F	Cb
Apple & Eve:			
100% Juice, No Sugar Added:			
Apple	**110**	0	26
Cranberry Blend/Raspberry	**110**	0	28
Cranberry Pomegranate	**120**	0	31
Strawb. Watermelon, 6.75 oz	**90**	0	24
Cool Waters, average, 6.75 fl.oz	**15**	0	4
Fruitables, av. all flav., 6.75 fl.oz	**50**	0	13
Organic Quenchers, all flav., 6.75 fl.oz	**40**	0	9
Bolthouse Farms: *Per 15.2 fl.oz Unless Indicated*			
B'fast Smoothie, Peach Parfait, 8 fl oz	**190**	2.5	34
Juice: 100% Carrot	**130**	0.5	29
100% Pomegranate, 8 fl.oz	**150**	0	38
Acai + 10 Superblend	**240**	0.5	60
Tropical + Carrot, 8 fl.oz	**90**	0.5	21
Fruit Smoothies: Amazing Mango	**230**	0	56
Berry Boost	**250**	0.5	61
Blue Goodness	**290**	0	72
C-Boost	**210**	0	52
Strawberry Banana	**250**	0.5	61
Tropical Goodness	**220**	1	51
Cactus Cooler, Orange Pineapple Blast, 12 fl oz can	**150**	0	40

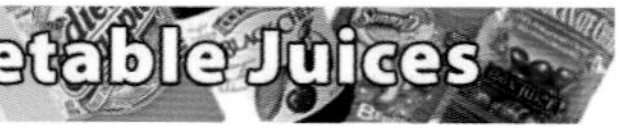

Juice Brands (Cont)

	C	F	Cb
Per 8 fl.oz Unless Indicated			
Campbell's:			
Tomato Juice: 11.5 fl.oz can	70	0	14
8 fl.oz	50	0	10
Califia Farms: *Per 8 fl.oz Unless Indicated*			
Ginger Limeade	80	0	21
Meyer Lemonade	80	0	21
Orange Juice, 10. 5 fl.oz	140	0.5	32
Tangerine	110	0	25
Tart Cherry Lemonade	110	0	27
Capri Sun: *Per 6 fl.oz*			
100% Juice, average,	85	0	21
Juice Drinks,			
(25% Less Sugar), all flavors	50	0	14
Refreshers, average, 6 fl.oz	45	0	11
Roarin' Waters, all flav., 6 fl.oz	30	0	8
Sport, average, 6 fl.oz	30	0	8
Sun Adventures, av., 6 fl.oz	50	0	13
Clamato: *Per 8 fl.oz*			
Original Tomato Cocktail	60	0	12
Picante	60	0	13
Coco Joy:			
Natural Coconut Water, 8.4 fl.oz	60	0	15
Sparkling Coconut Water, all, 11 fl.oz	80	2	20
Coco Libre, Flav. Coconut Water, 11 fl.oz	75	0	18
CocoZia, Coconut Water:			
100% Organic, 11.1 fl.oz pkg	70	0	16
Original, 8 fl.oz	40	0	10
Chocolate, 8 fl.oz	60	0.5	13
Dole: *Per 8 fl.oz*			
Canned: 100% Juice, 6 fl.oz	100	0	25
Jaya Juice, av. all flavors, 8 fl.oz	145	0	36
Florida's Natural: *Per 8 fl.oz*			
Apple Juice	120	0	29
Lemonades, all flavors	110	0	28
Orange, No Pulp	110	0	26
Light Orange Juice	50	0	12
Ruby Red Grapefruit	90	0	22
Fuze: *Per 12 fl.oz*			
Blueberry Lemonade	80	0	21
Pineapple + Mango	80	0	21
Goya: *Per 9.6 fl.oz Can*			
Cocktail, Passion Fruit	130	0	34
Juice, Pineapple	110	0	27
Nectar: Mango	180	0	47
Peach	140	0	36
Pear & Passion Fruit	140	0	36
Soursop	130	0	35

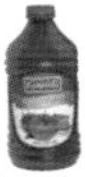
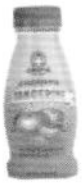
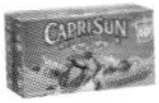
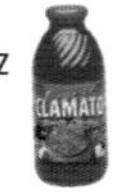
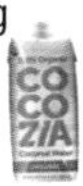
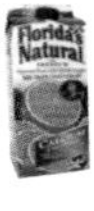
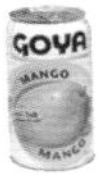

	C	F	Cb
Per 8 fl.oz Unless Indicated			
Great Value *(Walmart):*			
100% Juice: *Per 8 fl.oz*			
Apple	110	0	28
Cranberry Blend	120	0	30
Grape	150	0	38
Orange	110	0	27
White Grape	140	0	38
Hansen's:			
Junior Juice,			
100% Juice, av. of flavors,			
4.23 oz box	60	0	16
Natural, (64 fl.oz Bottles): *Per 8 fl.oz*			
Apple	120	0	28
Apple Strawberry	110	0	27
Cranberry Apple	110	0	27
Cranberry Grape	140	0	35
Grape	120	0	33
Orange Pineapple	110	0	27
White Grape	140	0	36
Hawaii's Own, Frozen Concentrate,			
100% Juice, average all flavors,			
8 fl.oz prepared	105	0	27
Hi-C Juice Drinks: *Per 6.75 fl.oz Box*			
Flashin' Fruit Punch	90	0	25
Orange Lavaburst	90	0	25
Poppin' Lemonade	100	0	27
Hood: *Per 8 fl.oz*			
Lemonade	110	0	29
Orange	120	0	30
Jamba Juice ~ *See Fast-Foods Section*			
Juicy Juice *(Nestle):*			
Juicy Waters, 6.75 fl.oz	0	0	0
Organic Juice : *Per 8 fl.oz Unless Indicated*			
100%, Apple Juice; Fruit Punch	120	0	28
Fruitfuls, all flavors	70	0	16
6.75 fl.oz box	50	0	13
Plus Protein, all flavors, 6 fl.oz	90	0	17
Splashers, all f lavors, 1 pouch	40	0	9
Kerns:			
Nectars: *Per 11.5 fl.oz Can*			
Apricot	210	0	52
Guava; Strawberry, av.	180	0	45
Pear; Strawb. Banana, av.	195	0	46
Pineapple Coconut	230	6	43
L & A: *Per 8 fl.oz*			
All Cherry	180	0	45
All Cranberry	60	0	14
Papaya Delight	130	0	32
Pineapple Coconut	140	3	28

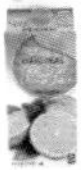
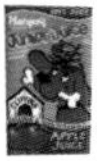
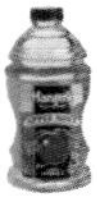
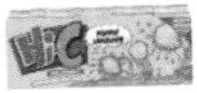
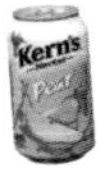
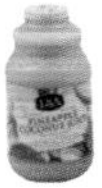

Juice Brands (Cont)

Per 8 fl.oz Unless Indicated

Lakewood Organic: *Per 8 fl.oz*

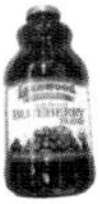
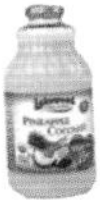

	C	F	Cb
Organic Blends:			
Black Cherry	130	0	32
Blueberry Blend	120	0	29
Pineapple Coconut	190	8	29
Pom Blue	120	0	29
Kale	80	0	19
Papaya	110	0	27
Tart Cherry	130	0	31
Veggie	80	0	17
Organic Pure: Beet	100	0	23
Blueberry	110	0	26
Carrot	90	0	20
Cranberry	80	0	19
Noni	5	0	1
Orange	120	0	28
Pineapple	130	0	31
Pink Grapefruit	110	0	26
Prune	180	0	43

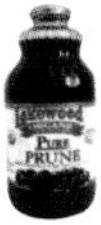

Langers: *Per 8 fl.oz*

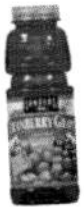

	C	F	Cb
100% Juice:			
Apple Juice	120	0	28
Red/White Grape Juice	160	0	40
Juice Cocktails (27% Juice):			
Blueberry Cranberry	135	0	34
Cranberry	140	0	35
Cranberry Grape	165	0	41
Cranberry Raspberry	140	0	35
20% Juice, all flavors	120	0	30

Martinellli's:

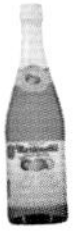

	C	F	Cb
Juice, 100% Apple, all varieties, 8 fl.oz	140	0	35
Sparkling: Apple Juice, 10 fl.oz	180	0	43
Apple Grape, 8 fl.oz	120	0	31
Apple-Pear, 8.4 fl.oz	130	0	31
Blush, 8 fl.oz	120	0	30
Cider, 8.4 fl.oz	150	0	37
Red Grape, 8.4 fl.oz	1270	0	42
White Grape, 8.4 fl.oz	170	0	42

Minute Maid:

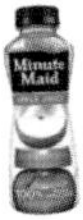

	C	F	Cb
12 fl.oz Bottles: *Per Bottle*			
Apple Juice	170	0	41
Cranb. Apple Raspberry	180	0	48
Cranberry Grape	190	0	50
Pineapple Orange	180	0	43

Per 8 fl.oz Unless Indicated

Minute Maid (Cont):

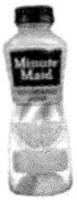

	C	F	Cb
Orange Juice,			
Original, 8 fl.oz	110	0	27
Just 15 Calories, Lemonade, 8 fl.oz	15	0	4
Kid's Juice Boxes, 100% Juice,			
Apple White Grape, 6.75 fl.oz	90	0	22
Light Juice, Cherry Limeade, 8 fl.oz	4	0	1
Soft Frozen Concentrate,			
Limeade, 8 fl.oz prepared	90	0	25

Mott's:

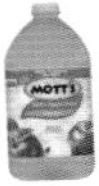

	C	F	Cb
100% Juice:			
Original Apple, 8 fl.oz	120	0	29
Apple Mango, 8 fl.oz	120	0	29
Apple White Grape, 6.75 fl.oz	130	0	31
Fruit Punch, 4.23 fl.oz	60	0	15
Juice Drink, Light Apple, 8 fl.oz	50	0	12
Mott's For Tots (47-54% Juice):			
40% Less Sugar: Fruit Punch, 8 fl.oz	70	0	16
Other flavors, 8 fl.oz	60	0	16
Sensibles, all flavors, 8 fl.oz	90	0	21

Naked Juice: *Per 15.2 fl.oz*

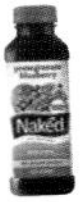
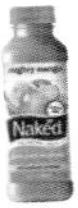
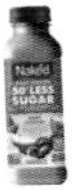
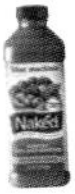

	C	F	Cb
100% Juice, No Sug. Added:			
O-J	210	0	51
Orange Mango	230	0	59
Pomegranate Blueberry	290	0	68
100% Juice Smoothie, No Sugar Added:			
Berry Blast	220	0.5	55
Mighty Mango	290	0	68
Orange Carrot	220	0	55
Pina Colada	310	3.5	66
Strawberry Banana	250	0	59
Half Naked 50% Less Sugar:			
Berry Almond	240	15	12
Lively Greens	150	0.5	32
Mango Orange	220	13	37
Watermelon with Passion Fruit	120	1	33
Machines: Blue	320	0	76
Power-C	220	0	55
Red	320	9	59
Vitamin D	230	0	55

Juice Brands (Cont)

Per 8 fl.oz Unless Indicated

	C	F	Cb
Nantucket Nectars:			
Juice: *Per 16 fl.oz*			
Orange Mango	220	0	59
Peach Orange	260	0	63
Pineapple Orange Banana	290	0	69
Pineapple Orange Guava	210	0	52
Pomegranate Cherry	230	0	57
Pomegranate Pear	230	0	57
Premium Orange Juice	220	0	51
Pressed Apple	240	0.5	59
Red Plum	220	0	55
Watermelon Strawberry	220	0	55
Juice Cocktail, Cranberry	240	0	59
Lemonade, Squeezed	180	0	47

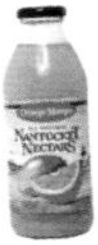
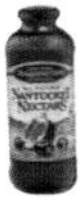

	C	F	Cb
Newman's Own: *Per 8 fl.oz*			
Lemonade, Regular; Pink	110	0	27
Limeade	140	0	34
Fruit Juice Cocktail:			
Grape	110	0	29
Orange Mango Tango	130	0	33

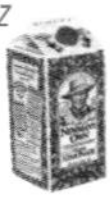

	C	F	Cb
Northland: *Per 8 fl.oz*			
100% Juice:			
Blueberry Blackberry Acaí	110	0	27
Cranb. Blackberry/Raspberry, av.	110	0	27
Cranberry Cherry	120	0	30
Cranberry Grape	110	0	28
Cranberry Mango	120	0	29

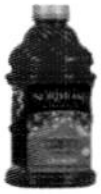

	C	F	Cb
Ocean Spray: *Per 8 fl.oz*			
Juice Cocktails:			
Cranberry	110	0	28
100% Juice Blends:			
Cranberry Concord Grape	130	0	36
Cranberry Mango	120	0	31
Cranberry Pineapple	110	0	31
Cranberry Raspberry	120	0	32
Juice Drinks:			
Cran-Apple	100	0	27
Cran-Grape	100	0	28
Cran-Tangerine	100	0	28
Diet Juice Drinks, all flavors	5	0	2
Growing Goodness, av., 6.75 fl.oz	45	0	12
Light Juice Drinks, av. all flavors	50	0	13
Sparkling, av. all flavors, 8.4 fl.oz	70	0	20

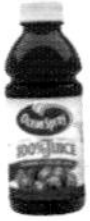
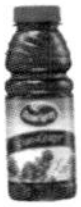

Per 8 fl.oz Unless Indicated

	C	F	Cb
Orange Julius:			
Originals:			
Medium: Mango Pineapple	320	0.2	78
Orange	260	0.5	63
Strawberry	300	0.2	75
Large: Mango Pineapple	470	0.3	117
Orange	400	0.5	98
Strawberry	450	0.3	113
Smoothies ~ *See Fast-Foods Section*			
Orangina, 10 fl.oz bottle	130	0	32
Pom Wonderful,			
100% Juice (8 fl.oz Bottle),			
Pom Blueberry/Cherry/Pomegranate	155	0	38

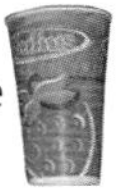

	C	F	Cb
R.W. Knudsen: *Per 8 fl.oz*			
Organic, 100% Juice: Apple	110	0	28
Acai Berry	110	0	26
Concord Grape	160	0	39
Cranberry Blueberry	110	0	27
Mango Nectar	120	0	29
Orange Carrot	110	0	27
Tomato	45	0	10
Natural, 100% Juice:			
Mango Peach	120	0	30
Papaya Nectar	130	0	32
Razzleberry	110	0	28
Rio Red Grapefruit	140	0	34
Just Juice:			
Just Blueberry	90	0	23
Just Black Cherry	190	0	45
Just Black Currant	110	0	24
Simply Nutritious:			
Lemon Ginger Echinacea	110	0	27
Average other flavors	115	0	28
Shots: Apple Cider Vinegar, 2.5 fl.oz	10	0	2
Beet , 2.5 fl.oz	25	0	5
Carrot, Black Pepper & Turmeric, 2.5 fl.oz	25	0	5
Pineapple Ginger, 2.5 fl.oz	30	0	9
Sparkling: Caramel Apple	110	0	28
Cranberry	110	0	27
Cherry; Pomegranate	130	0	32
Organic Pear	120	0	30

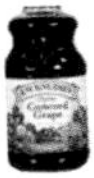

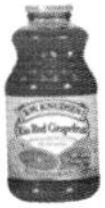
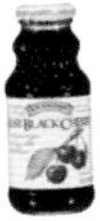
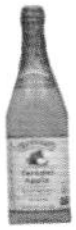

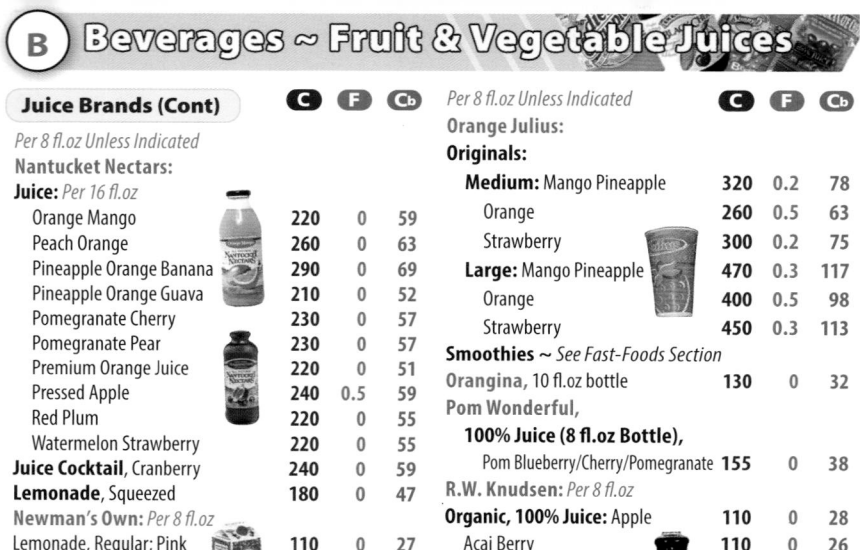

Juice Brands (Cont)

Per 8 fl.oz Unless Indicated

	C	F	Cb
R.W. Knudsen (Cont):			
Organic Veggie Blends:			
Beet, Carrot Orange	90	0	22
Carrot Ginger Turmeric	70	0	16
Celery Apple Cucumber	50	0	11
Sweet Potato	100	0	24
Very Veggie; Low Sodium	50	0	10
Spicy	45	0	10
ReaLemon – ReaLime:			
Lemon/Lime Juice (from concentrate):			
1 teaspoon	0	0	0
2 Tbsp, 1 fl.oz	.10	0	2.5
Santa Cruz: *Per 8 fl.oz*			
Organic, 100% Juice:			
Apple; Apricot Mango, average	115	0	29
Concord/White Grape	160	0	39
Orange Mango; Red Tart Cherry	120	0	29
Pear Nectar	140	0	34
Lemonade:			
Regular; Peach	90	0	22
Blueberry; Raspberry; Strawberry, av.	90	0	23
Cherry	100	0	25
Peach	80	0	21
Simply Orange Juice Company:			
Lemonade; Limeade, average	120	0	31
Lemonade, with Raspberry	110	0	28
Mixed Berry; Tropical	100	0	26
Orange Juice, with or without pulp	110	0	26
Snap•E•Tom,			
Tomato & Chili Cocktail, 11.5 fl.oz can	70	0	15
Snapple: *Per 16 fl.oz Bottle*			
Juice: Go Bananas.	230	0	55
Grapeade; Orangeade	190	0	46
Fruit Punch	200	0	48
Kiwi Strawberry	190	0	46
Mango Madness	190	0	45
Watermelon Lemonade	150	0	35
Diet, Cranberry Raspberry	20	0	5
Ssips, Juice Boxes, av. all flavors, 6 fl.oz box	80	0	21

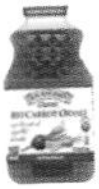
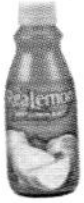
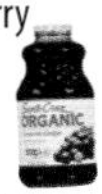
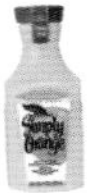
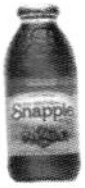
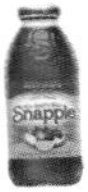

Per 8 fl.oz Unless Indicated

	C	F	Cb
SunnyD: *Per 8 fl.oz*			
Blue Raspberry	60	0	15
Fruit Punch	60	0	16
Lemonade	60	0	15
Orange Mango/Strawberry	60	0	16
Orange Peach	60	0	17
Orange Pineapple	60	0	16
Orange Strawberry	60	0	16
Smooth Orange	50	0	14
Tangy Original	60	0	16
Sunsweet: *Per 8 fl.oz*			
Plum Smart: Original	160	0	36
Light	60	0	15
Prune Juice: Original	180	0	42
Light	100	0	26
Trader Joe's:			
All Natural Pasteurized, 32/64 fl.oz Bottle: *Per 8 fl.oz*			
100% Cranberry	70	0	16
Blueberry Pomegranate	140	0	34
Just Blueberry	100	0	24
Just Pomegranate	150	0	37
Mango PassionFruit	130	0	32
Omega Orange Carrot	110	0	26
Organic, 32/64 fl.oz Bottle: *Per 8 fl.oz*			
Apple Juice	120	0	30
Concord Grape Juice	160	0	39
Cranberry	70	0	18
Grapefruit Sunset	120	0	30
jalapeno Limeade	100	0	25
Mango Nectar	130	0	32
Pink Lemonade	130	0	32
Strawberry Lemonade	120	0	29
White Grape Juice	160	0	40
Cold Presssed, 12 fl.oz:			
Coconut Carrot	70	0	16
Spiced Fuji Apple Cider	200	0	48
Spiced Cider	130	0	31
Winter Wassail	100	0	26
Joe's Kids: *Per 6.75 oz Box*			
From Concentrate: Apple	90	0	23
Apple Grape	100	0	24
White Grape	120	0	30
10% Juice, Lemonade	90	0	22
Sparkling Juices, 25.4 fl.oz Bottle: *Per 8 fl.oz*			
Blueberry	120	0	30
Cranberry	140	0	35
Pomegranate	130	0	31

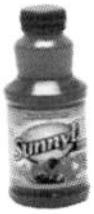
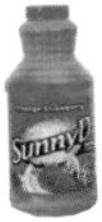
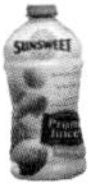
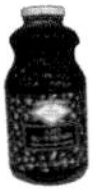
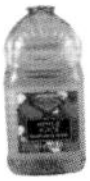
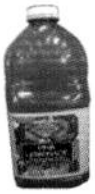
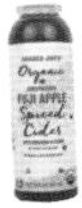
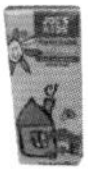

Juice Brands (Cont)

Per 8 fl.oz Unless Indicated	C	F	Cb
Tree Top:			
100% Juice, 64 fl.oz Bottle: *Per 8 fl.oz*			
Apple Berry/Grape, average	125	0	31
Mango Cherry	120	0	29
Orange Passionfruit ; P'apple Orange	120	0	30
5.5 fl.oz can, apple	80	0	19
6.75 fl.oz Box, Apple; Pear	100	0	24
Fruit & Water: Tropical, 6 fl.oz	45	0	11
All other Flavors, 6 fl.oz	50	0	12
Tropicana: *Per 8 fl.oz*			
Essentials Fiber,			
Strawberry Banana	140	0	35
Premium Drinks:			
Island Punch	90	0	21
Lemonade: Peach	110	0	27
Raspberry; Tangerine, average	100	0	25
Strawberry Peach	100	0	24
Pure Premium Orange Juice:			
Grovestand, Lots of Pulp	110	0	26
No Pulp	110	0	26
Trop 50: Pomegranate Blueberry	50	0	14
Orange Mango/Peach, av.	50	0	12
Tru Nopal:			
Cactus Water: 1 Cup, 8 fl.oz	25	0	6
16.9 fl.oz carton	50	0	12
Turkey Hill: *Per 12 fl.oz*			
All Natural Lemonade: Original	170	0	41
Blackberry; Watermelon	160	0	39
Pink	150	0	37
Watermelon	160	0	39
Fruit Punch	150	0	39
V8 Juices & Drinks *(Campbell's):*			
Original/Spicy 100% Vegetable Juice:			
5.5 fl.oz can	35	0	7
8 fl.oz cup	45	0	9
11.5 fl.oz can	70	0	14
12 fl.oz bottle	75	0	15
Blends: Peach Mango, 8 fl.oz	110	0	27
Healthy Greens; Carrot Mango, 8 fl.oz	60	0	14
Red Radiance, 8 fl.oz	70	0	17
Sparkling V8-Energy:			
Orange Pineapple, 11.5 fl.oz	140	5	20
Strawberry Kiwi, 11.5 fl.oz	50	0	12
Veryfine:			
100%: Apple, 8 fl.oz	120	0	29
Apple Strawb., Krazy Kiwi, 11.5 fl.oz	170	0	43
Orange, 8 fl.oz	120	0	30

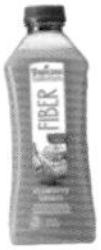
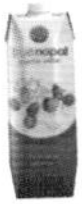
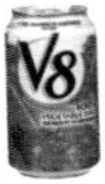
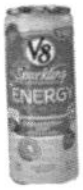

Per 8 fl.oz Unless Indicated	C	F	Cb
Vita Coco: *Per 8 fl.oz*			
Coconut Water: Regular	45	0	11
with Peach & Mango	90	3	16
with Pineapple	60	0	14
Walnut Acres: *Per 8 fl.oz*			
Organic: Apple	110	0	29
Apricot; Raspberry	130	0	32
Cherry	140	0	34
Concord Grape	120	0	31
Incredible Vegetable	50	0	12
Orange Carrot	110	0	27
Welch's: *Per 8 fl.oz Unless Indicated*			
100% Juice: Concord Grape	140	0	38
Red Sangria	140	0	34
White Grape	140	0	38
White Grape Peach	140	0	34
Juice Drink, Fruit Punch, 10 fl.oz	120	0	31
Refrigerated Cocktails: CherryBurst	100	0	23
Mango Twist	120	0	28
Peach Medley	100	0	25
Sparkling Juice Cocktail:			
Red/White Grape, av.	150	0	40
Rose; Mimosa, average	75	0	18
Zola:			
Acai: *Per 12 fl.oz Bottle*			
Original	185	3	38
with Blueberry/Pomegranate	180	3	38
Coconut Water, 17.5 oz Can:			
Original,	50	0	13
Chocolate, 8 fl.oz	50	0	12
Espresso, 8 fl.oz	60	0	13

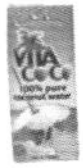
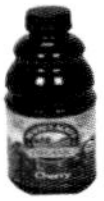
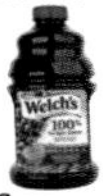
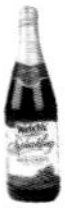
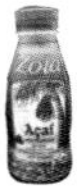
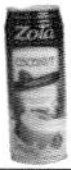

CALORIEKING PORTION WATCH

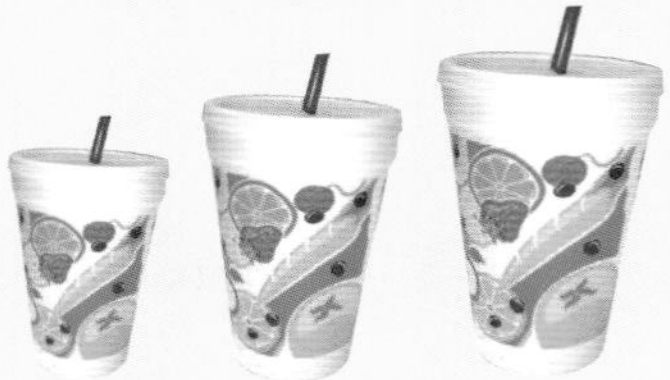

ORANGE JUICE	C	Cb
8 fl.oz	110	26
16 fl.oz	220	52
24 fl.oz	330	78
32 fl.oz	440	104

Quick Guide

Cow's Milk ~ Average All Brands

	C	F	Cb
Whole (3.25% fat):			
2 Tbsp, 1 fl.oz	20	1	1.5
1 Cup, 8 fl.oz	150	8	12
1 Large Glass, 12 fl.oz	220	12	17
1 Pint, 16 fl.oz	295	16	22
1 Quart, 946 ml	590	32	44
Reduced-Fat (2% fat):			
2 Tbsp, 1 fl.oz	15	0.5	1.5
1 Cup, 8 fl.oz	120	5	12
1 Large Glass, 12 fl.oz	180	7.5	18
1 Pint, 16 fl.oz	245	10	23
1 Quart, 946 ml	490	20	46
Light/Low-Fat (1% fat):			
2 Tbsp, 1 fl.oz	13	0.3	1.5
1 Cup, 8 fl.oz	100	2.5	12
1 Large Glass, 12 fl.oz	150	4	18
1 Pint, 16 fl.oz	205	5	25
1 Quart, 946 ml	410	10	49
Fat Free/Skim (0% fat):			
2 Tbsp, 1 fl.oz	10	0	1.5
1 Cup, 8 fl.oz	90	0.5	13
1 Large Glass, 12 fl.oz	135	0.5	19
1 Pint, 16 fl.oz	180	1	26

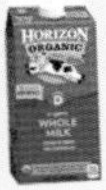
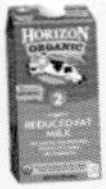
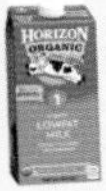
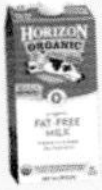

Half & Half ~ *See Page 89*

SWITCH & SAVE

Switch from whole milk to either 2%, 1% or 0% milk and save significant calories.

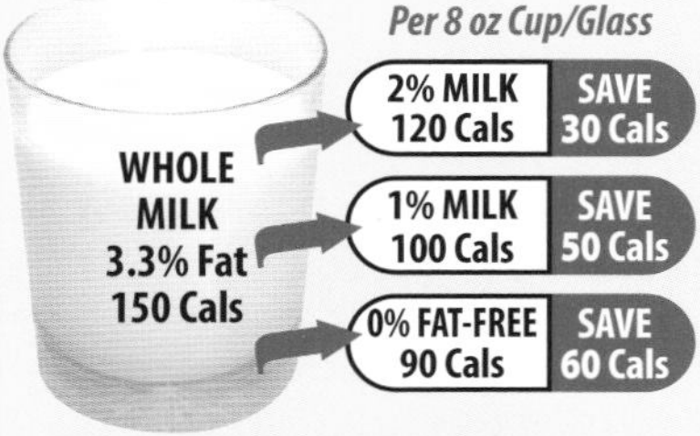

Switching to low-fat or fat-free milk also greatly reduces saturated fat.

Other Milks

	C	F	Cb
Buttermilk: *Average All Brands*			
Reduced-Fat (2%), 1 cup, 8 fl.oz	120	5	10
Low-Fat (1%), 1 cup, 8 fl.oz	100	2.5	12
Lactose Free:			
Lactaid 100: Whole	160	8	13
2% Reduced-Fat	130	5	12
1% Low-Fat	110	2.5	13
Fat Free; Calcium Enriched	90	0	13
Smart Balance,			
FF + Omega-3s & Vit. E	100	0	14
Lower Calorie/Carb Dairy Drinks: *Per 8 fl.oz Cup*			
Calorie Countdown (*Hood*):			
2% Reduced-Fat: Plain	70	4.5	3
Chocolate	80	4.5	6
Fat-Free	35	0	4

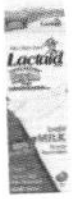
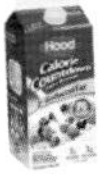

Goat/Sheep Milk, Kefir

	C	F	Cb
Goat's Milk (*Meyenberg*):			
Whole, 1 cup, 8 fl.oz	140	7	11
Low-Fat (1%), 8 fl.oz	100	2.5	11
Evaporated, reconst., 8 fl.oz	140	8	12
Kefir: *Per 8 fl.oz*			
Lifeway: Original, Plain	150	8	12
Greek, Plain, whole milk	210	14	12
Lowfat, average all flavors	140	1.5	20
Nancy's: Plain, low fat	140	3	17
Fruit flavors, average	205	2.5	38
Trader Joe's: Plain, 1%	110	2.5	8
Strawberry	160	2	21
Sheep's Milk, Whole, 1 cup	265	17	13

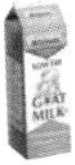
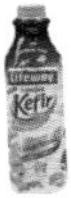
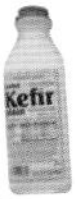

Canned & Dried Milk

	C	F	Cb
Condensed: Sweetened, 2 T., 1 fl.oz	130	3	22
Low Fat, 2 Tbsp	120	1.5	23
Fat-Free, 2 Tbsp	110	0	24
Evaporated: Whole, 2 Tbsp	40	3	3
Whole, ½ cup, 4 fl.oz	170	10	13
Carnation: Low Fat, 2 Tbsp, 1 oz	25	0.5	3
½ cup, 4 fl.oz	115	2.5	14
Fat-Free, 2 Tbsp, 1 oz	25	0	4
Dried: Whole, ¼ cup, 1 oz	160	9	12
Skim/Non-Fat, ⅓ cup	80	0	12
Made-up, 1 cup, 8 fl.oz	80	0	12
Buttermilk (sweet cream): 1 oz	110	2	14
Non-Fat, 1 Tbsp	25	0	3
Carnation, Malted, dry, 3 Tbsp, 0.7 oz	90	2	15
Horlick's, Malt Powder, dry, 1 oz	180	4	27

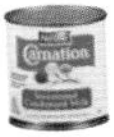
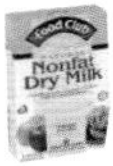

Soy/Non-Dairy Drinks ~ **See Page 49**

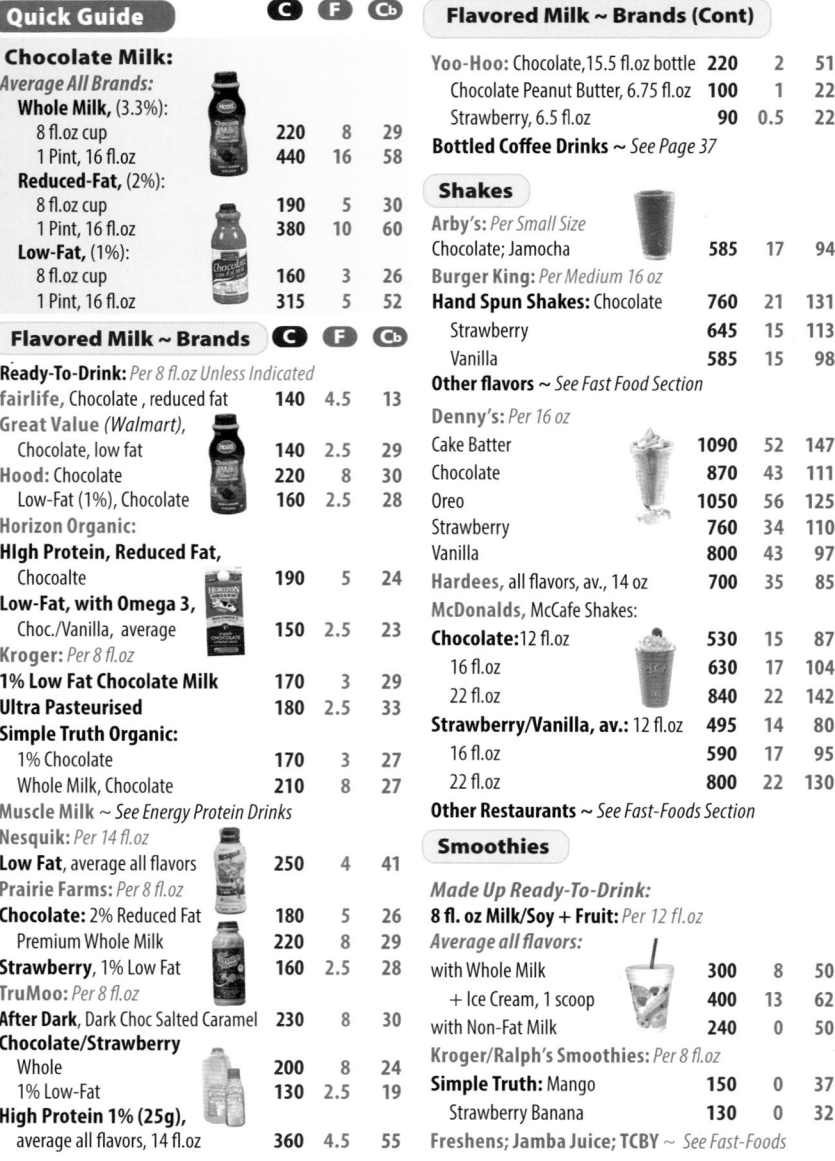

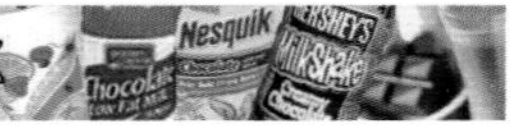

Quick Guide

	C	F	Cb
Chocolate Milk:			
Average All Brands:			
Whole Milk, (3.3%):			
8 fl.oz cup	220	8	29
1 Pint, 16 fl.oz	440	16	58
Reduced-Fat, (2%):			
8 fl.oz cup	190	5	30
1 Pint, 16 fl.oz	380	10	60
Low-Fat, (1%):			
8 fl.oz cup	160	3	26
1 Pint, 16 fl.oz	315	5	52

Flavored Milk ~ Brands

	C	F	Cb
Ready-To-Drink: *Per 8 fl.oz Unless Indicated*			
fairlife, Chocolate , reduced fat	140	4.5	13
Great Value *(Walmart),*			
Chocolate, low fat	140	2.5	29
Hood: Chocolate	220	8	30
Low-Fat (1%), Chocolate	160	2.5	28
Horizon Organic:			
HIgh Protein, Reduced Fat,			
Chocoalte	190	5	24
Low-Fat, with Omega 3,			
Choc./Vanilla, average	150	2.5	23
Kroger: *Per 8 fl.oz*			
1% Low Fat Chocolate Milk	170	3	29
Ultra Pasteurised	180	2.5	33
Simple Truth Organic:			
1% Chocolate	170	3	27
Whole Milk, Chocolate	210	8	27
Muscle Milk ~ *See Energy Protein Drinks*			
Nesquik: *Per 14 fl.oz*			
Low Fat, average all flavors	250	4	41
Prairie Farms: *Per 8 fl.oz*			
Chocolate: 2% Reduced Fat	180	5	26
Premium Whole Milk	220	8	29
Strawberry, 1% Low Fat	160	2.5	28
TruMoo: *Per 8 fl.oz*			
After Dark, Dark Choc Salted Caramel	230	8	30
Chocolate/Strawberry			
Whole	200	8	24
1% Low-Fat	130	2.5	19
High Protein 1% (25g),			
average all flavors, 14 fl.oz	360	4.5	55

Flavored Milk ~ Brands (Cont)

	C	F	Cb
Yoo-Hoo: Chocolate,15.5 fl.oz bottle	220	2	51
Chocolate Peanut Butter, 6.75 fl.oz	100	1	22
Strawberry, 6.5 fl.oz	90	0.5	22
Bottled Coffee Drinks ~ *See Page 37*			

Shakes

	C	F	Cb
Arby's: *Per Small Size*			
Chocolate; Jamocha	585	17	94
Burger King: *Per Medium 16 oz*			
Hand Spun Shakes: Chocolate	760	21	131
Strawberry	645	15	113
Vanilla	585	15	98
Other flavors ~ *See Fast Food Section*			
Denny's: *Per 16 oz*			
Cake Batter	1090	52	147
Chocolate	870	43	111
Oreo	1050	56	125
Strawberry	760	34	110
Vanilla	800	43	97
Hardees, all flavors, av., 14 oz	700	35	85
McDonalds, McCafe Shakes:			
Chocolate: 12 fl.oz	530	15	87
16 fl.oz	630	17	104
22 fl.oz	840	22	142
Strawberry/Vanilla, av.: 12 fl.oz	495	14	80
16 fl.oz	590	17	95
22 fl.oz	800	22	130
Other Restaurants ~ *See Fast-Foods Section*			

Smoothies

	C	F	Cb
Made Up Ready-To-Drink:			
8 fl. oz Milk/Soy + Fruit: *Per 12 fl.oz*			
Average all flavors:			
with Whole Milk	300	8	50
+ Ice Cream, 1 scoop	400	13	62
with Non-Fat Milk	240	0	50
Kroger/Ralph's Smoothies: *Per 8 fl.oz*			
Simple Truth: Mango	150	0	37
Strawberry Banana	130	0	32
Freshens; Jamba Juice; TCBY ~ *See Fast-Foods*			

Nut, Rice & Cereal Drinks

Per 8 fl.oz Cup Unless Indicated	C	F	Cb
Almond Breeze *(Blue Diamond):*			
Almond Milk: Original	60	2.5	8
Chocolate	100	2.5	21
Vanilla	80	2.5	14
Blended with Bananas	80	2	14
Red. Sugar: Original	45	2.5	6
Vanilla	60	2.5	8
Unsweetened: Chocolate	40	3	2
Original; Vanilla, average	30	2.5	1
Blends:			
Almond Cashew,			
Unsweetened, Plain; Vanilla	25	2	1
Almond Coconut: Original	60	3	7
Vanilla, unsweetened	40	3.5	1
Almond Dream ~ *See Dream*			
Amazake,			
Oh So Original, Rice Shake	150	0	31
Better Than Milk:			
Rice Vegan Powder Mix,			
Orig.; Van., 2 Tbsp, 0.7 oz	70	0	17
Cacique,			
Original Horchata, 12 fl.oz	230	5	46
Califia Farms: *Per 8 fl.oz Cup*			
Almond Milk: Original	60	4	6
Unsweetened	35	3	1
Vanilla	50	3	4
Barista Blend	70	4.5	7
Coconut: Chocolate	90	4.5	11
Toasted	45	4	1
Oatmilk, Barista Blend	130	7	14
Don Jose: *Per 8 fl.oz Cup*			
Horchata Rice Drink	140	4	25
Dream: *Per 8 fl.oz Cup*			
Almond Dream, unsweetened	50	3.5	3
Coconut Dream ~ *See page 50*			
Oat Dream: Original; Vanilla, av.	120	3.5	21
Unsweetened	70	3	8
Chocolate	170	3.5	32
Rice Dream: Classic Orig./Enriched	120	2.5	23
Enriched: Unsweetened	70	2.5	11
Vanilla	130	2.5	26
Horchata	160	2.5	33
Sprouted, unsweetened	70	2.5	11
Soy Dream ~ *See page 50*			

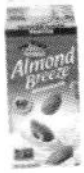
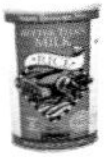
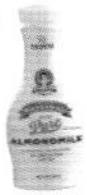
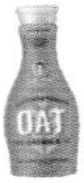

Note: Rice/Oat/Nut Drinks are very low in protein. Unless enriched with protein (and calcium), they are not suitable for infants as a substitute for milk or calcium-enriched soy drinks.

Nut & Rice Drinks (Cont)

Per 8 fl.oz Cup Unless Indicated	C	F	Cb
Milkadamia: *Per 8 fl.oz Cup*			
Macadamia Milk: Original	70	5	7
Unsweetened, Orig./Vanilla	50	5	1
Pacific Foods: *Per 8 fl.oz Cup*			
Cashew, Original	80	4.5	8
Hazelnut, Orig./Chocolate, av.	120	5	18
Hemp: Original	140	6	19
Unsweetened Orig./Vanilla	60	4.5	0
Chocolate	200	6	32
Vanilla	170	6	23
Organic Almond:			
Original; Vanilla, av.	65	3	10
Chocolate, single serve	110	3	19
Oat, Vanilla	130	2	25
Silk: *Per 8 fl.oz Cup*			
Almond: Original	60	2.5	8
Less Sugar	30	1.5	4
Unsweetened	30	2.5	1
Dark Chocolate	100	2	19
Vanilla: Regular	80	2.5	14
Unsweetened	30	2.5	1
Cashew: Unsweetned Orig; Vanilla	25	2	1
Chocolate	90	2	19
Coconut Milk: Original	70	4.5	6
Unsweetened	40	4	1
Protein:			
Almond & Cashew:			
Original	130	8	3
Unsweetened	110	7	2
Chocolate	150	5	18
Vanilla	140	7	8
Trader Joe's:			
Rice Drinks: *Per 8 fl.oz*			
Unsweetened: Original, Organic	120	2.5	23
Vanilla	130	2.5	26

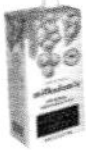
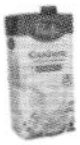
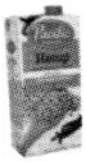

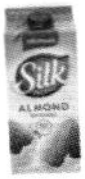
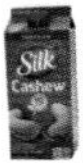
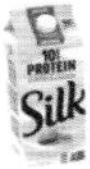

Soy Milk ~ Ready-To-Drink

	C	F	Cb
365 Organic *(Whole Foods): Per 8 fl.oz Cup*			
Original, unsweetened	70	3.5	3
Chocolate, unsweetened	40	3	1
8th Continent: *Per 8 fl.oz*			
Original	80	2.5	7
Vanilla	100	2.5	11
Edensoy: *Per 8 fl.oz Cup*			
Organic: Original	130	5	11
Unsweetened	120	6	4
Carob; Vanilla	150	3.5	23
Cocoa	200	4.5	32
Extra: Original	130	5	12
Vanilla	150	3	23
Great Value *(Walmart),* Orig. Soy	100	4	9

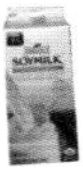
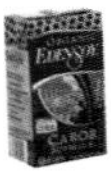

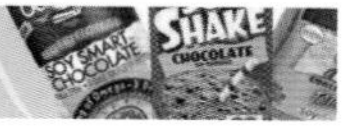

Soy Milk ~ Ready-To-Drink (Cont)

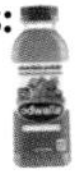
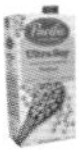
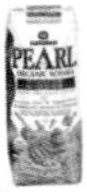
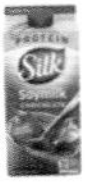
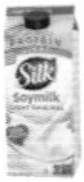
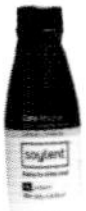
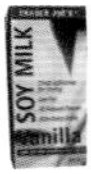
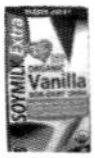

Per 8 fl.oz Unless Indicated	C	F	Cb
Odwalla: *Per 15.2 fl.oz Bottle*			
Soy & Dairy Protein Shakes:			
Chocolate	340	8	38
Strawberry	320	7	37
Vanilla	330	7	35
Pacific: *Per 8 fl.oz Cup*			
Soy, Organic, Orig., unswtnd	90	4	5
Ultra Soy, Original	140	5	13
Pearl *(Kikkoman): Per 8 fl.oz Cup*			
Organic: Original; Crmy Van.	130	4.5	13
Unsweetened	90	5	4
With Green Tea	140	4.5	18
Chocolate; Coffee, av.	135	3	21
Silk *(Whitewave): Per 8 fl.oz Cup*			
Organic: Original; Vanilla, av.	105	4	10
Chocolate	150	5	19
Very Vanilla	130	3.5	18
Light, Original	60	2	5
Unsweetened: Original	80	4	3
Vanilla	80	4	4
Slim-Fast ~ *See Page 40*			
Soy Dream *(Dream): Per 8 fl.oz Cup*			
Enriched: Original	100	4	8
Vanilla	120	4	14
Soylent:			
Ready To Drink Bottles: *Per 14 fl.oz*			
Original	400	24	37
Banana; Cacao; Strawberry	400	21	37
Creamy Chocolate; Vanilla	400	24	36
Mint Chocolate	400	24	36
Cafe, Chai; Mocha; Vanilla, average	400	22	36
Stacked, Chocolate, 11.15 fl.oz	180	10	12
Soy Slender *(Westsoy): Per 8 fl.oz Cup*			
Soy Milk,			
Cappuccino; Vanilla; Chocolate	70	3	4
Trader Joe's: *Per 8 fl.oz*			
Soy Milk: Original	110	2	13
Chocolate	130	2.5	23
Vanilla	100	2	16
Organic: Original	130	3.5	18
Chocolate	120	3	17
Vanilla	130	3	19

Soy Milk ~ Ready-To-Drink (Cont)

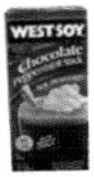
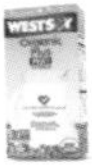

Per 8 fl.oz Unless Indicated	C	F	Cb
WestSoy:			
Soy Milk: Chocolate Peppermint Stick	180	3.5	30
Organic: Original	130	3.5	18
Unsweetened: Plain	100	5	4
Vanilla	100	4.5	5
Organic Plus, Plain/Vanilla	110	4.5	11
Low-Fat: Plain	90	2	15
Vanilla	120	2	23
Non-Fat: Plain	70	0	10
Vanilla	80	0	12

Soy Powder Mix

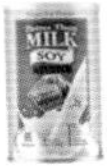
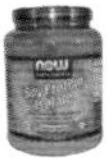

1 oz (¼ cup) mix makes 8 fl.oz Cup	C	F	Cb
Soy Protein Isolate, dry, 1 oz	95	1	2
Better Than Milk:			
Original, 2 Tbsp	90	1.5	18
Vanilla, 2 Tbsp	90	1.5	18
Now:			
Soy Protein Isolate:			
Plain, ⅓ cup, 0.8 fl.oz	90	0.5	0
Chocolate, 1 scoop, 1.6 oz	160	1.5	9
Vanilla, 1 scoop, 1.6 oz	180	2.5	13
Soylent:			
Meal Replacement Powders:			
Original, ⅔ cup, 3.2 oz	400	20	41
Cacao, 2 rounded scoops, 3.2 oz	400	20	41
Cafe Mocha, ⅔ cup, 3.2 oz	400	20	41
Whole Foods:			
Chocolate, with Spirulina, 1 oz	100	1	10
Vanilla, with Spirulina, 1 oz	100	0	11

Coconut Milk Drinks

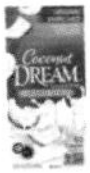
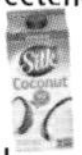
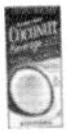

	C	F	Cb
Califia Farms: *Per 8 fl.oz Cup*			
Blend, Coconut Almond, Chocolate	90	4.5	11
Go Coconuts, Coconut Water Blend	45	4	2
Coconut Dream *(Dream): Per 8 fl.oz Cup*			
Enriched: Original	80	5	7
Unsweetened	60	5	1
Vanilla	90	5	9
Great Value *(Walmart),*			
Original Unsweetened	50	5	1
Pacific, Organic, Original Unsweetened	45	4	1
Silk: Original	70	4.5	6
Unsweetened	40	4	1
So Delicious: *Per 8 fl.oz cup*			
Organic, Unswtn'd Shelf Stable	45	4	2
Trader Joes: *Per 8 fl.oz cup*			
Unsweetened	60	5	1
Vanilla	90	5	9

(Enriched with calcium + vitamins D & B12)

Quick Guide

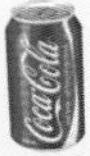
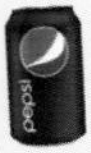

	C	F	Cb
Cola:			
Drinks: *Average all Brands*			
8 fl.oz Cup/Can	100	0	26
12 fl.oz Can	150	0	39
16 fl.oz Bottle	200	0	52
20 fl.oz Bottle	250	0	65
24 fl.oz (Pepsi)	300	0	84
1-Liter Bottle (34 fl.oz)	400	0	100
2-Liter Bottle (68 fl.oz)	800	0	200
Other Soda Drinks: *Per 12 fl.oz, average all brands*			
Club Soda	0	0	0
Cream Soda	190	0	48
Ginger Ale	125	0	31
Lemonade, Regular/Pink	180	0	45
Orange	180	0	45
Root Beer	150	0	39
Tonic Water	125	0	32
Mineral Water: Plain	0	0	0
Sweetened/flavored	150	0	37
with Fruit Juice	120	0	30
Soda Water/Seltzer: Plain/Diet	0	0	0
Sweetened/flavored	155	0	39
with Fruit Juice	160	0	40

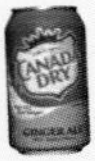
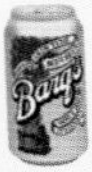

Fountain, Movie Theater & Take-Out

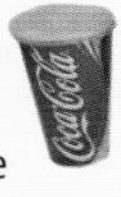

Average All Flavors	C	F	Cb
Small Cup, 12 fl.oz: No Ice	160	0	40
with ⅓ Ice	120	0	30
Regular, 16 fl.oz: No Ice	215	0	53
with ⅓ Ice	160	0	40
Medium, 22 fl.oz: No Ice	295	0	73
with ⅓ Ice	220	0	55
Large, 32 fl.oz: No Ice	430	0	105
with ⅓ Ice	320	0	80

Note: ⅓ Cup of Ice = ¼ Cup Liquid

Soft Drink ~ Brands

Per 12 fl.oz Unless Indicated

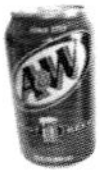
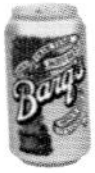

	C	F	Cb
A&W: Root Beer, 20 fl.oz	290	0	78
Cream Soda, 20 fl.oz	170	0	46
Albertson's:			
Signature Select: Cola	160	0	44
Diet Cola	0	0	0
Barq's: Root Beer	160	0	44
Creme Soda: Fr. Vanilla	160	0	45
Red	170	0	45
Big Red, Red Soda, 20 fl.oz	250	0	63
Blue Sky, Root Beer	130	0	32

Soft Drink Brands (Cont)

Per 12 fl.oz Unless Indicated

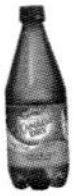
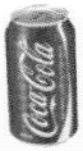
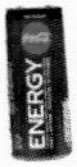
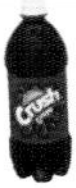
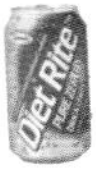
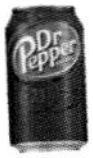

	C	F	Cb
Bubble Up,			
Lemon-Lime Soda	140	0	42
Cactus Cooler	150	0	40
Canada Dry:			
Club Soda; Diet Ginger Ale	0	0	0
Ginger Ale; Tonic Water, av.	140	0	36
Cheerwine	150	0	42
Coca-Cola:			
Classic; Orange/Cherry Vanilla	140	0	39
Vanilla	150	0	42
Diet Coke; Zero	0	0	0
Energy: Regular	140	0	39
Cherry	140	0	39
Zero Sugar	0	0	0
Life	140	0	39
Crush: *Per 20 fl.oz*			
Cherry; Strawberry	290	0	77
Grape; Orange	270	0	72
Peach; Pineapple, average	315	0	84
Dad's: Cream Soda, 12 fl.oz	200	0	51
Root Beer, 12 fl.oz	180	0	45
Diet Rite, Pure Zero	0	0	0
Dr Pepper: *Per 12 fl.oz Can*			
Regular	150	0	40
Cherry	160	0	43
Ten	10	0	3
Fanta: Orange	160	0	44
Zero, all flavors	0	0	0
Fresca, all flavors	0	0	0
Great Value *(Walmart)*, Cream Soda	180	0	49
GuS, Cola; Root Beer, av.	95	0	24
Hansen's: *Per 12 fl.oz*			
Natural Cane Sugar:			
Original Cola; Root Beer	160	0	41
Pomegranate	140	0	35
Diet, all flavors	0	0	0
Hawaiian Punch, all flavors	60	0	15
Henry Weinhard's: Root Beer	170	0	43
Orange/Vanilla Cream, av.	180	0	44
Hires, Root Beer	170	0	45
IBC: Cream Soda; Black Cherry	175	0	44
Root Beer; Cherry Limeade, av.	165	0	40
Icee: Cola; Orange; Lemon Lime, 6 fl.oz	80	0	20
Average other flavors	80	0	21
Jarritos, av. all flavors, 8 fl.oz	110	0	28
Jelly Belly, all flavors	180	0	42
Jolt, Cola, 16 fl.oz	190	0	50

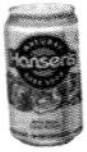
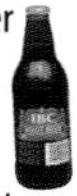
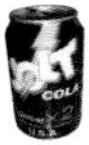

Soft Drink Brands (Cont)

Per 12 fl.oz Unless Indicated

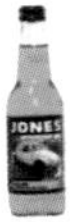

Per 12 fl.oz Unless Indicated	C	F	Cb
Jones Soda:			
Regular, all flavors, 12 fl.oz	160	0	36
Stripped, all flavors, 12 fl.oz	30	0	8
Zilch, sugar free, 12 fl.oz	0	0	0
Kool Aid, Bursts, av., 6.75 fl.oz	20	0	5
Mello Yello: Regular, 12 fl.oz can	170	0	47
Cherry; Peach, 20 fl.oz	290	0	78
Mountain Dew: All flavors, can	170	0	46
Diet, 20 fl.oz	10	0	0.5
Dewshine, 12 fl.oz can	160	0	42
Kickstart, all flavors, 16 fl.oz	80	0	20
Mug, Root Beer	160	0	43
Natural Brew: Draft Root Beer	170	0	43
Outrageous Ginger Ale	180	0	44
Vanilla Cream Soda	160	0	39
Nehi, Peach	190	0	51
Pepsi: *Per 12 fl.oz*			
Regular; Mango Flavor	150	0	41
Black Currant; Citrus Flavor	150	0	39
Zero	0	0	0
7.5 Fl.oz, Regular	100	0	26
Perrier, Carbonated Water	0	0	0
Pibb: Xtra	140	0	38
Zero	0	0	0
RC Cola: Regular, 12.fl.oz	160	0	43
Cherry, 12.fl.oz	160	0	45
Reed's: Ginger Beer, all varieties	145	0	35
Ginger Ale	140	0	35
7•UP: Lemon Lime; Cherry	140	0	39
Diet flavors	0	0	0
Safeway *(Albertson's): Per 12 fl.oz Can*			
Refreshe: Cherry Cola	160	0	44
Dr Dynamite	140	0	38
Grape	200	0	53
Root Beer	170	0	47
Signature Select, Ginger Ale, 12 fl.oz	140	0	37
Schweppes: Ginger Ale	120	0	33
Tonic Water	130	0	33
Shasta: Cream Soda	190	0	47
Cola	130	0	33
Club Soda; Diet, all flavors	0	0	0
Dr. Shasta	150	0	38
Ginger Ale; Orange	130	0	33
Lemon Lime	120	0	29
Tiki Punch	150	0	39
Average other flavors	170	0	41
Sierra Mist, Lemon Lime	120	0	30
Sprite: Original, 12 fl.oz	140	0	37
Zero, all flavors	0	0	0

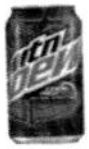
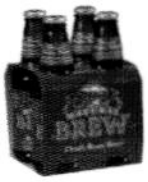
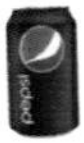
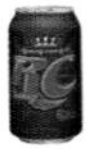
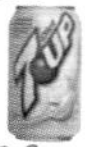
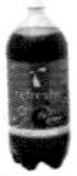
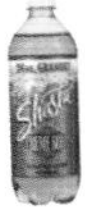
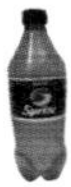

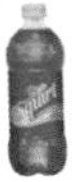

Per 12 fl.oz Unless Indicated	C	F	Cb
Squirt, Ruby Red	170	0	45
Stewarts: Cherries 'n Cream	190	0	46
Grape; Orange 'n Cream	180	0	45
Root Beer	150	0	38
Average Other Flavors	180	0	44
Sun Drop: Citrus Soda, 20 fl.oz	290	0	76
Diet Citrus Soda	10	0	1
Sunkist: Orange; Grape, av., 12 fl.oz	165	0	45
Pineapple, 12 fl.oz	190	0	51
Surge, Original 16 fl.oz	230	0	62
Tab, Original	0	0	0
Tampico: *Per 8 fl.oz*			
Lemonade, with Lime	50	0	14
Punch: Blue Raspberry	60	0	14
Pineapple Coconut	70	0	17
Average other flavors	55	0	14
Thomas Kemper: *Per 12 fl.oz*			
Black Cherry	170	0	44
Ginger Ale; Vanilla Cream	150	0	36
Root Beer	160	0	41
Trader Joe's:			
Sparkling:			
French Berry Lemonade:			
1 cup, 8 fl.oz	130	0	31
1 bottle, 33.8 fl.oz	520	0	124
Lime Ade: 1 cup, 8 fl.oz	110	0	28
1 bottle, 33.8 fl.oz	440	0	108
Pink Lemonade: 1 cup, 8 fl.oz	130	0	31
1 Bottle, 33.8 fl.oz	520	0	124
Vernors, Ginger Soda, 20 fl.oz	240	0	65
Virgil's, Root Beer	160	0	42
Walgreens: *Per 12fl.oz*			
Nice: Cherry Cola	170	0	45
Diet Cola	0	0	0
Root Beer	160	0	45
Zevia, all flavors,	0	0	0

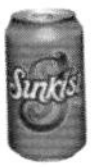
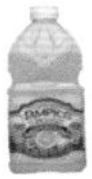
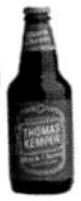
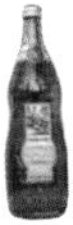

Powdered Soft Drink Mixes

Per 8 fl.oz Prepared, Unless Indicated	C	F	Cb
Country Time: *Per 12 fl.oz*			
Lemonade; Pink Lemonade	100	0	26
Strawberry Lemonade	130	0	33
Crystal Light *(Kraft):*			
Fruit Drinks, all flav., ½ tsp	5	0	0
On The Go, 1 pkt, 3 grams	10	0	3
Flavor Aid, ⅛ package	0	0	0
Kool-Aid, sweetened, 0.6 oz	60	0	16
Tang, Regular, 1 cap, 0.9 oz	90	0	22

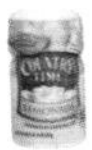
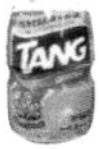

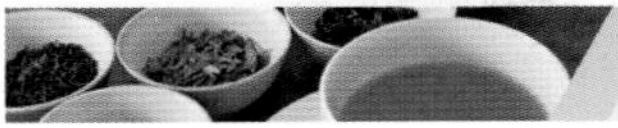

Quick Guide

	C	F	Cb
Teas			
Regular: Bag, Loose or Instant			
Brewed, 1 cup, 8 fl.oz	2	0	0.5
(Add extra for sugar/milk)			
Herbal, av. all flav., 1 cup	2	0	0.5
Bubble Milk Tea, w/ Pearls, 8 fl.oz	175	0	41
Chai Tea Latte Mix, 1 oz	110	1	24
Kombucha Tea, *Average all Brands:*			
Low Sugar, 1 cup, 8 fl.oz	30	0	7
Higher Sugar, 1 cup, 8 fl.oz	50	0	12
Iced Tea			
Average All Brands			
Sweetened: 8 fl.oz cup	90	0	22
12 fl.oz glass/can	140	0	35
16 fl.oz bottle	180	0	45
20 fl.oz bottle	225	0	55
Unsweetened, 8 fl.oz	0	0	0

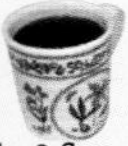

Iced Tea Mixes

	C	F	Cb
Per 8 fl.oz Made-Up Unless Indicated			
4C Iced Tea: *Per 12 fl.oz*			
Average all flavors, 0.9 oz	100	0	25
Light, all flavors, 1 Tbsp	25	0	6
Crystal Light, sugar free	5	0	0
Lipton:			
Sweetened: Lemon	70	0	18
Mango; Peach	80	0	19
Unsweetened	0	0	0
Diet, all varieties	5	0	0.5

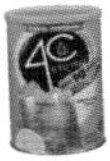

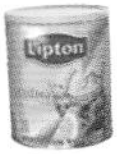

Bottled & Canned Teas

	C	F	Cb
Arizona: *Per 8 fl.oz*			
Brewed Tea,			
Southern Style, Sweet	130	0	33
Green Tea, with Ginseng & Honey	70	0	18
Half & Half, Mango	50	0	14
Iced Tea, Lemon Flavor	100	0	25
White Tea, Blueberry	70	0	19
Fuze: *Per 12 fl.oz*			
Lemon + Sweet Black Tea	80	0	22
Strawberry + Peach Green Tea	80	0	21
Watermelon + Lime Green Tea	80	0	21
Gold Peak, Lemon, 18.5 fl.oz	180	0	45
Health-Ade: *Per 8 fl.oz*			
Original Kombucha	30	0	7
Blood Orange Carrot Ginger	35	0	7
Ginger Lemonade	35	0	7
Pink Lady Apple; Bubbly Rose	40	0	9

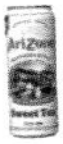

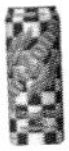

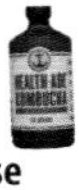

Bottled & Canned Teas (Cont)

	C	F	Cb
Honest Tea:			
Honey Green Tea, 16.9 fl.oz	70	0	19
Mango White Tea, 16 fl.oz	70	0	19
Peach Oolong, 16.9 fl.oz	70	0	19
Lipton:			
Green Tea, Citrus Flav. & Juice, 20 fl.oz	100	0	25
Half & Half	90	0	24
Flavored Iced Tea:			
Lemon Flavor, 12 fl.oz	70	0	19
Mango Flavor, 20 fl.oz	120	0	30
Peach Flavor, 12 fl.oz	70	0	18
Pear & Peach, 20 fl.oz	100	0	26
Tropical, 16.9 fl.oz	90	0	22
Sweet Tea, Black, 12 fl.oz	70	0	17
Nestea:			
Classics, all flavors, 8 fl.oz	50	0	13
Flash Brewed, all flavors, 17.6 fl.oz	100	0	25
POM:			
Antioxidant Super Tea: *Per 12 fl.oz*			
Pomegranate:			
Honey Green Tea	130	0	35
Lemonade Tea	140	0	35
Peach Passion White Tea	130	0	32
Sweet Tea	120	0	30
Snapple: *Per 16 fl.oz*			
Green Tea	120	0	31
Diet Green Tea	0	0	0
Half & Half	210	0	51
Lemon Tea; Raspberry Tea	150	0	37
Diet Lemon/Raspberry Tea	5	0	0
Straight Up Tea: *Per 18.5 fl.oz Bottle*			
Sorta Sweet	90	0	22
Sweet	180	0	45
SoBe, Elixir, Green Tea, 20 fl.oz	200	0	52
Ssips, Lemon Iced Tea, 8 fl.oz	100	0	24
Steaz, Iced Green Tea,			
lightly sweetened, av., 16 fl.oz	80	0	20
Tampico, Iced Tea,			
Peach, Lemon, 8 fl.oz	40	0	10
Tazo, Giant Peach, 13.8 fl.oz	150	0	37
TeaZazz, NaturalZ,all flav., 12.8 fl.oz	70	0	20
Trader Joe's:			
Org. Tea & Lemonade, 8 fl.oz	100	0	25
Hibiscus Tea & Lemonade, 16 fl.oz	40	0	9
Turkey Hill: Iced Tea, 12 fl.oz	120	0	31
Orange Tea, 12 fl.oz	150	0	38
Peach Tea, 12 fl.oz	140	0	34
365 Organic *(Whole Foods)*:			
Unsweetened: Black Tea	0	0	0
Green Tea	0	0	0

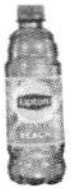

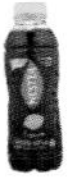

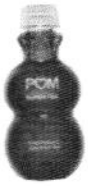

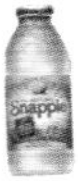

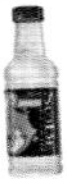

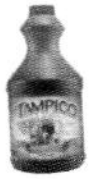

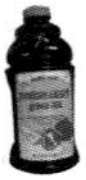

B Bread & Bread Products

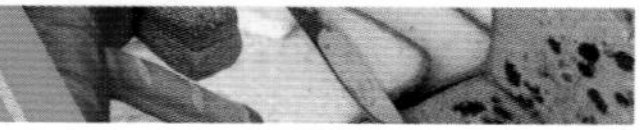

Note: Most breads have similar calories on a weight basis. However, volume may vary.

For example, 1 oz of bread may equal 1 slice regular bread or 2 slices of a lighter bread. It is best to weigh bread used and calculate using: 1 oz bread = 70 calories, 14g carb.

Quick Guide

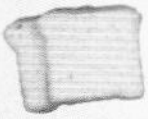
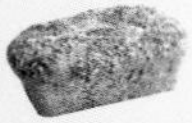
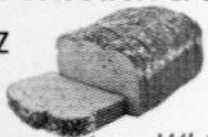

	C	F	Cb
Bread			
White or Wheat: *Average Per Slice*			
Thin or Light, 0.85 oz	**65**	0.5	12
Regular slice, 1 oz	**75**	1	14
Thick or Large, 1.5 oz	**115**	1.5	21
Thick, 2 oz	**150**	2	28
Extra Thick, 3 oz	**225**	3	42
Whole Loaf, 16 oz	**1200**	16	224
Multi Grain/Whole Wheat: *Per Slice*			
Regular Slice, 1.3 oz	**90**	1	16
Thick Slice, 1.5 oz	**110**	1.5	19
Toast: *Based on same counts as White/Wheat as above*			
1 Thick Slice (1.5 oz untoasted):			
with 1 tsp butter/margarine	**150**	5.5	21
with 1 tsp "light" butter/marg.	**135**	4	21
with 2 tsp butter/margarine	**185**	9.5	21
with 2 tsp "light" butter/marg.	**155**	6.5	21

Breads

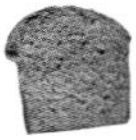
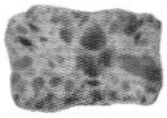
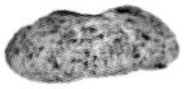

Per Slice Unless Indicated	C	F	Cb
12-Grain, 1.5 oz	**110**	1.5	22
Bran style/Dark, 1 oz	**70**	1	14
Buttermilk, average, 1.5 oz	**110**	1	22
Challah, 0.75 oz	**85**	1.5	17
Chapati, 1 oz	**110**	3	18
Ciabatta, 2 oz	**130**	1	26
Cornbread, average, 3 oz	**220**	6	37
Cracked Wheat Sourdough, 1.5 oz	**130**	0.5	27
Croissants ~ *See Page 134*			
Crustless Bread, regular, slice, 0.75 oz	**40**	0.5	8.5
Crusts Only, regular slice, 0.25 oz	**30**	0	7
English Toasting, 2 oz	**140**	1.5	27
Flax & Grain, 1.5 oz	**120**	3	19
Foccacia: Plain, 2 oz serve	**150**	2.5	28
Cheese & Garlic; Pesto, 2 oz serve	**160**	6	21
Tomato & Olive, 2 oz serve	**150**	5	21

Breads (Cont)

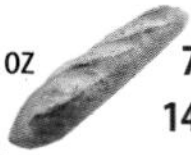
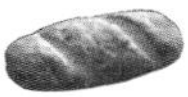
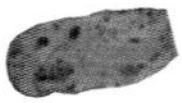
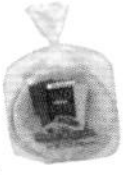
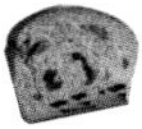
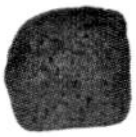
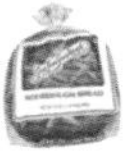

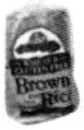

Per Slice Unless Indicated	C	F	Cb
French Stick/Baguette, 1 oz	**70**	1	15
French Toast: Slice, 1.5oz	**140**	2	26
Aunt Jemima, Sticks, av., 2 oz	**110**	2	18
Garlic Bread/Toast:			
Small slice + 1 tsp spread, 0.75 oz	**80**	5	7
Medium slice + 2 tsp spread, 1.5 oz	**160**	10	14
Thick slice + 3 tsp spread, 1.8 oz	**220**	14	20
Pepperidge Farm, Texas, 1 sl., 1.4 oz	**150**	8	15
Hawaiian Sweet Bread, 1.5 oz	**110**	2	19
Hemp Bread, 1.2 oz	**95**	2	12
Italian Bread, 2 oz	**140**	1	28
Lower Carb, (higher protein/fiber), average all brands, 1 oz	**50**	1.5	9
MultiGrain, 1.5 oz	**100**	2	21
Naan Flatbread, 2 oz	**160**	3.5	29
Nut/Health Nut, 1.35 oz	**90**	1.5	18
Oatmeal/Oatbran Bread, 1.5 oz	**90**	0.5	19
Pita, average all types:			
Small (4" diam), 1 oz	**90**	0	18
Large (6½" diam), 2 oz	**140**	1.5	27
Extra Large (9" diam), 4 oz	**300**	1.5	60
Popovers, (1), without butter	**130**	2	18
Pumpernickel:			
Cocktail/Party size	**30**	0.5	6
Large slice, 1.35 oz	**80**	0	15
Raisin Bread, 1 oz	**80**	1	15
Rye: 1 thin slice, av., 1 oz	**80**	1	14
1 thick slice, 2 oz	**150**	2	25
Cocktail size, 0.4 oz	**25**	0.5	4
Sandwich Pockets, 2 oz	**140**	1.5	27
Sourdough: Regular, 1.5oz	**120**	1	25
French Style, 1 oz	**75**	0	14
Spelt, 1.6 oz	**130**	1	26
Sprouted 7-Grain, 1.5 oz	**110**	0.5	18
Squaw, 1.1 oz	**85**	0.5	13
Tacos/Tortillas ~ *See Page 172*			
Turkish/Middle Eastern, 1 oz	**80**	1.5	16
Wheat-Free Breads: Spelt, 1.6 oz	**130**	1	26
Rice, with Fruit Juice, 1.5 oz	**110**	2	21
Healthseed Rye, 1.6 oz	**90**	1	20
Millet, 1.5 oz	**100**	1	20

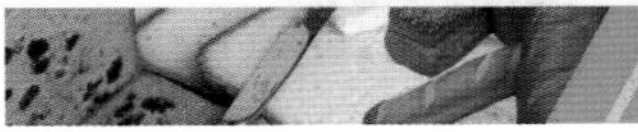

Bread ~ Brands

Per Slice Unless Indicated

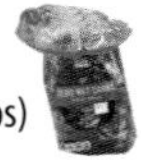
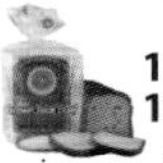
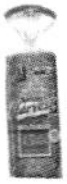
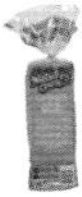
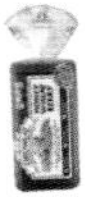

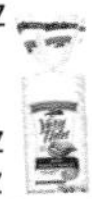
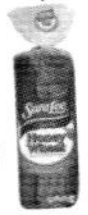

	C	F	Cb
Aldi: *Per 1 slice*			
Fit & Active: Whole Wheat	35	0.5	8
Keto Friendly (Zero Net Carbs) *(Contains 9g dietary fiber)*	50	2.5	9
Bimbo: 100% Whole Wheat, 1 slice	60	1	12
Pan Integral Grande Wheat, 1 slice	75	1	14
Soft Wheat, 1 slice	65	1	12
Ener-G, Gluten-Free: *Per 1 slice*			
Classic White, Reg., 1.4 oz	110	6	15
Multigrain: Regular, 1.4 oz	100	5	15
Light, 0.8 oz	60	3	9
Brown Rice: Brown Loaf, reg., 1.2 oz	100	3	16
White Rice, 1.34 oz	100	3.5	17
Home Pride: *Per 1 Slice*			
Butter Top, Wheat/White, 0.9 oz	70	1	13
Nature's Harvest: *Per 2 Slices*			
100% Whole Wheat	120	1.5	26
Honey 7 Grain	160	2.5	28
Light Multigrain, 0.7 oz	80	1	18
Nature's Own: *Per 1 Slice*			
100% Whole Wheat, 0.9 oz	60	0.5	11
Butterbread, 0.9 oz	60	1	12
Honey Wheat, 0.9 oz	70	0.5	13
Oroweat: *Per 1 Slice*			
100% Whole Wheat, 1.3 oz	100	1	19
Country Sourdough, 1.35 oz	100	1.5	18
Health Nut, 1.34 oz	100	1.5	18
Honey Wheat Berry, 1.2 oz	90	1	17
Organic 22 Grains & Seeds, Regular, 1.7 oz	140	3	23
Pepperidge Farm: *Per 1 Slice*			
100% Whole Wheat, 1.7 oz	120	2	23
15 Grain, 1.7 oz	130	2.5	22
Family, White Sandwich, 1 oz	75	1.5	13
Honey White Bread, 1.6 oz	130	1	24
Italian, w/ Sesame Seeds, 1.1 oz	90	1.5	17
Light Style Oatmeal, 0.7 oz	45	0	9
Oatmeal, 1.7 oz	130	2	25
Swirl, Brown Sugar Cinn., 1.34 oz	110	2	21
Very Thin, Whole Wheat, 0.52 oz	35	0.5	8
Roman Meal: 100% Whole Grain, 1 sl	80	1	16
Honey Split Top, 2 slices, 2 oz	130	1.5	25
Sara Lee: *Per 1 Slice*			
100% Whole Wheat, 0.9 oz	60	1	12
Artesano: Brioche, 1 sl., 1.34 oz	110	1.5	21
Golden Wheat, 1 slice	100	1.5	19
Delightful, Multi Grain, white, 0.77 oz	45	0.5	9
Honey Wheat, 0.9 oz	70	1	13
Trader Joe's: Gourmet White, 1.5 oz	120	3.5	19
Sprouted Wheat Cranberry, 1.2 oz	90	1	16
Wonder: 100% Wh. Wheat, 1 sl., 0.9 oz	60	0.5	11
Classic White, 1 slice, 1oz	70	1	14

Biscuits, Bread Rolls & Buns

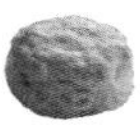
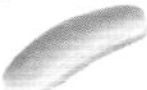

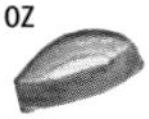
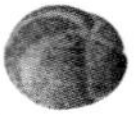
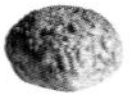

	C	F	Cb
Biscuits: *Average, 2½" diameter*			
Plain/Butter Milk:			
Prepared from Recipe	210	10	27
Refrig. Dough, Baked	95	4	13
Brown 'n Serve, av., 1 oz	70	1	13
Refrigerated Dough:			
Pillsbury, Buttermilk Biscuit, (3), 2.25 oz	150	2	30
Buns:			
Frankfurter/Hot Dog: 1.25 oz	110	1.5	21
1.5 oz	130	2	25
Hamburger: Regular, 1.5 oz	110	1.5	22
Large, 3 oz	210	3	40
Hoagie/Submarine, Plain, 2.3 oz	200	1	38
Rolls:			
Ciabatta Roll, 3.5 oz	230	4	41
Crescent Roll, Original, 1 oz	100	6	11
Dinner:			
1 small, 1 oz	90	1.5	17
1 medium (3" diam),1.5 oz	110	1	23
French: 1 medium 1.3 oz	110	1.5	22
1 large, 3 oz	230	2.5	42
Kaiser:			
Small, 2 oz	200	2.5	35
Large, 3.5 oz	350	4	61
Plain, 6", average all, 2.5 oz	200	1	38
Sourdough, 1.3 oz	110	1	21
Wheat Rolls: Small, 1.2 oz	100	1	17
Medium, 1.8 oz	130	1.5	23
Large, 3.5 oz	260	3	46

Breadsticks, Croutons

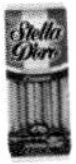

	C	F	Cb
Breadsticks:			
Salt Sticks, plain, 1 oz	110	1	20
Fresh baked (1), 2 oz	180	2.5	34
Stella D'oro: Original (1)	45	1	7
Sesame (1)	50	2	7
Croutons: Seasoned, 2 Tbsp, 0.3 oz	35	1.5	4
Pepp. Farm, Zesty Italian, 6 croutons	30	1	5

Bread Products

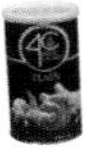
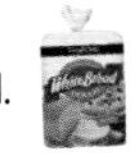

	C	F	Cb
Bread Crumbs, dry:			
Plain or seasoned: 1 oz	110	1.5	20
1 cup, 3.5 oz	385	5	70
Corn Flake Crumbs, 1 oz	120	0	29
Graham Cracker Crumbs *(Keebler)*,1 oz	110	2.5	20
Bread Dough, average:			
Frozen, 1 slice, 2 oz	140	2	26
Refrigerated: French, 1" sl.	60	1	13
Wheat; White, 1" slice	80	2	14
Coating Mixes, av., 2 Tbsp., 1 oz	100	0.5	20
Stuffing: Dry mix, average all,1 oz	110	1	10
Prepared, ½ cup, 4 oz	180	9	22

Quick Guide

	C	F	Cb
Bagels			
Average All Brands			
Plain/Onion:			
1 mini/bagelette, 1 oz	65	0.5	13
1 small bagel, 2 oz	145	1	29
1 medium bagel, 3 oz	220	1.5	43
1 large bagel, 4 oz	290	2	57
Bagel Chips, 1 oz	130	4.5	19
Pizza Bagel Bites (Bagel Bites), average all varieties., 4 pieces, 3 oz	190	5.5	27
Bagel Crisps *(New York Style),* average all varieties, 6 crisps, 1 oz	130	5	17
Bagel Thins *(Thomas'),* 1, 1.5 oz	110	1	25

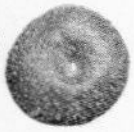

Bagel ~ Brands

Per Bagel			
Bubba's: Plain	220	1.5	45
Blueberry	230	2	49
Cinnamon Raisin	230	1.5	48
Costco Bakery: Plain	330	1.5	70
Cinnamon Raisin	340	1.5	73
Whole Grain	300	5	56
Lender's, Fresh, NY Style:			
Plain, 3.3 oz	240	2	46
Blueberry, 3.3 oz	240	2	46
Cinnamon, 3.3 oz	240	2	46
French Toast, 2.86 oz	220	1.5	45
Whole Wheat, 3.3 oz	240	2	46
Panera Bread: Plain	280	1	57
Cinnamon Swirl & Raisin, 3.8 fl.oz	310	1.5	65
Everything, 4 oz	290	1.5	58
Whole Grain, 4.3 oz	330	2.5	66
Sara Lee: Plain, 3.4 oz	260	1	52
Blueberry, 3.4 oz	260	1	54
Cinnamon Raisin, 3.7 oz	260	0.5	54
Everything, 3.4 oz	270	3	50
Onion, 3.4 oz	260	1	53
Western, The Alternatives, av., 2 oz	120	0.5	29

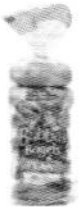
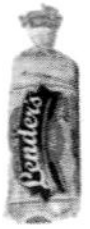
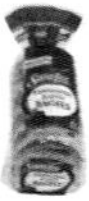

Bagel Spreads

Cream Cheese:			
Plain: 2 Tbsp, 1 oz	100	9	1
2 oz mini-tub	200	18	2
Reduced Fat: 2 Tbsp, 1 oz	60	5	2
2 oz mini-tub	120	10	4
Flavors: Lox, 1 oz	90	8	2
Honey Nut, 1 oz	80	7	4
Strawberry, 1 oz	90	7	5
Sundried Tomato, 1 oz	80	7	2
Vegetable, 1 oz	90	8	2

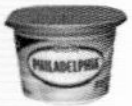

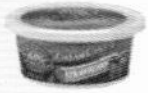

English Muffins

	C	F	Cb
Average All Brands			
Plain/Whole Wheat: Regular, 2 oz	135	1.5	26
Heavier, 2.5 oz	155	2	31
Super Size, 3.2 oz	190	2	38
Raisin-Cinnamon, 2.2 oz	150	1	30

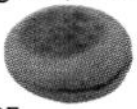

Note: Actual weight of packaged muffins can be 10-15% heavier than stated net weight.

Rice Cakes

Hain, Mini, White Cheddar (10), 1.2 oz	70	2.5	11
Lundberg:			
Minis, av. all flavors, 13 pieces	130	5	20
Thin Stackers, All flavors, (4)	110	1	24
Quaker: Apple Cinn., (1)	50	0	11
Butter Popcorn, (1)	35	0	7
Chocolate, (1)	60	1	12
Tomato & Basil, (1)	50	2	8
White Cheddar, (1)	45	1	8

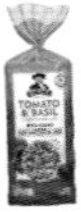

Tortillas & Shells

Tortillas: *Per Tortilla*			
Corn Flour, White/Yellow: 6", 1 oz	55	1	11
7", 1.2 oz	75	1	14
Wheat Flour:			
6", 1.2 oz	100	3	16
8", 1.4 oz	130	4	20
10", 2.3 oz	200	6	31
Shells: *Per Shell, without Fillings*			
Corn Taco Shells: Mini, 3", 0.2 oz	25	1	3
Medium, 5", 0.5 oz	60	2.5	8
Large, 6½", 0.7 oz	100	4.5	13
Salad Shell, 10"	310	17	34
Tostada Shells, fried:			
White Corn, 5½" diam., 0.4 oz	55	2.5	8
Yellow Corn, 5½" diam., 0.5 oz	80	3.5	11
Sopes, 1 shell, 4" 2 oz	110	1.5	23
La Tortilla Factory:			
Non GMO: Hand Made Style,			
White Corn & Wheat, 1.45 oz	90	1	15
Gluten Free, Casava Flour, 1.4 oz	190	3	20
Low Carb, Quinoa & Flax, 1.45 oz	60	2	15
Whole Wheat Protein, 1.76 oz	120	3.5	12
Traditional, Flour, Burrito Size, 2 oz	170	4.5	24
Mission Foods:			
Corn, Yellow, Super Soft:			
Low Fat, 2 Tortillas, 1.65 oz	100	1.5	20
Flour, Large Burrito Size (1), 2.47 oz	210	4	37
Ortego:			
Cauli/Corn: Taco Shell (1)	65	3	9
Tortillas (1)	120	2	22

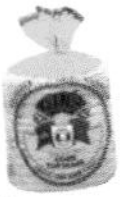
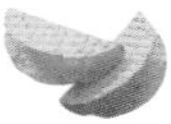
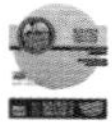
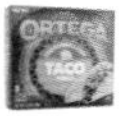

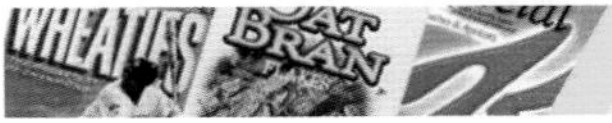

Quick Guide

Cooked Cereals

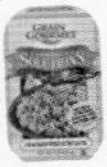
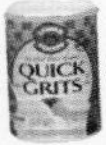
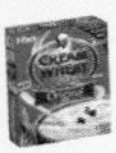
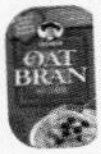

		F	Cb
Barley, pearled, cooked, 1 cup	195	0.5	44
Buckwheat Groats, roasted:			
Dry, ½ cup, 3 oz	285	2	61
Cooked, 1 cup, 6 oz	155	1	34
Bulgur: Dry, ½ cup, 2.5 oz	240	1	53
Cooked, 1 cup, 6.5 oz	150	0.5	34
Corn/Hominy Grits:			
Dry: Regular, ¼ cup, 1.4 oz	140	0.5	32
Instant: 0.8 fl.oz packet	75	0	18
w/ Imitation Bacon Bits, 1 oz	100	0.5	22
Cooked, ¾ cup, 6.5 oz	110	0.5	23
Cream of Rice, cooked, ¾ cup, 6.5 oz	95	0	21
Cream of Wheat:			
Cooked: Regular, ¾ cup, 6.5 oz	95	0.5	20
Instant, ¾cup, 6.5 oz	105	0.5	21
Quick, ¾ cup, 6.5 oz	100	0.5	22
Farina, cooked, ¾ cup, 6 oz	95	0.5	19
Millet, dry, ½ cup, 1.8 oz	190	2	36
Oat Bran: Raw, ⅓ cup, 1 oz	70	2	19
Cooked, ½ cup, 3.8 fl.oz	45	1	13
Oatmeal:			
Dry: Regular, ⅓ cup, 1 oz	100	1.5	18
Instant: Regular, average, 1 oz	105	1.5	18
Flavored, average, 1.5 oz	165	2	34
Cooked: Regular, ¾ cup, 6 oz	125	2.5	21
1 cup, 8 fl.oz	165	3.5	28
Whole Wheat, cooked, ¾ cup, 6.5 oz	115	0.5	25

Brans, Wheat Germ, Add-Ons

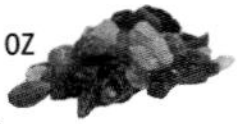

Bee Pollen Granules, 1 Tbsp, 0.3 oz	25	1	2
Bran:			
Oat Bran: Raw, 1 Tbsp, 0.2 oz	20	0.5	3
⅓ cup, 1 oz	100	2	17
Rice Bran: Raw, 1 Tbsp, 0.2 oz	15	1	2.5
¼ cup, 1 oz	95	6	15
Fruit: Dried, average, 1 oz	70	0	18
Banana, ½ medium	55	0	14
Prunes in Syrup (5), 3 oz	90	0	23
Honey, 1 Tbsp, 0.75 oz	65	0	17
Lecithin Granules, 1 Tbsp, 0.4 oz	55	4	0.5
Nuts, Almonds (6), 0.3 oz	40	4	1.5
Psyllium Husks, 1 Tbsp, 0.2 oz	10	0	4
Wheat, unprocessed, 1 Tbsp	5	0	2
Wheat Germ: Raw, 1 Tbsp, 0.3 oz	25	0.5	4
¼ cup, 1 oz	105	3	15

Hot/Cooked Cereals ~ Brands

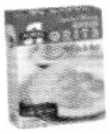
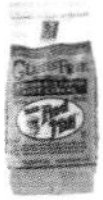
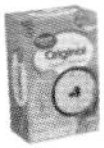
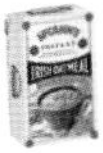
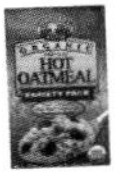
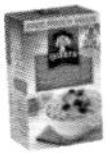

Per Serving, Dry Mix only	C	F	Cb
Albers,			
Quick Grits, ¼ cup, 1.4 oz	140	0.5	31
B&G:			
Cream of Wheat Instant:			
Original, 1 oz	100	0	20
Maple Brown Sugar, 1.3 oz	130	0	29
Bob's Red Mill:			
Brown Rice Farina, ¼ cup	150	1	32
Extra Thick Rolled Oats,			
½ cup, 1.7 oz	190	3.5	33
Dr. McDougall's:			
Stay Full,			
Organic Maple Hot Oatmeal, no sugar	250	3.5	46
Great Value *(Walmart):*			
Instant Oatmeal:			
Cinnamon Swirl, 1.6 oz	160	2	34
Original, 1 oz packet	100	2	19
McCann's:			
Instant Irish Oatmeal:			
Apples & Cinn., 1.3 oz	130	1	28
Maple & Brown Sugar, 1.5 oz	160	1.5	34
Malt-O-Meal: Orig.; Creamy, 3 tbsp	130	0	27
Maple Brown Sugar, ¼ cup	170	0	38
Natures Path:			
Oatmeal: Flax Plus, 1.76 oz	210	0	38
Apple Cinnamon, 1.76 oz	210	2.5	40
Maple Nut, 1.7 oz	210	4	38
NutriSystem,			
Oatmeal, Maple Brown Sugar, 1 pkg	150	1.5	29
Quaker:			
Gluten Free, Instant, Orig., 1.23 oz pkt	130	2.5	24
Instant Grits, Butter, 1.45 oz	150	1.5	32
Quick Grits, Original, ¼ cup, 1.3 oz	130	0.5	29
Instant Oatmeal:			
Maple & Brown Sug.,1.5 oz	160	2	33
Peaches & Cream, 1 oz	110	2	23
Old Fash'nd/Quick Oats, ½ c., 1.4 oz	150	3	27
Wegmans: *Per Packet*			
Instant Oatmeal: Original, 1 oz	110	2	19
Raisin & Spice, 1.5 oz pkt	160	2	32

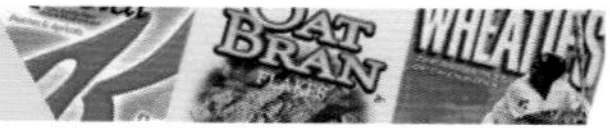

Quick Guide

Cold Cereals

Average All Brands

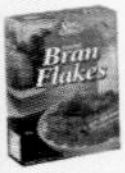

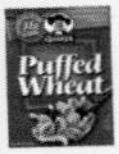

	C	F	Cb
Bran Flakes, ¾ cup, 1 oz	95	0.5	24
Corn Flakes, 1 cup, 1 oz	100	0	22
Frosted Flakes, ¾ cup, 1 oz	110	0	27
Granola, 100% Nat., ½cup, 1.7 oz	205	6	35
Oat Bran Cereal, ½ cup, 1.5 oz	145	3	25
Puffed Rice, 1 cup. 0.5 oz	55	0	13
Puffed Wheat, 1 cup, 0.5 oz	45	0	10
Raisin Bran, ½ cup, 1 oz	90	0.5	22
Rice Crisps, 1 cup, 1 oz	105	0.5	24
Shredded Wheat, 1 biscuit, 1 oz	85	0.5	20
Wheat Flakes, ¾ cup, 1 oz	105	1	24

Breakfast/Cereal Bars ~ *See Page 31*

Ready-To-Eat Cereal ~ Brands

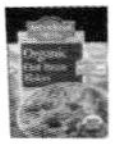

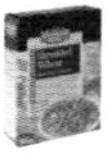

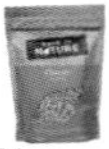

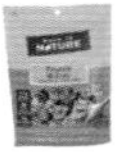

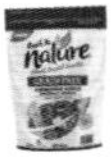

	C	F	Cb
Arrowhead Mills:			
Organic:b Bulgar Wheat, 1.5 oz	150	0.5	34
Flakes: Amaranth, 1.2 oz	140	2	26
Maple Buckwheat, 1.5 oz	170	1	35
Oat Bran, 1.2 oz	140	2.5	24
Spelt, 1 oz	120	1	24
Sprouted Corn, 1.3oz	110	1	25
Organic Puffed: Corn, 0.5 oz	60	1	12
Kamut, 0.5 oz	50	0	11
Millet, 0.5 oz	60	0.5	11
Rice, 0.5 oz	60	0	14
Wheat, 0.5 oz	60	0	12
Rise & Shine, 1.45 oz	150	1	32
Sprouted, Corn Flakes, 1.3 oz	110	1	25
Back to Nature: *Per ½ Cup*			
Granola: Apple Blueberry, 1.76 oz	200	3	39
Chocolate Delight, 1.76 oz	210	5	37
Classic, 1.76 oz	200	2.5	40
Cranberry Pecan, 1.65 oz	190	5	36
Dark Chocolate Coconut, 1.76 oz	230	11	32
Granola Clusters:			
Almond Chia, 1.8 oz	200	5	33
Banana & Walnut, 1.8 oz	210	5	36
Peanut Butter, 1.8 oz	220	9	27
Granola Crunch:			
Cinnamon Apple, 1 oz	170	13	8
Cocoa, 1 oz	170	12	7
Vanilla Almond, 1 oz	160	12	8

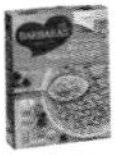

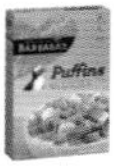

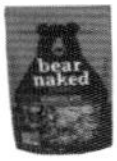

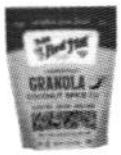

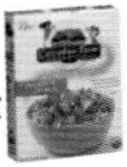

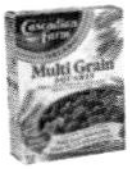

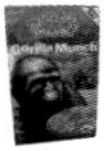

	C	F	Cb
Barbara's Bakery:			
Classics, Organic & Sweetened:			
Brown Rice Crisps, 1.4 oz	160	1	35
Corn Flakes, 1.4 oz	150	0	34
Honest O's, Orig., 1.4 oz	150	2	30
Morning Oat Crunch, Original, 2 oz	210	2.5	45
Puffins:			
Original; Cinnamon, 1.4 oz	130	1	32
Honey Rice, 1 oz	150	1	34
Multigrain, 1.4 oz	130	0.5	33
PB/PB & Choc., av.,1.3 oz	150	2	30
Snackimals, all var., 1¼ cup, 1.4 oz	145	0.5	35
Shredded Wheat, 2 biscuits, 1.8 oz	170	1	41
Spoonfuls, Multigrain, 1.4 oz	140	1.5	31
Squarefuls, Multigrain, 1.95 oz	200	1	48
Bear Naked:			
Granola: Chocolate, 1.83 oz	210	7	36
Fruit & Nut, 2 oz	270	12	39
Maple Pecan, 2 oz	260	9	43
Original Cinnamon, 2 oz	260	12	31
Peanut Butter, 2.2 oz	290	13	42
V'nilla Almond, 2 oz	210	5	40
Bob's Red Mill:			
Granola:			
Coconut Spice; Maple Sea Salt, 1 oz	150	7	17
Lemon Blueberry, 1 oz	140	6	19
Muesli: Old Country Style, ¼ c.,1.23 oz	140	3	23
Paleo Style, ¼ cup, 0.85 oz	140	10	9
Cascadian Farm:			
Buzz Crunch, 21.9 oz	210	2.5	44
Cinnamon Crunch, 1.3 oz	140	3	29
Graham Crunch, 1.3 oz	150	3	30
Granola: Ancient Grains, 2 oz	250	6	42
Coconut Cashew, 2.2 oz	330	19	37
Dark Chocolate Almond, 2.2 oz	260	8	45
French Vanilla Almond, 2 oz	240	7	42
Lemon Blueberry, 2 oz	240	7	38
Honey Nut O's, 1.5 oz	160	1.5	35
Multi Grain Squares, 1 cup, 2 oz	260	1.5	54
Raisin Bran, 2.2 oz	210	1.5	50
EnviroKidz: *Per 1 oz*			
Amazon Frosted Flakes, 1.4 oz	160	0	36
Gorilla Munch, 1.4 oz	150	1	35
Leapin' Lemurs, 1.4 oz	160	2	33
Panda Puffs, 1.4 oz	170	4.5	31

Ready-To-Eat Cereal (Cont)

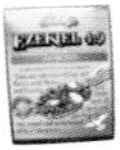

Ezekiel 4.9:	C	F	Cb
Sprouted Whole Grain Cereal:			
Original, ½ cup, 2 oz	190	3	35
Almond, ½ cup, 2 oz	200	3	34
Cinnamon Raisin, 2 oz	190	1	38
Sprouted Flakes: Almond, ¾ c., 1.94 oz	200	2.5	40
Flax & Chia, ¾ cup, 1.94 oz	200	1.5	41
Original, ¾ cup, 1.94 oz	210	21	42
General Mills:			
Cheerios: *Per Cup Unless Indicated*			
Original, 1½ cups1.4 oz	140	2.5	29
Apple Cinnamon, 1.3 oz	150	2.5	30
Banana Nut, ¾ cup, 1 oz	110	1.5	22
Chocolate, 1.3 oz	140	2	28
Cinnamon, 1.3 oz	140	3	29
Frosted, 1.3 oz	140	1.5	29
Fruity, 1.3 oz	140	2	29
Multi Grain, 1⅓ cups, 1.4oz	150	1.5	32
Very Berry, 1.3 oz	140	2	29
Chex: Choc., 1.5 oz	180	3.5	36
Cinnamon, 1.4 oz	170	4	33
Corn, 1 oz	120	0.5	26
Honey Nut, 1 ¼ cups, 1.4 oz	150	1	33
Rice, 1⅓ cups, 1.4 oz	160	1	35
Vanilla, 1.4 oz	170	3.5	33
Wheat, 2 oz	210	1	51
Crunch: Blueberry, 1 oz	120	3	22
Cinnamon Toast, 1.1 oz	130	3	25
Fiber One: Original, ⅔ cup, 1.4 oz	90	1	34
Honey Clusters, 1.8 oz	170	1.5	43
Strawberry & Vanilla Clusters, 2 oz	190	3	45
French Toast Crunch, 1.3 oz	150	1.5	32
Kix: Original, 1¼ cups1 oz	120	1	27
Berry Berry; Honey, av., 1¼ cups, 1.2 oz	120	1.5	27
Lucky Charms:			
Original, 3/4 cup, 1 oz	110	1.5	23
Honey Clovers, 1.25 oz	140	1	31
Monster: Berry varieties, 1 cup 1.2 oz	130	1.5	28
Count Chocula, 3/4 cup, 1 oz	100	1.5	23
Total, Whole Grain, ¾ cup1 oz	110	0.5	25
Wheaties, 1.4 oz	130	0.5	30

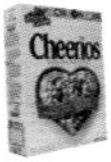
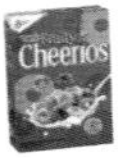
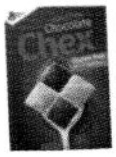
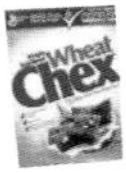
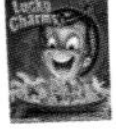
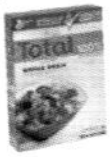

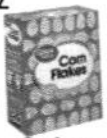
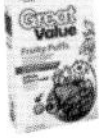

Great Value *(Walmart)*:	C	F	Cb
Apple Blasts, 1⅓ cups, 1.4 oz	150	1	34
Awake, Fruit & Yogurt, 1 cup, 1.94 oz	210	1.5	46
Cinnamon Crunch, 1 cup, 1.4 oz	180	5	32
Corn Flakes, 1⅓ cups	160	0	35
Crunchy Nuggets, ½ cup, 2 oz	200	1	47
Extra Raisin Raisin Bran, 1 cup, 2.1 oz	200	1	48
Frosted Shredded Wheat (21), 2 oz	210	1	50
Fruit Spins, 1½ cups, 1.4 oz	170	1.5	36
O's Oat, 1½ cups1 oz	150	2.5	30
Kashi:			
7 Whole Grain: Flakes, 1¼ cups, 1.8 oz	210	1	51
Whole Grain Puffs, 1½ cups, 1.4 oz	150	1.5	32
Go: Original, 1¼ cups, 2 oz	180	2	40
Cinnamon Crisp, 1 cup, 2.1 oz	230	5	39
Crunch: Original, ¾ cup, 2 oz	190	3	38
Chocolate, ¾ cup, 1.83 oz	210	7	32
Coconut Almond, ¾ cup, 1.85 oz	210	8	32
Honey Almond Flax, ¾ cup, 1.86 oz	200	5	35
Peanut Butter, ¾ c., 1.87 oz	220	9	31
Toasted Berry Crisp, ¾ cup, 1.87 oz	200	4.5	36
Organic:			
Honey Toasted Oat, 1 cup, 1.45 oz	150	2.5	34
Indigo Morning, 1 cup, 1.4 oz	140	1.5	32
Sprouted Grains, 1⅓ cups, 2 oz	210	1.5	48
Strawberry Fieldfs, 1 cup, 1.8 oz	200	1	47
Whole Wheat Biscuit:			
Autumn Fruit, 32 biuscuits	200	1	47
Cinnamon Crunch, 31 biscuits	200	1	48
Island Vanilla, 29 biscuits	200	1	47
Kellogg's:			
All-Bran: Original, ½ cup, 1 oz	80	1	23
Bran Buds, ⅓ cup, 1 oz	80	1	24
Compl. Wheat Flakes, 1.3 oz	90	1	30
Apple Jacks, 1 cup, 1 oz	110	1	25
Choco Krispis, 1.4 oz	160	0.5	37
Corn Flakes, Original, 1½ cups, 1.4 oz	150	0	36
Cracklin' Oat Bran, ¾ cup, 2 oz	230	8	41
Crispix, Original, 1⅓ cups, 1.4 oz	150	0	34

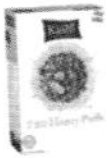
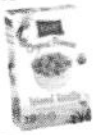
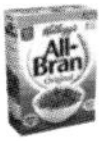
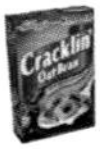

continued next page...

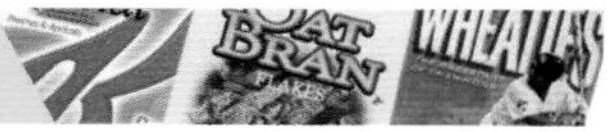

Ready-To-Eat Cereal (Cont)

Kellogg's (Cont):	C	F	Cb
Despicable Me 3 Minion, 1 c., 1.2 oz	120	1	27
Froot Loops: Original, 1 ⅓ cups, 1.4 oz	150	1.5	34
Marshmallow, 1 ⅓ cups, 1.4 oz	150	1	35
Frosted Flakes: *Per 1 oz*			
Chocolate, 1 cup, 1.4 oz	150	1	33
Cinnamon, 1 cup, 1.4 oz	140	0	34
Honey Nut, 1 cup, 1.4 oz	140	0	33
Original Flakes, 1 cup, 1.4 oz	140	0	34
w/ Marshmallows, 1¼ cups, 1.4 oz	150	0	36
Happy Inside, all flavors, 1.94 oz	210	4	44
Honey Smacks, 1 cup, 1.3 oz	130	0.5	32
Krave, Double Choc., 1 cup,1.45 oz	170	5	31
Krispies:			
Original, 1½ cups, 1.4 oz	150	0	36
Cocoa, 1 cup, 1.4 oz	160	1	35
Frosted, 1 cup, 1.38 oz	150	0	35
Mini-Wheats, Frosted:			
Original (25), 2 oz	210	1.5	51
Blueberry (25), 2 oz	210	1	51
Strawberry (25), 2 oz	210	1	51
Little Bites, Orig., 1 c., 2 oz	190	1	47
Mini Wheats, unfrosted:			
Bite Size (30), 1.8 oz	190	1	45
Mueslix, 1 cup, 2.36 oz	250	3.5	50
Raisin Bran: Reg., 1 c., 2 oz	190	1	47
Crunch, 1 cup, 1.94 oz	190	1	46
Smart Start,			
Orig. Antioxidants, 1¼ cups, 2.25 oz	240	1	56
Special K: Orig., 1¼ cups, 1.4 oz	150	0.5	29
Apple Cinnamon Crunch, 1.5 oz	160	1.5	35
Banana, 1 cup, 1.4 oz	160	2.5	35
Chocolate Strawberry, 1 cup, 1.5 oz	160	2	35
Chocolatey Delight, 1 cup, 1.48 oz	170	3	34
Fruit & Yogurt, 1 cup, 1.48 oz	160	1	36
Red Berries, 1¼ cups, 1.4 oz	140	0.5	34
Vanilla & Almond, 1.4 oz	150	1.5	33
Kind:			
Clusters: *Per ⅓ Cup*			
Almond & Coconut Nut,1 oz	140	10	11
Almond Cashew Sunflower, 1 oz	140	13	10
Dark Choc. Nuts & Sea Salt, 1 oz	140	11	11
Peanut Butter Dark Choc. Nut, 1 oz	150	12	10

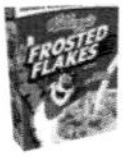

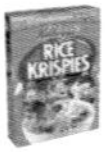

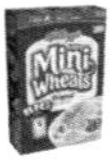

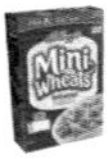

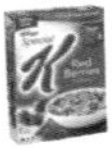

Malt-O-Meal:	C	F	Cb
Apple Zings, 1⅓ cups, 1.4 oz	140	1	34
Cocoa Dyno-Bites, 1.4 oz	170	1.5	37
Coco Roos, 1¼ cups, 1.45 oz	170	2	38
Frosted Flakes, 1¼ cups, 1.4 oz	160	0	37
Fruity Dyno-Bites, 1 cup, 1.27 oz	140	1	32
Frosted Mini Spooners, 21 biscuits	210	1	50
Golden Puffs, 1 cup, 1.35 oz	150	0.5	34
Honey Nut Scooters, 1.4 oz	160	2	33
Marshmallow Mateys, 1.4 oz	160	1.5	35
Peanut Butter Cups, 1.4 oz	170	4.5	31
Raisin Bran, 1¼ cups, 2.1 oz	190	1	48
Nature's Path:			
Flax Plus: *Per 1 Cup*			
Maple Pecan Crunch, 2.1 oz	240	8	41
Multibran Flakes, 1.4 oz	150	2	31
Granola: Coconut Chia, ¾ c., 1.94 oz	270	11	36
Honey Almond, ⅓ cup, 1 oz	140	4.5	21
Maple Almond, Grain Free, ⅓ cup, 1 oz	170	14	8
Heritage Flakes, 1.4 oz	160	1.5	31
Love Crunch Granola: *Per ¼ Cup Unless Indicated*			
Apple Chia Crumble, 1 oz	140	4	22
Espresso Vanilla Cream, 1 oz	130	4.5	21
Salted Caramel Pretzel, 1 oz	140	5	21
Sunrise: *Per ⅔ Cup*			
Crunchy Honey, 1 oz	120	1	26
Crunchy Maple, 1 oz	110	1	25
Superflakes,			
Qi'a Cocoa Coconut, 1.94 oz	240	7	39
New England Natural Bakers:			
Organic Granola:			
Berry Coconut, unswtnd, 2 oz	290	13	37
Blueberry Harvest, ⅔ cup, 2 oz	270	7	41
Chocolate Peanut, ⅔ cup, 2 oz	270	9	42
Cranberry Almond, ⅔ cup, 2 oz	240	9	36
Granny Smith Apple ⅔ cup, 2 oz	260	7	41
Salted Caramel Apple, ⅔ cup, 2 oz	260	7	43
Strawberry, ½ cup, 2 oz	290	16	34
Toasted Coconut, ⅔ cup, 2 oz	270	10	42
NutriSystem,			
NutriFlakes, 1 pkt	90	1	22

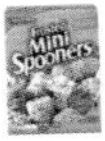

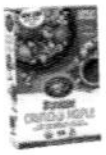

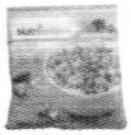

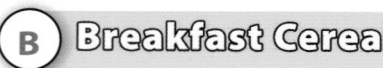

Ready-To-Eat Cereal ~ Brands (Cont)

	C	F	Cb
Post:			
Alpha Bits, 1 cup, 1.3 oz	140	1.5	29
Bran Flakes, 1 cup, 1.3 oz	110	1	29
CoCo Wheats, 1.1 oz	110	0	24
Golden Crisp, 1 cup, 1.34 oz	150	0.5	34
Grape-Nuts: Original, 2 oz	200	1	47
Flakes, ¾ cup, 1.45 oz	150	1.5	34
Great Grains:			
Banana Nut Crunch, 1 cup, 2 oz	230	4.5	45
Cranb. Alm. Crunch, 1 cup,1.9 oz	210	3	44
Crunchy Pecan, ¾ cup, 1.8 oz	210	5	39
Honey Bunches of Oats:			
Frosted; Honey Roasted, 1.4 oz	160	2	34
Honey Roasted Granola, 1.92 oz	230	7	40
Pecan & Maple Brown Sugar, 1 oz	160	3.5	33
With Almonds, 1.42 oz	170	3	34
W/ Cinnamon Bunches, 1.4 oz	160	2	34
Malt O Meal ~ *see Page 60*			
Nutter Butter, 1¼ cups, 1.4 oz	180	5	31
Oreo O's, 1⅓ cups, 1.4 oz	160	2	34
Pebbles, Marshmallow, 1.4 oz	160	1	36
Raisin Bran, 1¼ cups, 2 oz	190	1	48
Shredded Wheat, Spoon Size:			
Original, 1⅓ cups, 2 oz	210	1.5	49
Wheat & Bran, 2 oz	210	1.5	49
Shredded Wheat, Frosted,			
Choc. Strawb., 21 bisc., 2 oz	210	1	49
Quaker:			
Life, all types, 1 cup, 1.4 oz	160	2	33
Oatmeal Squares,			
all varieties,1 cup., 1.58 oz	210	3	44
Multigrain Flakes, av., ¾ cup, 2.1 oz	240	3.5	49
Real Medleys:			
Granola, Summer Berry, ⅔ c., 1.83 oz	210	5	39
Multigrain, Cherry Alm. Pecan, ¾ c., 1.9 oz	240	7	41
Supergrains, all flavors, ½ c., 1.83 oz	220	8	37
Simply Granola:			
Apple Cranberry Almond, 2.2 oz	260	7	49
Oats, Honey, Raisins & Alm., 2.4 oz	270	7	51
Sweet Home Farm:			
Granola: Blueberry, w/ Flax, 1.94 oz	240	8	40
Cinnamon with Raisins, 1.94 oz	200	3	43
French Vanilla with Almond, 1.94 oz	250	8	41
Honey Nut with Almonds, 1.87 oz	240	10	36
Maple Pecan with Syrup, 2 oz	260	9	42
Pumpkin Flax, 1.94 oz	240	9	37

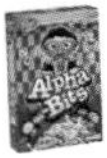

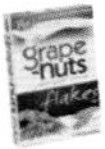

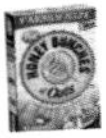

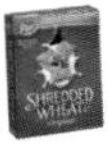

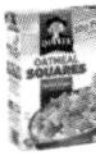

Trader Joe's:	C	F	Cb
Bran Flakes, 1¼ cups cup, 1.4 oz	170	1	37
Cinnamon Squares, ¾ cup, 1.1 oz	130	2.5	24
Cocoa Crunch, 1 cup, 1.4 oz	150	1	33
Cornflakes, 1 cup, 1 oz	110	0	26
Frosted Flakes, ¾ c., 1 oz	110	0	24
High Fiber Cereal: Reg., ⅔ cup, 1 oz	80	0.5	23
Fruit & Nut, Multigrain, ⅔ cup, 1 oz	90	1.5	25
Granola: Ancient Grains & Nuts, 1.8 oz	220	10	29
Low Fat, av., ¾ cup, 2 oz	210	3	44
Org., Apple/Mango, av., ⅔ cup, 2 oz	240	8	37
Joe's O's, 1 cup, 1 oz	110	2	20
Just The Clusters, av., ⅔ cup, 2 oz	240	9	36
O's, av. all flavours, ¾ - 1 cup, 1 oz	120	2	24
Oatmeal (Instant): *Per 1.4 oz Pkt*			
Ancient Grains	160	6	24
Mango; Maple & Brown Sugar, av.	160	2	32
Unsweetened	160	3.5	27
Oatmeal Complete: Plain, 1.4 oz pkt	170	3	29
Maple Brown Sugar, 1.4 oz pkt	210	3	38
Raisin Bran: Regular, 1 cup, 1 oz	170	1	44
Clusters, 1 cup, 2 oz	190	3	41
w/ Pomegr. Blue. Flakes/Clusters, 1 c.	210	2	44
Shredded Wheat, 1 cup, 1.7 oz	180	1	38
Toasted Oatmeal Flakes, ¾ c.,1 oz	110	1	23
Udi's:			
Simple Gluten Free:			
Original; Cranb., av., 2 oz	270	11	42
Almond Butter, ½ cup, 2 oz	280	12	36
Au Naturel Honey; Vanilla, av., 2 oz	275	10	39
Uncle Sam:			
Original, Wheat Berry, ¾ cup, 2 oz	220	6	43
Skinner's Raisin Bran, 1 cup, 2 oz	200	1	48
Weetabix, 3 bisc., 1.84 oz	180	1	43
Wegmans:			
Chocolaty Rice Crisps, 1 cup,1.5 oz	170	1.5	37
Crunchy Raisin Bran, 1 cup, 1.8 oz	230	0	50
Granola:			
Oats & Honey, with Alm., ⅔ cup, 2.3 oz	270	8	46
Vanilla & Almonds, ⅓ cup, 1.1 oz	130	4	21
Shredded Wheat,			
Frosted Bite Size, 21 biscuits	210	1	50
Toasted Grains, 1 cup	150	0	29
Whole Foods 365:			
Organic: Bran Flakes, ¾ up, 1.1 oz	100	0	24
Blueberry Almond Granola, 2 oz	240	9	38
Brown Rice Crisps, 1.1 oz	110	1	25
Fruit & Nut Granola, ½ cup, 1.9 oz	250	10	36
Honey Almond Flax, ¾ cup, 1.87 oz	210	5	35
Honey Flakes & Oat Clusters, 1.1 oz	120	1	25
Morning O's, Honey & Nut, 1.4 oz	150	2	32

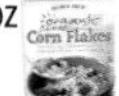

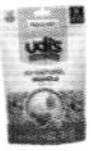

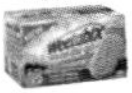

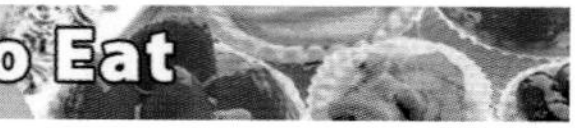

Ready-to-Eat

Per Piece/Slice

	C	F	Cb
Angel Food, Plain: without oil, 2 oz	**145**	0	33
with oil, 2 oz	**145**	1	27
with Cream Frosting	**255**	7	45
Almond Croissant, 5 oz	**620**	35	67
Apple Danish, 5 oz	**450**	18	67
Apple Pie ~ *See Pies/Tarts Page 134*			
Baklava, 1½" square, 1.75 oz	**200**	10	27
Banana Cake, with Butter Cream, 2 oz	**230**	9	37
Banana Walnut Cake, 3 oz	**270**	11	40
Bear Claw, 4.5 oz	**540**	24	71
Black Forest, 3 oz	**345**	11	59
Brownie: Small, 2" Square, 1 oz	**130**	8	14
Large, 3 oz	**390**	24	42
Bundt Cakes, av. all types:			
3 oz slice	**300**	13	42
Mini-Bundt, 5 oz	**500**	22	70
Cannoli's: Mini, 1 oz	**85**	3	11
Regular, 2.5 oz	**215**	8	28
Carrot Cake: Plain, 3 oz	**300**	16	37
with Cream Cheese Frosting	**400**	22	48
Cheesecake:			
Small serving, 3 oz	**240**	13	26
Large serving, 5 oz	**400**	21	44
with Low-Fat Cheese/Fruit, 3 oz	**170**	4	28
Denny's, NY Style, 5oz	**510**	34	43
Chocolate Cake:			
with Choc. Frosting, 4 oz	**415**	18	62
without Frosting, 1⁄12 of 9", 3.5 oz	**340**	14	51
Chocolate Croissant, 4.25 oz	**470**	26	54
Chocolate Eclair, w/ custard, 3.5 oz	**260**	16	24
Chocolate Fudge Cake, 3 oz	**270**	12	40
Chocolate Meringue, 2.5 oz	**320**	13	48
Churros, 1 stick, 1.5 oz	**165**	8	21
Cinnamon Crumb Cake, 2.5 oz	**260**	9	40
Cinnamon Rolls: Small, 2 oz	**220**	8	34
Regular, 4 oz	**440**	16	68
Large, 6 oz	**660**	24	102
Brands ~ *See Page 67*			
Coffee Cake, 2 oz	**180**	6	30
Concha: Small, (3") 2.5 oz	**250**	8	38
Large (5" diam.), 5.5 oz	**550**	18	84
Cream Puff, custard filled, 4.6 oz	**335**	20	30
Cream Horn, 3 oz	**210**	5	36
Crumble Coffee Cake, 4.5 oz	**500**	25	65
Danish Pastries:			
Small, 2.5 oz	**250**	14	25
Large, 5 oz	**500**	28	50
Donuts ~ *See Page 66*			
Eclair, Chocolate, custard filled, 3.5 oz	**260**	16	24
Fig Bars, average	**160**	3	31

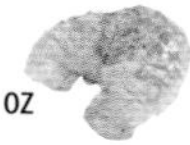
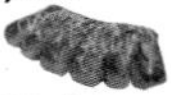
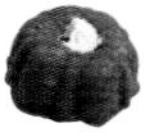
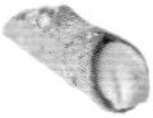
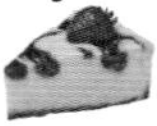
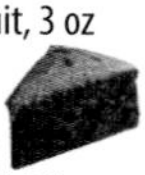
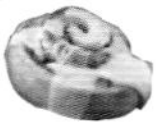

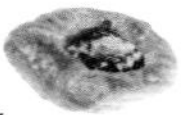

Ready-to-Eat (Cont)

Per Piece/Slice

	C	F	Cb
Fruit Cake, Dark/Light, 2 oz	**185**	5	34
Fudge Nut Brownie, 3.5 oz	**380**	18	54
Gingerbread, from mix, 3" square	**210**	4	41
Honey Bun, glazed, large, 4.75 oz	**560**	29	68
Jelly Roll, 1⁄12 roll, 1.8 oz	**150**	2	32
Key Lime Pie, 4.3 oz	**400**	25	41
Kringles: Almond; Pecan, average	**205**	12	24
Blueberry: Cherry; Raspberry, av.	**165**	8	24
Lady Finger, 3 oz	**310**	4.5	59
Lemon Cake, 4 oz	**440**	24	49
Marble Cake, 4 oz	**430**	23	50
Mississippi Mud Pie, 4 oz	**480**	22	67
Mud Cake, 4.5 oz	**380**	20	44
Muffins ~ *See Page 67*			
Palmier Cookie, large, 4.5 oz	**490**	25	62
Pineapple Upside Down Cake, 2.5 oz	**230**	9	36
Peach Melba, 3.5 oz	**300**	8	52
Pecan Sticky Roll, 6.5 oz	**690**	22	91
Pecan Twirls, 1.3 oz	**170**	7	26
Pies & Tarts ~ *See Page 134*			
Pound Cakes: Iced Lemon, 3.5 oz	**360**	17	50
Marble, 3.75 oz	**350**	13	53
Raspberry Rugulah, 1.2 oz	**110**	9	7
Scone, fruit, 2 oz	**200**	9	30
Sponge Cake: Plain, 2.5 oz	**220**	10	33
with Chocolate Frosting	**290**	12	45
with Cream & Strawberry Jam	**390**	12	69
Starbucks Cakes ~ *Page 244*			
Strawberry Cream Cake, 4.7 oz	**400**	27	33
Strudel Bites, 0.75 oz	**60**	2.5	9
Strudel, fruit, av., 4.5 oz	**300**	17	32
Swiss Rolls, 1 oz	**135**	6	19
Tiramisu, 4.5 oz	**440**	22	34
Turnovers, fruit, average, 3 oz	**290**	15	35

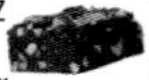
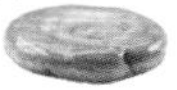
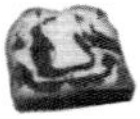
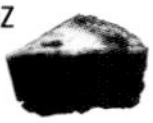
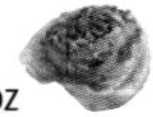
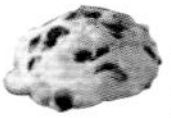
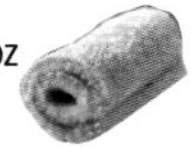

Cupcakes

Average all Varieties

	C	F	Cb
Regular:			
Cake only, 1.5 oz	**140**	5.5	20
Cake + Icing, 2.5 oz	**260**	13	34
Large, (Muffin Size):			
Cake only, 2.5 oz	**235**	9	34
Cake + Icing, 5 oz	**520**	27	67
Mini, (2-Bite):			
Cake only, 0.4 oz	**40**	1.5	5.5
Cake + Icing, 1 oz	**110**	5.5	13
Icing Only: Per 1 oz	**115**	7	13
Thick/Tall amount, 2.5 oz	**290**	17	32

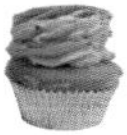
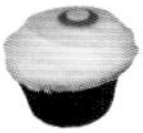
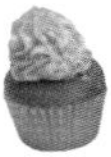

Cakes ~ Brands

	C	F	Cb
Albertson's Bakery:			
Ring Cakes: *Per 1/10 Cake*			
Angel Food	135	0	27
Cake Slices: *Per Slice Unless Indicated*			
Banana Nut Loaf	330	17	39
Creme Cake (2), 3.2 oz	300	12	43
Cinn. Streusel (2), 3.2 oz	350	18	43
Bimbo Bakery:			
Conchas, Vanilla, 2.12 oz	230	9	32
Pound Cakes: *Per Slice*			
Panque/Chocolate, 2.2 oz	240	10	35
Panqecitos, 3.5 oz	410	18	54
Bon Appetit Bakery:			
Banana Bread, 4 oz	440	25	49
Cream Cheese Cake, 4 oz slice	430	24	49
Danish: Apple (1), 5 oz	210	11	25
Bear Claw (1), 5 oz	240	13	27
Cheese & Berries (1), 5 oz	250	14	26
Vienna Cream (1), 5 oz	240	14	27
Slices: Cheesecake, 4 oz	430	24	49
Lemon Cake, 4 oz	430	24	49
Marble Cake, 4 oz	430	24	50
Walnut Brownie, 3.5 oz	380	18	54
Cheesecake Factory ~ *See Fast-Foods Section*			
Entenmann's: *Per Slice*			
Crumb Cakes: Butter French, 2.3 oz	280	14	36
Cheese-Filled Coffee, 2 oz	200	9	27
NY Style, 1/9 cake, 2 oz	230	10	34
Danish: Apple, ½, 2.5 oz	250	10	37
Cheese, ½, 2.5 oz	270	12	35
Cheese, Minis, 1, 2 oz	210	5	35
Cherry Cheese, ½, 2 oz	225	12	26
Pecan Twist, 1/6, 2 oz	260	16	27
Raspberry Twist, 1/8, 1.86 oz	220	11	29
Iced Cakes:			
Chocolate Fudge, 1/6, 3.17 oz	330	13	53
Lemon, 1/6, 3 oz	370	19	48
Marshmallow Devil's Food, 3.17 oz	370	17	52
Loaf Cakes: Banana Bread, 2.2 oz	210	7	32
Blueberry Crumb, 1.76 oz	200	9	28
Chocolate, 1.9 oz	190	8	29
Choc. Chip Crumb, 1.7 oz	190	9	27
Lemon, 1.9 oz	210	10	28

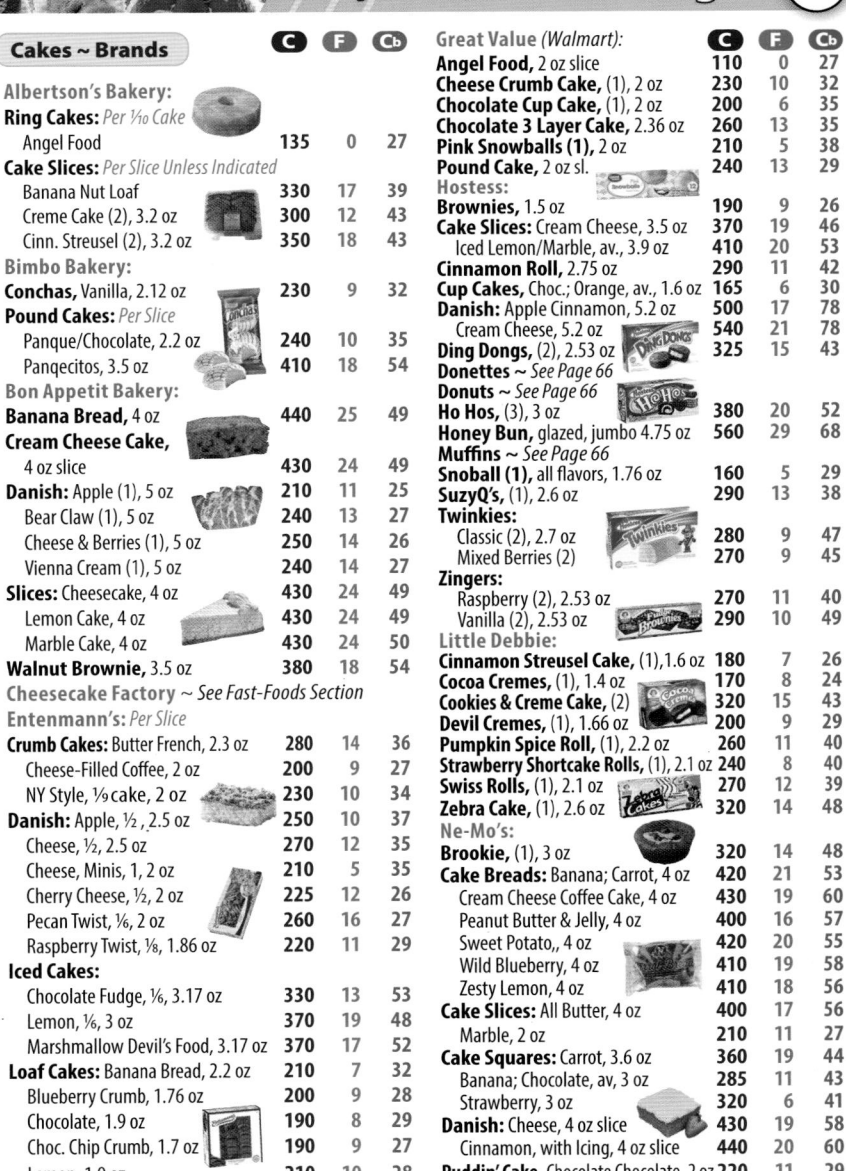

	C	F	Cb
Great Value *(Walmart):*			
Angel Food, 2 oz slice	110	0	27
Cheese Crumb Cake, (1), 2 oz	230	10	32
Chocolate Cup Cake, (1), 2 oz	200	6	35
Chocolate 3 Layer Cake, 2.36 oz	260	13	35
Pink Snowballs (1), 2 oz	210	5	38
Pound Cake, 2 oz sl.	240	13	29
Hostess:			
Brownies, 1.5 oz	190	9	26
Cake Slices: Cream Cheese, 3.5 oz	370	19	46
Iced Lemon/Marble, av., 3.9 oz	410	20	53
Cinnamon Roll, 2.75 oz	290	11	42
Cup Cakes, Choc.; Orange, av., 1.6 oz	165	6	30
Danish: Apple Cinnamon, 5.2 oz	500	17	78
Cream Cheese, 5.2 oz	540	21	78
Ding Dongs, (2), 2.53 oz	325	15	43
Donettes ~ *See Page 66*			
Donuts ~ *See Page 66*			
Ho Hos, (3), 3 oz	380	20	52
Honey Bun, glazed, jumbo 4.75 oz	560	29	68
Muffins ~ *See Page 66*			
Snoball (1), all flavors, 1.76 oz	160	5	29
SuzyQ's, (1), 2.6 oz	290	13	38
Twinkies:			
Classic (2), 2.7 oz	280	9	47
Mixed Berries (2)	270	9	45
Zingers:			
Raspberry (2), 2.53 oz	270	11	40
Vanilla (2), 2.53 oz	290	10	49
Little Debbie:			
Cinnamon Streusel Cake, (1),1.6 oz	180	7	26
Cocoa Cremes, (1), 1.4 oz	170	8	24
Cookies & Creme Cake, (2)	320	15	43
Devil Cremes, (1), 1.66 oz	200	9	29
Pumpkin Spice Roll, (1), 2.2 oz	260	11	40
Strawberry Shortcake Rolls, (1), 2.1 oz	240	8	40
Swiss Rolls, (1), 2.1 oz	270	12	39
Zebra Cake, (1), 2.6 oz	320	14	48
Ne-Mo's:			
Brookie, (1), 3 oz	320	14	48
Cake Breads: Banana; Carrot, 4 oz	420	21	53
Cream Cheese Coffee Cake, 4 oz	430	19	60
Peanut Butter & Jelly, 4 oz	400	16	57
Sweet Potato,, 4 oz	420	20	55
Wild Blueberry, 4 oz	410	19	58
Zesty Lemon, 4 oz	410	18	56
Cake Slices: All Butter, 4 oz	400	17	56
Marble, 2 oz	210	11	27
Cake Squares: Carrot, 3.6 oz	360	19	44
Banana; Chocolate, av, 3 oz	285	11	43
Strawberry, 3 oz	320	6	41
Danish: Cheese, 4 oz slice	430	19	58
Cinnamon, with Icing, 4 oz slice	440	20	60
Puddin' Cake, Chocolate Chocolate, 2 oz	220	11	29

Cakes ~ Brands (Cont)

	C	F	Cb
Pepperidge Farm:			
Layer Cakes (Frozen): *Per ⅛ Cake, 2.43 oz*			
Chocolate Fudge	240	13	32
Chocolate Fudge Stripe	250	13	32
Coconut	250	12	34
Creamy Red Velvet	240	13	30
German Chocolate	240	12	31
Lemon; Tangy Key Lime; Vanilla	240	12	34
Turnovers (Frozen):			
Apple; Cherry; Raspberry (1), av.	245	13	30
Peach (1)	270	13	34
Pop-Tarts *(Kellogg's):*			
Brown Sugar Cinnamon, (2)	400	13	68
Chocolate Fudge, (2)	400	10	74
Cherry, (2)	370	9	70
Fruit, Unfrosted, average (2)	380	10	69
Bites, Strawberry, 1.4 oz pouch	150	3	30
Prairie City:			
Brownie, Big n' Fudgy, 3.5 oz pkg	440	23	58
Cinnamon Roll, Bigger Big, 6 oz	630	34	76
Danish: Ooey Gooey Cheese (1)	470	24	57
Raspberry (1)	420	17	64
Turnovers: Apple & Maple Strudel (1)	500	23	67
Blueberry Cheese (1)	430	20	56
Cherry/Strawberry Cheese (1)	500	23	67
Safeway Select,			
Molten Chocolate Lava Cake (1)	390	23	43
Sara Lee:			
Butter Streusel Coffee Cake,			
⅙ Cake, 1.9 oz	200	9	26
Cheesecakes:			
Classic: Cheesecake, 4.27 oz	330	17	37
Cherry, 4.76 oz	360	12	55
Strawberry, 4.76 oz	330	12	50
French Style: Classic, 4.7 oz	410	26	38
Strawberry, 4.34 oz	310	18	35
NY Style, 4.73 oz	460	27	47
Pecan Coffee Cake,			
⅙ Cake, 1.9 oz	190	9	25
Pound Cakes: *Per ¼ Cake*			
All Butter, 2.68 oz	340	21	34
Blueberry, 2.57 oz	210	7	36
Lemon, 2.68 oz	240	8	39
2 Slices: Original, 2.8 oz	250	8	41
Double Chocolate, 3 oz	280	10	45
Special K, Pastry Crisps,			
all varieties, 1 pouch, 0.9 oz	100	2	20

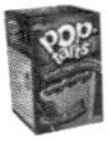

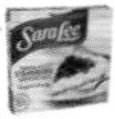

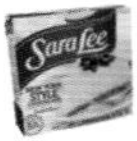

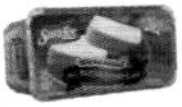

	C	F	Cb
Tastykake:			
Creme Filled Cupcakes:			
Chocolate (2), 2.4 oz	270	10	42
Koffee Cake (2), 2.1 oz	240	9	38
Swirly Choc. (1), 2 oz	200	6	35
Kandy Kake: Choc. (2), 1.3 oz	180	9	24
Peanut Butter (2), 1.3 oz	190	10	20
Krimpets: Butterscotch (2), 2 oz	220	6	39
Creme Filled (2), 2.4 oz	280	11	44
Jelly (2), 2 oz	190	3.5	37
Lemon Flavored (2), 2 oz	220	6	40
Toaster Strudel *(Pillsbury): Per 1.9 oz*			
Boston Cream Pie	180	7	26
Cream Cheese,			
average all varieties	190	9	25
Fruit flavors, all var.	180	7	27
Trader Joe's:			
Bakery Fresh:			
Apricot Almond Tart,			
4 oz slice	450	24	56
Cheesecake Brownie Bites (1)	110	7	9
Chocolate Ganache Cake, 3 oz slice	390	22	44
Flourless Chocolate Cake,			
1 slice, 2 oz	260	17	23
I Dream of Chocolate, 2.68 oz slice	250	13	31
Lemon Cake, 3.3oz slice	350	19	43
Mini Carrot Cake, 5 oz	450	19	68
Whoopie Pie (1), 2.5 oz	350	14	54
Bread Cake:			
Banana Bonanza, 2.6 oz slice	250	9	39
Pumpkin Nut, 2.6 oz slice	270	10	43
Walnut Streusel Coffee, 2 oz slice	180	8	25
Zucchini Carrot, 2 oz slice	200	7	32
Loaf Cake:			
Cranberry Pumpkin, 2 oz slice	140	2	30
Pumpkin Nut, 2.6 oz slice	270	10	43
Frozen:			
Apple Raspberry Turnover, 3.2 oz	280	14	34
Chocolate Dilemma Cheesecake:			
Plain, 3.5 oz	320	19	30
Choc. Chip; Triple Choc, av., 3.5 oz	345	20	35
Tuxedo, 3.5 oz	320	17	34
Choc Lava Cake, 4 oz	360	23	40
Karat Cake, 3 oz slice	320	19	37
N.Y. Style Cheesecake, 4.5 oz slice	400	28	32
Tiramisu Torte, 3.2 oz slice	230	12	24
Tarts:			
Pear, 3.5 oz slice	250	9	39
Raspberry, 5 oz slice	290	10	51
Wild Blueberry, 3.5 oz slice	260	6	52

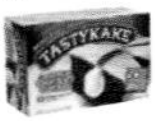

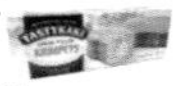
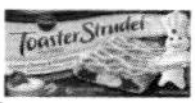

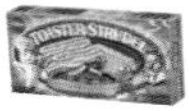
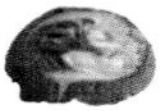
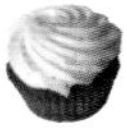
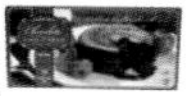
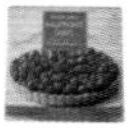

Cakes ~ Mixes

	C	F	Cb
Arrowhead Mills: *Dry Mix Only*			
All Purpose Mix, 1.4 oz	130	1	28
Betty Crocker: *Dry Mix Only*			
Brownie Mix:			
Dark Chocolate, 1 oz	110	1	24
Fudge, 0.9 oz	100	1	22
Milk Chocolate, 1 oz	110	1	25
Salted Caramel, 1.15 oz	120	1.5	26
Supreme:			
Chocolate Chunk, 1.1 oz	130	2	26
Fudge, 1.2 oz	120	1.5	26
Triple Chunk, 1.1 oz	130	2.5	26
Walnut, 1.1 oz	120	2.5	23
Cake Mix: Gingerbread, 1.8 oz	220	6	38
Pound Cake, 2 oz	220	2.5	47
Fat Free Cake Mix: Angel Food, 1.34 oz	140	0	32
Pineapple Upside Down Cake, 3.6 oz	140	0	32
Super Moist Delights Cake Mix: *Per 1.5 oz Dry Mix*			
Butter Recipe Yellow	160	1.5	36
Butter Pecan	160	1.5	36
Carrot; Devil's Food	160	1.5	35
Cherry Chip	160	1.5	36
French Vanilla	160	1	36
German Chocolate	160	1.5	35
Lemon	160	1.5	36
Red Velvet	160	1.5	35
Strawberry	160	1.5	36
Triple Chocolate Fudge	160	2	34
Dessert Bars: *Dry Mix Only*			
Coconut White Chip Oat Bar, 1.1 oz	150	6	22
Reese's PB & Chocolate, 1.1 oz	130	1.5	27
Duncan Hines: *Dry Mix Only*			
Brownie Mix: Chewy Fudge, 0.9 oz	110	1.5	22
Decadent, Choc. Peanut Butter, 1 oz	130	3.5	24
Perfectly Moist Cake Mix:			
Classic: Butter Golden, 1.5 oz	170	3	35
Dark Choc. Fudge, 1.5 oz	170	4	33
White, 1.5 oz	170	4	34
Signature Cake Mix:			
French Vanilla, 1.5 oz	180	4	34
German Chocolate, 1.5 oz	180	4	34
Orange, 1.5 oz	180	4	34
Triple Chocolate, 1.5 oz	170	3.5	34

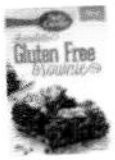

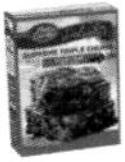
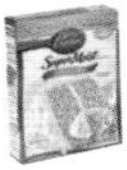
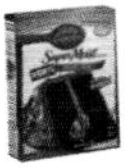
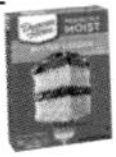
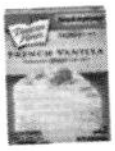

	C	F	Cb
Jell-O: *Dry Mix Only*			
No Bake: Classic Cheesecake, 1.83 oz	210	5	41
Double Choc. Cheesecake, 1.5 oz	180	5	33
Strawberry Cheesecake, 2.2 oz	210	4	42
Krusteaz: *Dry Mix Only*			
Bars: Meyer Lemon, 1.1 oz	130	3	26
Pumpkin Pie, 1 oz	110	1	24
Raspberry, 1.2 oz	100	0.5	22
Cakes: Lemon Pound Cake, with Glaze, 1.87 oz	180	1	41
Pumpkin Spice Cake Bread, 1.23 oz	140	1.5	30
Gluten Free Cakes: Choc., 1.24 oz	130	1	29
Yellow Cake, 1.5 oz	170	1	37
Pillsbury: *Per 1 oz Dry Mix Only*			
Classic Brownie Mix: Choc Fudge	110	0.5	25
Classic Fudge	120	1	28
Dark Chocolate	110	1	25
Milk Chocolate	110	0.5	25
Funfetti Brownie Mix: Blondie, 1.1 oz	120	2	26
Chocolate Fudge, 1 oz	110	1	24
Premium Brownie Mix:			
Caramel Swirl, 1.2 oz	120	1	28
Cheesecake Swirl, 1 oz	110	1.5	25
Chocolate Chunk, 1 oz	120	2.5	24
Chocolate Walnut, 1.1 oz	130	3	25
Toffee Flavored Brownie Bark, 1 oz	110	1	25
Moist Supreme Cake Mix:			
Devils Food, 1.5 oz	160	2	35
White/Yellow, 1.5 oz	160	1.5	35
Traditional Cake Mix, Vanilla Flavored, 1.5 oz	160	1.5	35

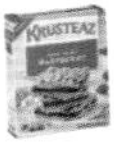

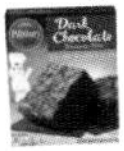

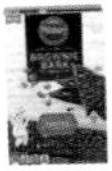
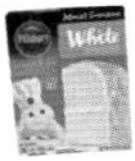

Cake Frostings

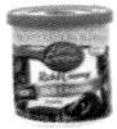

	C	F	Cb
Betty Crocker: *Per 2 Tbsp*			
Rich & Creamy: Coconut Pecan, 1.23 oz	140	8	18
Av. other flavors, 1.23 oz	135	5	23
Whipped, av. all flavors., 0.9 oz	100	4.5	15
Cool Whip, Original, 2 Tbsp, 0.3 oz	25	1.5	3
Duncan Hines: *Per 2 Tbsp*			
Creamy, average all flavors, 1.23 oz	140	6	23
Whipped, av. all flavors, 0.9 oz	100	5	15
Pillsbury: *Per 2 Tbsp*			
Creamy Supreme:			
Choc Fudge; Milk Choc., 1.2 oz	130	6	21
Strawb.; Vanilla; White, 1.2 oz	140	5	22
Funfetti, av. all flavors, 1.2 oz	140	5	23
Sugar Free, average, 1.1 oz	100	6	16

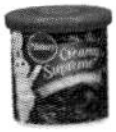

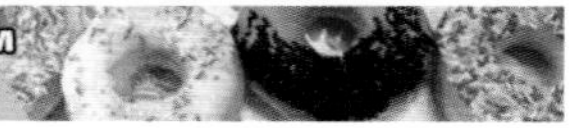

Quick Guide

	C	F	Cb
Donuts			
Average All Brands			
Cake: Plain, 1.8 oz	205	12	23
Chocolate Iced, 2 oz	255	14	29
Sugared, 0.8 oz	205	10	29
Non-Cake, Glazed, 2 oz	225	11	29
Croissant-Donuts			
(Includes Cronuts/Frissants)			
Average all Brands			
Cream-filled, 3.5 oz	430	26	45
Custard-filled, 3.5 oz	360	19	45

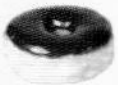

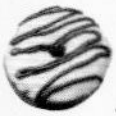

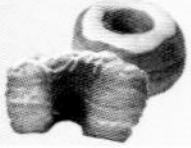

Extra Listings ~ *See CalorieKing.com*

(Cronut is a trademark of Dominique Ansel Bakery, New York)

Donuts ~ Brands

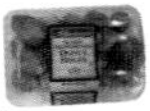

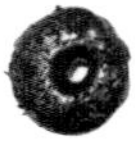

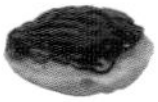

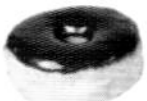

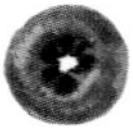

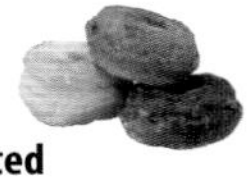

	C	F	Cb
Albertson's:			
Donut Holes:			
Glazed Old Fashioned (4)	240	12	31
Powdered Sugar (4)	210	12	24
Gem Donuts: Plain Cake (3)	190	12	20
Cinnamon Sugar (3)	240	15	23
Glazed (1)	140	6	21
Bon Appetit:			
Mini Donuts:			
Chocolate (4)	270	16	29
Crumb (4)	240	12	32
Powdered (4)	250	12	34
Dunkin':			
Apple Crumb	290	11	44
Apple N' Spice	230	10	31
Barvarian Kreme	240	11	31
Boston Kreme	270	11	39
Chocolate Frosted Cake	260	11	34
Chocolate Headlight	310	14	41
Coconut	410	21	50
Glazed Chocolate	240	11	33
Jelly Filled	250	10	36
Lemon	230	10	31
Powdered	330	20	34
Strawberry Frosted	260	11	35
Sugared	210	11	24
Vanilla Creme	300	15	37

Extra Listings ~ *See Fast Food Section*

Donuts ~ Brands (Cont)

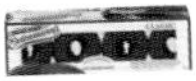

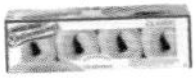

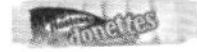

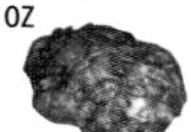

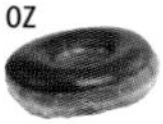

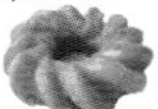

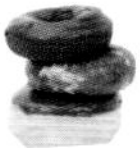

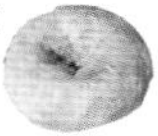

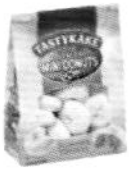

	C	F	Cb
Entenmann's:			
8 Pack: *Per Donut*			
Apple Cider, 2 oz	240	11	34
Crumb Topped, 1.94 oz	240	11	33
Frosted: Devil's Food, 2.1 oz	290	17	33
Rich Frosted, 2 oz	290	18	30
12 Count Softees Variety Pack: *Per Donut*			
Glazed, 1.4 oz	180	11	19
Plain, 1.4 oz	180	11	19
Cinnamon; Powdered, 1.5 oz	210	12	24
Pop'ems Donut Holes: Glazed (4)	240	13	28
Party Sprinkled Devil's Food (4)	230	12	31
Rich Frosted (4)	330	26	24
Hostess:			
Mini Donettes: Crumb, 6-pack, 4 oz	430	18	63
Frosted, 6-pack, 3 oz	360	22	38
Powdered, 6-pack, 3 oz	340	17	43
Krispy Kreme:			
Apple Fritter, 3.5 oz	350	19	42
Chocolate: Iced Cake, 2.5 oz	280	13	37
Iced Custard Filled, 3 oz	300	15	37
Iced Glazed Cruller, 2.5 oz	260	10	40
Iced Glazed, 2.2	240	11	33
Iced Kreme Filled, 3 oz	350	19	41
Iced Glazed w/ Sprinkles, 2.3 oz	250	11	36
Cinnamon Twist, 1.9oz	210	11	26
Glazed Cruller, 1.9 oz	210	10	29
Glazed Doughnut Holes:			
Original (5)	220	11	25
Blueberry (4)	190	7	28
Cake (4)	190	8	28
Chocolate Cake (4)	180	7	27
Glazed Kreme Filled, 3 oz	340	19	40
Maple Iced Glazed, 2.2 oz	240	11	34
New York Cheesecake, 3.3 oz	310	17	35
Original Glazed, 1.7 oz	190	11	22
Powdered Cake, 2.3 oz	240	11	29
Traditional Cake, 2 oz	230	12	26
Little Debbie,			
Donut Sticks, 1.9 oz	270	16	29
Tastykake: *10 oz Bags*			
Mini: Black & White (4), 2 oz	220	10	33
Blueberry (4), 2 oz	260	14	31
Cinnamon (4), 1.9 oz	230	10	31
Lemon (4), 2 oz	260	14	30
Orange (4), 2 oz	260	14	31
Salted Caramel Flavored (4), 2 oz	260	10	39

Quick Guide

	C	F	Cb
Muffins: Ready-To-Eat			
Average All Brands			
Small, 1 oz	90	3.5	14
Medium, 2 oz	185	6.5	28
Large, 3 oz	275	10	42
Extra Large, 4 oz	365	13	57
Giant, 6 oz	550	20	84
Super Size, 8 oz	730	27	112

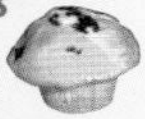
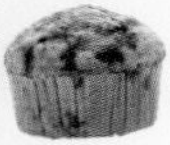

Muffins Ready-To-Eat ~ Brands

	C	F	Cb
Albertsons: *Each*			
Banana Nut	450	23	54
Blueberry	420	21	53
Entenmann's,			
Blueberry; Corn (2), average, 3.5 oz	380	18	50
Garden Lites: *Per 2 oz Muffin*			
Banana Choc. Chip	120	3	22
Blueberry Oat	110	2	21
Double Chocolate	110	2	21
Great Value *(Walmart):*			
Banana Nut Filled, (4), 4 oz	410	19	56
Blueberry Filled, (1), 4 oz	430	17	65
Chocolate Filled, (1), 4 oz	430	19	62
Hostess:			
Mega Muffin: Banana/Blueb., av., 5.5 oz	540	27	69
Double Choc, 5.5 oz	580	33	71
Mini Muffins (4): Blueberry/Choc., av.	220	11	30
Fudge	220	11	48
Little Debbie:			
Mini Muffins: Blueberry (1), 1.9 oz	170	6	28
Chocolate Chip (1), 1.9 oz	190	8	27
My Favorite Muffin: *Per Large*			
Banana Nut	650	38	71
Blueberry	590	28	78
Boston Cream Pie	740	33	105
Chocolate Chip	790	39	100
Lemon Poppyseed	670	32	90
Otis Spunkmeyer:			
Banana, 2 oz	220	10	30
Banana Minis (3), 2.2 oz	260	12	35
Blueberry, 2 oz	210	9	29
Starbucks ~ *See Fast-Foods Section*			
Trader Joe's: *Per Muffin*			
Apple Cranberry, 4.8 oz	220	5	38
Banana Chocolate Chip, 4 oz	400	18	57
Carrot, 4 oz	320	11	52
Triple Berry, 4 oz	310	11	49
Vitalicious:			
VitaTops: Banana Choc. Chip, 2 oz	130	2	25
Deep Chocolate, 2 ozimage	100	2	26
Wild Blueberry, 2 oz	120	1.5	27
Weight Watchers,			
Blueberry, 1.9 oz	150	1.5	35

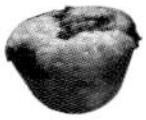
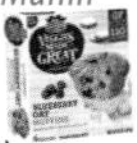
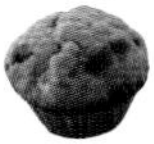

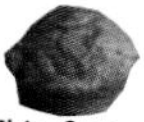
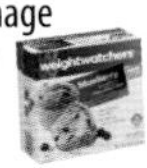

Muffin Mixes

	C	F	Cb
Dry Mix Only			
Betty Crocker: *Makes 2 Muffins*			
Boxed: Banana Nut, 2 oz	230	4.5	44
Cinnamon Streusel, 2.3 oz	270	6	51
Wild Blueberry, 2.8 oz	230	2.5	49
Pouch Mix:			
Banana Nut, 2.1 oz	240	5	45
Blueberry, 2.1 oz	250	5	46
Chocolate Chip, 2.1 oz	250	6	46
Krusteaz: *Dry Mix Only*			
Almond Poppy Seed, 1.4 oz	150	1.5	35
Choc Chunk, 1.5 oz	180	3.5	35
Cranb. Orange, 1.23 oz	140	0	33
Trader Joe's, Triple Berry	150	2	28

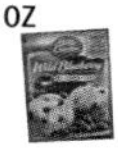
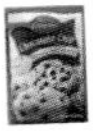
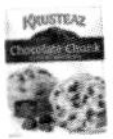

Sweet Rolls & Buns

Note: It is best to weigh for accuracy as actual weight can be 10-50% higher than label weight.

	C	F	Cb
Per Sweet Roll or Bun Unless Indicated			
Bimbo, Crispy Wheels, 4 pcs, 2.33 oz	360	22	41
Bon Appetit, Super Cinn. Roll, 5 oz	480	16	72
Cinnabon: Classic	880	37	127
Caramel Pecanbon	1080	51	146
Cloverhill Bakery,			
Big Texas Cinnamon Roll, 4 oz	430	18	62
Entenmann's, Iced Honey Bun, 4 oz	450	19	62
Hostess, Honey Bun, 4.75 oz	560	29	68
Little Debbie:			
Honey Bun: 1.5 oz	230	13	26
Individual, 3 oz Bun	360	20	41
Pecan Spinwheels: Single, 1 oz	110	3.5	18
2 Pack, 2.1 oz	210	7	32
O&H Danish: *Per 1.95 oz*			
Kringles: Apple: Wisconsin, av.	185	9	26
Almond; Turtle, average	215	13	27
Cinn. Roll; Cream Cheese, average	220	14	25
Pillsbury:			
Sweet Rolls, Refrigerated: *Per Roll Unless Indicated*			
Orig; Cinnamon, w/ Crm Cheese Icing	140	4.5	24
Cinn., Flaky w/ Butter Cream Icing	160	7	23
Orange, with Orange Icing	160	5	26
Grands, Refrigerated: *Per Roll*			
Cinnabon: Cinnamon Roll,			
with Cream Cheese Icing	300	7	54
w/ Extra Rich Butter Icing, 3.5 oz	300	7	56
Flaky Supreme Cinnamon Roll,			
with Icing, 3.5 oz	360	16	50
7-Eleven: Iced Honey Bun, 6 oz	820	58	68
Glazed Honey Bun, 5 oz	620	35	70

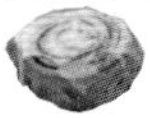
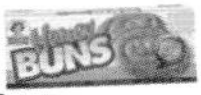

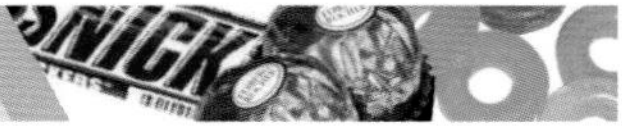

Quick Guide

	C	F	Cb
Chocolate:			
Average All Brands			
Milk Chocolate, regular:			
Plain/Nuts/Fruit, average, 1 oz	150	9	17
1.5oz Bar	230	13	25
2 oz Bar	305	17	34
4 oz Block	610	34	68
8 oz Block	1220	68	136
1 Pound, 16 oz	2440	136	272
Dark/White Chocolate: 1 oz	155	9	17
Hershey's, Sugar Free, 5 pieces	110	13	24
Milk Chocolate-Coated:			
Almonds, 5-6, 1 oz	150	10	15
Cherry Cordial Centers, 2 pcs, 1 oz	145	6	21
Clusters, Nut, 3 pieces, 1.2 oz	210	14	20
Coffee Beans, 1.4 oz	220	13	22
Macadamias, 10 pieces, 1.4 oz	220	16	21
Mints, 1 medium, 0.5 oz	55	1	11
Nougat & Caramel, 1 oz	150	9	15
Peanuts, 12 medium, 1 oz	145	10	14
Raisins, 28 medium, 1 oz	110	4	19
Baking Chocolate:			
Baker's: Bittersweet, 1 oz	140	12	14
Semi-sweet, 1 oz	140	9	16
Nestle, Chips: Dark, 1 Tbsp. 0.5 oz	70	5	3
Semi-Sweet, 1 Tbsp. 0.5oz	70	4	9
Unsweetened, 1 oz	140	14	8
Carob, Plain, 1 oz	155	9	16

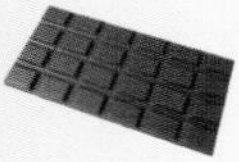

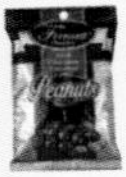

Candy ~ Brands & Generic

Per Piece/Serving

	C	F	Cb
3 Musketeers: Orig., 1 bar, 1.9 oz	240	7	42
2 To Go, 1.7 oz Bar	200	6	36
Fun Size, 3 bars, 1.6 oz	190	6	34
Minis, 7 pieces, 1.4 oz	170	5	32
100 Grand: 1.5 oz bar	190	8	30
Snack Size (1), 0.8 oz	95	4	15
Super Size, 2.8 oz	360	14	58
Abba Zabba, 2 oz bar	250	5	48
After Dinner Mints, 1 small	25	1.5	3
After Eight Mint, each	35	1.5	4
Airhead, 1 bar, 0.5 oz	60	1	14
Almond Joy: 2 bars, 1.6 oz	220	13	26
King Size, 4 bars, 3.2 oz	440	26	53
Snack Size, 2pieces, 1.2 oz	160	9	20
Miniatures, 2 pieces, 1 oz	130	7	15

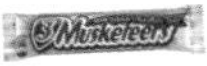

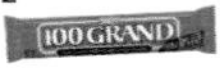

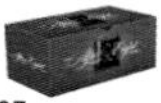

Per Piece/Serving

	C	F	Cb
Almond Roca, 3 pieces, 1.3 oz	200	15	17
Almonds: Sugar-coated (15), 1.4 oz	190	7	27
Jordan, 15 pieces, 1.4 oz	180	8	28
Almond Clusters:			
True North, 5 pieces, 1 oz	170	12	9
Trader Joe's, 2 pieces, 1.2 oz	190	14	13
Almond Pecan Crunch:			
True North, 5 pieces, 1.2 oz	150	11	10
Altoids: Original, 3 mints	10	0	2
Artic, 3 mints	5	0	2
Andes, Thins (8), av. all var., 1.4 oz	205	13	22
Anthon Berg:			
Creamy Mint (4), 1.4 oz	180	6	31
Marzipan with Plum, in Madeira	120	6	14
Atomic Fireball, 1 piece, 0.3 oz	35	0	9
Baby Ruth: King Size, 3.5 oz bar	500	24	66
2 oz bar	280	14	39
Fun size, 2 bars	170	8	24
Minis, 4 bars	210	11	28
Baci *(Perugina),*			
1 piece, 0.5 oz	75	6	7
Bark Thins, Snacking Chocolate,			
Dark Choc. Mint/Pretzel, av., 1 oz	140	6	20
Baskin-Robbins: Sugar Candy, 3 pcs	60	1	12
Sugar Free, 4 pieces, average, 0.6 oz	40	1	16
Note: Carb figure includes 16g sugar alcohol			
Big Hunk, 2 oz Bar	230	3	47
Bit-O-Honey:			
1.7 oz bar	180	3.5	39
Chews, 6 pcs, 1.4 oz	150	3	32
Blow Pops, each, 0.6 oz	60	0	17
Bon Bons, 3 pieces	65	0	15
Boston Baked Beans, (11)	70	2	11
Brach's: Almond Supremes (10)	200	14	20
Bridge Mix (15)	190	10	26
Double Dippers (15)	210	14	22
Gummi Bears (14)	130	0	30
Lemon Drops, Sugar Free, 4 pieces	35	0	17
Note: Carb figures include 17g Sugar Alcohol			
Mandarin/Orange Slices (3), 1.6 oz	150	0	37
Maple Nut Goodies (8)	190	9	27
Milk Maid Crmls (4)	150	4	25
Peanut Cluster (3)	210	15	20
Breath Savers, (1),all var.	5	0	2
Bubble Gum ~ *See Page 75*			
Bulls Eyes, 3 pieces, 1.2 oz	130	3	23
Buncha Crunch: 1.4 oz	180	9	25
Movie Box, 3.2 oz	450	20	65
Burnt Peanuts, 1.4 oz	170	6	29

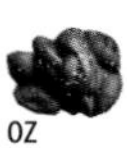

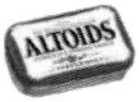

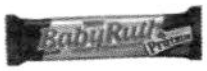

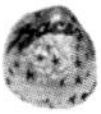

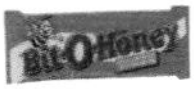

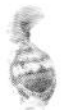

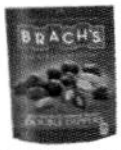

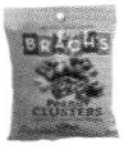

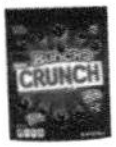

Candy ~ Brands & Generic (Cont)

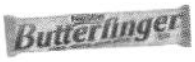
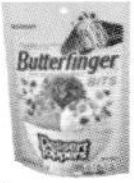
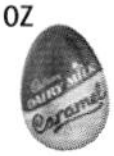
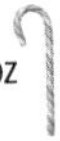

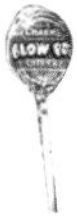
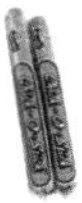
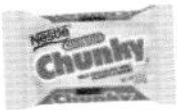

Per Piece/Serving	C	F	Cb
Butterfinger:			
Bars: 1.9 oz bar	250	10	36
Fun Size Bars (2), 1.3 oz	170	7	25
Minis, 1.1 oz	140	6	20
Bites, 6 pieces, 1.1 oz	140	6	20
Crisp Bar, 1 pkg, 2 oz	300	17	35
Dessert Toppers, 2 Tbsp, 1.3 oz	180	7	25
Butter Mints, 7 pieces, 0.5 oz	50	0	12
Butterscotch: 3 pieces	60	0	15
Discs (*Walgreens*), 3 pieces, 0.6 oz	70	0	17
Cadbury: Caramello Bar, 1.6 oz	220	10	29
Caramel Egg, 1.2 oz	170	8	22
Dairy Milk Bar, 7 pcs, 1.4 oz	200	11	23
Mini Eggs (Candy), 12 pcs, 1.4 oz	190	8	28
Candy Apple, medium, 6.5 oz	280	0	60
Candy Cane, medium, 5", 0.5 oz	40	0	14
Candy Corn, 20 pieces, 1.4 oz	150	0	38
Candy Jar Mix (*Jewel*), 3 pcs, 0.6 oz	60	0	14
Candy Necklace (*Smarties*), (1), 0.8 oz	90	0.5	20
Caramels: Each, 0.4 oz	40	1	8
Chocolate, each, 0.3 oz	25	0.3	6
Creams (3), 1.3 oz	130	3	23
Caramel Popcorn, ⅔ cup	150	6	23
Cella's,			
Milk Choc. Cherries, 3 pieces, 1.5 oz	160	6	27
Certs, Breath Mints, 1 piece	5	0	2
Charleston Chew:			
Chocolate Bar (1), 1.4 oz	160	4.5	30
Mini Bars, 13 pieces	190	6	34
Charms: Blow Pop	60	0	17
Flat Pop, 0.5 oz	50	0	14
Chew-ets, Peanut Chews,			
Original (4), 1.6 oz	230	12	29
Chewz, 1 roll, 1 oz	120	1	28
Chick O Stick, 2 oz	240	9	42
Chunky Bar (*Nestlé*),			
King Size, 2.5 oz	340	19	44
Chupa Chups, 1 Pop	50	0	12
Cinn. Buttons (*Walgreens*), 3 pieces	60	0	16

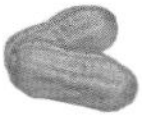
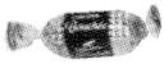
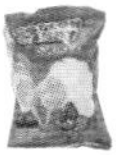
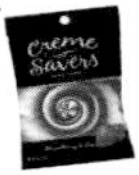
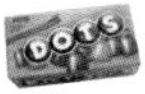
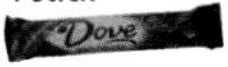

Per Piece/Serving	C	F	Cb
Cinnamon Disks (*Walmart*), 3 pieces	70	0	18
Circus Peanuts (*Spangler*),			
6 pieces, 1.3 oz	165	0	41
CocoaVia, Orig., 0.8 oz	100	6	12
Coconut Stacks, (8)	320	16	46
Coffee Go, Candy, (4)	60	1	12
Conversation Hearts (*Necco*):			
Small (40), 1.4 oz	160	0	39
1 large	10	0	3
Cookie Dough Bites, 1.4 oz	200	10	27
Cote d'Or: Dark 86% Coca, 4 pcs	270	22	14
Dark, 70%, Orange, 3.5 oz	575	46	34
Dark, Raspberry, 3.5 oz	580	46	34
Milk, Intense, 3.5 oz	575	40	45
Cotton Candy, 1 oz	110	0	28
Cough Drops ~ *See Page 75*			
Cracker Jack, ½ cup, 1 oz	120	2	23
Creme Savers:			
3 pieces, 0.5 oz	60	1	11
Sugar-Free, 3 pieces	30	1	8
Crisped Rice, Choc Chip, 1 bar, 1 oz	115	4	20
Crows, 11 pieces, 1.4 oz	130	0	33
Crunch Bar ~ *See Nestle*			
Dots, 11 dots, 1.4 oz	130	0	33
Double Dip Stick, 1 stick	15	0.5	3
Dove:			
Milk Choc: Singles Bar, 1.4 oz	220	13	24
Large Tablet Bar, 9 pcs, 1.5 oz	230	13	25
Choc. Cov. Almonds, 13 pcs, 1.4 oz	220	15	19
Promises: Milk Choc., 1 pce, 0.3 oz	45	2.5	5
w/ Caramel, 1 piece, 0.3 oz	40	2	5
w/ Peanut Butter, 1 pce, 0.3 oz	45	3	4
Swirls, all var., 9 pieces 1.5 oz	230	14	25
Dark Choc: Singles Bar, 1.3 oz	220	13	24
Large Tablet Bar, 9 pcs, 1.5 oz	220	14	25
Choc. Cov. Almds, 13 pcs, 1.4 oz	210	15	19
Promises, Almond, 1 piece, 0.3 oz	40	3	4
Swirls, Raspberry, 9 pcs, 1.4 oz	220	14	24
Sugar Free, all flav., 5 pcs, 1.4 oz	195	15	21
Dum Dum Pops (*Spangler*), 1 pop	25	0	7
Drops (*Hershey's*):			
Cookies 'n' Creme, 14 pieces, 1.5 oz	210	11	26
Milk Chocolate, 15 pieces, 1.4 oz	200	12	25

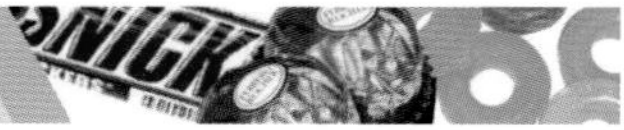

Candy ~ Brands & Generic (Cont)

Per Piece/Serving	C	F	Cb
English Toffee, 1 piece, 0.4 oz	70	4	6
5th Avenue:			
Bars: 2 oz	260	12	38
King Size, 3.5 oz	440	20	64
Fannie May:			
Mint Meltaway, (1)	240	16	24
Pixie (1), 1.5 oz	210	13	23
Trinidad (1), 1.5 oz	200	12	23
Fast Break (Reese's):			
Bars: 1.8 oz bar	230	11	32
King Size, 3.5 oz	460	22	63
Ferrero Rocher:			
Pieces: 1 piece	75	5	5
3 pieces, 1.3 oz	220	16	16
Rondnoir, 3 pieces, 1 oz	180	13	14
Fifty 50 Snack Bars:			
Milk Chocolate: 5 pieces, 1 oz	135	11	14
Almond, 5 pieces, 1 oz	135	12	14
Crunch Bar, 7 pcs, 1 oz	140	12	16
Dark Chocolate, 5 pieces, 1 oz	120	11	15
Note: Carb figures include 9-12g Sugar Alcohol			
Fluffy Stuff *(Charms)*,			
Cotton Candy, 1.4 oz	150	0	40
Fondant: Choc-coated, 1.2 oz	125	3	27
Mint, 1 oz	105	0	25
Fran's: Gold Bar, Macadamia (1)	250	14	27
GoldBite, Almond (1)	120	7	13
Fruit Drops, (1), ¼ oz	20	0	4
Fruit Gems *(Sunkist)*, (4), 1.4 oz	130	0	33
Fruit Leathers, average, 0.5 oz	50	0.5	12
Fruit Pastilles *(Rowntree)*, 1 roll	185	0	45
Fruit Roll-Ups *(Betty Crocker/Sunkist)*,			
1 roll, 0.5 oz	50	1	12
Fruit Runts *(Walgreens)*,			
12 pieces	60	0	14
Fruit Flavored Shapes *(Betty Crocker)*,			
all varieties, 0.8 oz	80	0	19
Fudge:			
Chocolate; Mint, 1 oz	130	8	14
P'nut Butter & Choc., 1 oz	130	8	13
Brevin's: Cashew, 1 oz	195	9	28
Triple Decker, 1 oz	165	7	25
Ghirardelli:			
Intense Dark Chocolate Bars: *Per 3 oz Bars*			
60% Cocoa, 3 squares	160	12	17
72% Cocoa, 3 squares	170	15	14
86% Cocoa, 2.5 squares	170	17	10
92% Cocoa, 3 squares	180	19	9

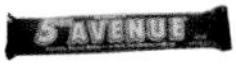
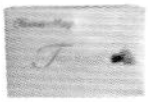
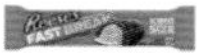

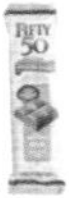
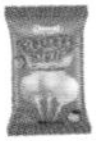
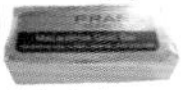
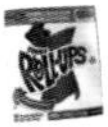
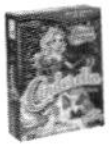
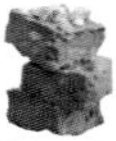
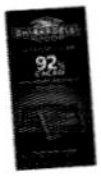

Per Piece/Serving	C	F	Cb
Godiva:			
Bars: Milk/Dark, av., 1.5 oz	230	14	26
Extra Dark: 75%, 1.5 oz	230	17	18
85%, 1.4 oz	260	21	14
Chocoiste: Dk Choc. Cherries (12)	190	7	30
Milk Chocolate Cashews (14)	230	15	19
Hearts: Dark Ganache (4)	200	12	23
Milk Praline (4)	220	13	23
Go Lightly:			
Assorted Toffee, 5 pieces, 1 oz	85	2	24
Fruit Chews, 5 pieces, 1 oz	95	2	26
Hard Candy, Assorted (4), 0.5 oz	45	0	15
Note: Carb figures include 15-25g sugar alcohol			
Goobers Peanuts, 1 package, 1.4 oz	200	13	21
Good & Plenty *(Hershey's)*, (33), 1.8 oz	180	0	46
GooGoo Clusters, 1 piece, 1.8 oz	240	12	30
Gum ~ *See Page 75*			
Gum Drops: 1 small, 0.1 oz	15	0	3
5 pieces, 0.5 oz	75	0	15
Gummi *(Shur Fine)*:			
Bears (15), 1.4 oz	130	0	29
Chewy Sweet Tarts (4)	160	0	36
Worms (9), 1.5 oz	140	0	31
Guylian:			
Bars: Dark Chocolate (3), 1 oz	150	12	11
Milk Choc. w/ Hazelnuts (3),1 oz	170	11	15
No Sugar Added Bars:			
Milk Chocolate, 3 squares	150	11	16
54% Cocoa, Dark Choc., 3 sqrs.	140	11	16
Seashells:			
Bar, 1.4 oz	210	13	21
Boxed, Originals (1), 0.4 oz	60	4	6
Truffles, (1), 0.4 oz	70	5.5	5
Heath: Original (1), 1.4 oz	210	13	24
King Size, 2.8 oz	410	22	49
Miniatures, 4 pieces, 1 oz	150	9	17
Hershey's:			
Cookie Layer Crunch, 2, 1.4 oz	190	11	24
Cookies 'n' Creme: 1.55 oz Bar	230	12	28
Snack Size, 2 pieces, 0.95 oz	130	7	17
Milk Chocolate:			
Bars: 1.55 oz	220	13	26
with Almonds, 1 bar, 1.45 oz	210	14	20
Golden Almond			
Kisses, 7 pieces, av., 1.2 oz	160	9	19
Nuggets: Milk Choc., 3 pieces	150	9	19
with Almonds, 3 pcs, 1 oz	150	10	15
Special Dark Choc., 1.45 oz bar	200	13	24

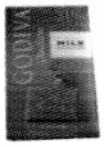
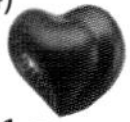
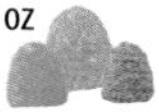
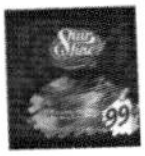
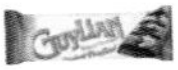
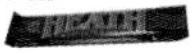
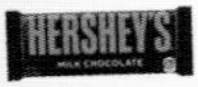

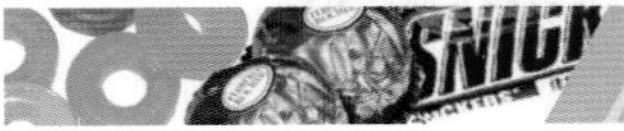

Candy ~ Brands & Generic (Cont)

Per Piece/Serving	C	F	Cb
Hershey's, (Cont):			
Candy-Coated Eggs, 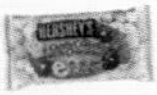			
Milk Chocolate, (5)	140	9	17
Pot of Gold Chocolate Asstd:			
Milk Choc: Carmel, 4 pieces, 1.4 oz	190	10	26
Av. other var., 4 pieces, 1.4 oz	210	12	24
Honeycomb: Plain, 1 oz	115	0	27
Choc-coated, 2 pieces	180	7	31
Hot Tamales, 20 pieces, 1.4 oz	150	0	36
Hugs ~ *See Kisses*			
Jawbreakers *(Sathers)*, (15), 0.6 oz	60	0	16
Jells *(Joyva)*, Raspb., 3 pieces, 1.6 oz	160	0	38
Jelly Beans, average all brands:			
Small Size (Jelly Belly): 1 bean	5	0	1
12 beans, 0.5 oz	50	0	13
Regular Size: 1 bean 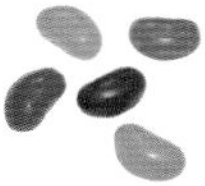	10	0	2
10 beans, 1 oz	105	0	26
Large Size: 1 bean	15	0	38
10 beans, 1.5 oz	150	0	38
Sugar Free, av. all brands, (25), 1 oz	60	0	26
Note: Carb figure include 26g sugar alcohol			
Jelly Belly: 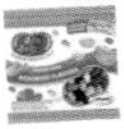			
25 beans, 1 oz	105	0	26
Sugar Free, 25 beans, 1 oz	60	0	26
Note: Carb figure include 26g sugar alcohol			
Chocolate Dips, all flavors: 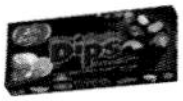			
1 bean	4	0	1
10 beans	40	1	8
2.8 oz bag	300	8	62
Jolly Rancher: 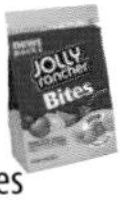			
Bites: Filled, 11 pieces	140	0	32
Sours, 16 pieces	130	0	34
Crunch 'N Chew, 1 oz pkg	160	0.5	40
Filled Fruity Bites, 22 pieces	140	1	31
Gummies, 9 pieces 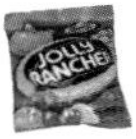	120	0	28
Hard Candy, 3 pieces	70	0	17
Jelly Beans/Sours, 1.4 oz	140	0	36
Lollipops (1), 0.55 oz	60	0	15
Triple Pop, 1 pop	80	0	19
Jujubes, all varieties (52), 1.4 oz	110	0	28
Juju Bears, 5 pieces	130	0	34
Juju Mix (Sathers), 11 pieces, 1.5 oz	150	0	36
Jujyfruits, 16 pieces, 1.4 oz	120	0	32
Junior Caramels: 13 pieces, 1.5 oz	190	6	33
Mini, 2 boxes, 1 oz	130	4	23
Junior Mints, 5 pieces 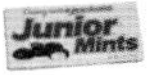	55	1	11

Per Piece/Serving	C	F	Cb
Justin's:			
Peanut Butter Cups: Dark Choc (1)	230	15	20
Milk Choc, (1)	230	15	20
Kinder Joy, 1 egg, 0.7 oz 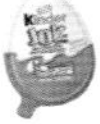	110	6	12
Kisses *(Hershey's)*:			
Candy Cane Mint, (6)	140	8	18
Dark Chocolate, Mint Truffles (7)	160	10	19
Milk Chocolate: 1 Kiss 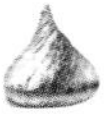	20	1	3
7 Kisses	160	9	19
With Almonds (7)	160	10	16
Filled with: Cherry Cordial (6)	120	5	19
Vanilla Creme (9)	210	13	24
Hot Cocoa (7) 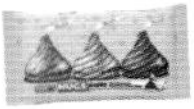	160	10	19
Hugs (9)	210	12	24
Kit Kat *(Hershey's)*:			
Dark Chocolate: 1.5 oz pkg	200	12	27
Mint & Dark Chocolate, 1.5 oz pkg	210	12	27
Milk Chocolate: 4 pce bar, 1.5 oz	210	11	28
Miniatures (4), 1.2 oz 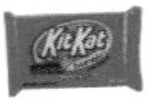	170	9	22
Snack Size (3), 1.5 oz	210	11	27
Apple Pie, 1.5 oz pkg	220	12	27
Halloween: 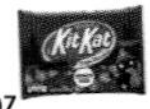			
1.5 oz package	210	11	28
White Choc., 1.48 oz	220	11	27
White Chocolate, Snack (3), 1.5 oz	220	11	27
Lemon Drops: (4), 0.6 oz	60	0	16
Walgreens, Sugar Free (3), 0.6 oz	50	0	17
Lemonhead, (26), 1.4 oz 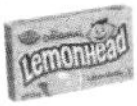	140	0	36
Lance, Peanut Bar, 2.2 oz	340	19	29
Licorice:			
Average all varieties, 1oz	100	0	25
Chews *(Panda)*, (1) 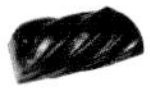	10	0	3
Tid Bits (1)	10	0	2
Twists: Black/Red, av., 1 pc	35	0	8
Sugar Free, 1 piece	15	0	2.5
American Licorice Co.:			
Natural Vines: Black (9), 1.4 oz	140	1	33
Strawberry (9), 1.4 oz	150	1	34
Red Vines (4), 1.4 oz	140	0	34
Sip-n-Chew, 1 oz package 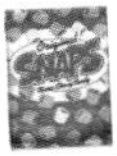	100	1	23
Snaps (31), 1.4 oz	140	0.5	33
Sour Punch (6), 1.4 oz	150	0.5	34
Super Ropes (1), 2 oz	200	0	46
Lifesavers: Large size, 1 candy	15	0	3
Regular: All flavors, 1 candy	10	0	3
1 Roll (14 candies), 1.2 oz	140	0	35
Creme Savers, 3 pcs, 0.5 oz 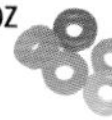	60	1	11
Fruit Splosion (10), 1.4 oz	130	0	31
Pep-o-mint: (3), 0.2 oz	20	0	5
Sugar-Free (4), 0.5 oz	35	0	14
Note: Carb figure includes 14g sugar alcohol			

Candy ~ Brands & Generic (Cont)

Per Piece/Serving	C	F	Cb
Lik-m-aid *(Nestle)*, Fun Dip, 1 package	50	0	13
Lindt (Excellence Bars):			
Dark Chocolate Bars:			
70% Cocoa, 2 squares	125	9	9
78% Cocoa, 2 squares	115	9	5
85% Cocoa, 2 squares	115	9	4
90% Cocoa, 2 squares	120	11	3
95% Cocoa, 2 squares	100	9	2
Extra Creamy Milk Choc., 2 squares	110	8	11
Coconut White Choc., 2 squares	120	9	9
Lollipops: Mini, 0.3 oz	25	0	6
Small, 0.5 oz	50	0	12
Medium, 1 oz	100	0	25
Giant (4" diam), 7 oz	790	0	198
M & M's:			
Dark Chocolate/Mint, 1.5 oz pkg	210	10	29
Milk Chocolate: 28 pieces, 1 oz	145	6.5	21
1.5 oz package	210	9	30
Minis, 1 tube, 1 oz	150	6	21
Almond, 1.5 oz	220	12	25
Coffee Nut, 1.1 oz	160	8	19
Crispy, 1.5 oz	200	7	31
Fudge Brownie, 11 pieces, 1 oz	140	6	20
Halloween, Popcorn Candy, 1 oz	130	5	21
Peanut 12 pieces, 1 oz	140	7	17
Peanut Butter, 1.62 oz pkg	240	13	26
Pretzel, 1.3 oz package	150	5	24
Red, White & Blue, 1 oz	140	5	20
White Chocolate, 1.5 oz pkg	210	11	29
Mamba Sours, Fruit Chews, 6 pcs, 1 oz	100	1	22
Marshmallow Egg, 1 egg, 1 oz	120	3	22
Mary Jane *(Necco)*, 5 pieces, 1.4 oz	160	3.5	32
Marshmallows: Firm/Soft, 1 oz	90	0	23
Regular size, 4 pieces, 1 oz	100	0	24
Mini-Marshmallow, ⅔ cup, 1 oz	95	0	24
Joyva, Choc-coated Twists	95	2	10
Fluff, 2 Tbsp, 0.6 oz	60	0	15
Kraft: Creme, 0.5 oz	45	0	11
Funmallows, ⅔ cup, 1 oz	100	0	24
Jet-Puffed, 5 pieces, 1 oz	100	0	24
Mini, 1 oz	90	0	23
Marzipan, 2 Tbsp, 1.4 oz	160	4	29
Mauna Loa, Mountains, 4 pcs	230	17	21
Mexican Hats, (7), 1.4 oz	120	0	30
Mentos: Regular	10	0	3
Sugar Free	5	0	2
Mike & Ike:			
Original: 2.1 oz package	220	0	55
23 pieces, 1.4 oz	140	0	36
Milk Duds, 1 box, 1.8 oz	230	8	38

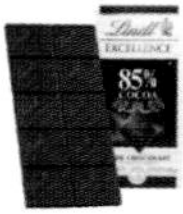

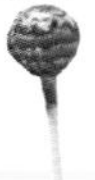
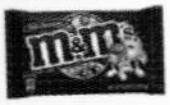

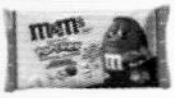

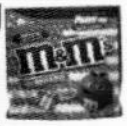

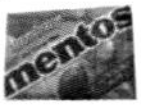

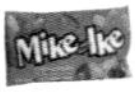

Per Piece/Serving	C	F	Cb
Milky Way *(Mars):*			
Bars: Single, 2 oz	240	9	37
Fun Size, 2 bars, 1.2 oz	160	6	24
To Go, 1.8 oz	230	9	36
Minis, 5 pieces, 1.5 oz	190	7	30
Midnight Bars: 1.8 oz	230	8	36
Minis, 5 pieces, 1.4 oz	190	7	30
Simply Caramel, 1.9 oz	250	11	37
Mints: *Average All Brands*			
1 mint , medium	7	0	1
1 large mint	15	0	3
Mon Cheri *(Ferrero)*, 4 pieces, 2 oz	260	18	20
Mounds: 1.75 oz bar	240	13	28
King Size, 4 pces, 3.5 oz	480	26	56
Snack Size, 1 piece, 0.6 oz	80	4.5	10
Mr Goodbar: 1.8 oz bar	250	17	26
King Size, 2.6 oz bar	380	26	38
Munch Bar, 1.4 oz	220	15	18
Necco, Candy Wafers (40), 2 oz	220	0	56
Nestle: Original,1.6 oz bar	220	11	30
Fun Size, 3 bars, 1.4 oz	180	9	26
Miniatures, 4 bars, 1.4 oz	200	10	27
Buncha Crunch, ⅓ cup, 1.2 oz	180	9	25
Crunch Crisp, 1.8 oz	240	13	32
Newman's Own:			
Milk Choc.: Caramel Cups (3)	160	8	21
Peanut Butter Cups (3)	180	12	17
Dark Choc.: Caramel Cups (3)	160	9	20
Peanut Butter Cups (3)	180	13	16
Nips, all varieties, 2 pieces, 0.5 oz	60	2	11
Nougat: 3 pieces, 1.5 oz	170	1	39
Chocolate Covered, 1 oz	125	4	22
Nutrageous Bar *(Reese's)*, 1.8 oz	260	16	28
Oh Henry!: Fun Size, 0.9 oz	120	5	16
1.8 oz bar	230	11	33
Orange Slices:			
Jewel, 3 pieces, 1.5 oz	140	0	35
Walgreens, 4 pieces, 1.6 oz	160	0	39
Oreo Choc. Candy Bars *(Milka)*:			
Regular, 1.44 oz bar	230	14	24
Big Crunch, 3.5 oz	550	35	57
Cookies & Creme, 1.44 oz bar	230	14	25
Fun Size, 2 pieces	170	10	18
Mint, 1.44 oz bar	230	13	24
Pastel Mints *(Walgreens)*, 20 pieces	60	0	14
PayDay Bar: 1.8 oz bar	240	13	27
King Size, 3.5 oz bar	440	24	50
Snack Size, 0.7 oz	90	5	10
Avalanche, 1.8 oz bar	250	13	29
Peanut Bar *(Planter's)*, 1.6 oz	240	14	21
Peanut Butter Cups ~ *See Reese's; Newman's Own*			
Peanut Brittle: 1 piece, 1.5 oz	190	5	32
Sugar Free *(Russell Stover)*, 4 pieces, 1.3 oz	140	10	24

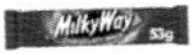

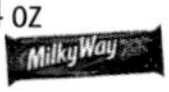

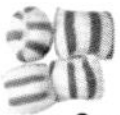
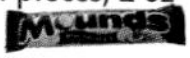

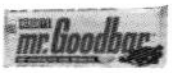

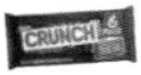

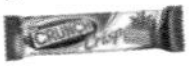
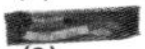
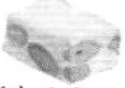
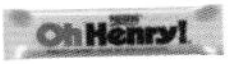

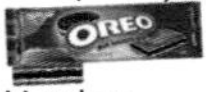

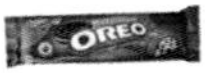

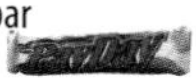

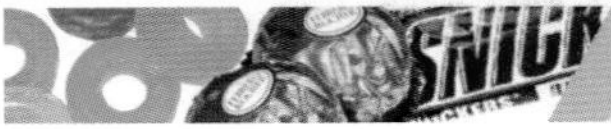

Candy ~ Brands & Generic (Cont)

Per Piece/Serving	C	F	Cb
Peanuts, choc-covered, 14 pieces	230	14	23
Pearson's, Mint Patties, (5), 1.3 oz	150	2.5	31
Peppermints: 7 small, 0.5 oz	60	0	15
Brach's, Star Brites (3)	60	0	16
Pez, 1 roll	35	0	9
Planters,			
Double Peanut Bar, 1.6 oz	240	14	21
Pop Rocks, 0.4 oz package	35	0	9
Pot of Gold *(Hershey's):*			
Assortment: Caramel, 4 pieces	190	10	25
Nut, 4 pieces	210	13	23
Pretzels: Choc-covered, Mini (6)	200	9	25
White Chocolate Bites (23), 1.4 oz	200	9	25
Pretzel Flipz *(Nestlé)*, 8 pcs, 1 oz	130	5	20
Raisinets:			
Milk Choc: 1.58 oz pkg	190	8	32
Movie Pack, 3.5 oz	380	16	64
Dark Chocolate, 1/4 cup, 1.6 oz	180	8	32
Reese's:			
Peanut Butter Cups:			
Dark Chocolate, (2), 1.5 oz	210	14	23
Milk Choc:			
1.5 oz Pkg	210	12	24
Big Cup, King Size, 2.8 oz pkg	400	22	46
King Size (2), 1.4 oz	200	12	22
Minis, 2 packages, 1.23 oz	180	11	20
Snack Size (1), 0.8 oz	110	6	12
Crunchy, 1.4 oz pkg	220	13	22
Outrageous Stuffed,			
Snack Size (1), 0.7 oz	100	4.5	13
Pieces: 3 pieces, 0.9 oz	130	7	16
2 pkgs, 1.4 oz	210	12	25
Thins (3), 1.25 oz	170	10	20
White Cups, 1.5 oz pkg	220	13	23
Rice Krispies Treats *(Kellogg's)*,			
1 bar, average all varieties, 0.8 oz	95	2.5	17
Riesen, Choc. Chew, 4 pcs, 1.3 oz	170	6	28
Rocky Road, Milk/Dark, 1.8 oz bar	240	11	34
Roca Thins, 3 pieces, av. all var.	210	14	24
Rolo:			
Regular, all var., 1.7 oz roll	220	10	33
Mini Chews, Caramel in milk choc. (11)	190	9	26
Root Beer Barrels, (3), 0.6 oz	60	0	17

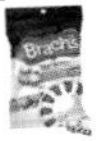
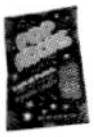
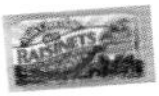
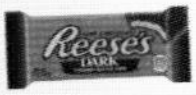
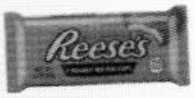
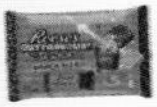
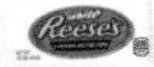

Per Piece/Serving	C	F	Cb
Russell Stover Candy:			
Boxed Chocolates Choc. Coated:			
Assorted (2), 1.2 oz	150	7	22
Cherry Cordials (3), 0.4 oz	150	5	25
Dairy Crm Caramels (2), 1.2 oz	160	7	22
Elegant Collection (3), 1.6 oz	210	10	25
French Choc. Mints (4), 1.4 oz	220	13	22
Nut, Chewy & Crisp Centers (2)	160	8	21
Sugar Free: Ass'td Hard Candies (3)	210	16	24
Bags: Caramel (3), 1.3 oz	180	8	25
Coconut (3), 1.5 oz	160	10	28
Mint Patty (3), 1.5 oz	180	12	26
Peanut Butter Cups (2), 1.2 oz	160	12	17
Pecan Delight (2), 1.2 oz	160	12	19
Note: Carbohydrate figures include sugar alcohol			
Salt Water Taffy *(Brach's)*, (5)	170	2.5	36
Seashells *(Guylian)*, (4), 1.6 oz	260	17	24
See's Candies:			
Almond Royal (5)	190	13	18
Butterscotch Chews (5)	210	12	27
Krispy's: Caffe Latte (5)	180	8	27
Mint (5)	170	8	27
Little Pops:			
Butterscotch (4), 0.5 oz	60	2	12
Av. other flavors (4)	55	3	10
Lollypops, average, 0.7 oz	90	3	17
Milk Molasses Chips (6), 1.4 oz	180	8	27
Milk Peppermints, 2 pieces, 1.3 oz	150	4	28
Peanut Brittle Bar, 1 oz	150	10	15
Peanut Butter Patties (2), 1.2 oz	170	10	16
Peppermint Twists, (3)	60	0	15
Toffee-ettes, 3 pieces	270	21	18
Sugar Free: Dark Bar, 1.5 oz	180	16	24
Dark Walnut Clusters (4), 1.5 oz	230	21	17
Peanut Brittle, 1.5 oz	170	14	17
Note: Carbohydrate figures include 12-18 g sugar alcohol			
Skinny Cow:			
Dreamy Clusters, all var., 1 pouch	120	6	20
Heavenly Crips, all varieties, 1 bar	110	6	14
Skittles:			
Original, 2 oz	230	2.5	52
Sour, 1.8 oz	200	2	44
Tropical; Wild Berry, 2.2 oz	250	2.5	56
Fun Size, 1 bag, 0.5 oz	60	1	14
Tear & Share, 4 oz bag	420	4.5	93
Skor, Toffee Bar (1), 1.4 oz	200	12	25
Smarties: Candy Rolls (1), 0.3 oz	25	0	6
Giant, 1 roll, 1 oz	100	0	25

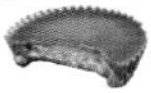
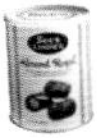
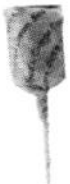
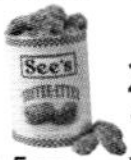
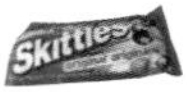
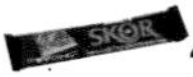

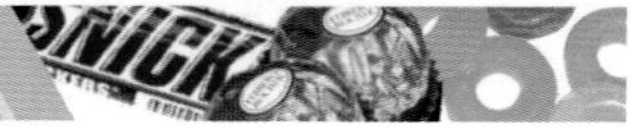

Candy ~ Brands & Generic (Cont)

Per Piece/Serving	C	F	Cb
Snickers:			
Milk Chocolate Bar:			
Original, 1.9 oz bar 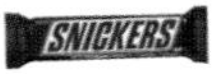	250	12	33
Fun Size, 2 bars, 1.2 oz	160	7	22
Minis, 3 pieces, 0.9 oz	130	6	17
Almond Bar, 1.8 oz 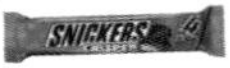	230	10	33
Crisper (2)	190	9	26
Crunchy Peanut Butter (2)	250	14	29
Hazelnut, 1 bar 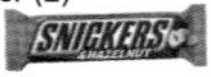	240	11	31
Sno Caps, ¼ cup, 1.4 oz	180	8	30
Soft 'N Chewy, Butter Toffee, 1 piece	30	0.5	5
Sorbee, Crystal Light Hard Candy (4)	25	0	13
Note: Carb figure includes Isomalt which has fewer calories than sugar.			
Sour Patch: Kids, average, 2 oz	210	0	52
Extreme, 1.8 oz	190	0	47
Spearmint Leaves: 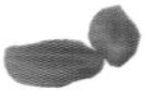			
Jewel, 5 pieces, 1.4 oz	140	0	35
Walgreens, 4 pieces, 1.6 oz	160	0	39
Spree Candies: Original, 15 pieces	50	0	13
Chewy, 8 pieces	60	0	13
Starburst: 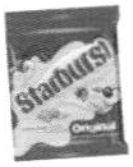			
Candy Canes, 0.5 oz	70	0	18
Fruit Chews: Original (1)	20	0.5	4
8 pieces, 1.4 oz	160	3.5	33
Gummibursts, 9 pieces, 1.4 oz	130	0	31
Jellybeans, 1.5 oz	150	0	37
Starlight Mints, 3 pieces, 0.5 oz	60	0	15
Suckers *(Walgreens)*, 1 piece, 0.4 oz	45	0	11
Sugar Babies, Original, 1.4 oz	160	1.5	37
Sugar Coated Peanuts, 1 oz	120	8	10
Sunbursts Sunflowers *(Kimmie)*:			
ChocoRocks Milk, 3.5 oz	525	25	67
Habanero Corn, 3.5 oz	500	23	70
Sunburst Mix, Milk, 3.5 oz	500	28	55
Swedish Fish, 7 pieces, 1.5 oz	150	0	38
SweeTARTS: 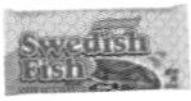			
Orig., 8 pieces, 0.5 oz	50	0	13
Mini Chewy, 23 pieces, 0.5 oz	50	0.5	12
Symphony *(Hershey's)*: 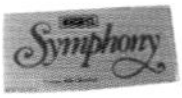			
Milk Choc: 1.5 oz bar	220	14	23
Large Block: 5 pieces, 1.4 oz	200	12	22
w/ Almond & Toffee, 5 pcs, 1.3 oz	200	13	21

Per Piece/Serving	C	F	Cb
Taffy, Fruit Chews, 1 piece	20	0.5	4
Take 5 *(Hershey's)*: 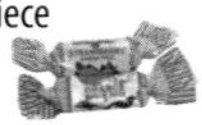			
Bars: Original, 1.5oz	200	11	25
King Size, 2.3 oz 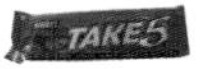	300	16	37
Snack Size, 2 pcs, 1 oz	150	8	19
3 Musketeers:			
Original, 1.9 oz 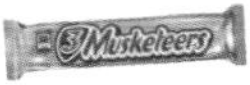	240	7	42
2 To Go, 1 bar, 1.6 oz	200	6	35
Fun Size, 3 bars, 1.6 oz 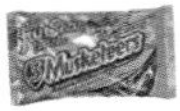	190	6	34
Minis, 7 pieces, 1.4 oz	170	5	32
Tang-a-Roos, 1 roll	25	0	6
Terry's:			
Chocolate Orange (5), 1.5 oz	230	12	27
Dark Chocolate Orange (5), 1.5 oz	240	13	28
Tic Tac, all flavors, 1 piece	2	0	0
Toblerone: 1.23 oz bar	190	10	22
Pieces, 5.3 oz pkg, 5 pieces, 1.5 oz	230	13	27
Fruit & Nut, ⅓ bar, 1.2 oz	170	8	21
Dark/White Chocolate, ⅓ bar 1.2 oz	180	10	20
Toffees, Regular, 1 oz	160	9	18
Tootsie Pops, (1), 0.6 oz	60	0	15
Tootsie Roll: 2.25 oz roll 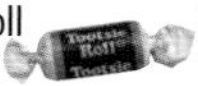	220	5	45
Midgees, 1.4 oz	140	3	28
Truffles: Reg., 1 piece, 0.4 oz	60	4	6
Large *(Godiva)*, 0.8 oz	110	6.5	12
Extra Large *(J.Schmidt)*, 1.5 oz	220	13	24
Turtles: Original, 1 piece, 0.6 oz	85	5	10
Sugar Free, 1 piece, 0.4 oz	50	3.5	7
Twists, Licorice; Strawb., sugar free, 7 pieces, 1.4 oz 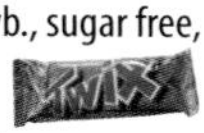	90	0	25
Twix:			
Caramel: 2 cookies, 1.8 oz	250	12	34
Fun Size, 1 cookie, 0.6 oz	80	4	11
4 To Go, 1 cookie, 0.8 oz	110	5	15
Minis, 3 pieces, 1 oz	150	7	20
Milk Chocolate, Bites, 5 pcs, 1 oz	140	7	18
White Chocolate, 2 cookies, 1.6 oz	110	12	29
Twizzlers:			
Cherry Bites, (13), 1.4 oz	110	0.5	25
Cherry Twists, 3 pieces, 1.2 oz	120	0.5	27
Pull 'n' Peel, Cherry, 1 piece, 1.2 oz	110	0.5	26
Twists, Strawberry, 1 twist	25	0	6
Watermelon Soft Bites, 11 pieces	150	1.5	33
U-No Bar, 1.5 oz	250	17	22
Weight Watchers *(Whitman's)*:			
Caramel Medallions, (3)	160	9	24
Coconut, (3)	150	9	23
English Toffee Squares, (3)	150	9	21
Mint Patties, (3) 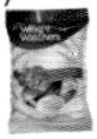	150	9	23
Peanut Butter Cups, (4)	180	8	31
Pecan Crowns, (3)	160	10	24

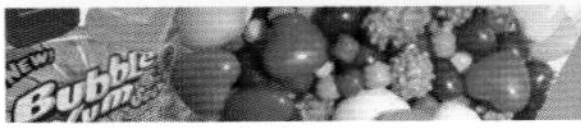

Candy ~ Brands & Generic (Cont)

Per Piece/Serving

	C	F	Cb
Werther's:			
Hard Candy: Original (3), 0.5 oz	70	1.5	14
Sugar-Free Original (5)	40	1.5	15
Note: Carb figure includes 14g sugar alcohol			
Soft, Chocolate Caramel (4), 1.4 oz	190	8	28
Whatchamacallit: 1.5 oz Bar	230	12	28
King Size Bar, 2.5 oz	370	20	45
Whitman's:			
Boxed Chocolates: Sampler (4)	220	12	27
12 oz Box, 3 pieces, 1.2 oz	170	9	21
Reserve, 7 oz Box, 2 pieces, 1.2 oz	160	9	21
Sugar Free, 10 oz Box, 3 pcs, 1.5 oz	190	13	25
Whoppers, av. all varieties, 18 pcs	190	7	31
Wonka:			
Bar, 2.5 oz	360	19	49
Exceptional Bars, average, 4 pieces	200	13	23
Gobstopper, 9 pieces, 0.5 oz	60	0	14
Laffy Taffy: Ropes, all var., 0.8 oz	80	1.5	18
Stretchy & Tangy, all var., 1.5 oz	150	3.5	29
Nerds, Giant, Chewy, 1.8 oz package	180	0	42
Yogurt Candy, Coated Raisins,1.4 oz	180	8	28
York: Mints, (3)	10	0	3
Peppermint Pattie, reg, 1.4 oz	140	2.5	31
Pieces (50)	170	8	28
Zagnut, 1.75 oz bar	220	9	35
Zero Bar: 1.8 oz bar	230	8	37
King Size, 3.5 oz	400	14	68

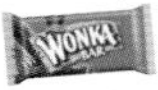

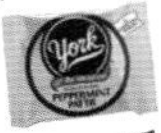

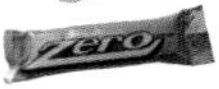

Gum

Per Piece

	C	F	Cb
Bazooka	15	0	4
Beechies	6	0	2
Big League Chews	10	0	2
Bubble Yum: Original	25	0	6
Sugarless	10	0	3
Candilicious	30	0	2
Carefree, Sugarless/Regular	5	0	2
Chiclet	5	0	1
Dentyne	5	0	0.5
Double Bubble Ball	20	0	5
Estee, Bubble/Regular	5	0	2
Extra *(Wrigley's)*, Sugar-Free	5	0	2
Freshen-Up	10	0	3
Hubba Bubba: Regular	25	0	6
Sugar-free, average	14	0	0.5
Ice Breakers	5	0	2
Jolt Gum	5	0	2
Super Bubble	15	0	4
Trident, Orig.; White	5	0	1
Wrigley's, all flavors	10	0	2

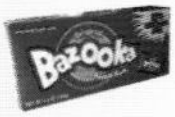

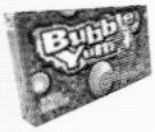

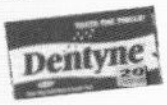

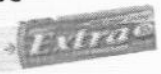

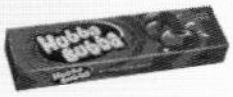

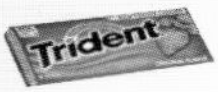

Carob Candy

Per Piece/Serving

	C	F	Cb
Carob, Plain/Natural, 1 oz	155	9	15
Carob Coated: Raisins, 1 oz	130	8	15
Almonds/Peanuts, 1 oz	150	10	14
Caramels, 1 oz	110	4	18
Dates, 1 oz	125	5	20
Malt Balls, 1 oz	135	8	15
Soybeans	145	9	16
Trail/Party Mix, 1 oz	150	9	15

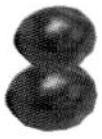

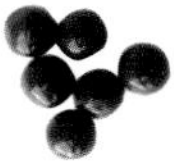

Cough Drops

Per Drop/Piece

	C	F	Cb
Beech Nut, 1 drop	10	0	2
CVS, Honey Lemon Cough Drops	15	0	4
Diabetic Tussin	0	0	0
Halls, Defense Vitamin C:			
Regular	15	0	4
Sugar Free	5	0	3
Fruit Breezers	15	0	4
Menthol Drops: Regular	15	0	4
Sugar Free	5	0	4
Plus	20	0	5
Listerine *(Amer. Chicle)*, Lozenge	10	0	2
Luden's, Throat Drops: Reg., all var.	10	0	2
Sugar Free	0	0	0
Pine Bros, Cough Drops	10	0	2
Ricola:			
Cough Drops:			
Natural Herbs	10	0	3
Sugar-Free Lemon Mint	0	0	1
Rolaids, Sodium Free	5	0	1
Sathers, Peppermint Lozenges	15	0	3
Sucrets *(Beecham)*, Lozenges	10	0	2.5
Wintergreen, Lozenges	15	0	3

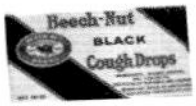

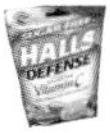

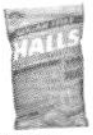

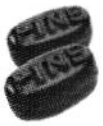

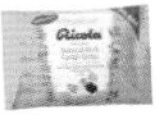

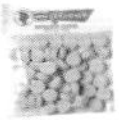

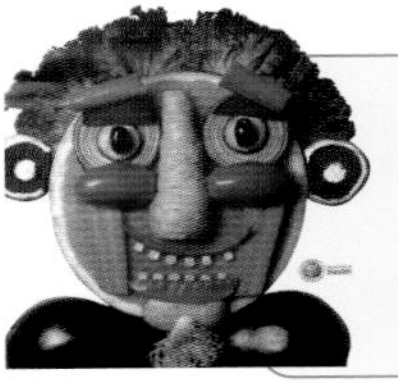

Eat at least 5 servings of fruit and vegetables every day . . . and Enjoy Better Health!

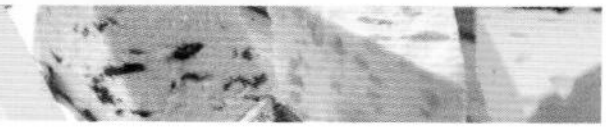

Quick Guide

Firm/Hard Cheeses

American, Cheddar, Jack, Swiss:
Average All Brands

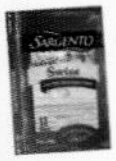

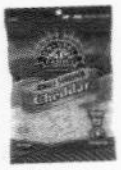

	C	F	Cb
Regular Cheese:			
Thin Deli slice, 0.8 oz	80	6	0.5
1 oz slice/piece	110	9	0.5
8 oz package	880	72	3
Cubes: 1" cube, 0.6 oz	70	5.5	0.5
1¼" cube, 1 oz	115	9	0.5
Diced, 1 cup, 4.5 oz	510	41	3
Melted, ¼ cup, 2 oz	245	20	1
Shredded: ¼ cup, 1 oz	110	9	0.5
1 cup, 4 oz	440	36	2

Cheese & Cheese Products

Per 1 oz Unless Indicated

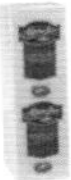

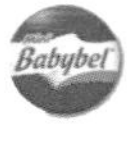

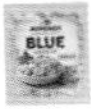

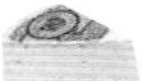

	C	F	Cb
Almond, *(Lisanatti)*, Chunks/Shreds, av.	70	4	3
American:			
Regular: 1 slice, 1 oz	105	9	0.5
Borden, Singles, 0.67 oz slice	70	4.5	2
Kraft, Singles, 0.67 oz slice	50	3.5	2
Land O'Lakes, Yellow, 0.67 oz slice	70	6	1
Reduced Fat:			
Alpine Lace, Yellow/White, 1 oz	90	6	2
Kraft, 2% Milk, 0.67 oz	45	2.5	2
Land O Lakes, White, 2% Milk, 1 oz	90	6	2
Babybel *(Laughing Cow)*, Mini:			
Original (1), 0.75 oz	70	6	0
Light (1), 0.75 oz	50	3	0
Gouda (1), 0.75 oz	70	6	0
White Cheddar (1), 0.75 oz	70	6	6
Blue/Bleu: Average all Brands			
Crumbled, ¼ cup, 1 oz	100	8	0
Castello, Blue Danish, 1 oz	110	10	0
Light, 0.8 oz	35	1.5	2
Brie: Average, 1 oz	95	8	0
Alouette, Original Creme, 1 oz	100	9	1
Camembert, 1 oz	85	7	0
Caraway, 1 oz	105	8	1
Cheddar:			
Regular: Medium/Sharp, av., 1 oz	110	9	1
Shredded, ¼ cup, 1 oz	110	9	1
Cracker Barrell: Extra Sharp, 1 oz	110	10	0
Vermont Sharp White, 1 oz	110	10	0

Cheese & Cheese Products (Cont)

Per 1 oz Unless Indicated

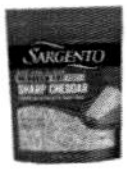

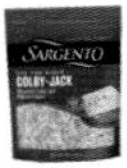

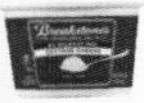

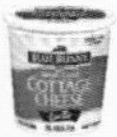

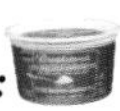

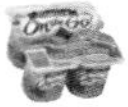

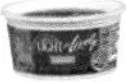

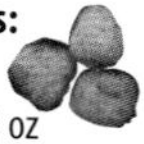

	C	F	Cb
Cheddar (Cont):			
Reduced Fat, 2% Milk, *Kraft,* Shredded, 1 oz	90	6	2
Curds, Cheddar Cheese,			
Cheese Curds ~ *See Cottage Cheese*			
Cheese Logs *(Kaukauna)*, average	100	7	4
Cheez Whiz ~ *See Dips*			
Cheshire, 1 oz	110	9	1.5
Colby, Regular, 1 oz	110	8	0
Colby-Jack:			
Big Slice, 0.8 oz	90	7	0
Cottage Cheese (Curds): *Average All Brands*			
Creamed (4% milk fat):			
2 Tbsp, 1 oz	30	1	1.5
½ cup, 4 oz	110	5	4
with fruit, ½ cup, 4 oz	115	4	5
Reduced-Fat (2%): 2 Tbsp, 1 oz	25	0.5	1
½ cup, 4 oz	100	3	4
Low-Fat (1%): 2 Tbsp, 1 oz	20	0.5	1
½ cup, 4 oz	80	1	3
Fat-Free/Non-Fat: 2 T., 1 oz	20	0	1
½ cup, 4 oz	80	0	5
Cottage Cheese (Curds): *Brands*			
Friendship:			
1% Low-Fat with Pineapple, 5 oz	120	1.5	12
Nonfat with Pineapple, ½ cup, 4 oz	110	0	18
Pot Style, 2%, ½ cup, 4 oz	100	2.5	4
Hood, Low Fat, 4 oz	90	1.5	5
Knudsen/Breakstone's:			
Free, Non-Fat, ½ cup, 4.25 oz	80	0	8
2% Milk Fat, ½ cup, 4 oz	90	2.5	6
On the Go!, Low-Fat, 4 oz carton	90	2.5	7
Lactaid, 4% Lowfat, ½ cup, 4 oz	110	5	5
Light n' Lively:			
Fat-Free, ½ cup, 4.4 oz	80	0	8
Low-Fat, ½ cup, 4.4 oz	80	1.5	6
Breaded & Fried Curds:			
A&W, 5 oz	570	40	27
Culver's, Wisconsin, 5.3 oz	510	25	51

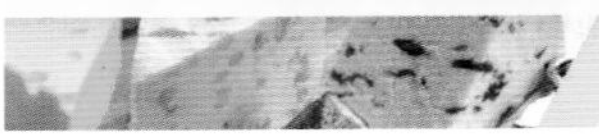

Cheese & Cheese Products (Cont)

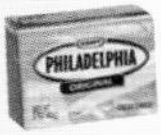
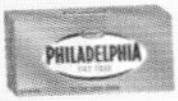
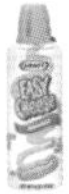
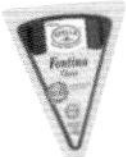
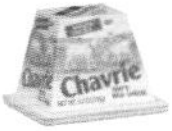
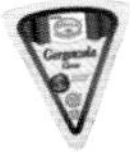
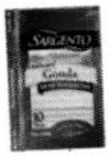

Per 1 oz Unless Indicated	C	F	Cb
Cream Cheese: *Average All Brands*			
Regular/Soft:			
2 Tbsp, 1 oz	**95**	10	1
3 oz package	**290**	29	3.5
8 oz package	**780**	78	9
Light, Plain, 1 oz	**60**	4.5	2.5
Fat-Free, Plain, 1 oz	**30**	0	2
Better Than Cream Cheese (Tofutti),			
all varieties, 1 oz	**85**	5	9
Easy Cheese *(Kraft),*			
American, 2 Tbsp, 1.2 oz	**80**	6	2
Edam, 1 oz	**100**	8	0.5
Farmer, Low-Fat, 1 oz	**40**	2.5	0
Feta: Regular, 1 oz	**75**	6	1
Crumbled, ½ cup, 2.5 oz	**190**	15	3
Athenos, Reduced-Fat,			
1 oz	**50**	3	1
Fontina, 2 Tbsp, 1 oz	**110**	9	0.5
Galaxy, Go Vegan Cheese Substitute:			
Grated Parmesan Flavor, 2 tsp, 0.2 oz	**20**	1	3
Slices: Cheddar, 1 slice, 0.6 oz	**40**	3	0.5
Mozzarella, 1 slice, 0.6 oz	**40**	2.5	0.5
Goat's Milk Cheese:			
Chevre: Original, 2 Tbsp	**80**	7	0
Semi-Soft, 1 oz	**100**	8.5	1
Hard, 1 oz	**130**	10	0.5
Chavrie, Logs:			
Original, 2 Tbsp, 1 oz	**80**	7	0
Honey, 1 oz	**80**	5	6
Sundried Tomato & Garlic, 1 oz	**80**	6	2
Gjetost, fresh, 1 oz	**130**	8	12
Myzithra, grated, 1 oz	**80**	4	2
Gorgonzola, 1 oz	**100**	8	0.5
Galbani, Dolcelatte, 1 oz	**95**	8	1
Gouda, 1 oz slice	**100**	8	0.5
Gruyere, 1 oz	**115**	9	1
Havarti *(Sargento),* 0.7 oz	**80**	6	0
Jarlsberg: Average, 1 oz	**100**	8	0
Reduced Fat, shredded, 1 oz	**70**	3.5	0
Labneh, (Lebanese Cream Cheese), 1.8 oz	**70**	4	4

Cheese & Cheese Products (Cont)

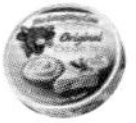
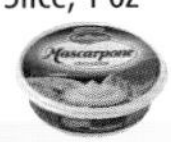
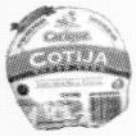
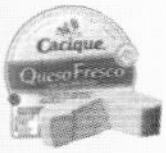
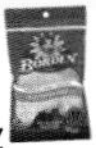
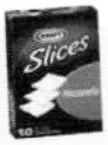
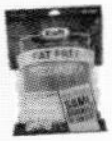
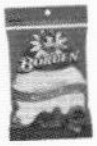
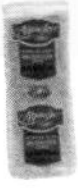

Per 1 oz Unless Indicated	C	F	Cb
Laughing Cow, Wedges:			
Creamy Asiago (1)	**30**	1.5	1
Creamy: Original (1)	**50**	4	1
Light (1)	**30**	1.5	1
Lifetime, Cholesterol Reducing,			
Fat Free, all varieties, 1 Slice, 1 oz	**40**	0	1
Limburger, 1 oz	**95**	8	0
Mascarpone, av., 1 oz	**125**	13	0.5
Mexican:			
Cacique: Asadero, sliced	**70**	4.5	1
Cotija	**90**	7	0
Enchilado; Manchego	**90**	7	0
Panela	**80**	8	0
Queso Blanco Fresco	**80**	6	0
Queso Quesadilla	**90**	7	0
Ranchero	**80**	6	0
Chi-Chi's, Salsa Con Quéso, Mild	**45**	3	4
El Mexicano: Cotija, 1 oz	**90**	6	0
Oaxaca, 1 oz	**90**	7	1
Kraft, Mexican Four Cheese; Taco,			
Shredded,	**100**	8	1
Sargento, 4 Cheese Mexican	**110**	9	2
Supremo, Quéso Chihuahua, 1 oz	**100**	8	0
Verole, Quéso Oaxaca, 1 oz	**80**	6	1
Monterey Jack:			
Regular, shredded, 1 oz	**100**	8	1
Land O Lakes, Co-Jack, 0.7 oz	**80**	7	0
Kraft, 1" cube, 1 oz	**100**	8	0
Mozzarella:			
Whole Milk: Average 1 oz	**85**	6.5	0.5
Land O'Lakes, String, 1 oz	**80**	6	2
Polly-O, Slice, average, 1 oz	**80**	6	1
Fat-Free,			
Kraft, Shredded, 1 oz	**45**	0	2
Reduced Fat,			
Kraft, 2% Milk Fat, Shredded, 1 oz	**80**	4	2
Part Skim:			
Borden, Shredded, 1 oz	**90**	6	2
Kraft, Shredded, 1 oz	**80**	5	2
Kraft, String, 1 oz	**80**	5	1
Polly-O, Shredded, 1 oz	**80**	5	0
Muenster:			
Alpine Lace, 1 oz slice	**100**	9	0
Wisconsin, 1 oz slice	**100**	8	0

Cheese & Cheese Products (Cont)

Per 1 oz Unless Indicated	C	F	Cb
Parmesan:			
Fresh/Block, Dry, 1 oz	**110**	7.5	1
Grated (Packaged): 2 tsp	**20**	1.5	0
½ cup, 1.8 oz	**215**	14	2
Kraft: Shaker Bottle, 1 oz	**110**	8	1
Reduced-Fat Topping, 1 Tbsp	**20**	1	2
Philadelphia:			
Cream Cheese Brick:			
Original: 1 oz	**100**	10	0.5
8 oz package	**800**	80	4
⅓ Less Fat, 1 oz	**70**	6	0.5
Flavored Spread:			
Chive & Onion, 1 oz	**80**	7	2
Cracked Pepper & Olive Oil, 1.1 oz	**70**	6	2
Smoked Salmon, 1.1 oz	**70**	5	2
Strawberry, 1.1 oz	**80**	6	5
⅓ Less Fat: Plain, 2 T., 1 oz	**70**	5	3
Neufchatel, 2 T., 1 oz	**70**	6	1
Fat-Free, Plain, 1 oz	**30**	0	3
Cheesecake Filling, 3 oz	**240**	17	18
Milk/White Chocolate:			
2 Tbsp, 1.27 oz	**110**	6	13
Dark Chocolate, 2 T., 1.23 oz	**100**	5	11
Whipped:			
Plain, 0.77 oz	**50**	4	2
Mixed Berry, 0.77 oz	**50**	3	5
Port de Salut, 1 oz	**100**	8	0
Port Wine *(Kaukauna/WisPride):*			
10 oz Ball, 1 oz	**100**	7	5
10 oz Log, 2 Tbsp, 1 oz	**100**	7	5
11.3 oz Tub, 0.85 oz	**80**	6	3
Provolone: Regular, 1 oz	**100**	7.5	0.5
Alpine Lace, Reduced-Fat, 1 oz	**80**	6	1
Sargento, 1 slice, 0.67 oz	**70**	5	0
Pub *(President),* average all varieties	**75**	7	1
Quark: 40% fat	**45**	3	1
20% fat	**30**	1.5	1
Skim/Non-Fat	**20**	0	1.5
Rice Cheese Chunks *(Lisanatti),*			
average, 1 oz	**60**	3	2

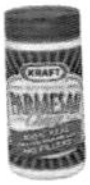
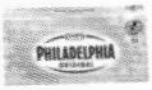

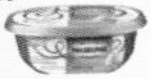
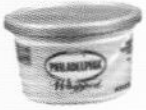
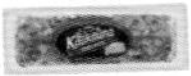
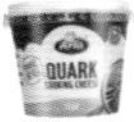

Cheese & Cheese Products (Cont)

Per 1 oz Unless Indicated	C	F	Cb
Ricotta Cheese:			
Whole Milk: 1 oz	**50**	3.5	1
½ cup, 4.5 oz	**215**	16	4
Part Skim: 1 oz	**40**	2	1.5
½ cup, 4.5 oz	**170**	10	6
Light/Low-Fat: 1 oz	**25**	1	1.5
½ cup, 4.5 oz	**125**	5	6
Fat-Free, ½ cup, 4.5 oz	**100**	0	10
Baked Ricotta, 2 oz	**130**	9	3
Romano: Block/Loaf	**110**	8	1
Grated: 1 oz	**120**	9	1
1 Tbsp, 0.2 oz	**20**	1.5	0
Roquefort, 1 oz	**105**	9	0.5
Sheep's Milk, (Manchego),			
Trader Joes/Wegman's, 1 oz	**120**	10	0
Soy Cheese:			
Trader Joe's, Mozzarella Style, 1 oz	**70**	4	3
Soya Kaas: Cheddar, 1 oz	**50**	2	8
Monterey Jack, 1 oz	**60**	4	0
Soy Sation, Cheddar,			
1 slice, 0.67 oz	**50**	4	2
Smoked Cheddar, average, 1 oz	**110**	10	0
Stilton, average, 1 oz	**110**	10	0
String:			
Regular, average all brands	**80**	6	0.5
Kraft: Twists/Strings,			
Mozzarella & Cheddar (1), 0.75 oz	**60**	4	0
Frigo, 1 oz	**80**	6	1
Light/Lite:			
Polly-O, String,			
2% Red-Fat, 1 oz	**70**	4.5	0
Sargento: 1 piece, 1 oz	**80**	6	1
Light, , 0.75 oz	**50**	2.5	1
Swiss: Regular, 1 oz	**110**	8	1.5
Alpine Lace, Reduced-Fat, 1 oz	**90**	6	1
Kraft, Slim Cut 2% Milk, 3 slices, 1.2 oz	**110**	7	0
Tilsit, 1 oz	**100**	7.5	0.5
Tofutti, Better Than Cream Cheese,			
all flavors, 2 Tbsp	**60**	5	2
Tybo, 1 oz	**100**	7	0.5
Velveeta *(Kraft): Per Slice*			
Original, 0.74 oz	**40**	2	3
3 Cheese Blend, 0.74 oz	**40**	2	3
Jalapeno, 0.74 oz	**40**	2	3
Queso Blanco, Mild, 0.74	**40**	2	3

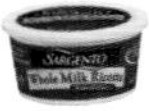
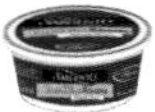
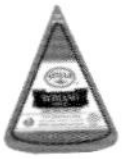
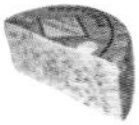
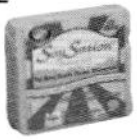
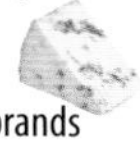
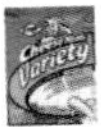
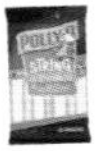

Dips/Spreads

Per 2 Tbsp, 1 oz, Unless Indicated	C	F	Cb
Average All Brands			
Avocado/Guacamole	45	4	2
Baba Ghanoush (Eggplant/Sesame)	70	6	2
Cheese Fondue, ½ cup, 4 oz	260	15	4
French Onion Dip	60	4.5	3
Hummus: 2 Tbsp	50	1	5
½ cup, 4.5 oz	220	4.5	23
Tzatziki (Cucumber/Yogurt)	30	2.5	2
Clearman's, Original Spread	150	16	0
De La Casa, 5 Layer Party Dip	45	2.5	4
Fritos: *Per 2 Tbsp*			
Dips: Bean; Hot Bean w/ Jalapeno	35	1	5
Jalapeno Cheddar Cheese	40	2.5	3
Mild Cheddar	40	3	3
Great Value *(Walmart)*:			
Cheddar Jalapeno	60	4.5	4
Original Cheddar Cheese Dip	80	7	5
Melt & Dip, Easy Melt Cheese, 1 oz	80	6	3
Guiltless Gourmet,			
Black Bean/Spicy Black Bean Dip	40	0	7
Heluva Good Cheese,			
Jalapeno Cheddar; White Chedd. Bacon	60	4.5	3
Kaukauna *(Wisconsin)*:			
Spreadable Cheddar,			
Sharp/Smokey Cheddar	80	6	3
Kemps: *Per 2 Tbsp*			
Dips: French Onion; Ranch Style	60	5	2
Top The Tater,			
Taco Fiesta; Veggie Ranch, av.	60	5	3
Kroger, Dips, all varieties	60	5	2
Kraft: *Per 2 Tbsp*			
Dips: Average all varieties	60	5	3
Cheez Whiz: Orig., 1.2 oz	80	5	6
Salsa Con Queso ~ See Velveeeta			
Spreads: Light Cheez Whip, 1 Tbsp	30	1.5	2
Pimento, 1.1 oz	80	6	3
Old English Sharp; Roka Blue, av	90	7	0.5
Marie's: *Per 1.5 oz Cup,*			
Dips: Blue Cheese	250	27	1
Creamy Ranch	270	29	1
Marzetti:			
Dips: Chocolate Fruit, 2 oz Tub	180	2	36
Classic Caramel, 1.25 oz	140	4.5	24
Veggie: Dill; Ranch, 1.1 oz	80	7	2
French Onion; Spinach, 1.1 oz	80	7	3
Southwest Ranch, 1 oz	110	10	2
Old Dutch:			
Dips: French Onion, 1 oz	50	3	5
Mild Cheddar, 1 oz	40	3	2
Nacho Cheese, 1 oz	35	2.5	2

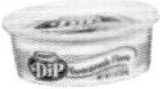
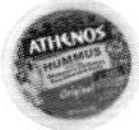
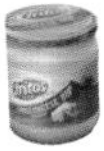
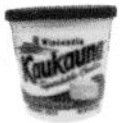
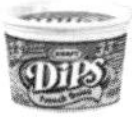
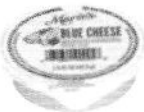
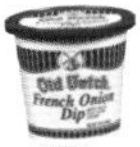

Dips/Spreads (Cont)

Per 2 Tbsp, 1 oz, Unless Indicated	C	F	Cb
On The Border,			
Dip, Salsa Con Queso, 2 Tbsp	45	3	4
Philadelphia: *Per 2 Tbsp, 1 oz*			
Dips:			
Buffalo Style with Celery	50	4	1
Caramelised Onion & Herb	60	5	2
Jalapeno & Cheddar,	70	6	2
Spinach & Artichoke	70	5	3
Spreads: Chive & Onion,	80	7	2
Honey Butter Cream Cheese	70	5	4
Whipped Mixed Berry, 0.78 oz	50	3	5
Price's: *Per 2 Tbsp*			
Dips: Fiesta; Green Chili, 1 oz	60	6	2
French Onion; Ranch Style, av., 1 oz	60	5.5	2
Spreads: French Onion, 1 oz	60	6	2
Pimiento Cheese , 1.1 oz	90	7	4
Stop & Shop: *Per 2 Tbsp*			
Dips: Veggie	100	10	3
Sour Cream French Onion	60	4.5	2
TGI Fridays,			
Spinach & Artichoke Cheese Dip, 1 oz	30	2	2
Toby's: Blue Cheesse Dip, 2 Tbsp	140	15	1
Honey Mustard, 2 Tbsp	120	10	5
Tostitos: *Per 2 Tbsp*			
Dips: Avocado Salsa, 1 oz	45	4	1
Salsa con Queso, 1.16 oz	40	2.5	5
Southwest Cheese & Corn, 1.3 oz	50	2.5	5
Wise: *Per 2 Tbsp*			
Dips: French Onion, 1.16 oz	60	5	3
Salsa con Queso, 1.2 oz	45	3	3

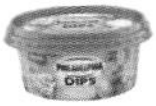
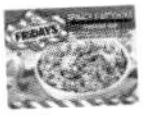
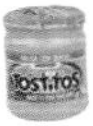
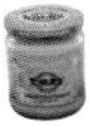

New Diet Aid - The Refrigerator Air Bag!

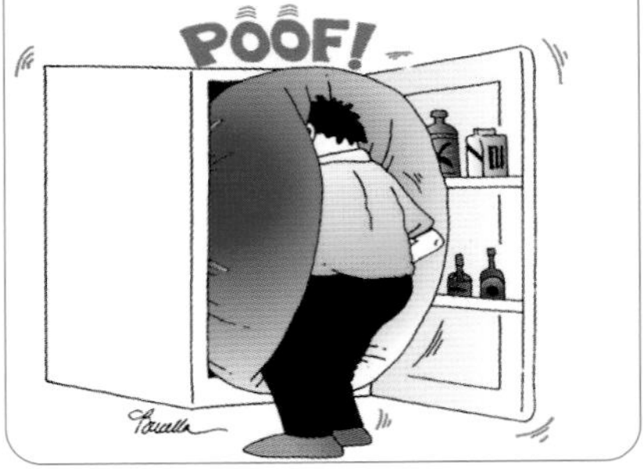

C Condiments ♦ Salsa

Condiments, Sauces

Average of Brands & Homemade

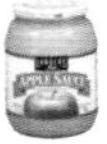
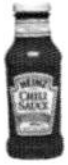
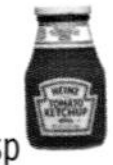
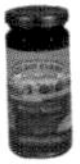
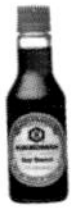
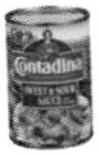
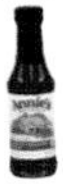

	C	F	Cb
Apple Sauce:			
Sweetened, ¼ cup, 2.5 oz	55	0	13
Unsweetened, ¼ cup, 2 oz	25	0	7
Barbecue Sauce:			
Regular, av. all flavors, 2 Tbsp, 1 oz	40	0	10
Bull's Eye, Original, 1 oz	60	0	14
Bearnaise Sauce, ¼ cup, 2.5 oz	190	19	5
Buffalo Wing Sce: Hon. Mustard, 1 T.	40	3	3
Average other varieties, 1 Tbsp	25	2	2
Cheese, h/made, ¼ cup, 2.5 oz	150	10	12
Chef-Mate, Hot Dog, ¼ cup	70	2.5	9
Chili Sauce *(Heinz),* 1 Tbsp	20	0	5
Cocktail Sauce: ¼ cup	110	0	15
Walden Farms, Fat-Free, 1 Tbsp	0	0	0
Cranberry Sauce, av. all varieties: 2 T.	45	0	11
¼ cup, 2.5 oz	110	0	27
Demi Glaze Gold, 2 tsp	30	0.5	3
Honey Mustard *(French's),* 2 Tbsp	60	0.5	12
Horseradish: 1 tsp	2	0	0
Kraft, 1 tsp	15	1.5	1
Ketchup: Regular, 1 Tbsp	15	0	4
Heinz: Reduced Sugar, 1 Tbsp	5	0	1
Simply Heinz, 1 Tbsp	15	0	4
Mole:			
Dona Maria, av. all varieties., 2 T.	150	10	10
Rogelio Bueno, 2 Tbsp, 1 oz	160	11	12
Mushroom Sce, ½ cup, 2 oz	50	2	5
Mustard, average, 1 tsp	5	0	0.5
Pesto Sauce, ¼ cup, 2 oz	270	28	2
Pizza Sauce, ¼ cup, 2 oz	30	0	6
Seafood Cocktail Sce, ¼ cup	60	0	15
Soy Sauce: Average all, 1 Tbsp	10	0	1
Kikkoman, Lite Soy, 1 Tbsp	10	0	1
Spaghetti Sce, ½ cup, 4.5 oz	135	6	19
Steak Sauce:			
Kraft, A1, 1 Tbsp, 0.5 oz	15	0	3
Lea & Perrins, 1 Tbsp, 0.5 oz	20	0	5
Strawb. Puree Sauce, Unsweet., 2 T.	10	0	2
Sweet & Sour Sauce:			
Contadina, 1.2 oz	40	1	8
Kraft, 1 Tbsp	60	0	13
Tabasco Sauce, 1 tsp	2	0	0
Taco Sauce, average all, 2 Tbsp, 1 oz	10	0	1
Tartar Sauce: *(Heinz),* 2 Tbsp, 1 oz	120	11	4
Hellmann's, Regular, 2 Tbsp, 1 oz	80	7	4
McCormick, Fat-Free, 2 Tbsp, 1 oz	30	0	7
Teriyaki Sauce *(Kikkoman),* 1 T., 0.5 oz	15	0	2
Vinegar, White or Wine, 2 T.	4	0	1
White Sauce, ½ cup, 5 oz	130	7	10
Worcestershire Sauce, 1 tsp	5	0	1

Pickles & Relish

Average All Brands

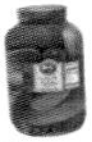
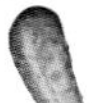
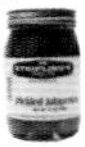
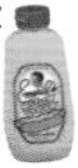
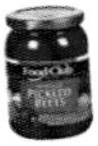
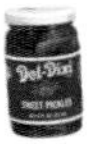
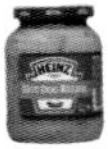
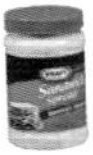
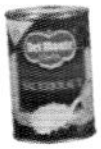

	C	F	Cb
Bread & Butter Pickles, 4 sl.,1 oz	25	0	6
Chutney, 2 Tbsp, 1.25 oz	50	0.5	11
Dill Pickles:			
Slices, 4 slices, 1 oz	4	0	1
1 large, (3¾"x 1¼" diam.), 2.25 oz	12	0	3
Extra large (4"x 1¾" diam.), 5 oz	30	0	6
Halves: Small, 1 oz	3	0	0.5
Large, 2.5 oz	8	0	2
Gherkins, sweet, 1 medium, 1 oz	30	0	7
Green Chiles, chopped, 2 Tbsp	5	0	1
Horseradish, 1 Tbsp	10	0	2
Jalapenos, pickled (2), 2 oz	10	0.5	2
Jalapeno Relish, 1 Tbsp, 0.5 oz	5	0	1
Mustard, av. all brands, 1 tsp	5	0	0.5
Peppers, Hot/Mild (1), 1.5 oz	20	0	4
Pickled: Beets, ½ cup, 4 oz	75	0	19
Cocktail Onion, 1 onion	2	0	0
Red Cabbage, ½ cup, 3 oz	65	0	15
Pickles: Sweet, 2 Tbsp, 1 oz	35	0	8
Large (3" x ¾ diam.),1.25 oz	40	0	10
Pickle in a Pouch, 1 large	12	0	3
Relishes:			
Cranberry-Orange, 1 Tbsp	30	0	7
Hot Dog *(Heinz),* 1 T., 0.5 oz	17	0	3
S'wich Spread, 1 tsp	20	1	5
Sweet Pickle, 1 Tbsp, 0.5 oz	20	0	5
Sweet Cauliflower, 1 oz	35	0	8
Sugar Free Relish, 1 tsp	5	0	1
Sweet Gherkins (2), 1 oz	5	0	1
Sauerkraut,			
Drained, 1 cup, 5 oz	25	0	6

Salsa

Average all Types:

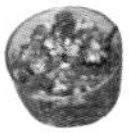
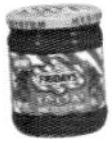

	C	F	Cb
Regular, w/out oil, 2 T., 1 oz	15	0	3.5
Made with oil, 2 Tbsp, 1 oz	40	3	8
La Victoria, 2 Tbsp, 1 oz	10	0	2
Old El Paso, 1 Tbsp, 1 oz	10	0	3
TGI Friday's, 1.2 oz	15	0	4

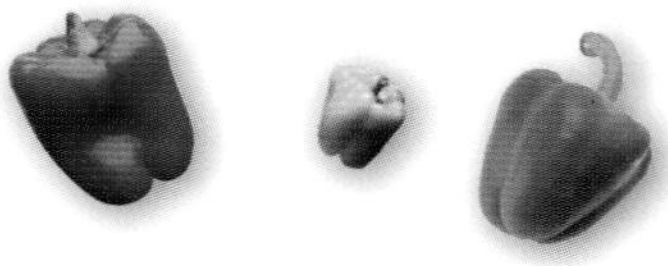

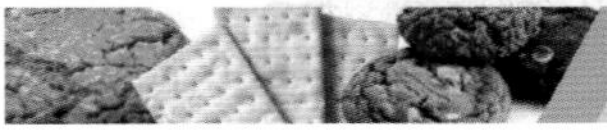

Cookies ♦ Crackers

Quick Guide

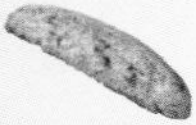
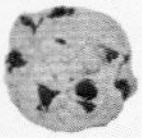
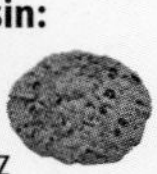
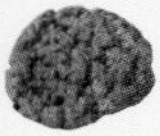
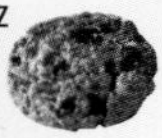

Cookies:	C	F	Cb
Average All Brands: *Per Cookie*			
Biscotti: Small, 0.5 oz	70	3	10
Regular, 1 oz	140	6.5	18
Chocolate Chip:			
Small/Thin, 0.5 oz	70	3.5	9
Regular, 1 oz	140	7	18
Large *(Mrs Fields)*, 3 oz	350	17	45
Extra Large, 4 oz	555	28	73
Oatmeal/Oatmeal Raisin:			
Small/Thin, 0.5 oz	65	2.5	10
Regular, 1 oz	130	5	20
Large *(Mrs Fields)*, 2.5 oz	330	14	44
Extra Large, 4 oz	510	20	78
Peanut Butter:			
Small/Thin, 0.5 oz	70	3.5	9
Regular, 1 oz	135	7	17
Large *(Mrs Fields)*, 2.5 oz	330	17	41
Extra Large, 4 oz	540	27	67
Low-Fat Cookies:			
Choc Chip (Low-Fat), (1), 0.5 oz	65	2	10
Oatmeal Raisin (Fat-Free), (1), 1 oz	95	0.5	22
Peanut Butter (Low-Fat), (1), 1 oz	105	5	15

Quick Guide

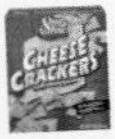
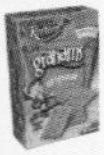
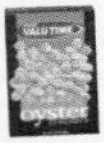
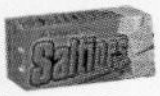
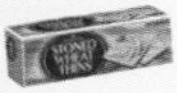

Crackers	C	F	Cb
Average All Brands: *Per Cracker Unless Indicated*			
Cheese Crackers:			
Plain: 1" square	5	0	0.5
Bag, single serving, 1 oz	140	7	16
Cheese/P'nut Butter filled	30	1.5	4
Crispbread, Rye	35	0	8
Grahams, 2½" square	30	0.5	5
Melba Toast, Plain, 1 piece	20	0	4
Matzo, Plain, 1 oz	110	0.5	23
Oyster/Soup, ½ cup	95	2	17
Rice: 1 crackers	70	1.5	11
Oriental Style, 1 oz	130	3.5	23
Saltines, 5 crackers	65	2	11
Snack-type, 1 round cracker	15	1	2
Soda Crackers *(Saltine)*, 2	25	1	4.5
Water Cracker *(Carr's)*, Original	15	0.5	2.5
Wheat:			
Wheat Thins	10	0.5	1.5
Cheese/Peanut Butter filled	35	2	4

Cookies & Crackers ~ Brands

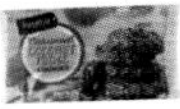
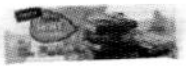
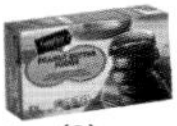
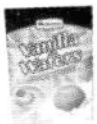
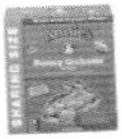
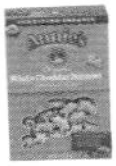
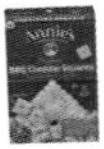
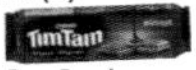

Per Cookie/Cracker, Unless indicated	C	F	Cb
Albertsons:			
Fresh Baked: PB Jumbo Cookie (1)	340	18	39
Rainbow Chip Jumbo Cookie (1)	320	14	46
Signature Select:			
Fudge:			
Caramel Coconut Stripes (2)	130	6	18
Graham (3), 1 oz	140	6	19
Mint (2)	180	9	25
Marshmallow (2)	150	5	25
Peanut Butter (2)	140	8	15
Stripes (3)	170	8	25
Swiss Milk Chocolate, (2)	130	6	17
Treasure Chips Chewy Cookie, (2)	140	6	20
Tuxedos, Double Flled Choc. (2)	140	6	21
Wafers: Chocolate Creme (3)	180	10	20
Strawberry Creme (3)	180	6	20
Vanilla (10)	140	5	22
Vanilla Creme (3)	180	10	20
Annie's (Organic):			
Bites, Choc. Chip Cookie (6)	150	8	19
Bunny Grahams:			
All Varieties, 1 oz	130	4.5	22
Gluten Free: Cocoa & Vanilla, 1 oz	120	4.5	23
SnickerDoodle, 1 oz	140	5	22
Sandwich Cookies, all varieties, (3)	160	7	24
Cheddar Bunnies Crackers:			
Regular (51), 1 oz	140	6	19
Super Cheesy (48), 1 oz	150	8	18
White Cheddar (48), 1 oz	150	7	17
Whole Wheat (51), 1 oz	140	5	20
Gluten Free, Bunny Tails (30), 1 oz	160	9	17
Squares: BBQ Cheddar (26), 1 oz	150	8	18
White Cheddar (26), 1 oz	150	7	18
Saltine Classics, (14), 1 oz	140	5	20
Arnott's:			
Tim Tams: Original; Chewy C'rml (2)	190	9	26
Classic Dark; Dark Mint (2)	190	10	25
Austin *(Kellogg's)*:			
Sandwich Crackers: *Per Package*			
Cheese: with Cheddar Cheese	190	9	24
with Peanut Butter	190	9	24
Peanut Buter on Toasty Crackers	190	9	24

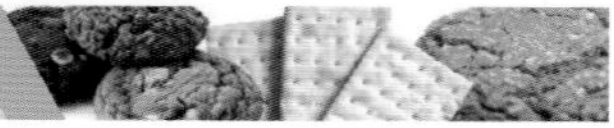

Cookies & Crackers ~ Brands (Cont)

Per Cookie/Cracker, Unless Indicated	C	F	Cb
BelVita *(Nabisco):*			
Breakfast Biscuits:			
Crunchy, 1 pack (4 biscuits), average	230	8	35
Soft Baked, 1 biscuit, average	200	8	32
Bites, (46), av., 1.8 oz	230	8	37
Blue Diamond:			
Nut Thins:			
Almond; Hint of Sea Salt (19), 1 oz	130	2	24
Average other varieties (19), 1 oz	130	3	24
Carr's:			
Crackers: Rosemary (4)	80	3.5	10
Toasted Sesame (4)	60	1.5	10
All other Varieties (4)	50	1	10
Cheez•It ~ *See Sunshine, Page 87*			
Chips Ahoy! ~ *See Nabisco, Page 85*			
Dr. Kracker:			
Crispbread: Klassic 3 Seed (2)	110	5	14
Multi Grain (2)	100	3.5	16
Pumpkin Seed Cheddar (2)	100	4.5	12
Flats: Robustica (4)	110	3.5	19
Roasted Red Pepper & Asiago (4)	100	3	18
Rosemary Parmesan (4)	110	4	17
Seed Power Snack Crackers, (8)	110	4	17
Seeds & Seasalt, (12)	120	4.5	19
Snackers, Pumpkin Seed Cheddar (8)	110	5	15
Ener-G Foods: (Gluten Free):			
Cinnamon Crackers, (7)	110	4.5	19
Flax Crackers, (9)	90	4.5	11
Erin Baker's:			
Original Breakfast: *Per 3 oz*			
Banana Walnut	310	8	55
Double Choc.; Oatmeal Raisin	300	7	57
Peanut Butter	320	11	51
Minis: Per 1 oz Cookie			
Caramel Apple, 1 oz	100	1.5	19
Double Chocolate, 1 oz	100	2.5	18
Grain free, Salted Choc. Cashew (2), 1 oz	130	9	14
Famous Amos:			
Bite Size: Chocolate Chip (4)	150	7	0
Chocolate Chip & Pecans (4)	150	8	19
Double Chocolate Chip (3)	145	7	18
fifty50:			
Chocolate Chip, (4)	170	9	22
Hearty Oatmeal, (4)	160	7	24

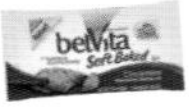

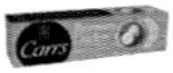

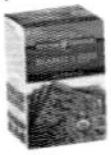

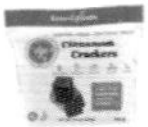

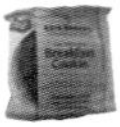

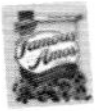

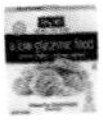

Per Cookie/Cracker, Unless Indicated	C	F	Cb
Fig Newtons ~ *See Nabisco, Page 85*			
Gamesa:			
Arcoiris Marshmallow, 2 oz pkg, 6 cookies	220	5	38
Barras de Coco, 1 cookie	120	3	22
Chokis, Chocolate Chip, 1.4 oz pkg	190	8	27
Emperador: Chocolate, (1), 1.15 oz	160	6	23
Lime Flavor (3), 1.1 oz	140	5	23
Florentinas, (8), 1 oz	120	2	23
Giro, 3 cookies, 1 oz	140	6	20
Mamut, 1 cookie, 1 oz	130	5	21
Maravillas, (6), 1 oz	120	3.5	21
Marias, 8 cookies, 1 oz	120	2	23
Ricanelas, (2)	140	4.5	24
Sugar Wafers, (3), average, 1.2 oz	180	9	25
Girl Scouts Cookies:			
Caramel DeLites/Samoas, (2), av.	145	7	18
Girl Scout S'Mores, (2)	150	7	21
Peanut Butter S'wich, (3)	170	7	21
Shortbread, (4)	120	4.5	19
Thanks-A-Lo, (2)	140	6	22
Thin Mints, (4)	160	7	22
Trefoils, (5)	160	7	21
Goldfish Crackers ~ *See Pepperidge Farm, Page 86*			
Goya:			
Lady Fingers , (4),1 oz	130	1	25
Marias, (5), 1 oz	130	3	23
Chocolate (5), 1 oz	130	3.5	23
Strawberry Wafers, (5), 1.15 oz	170	8	22
Grandma's *(Fritolay): Per Cookie*			
Chocolate Brownie	190	8	27
Chocolate Chip	200	10	25
Minis, 1 pkg	210	8	31
Oatmeal Raisin	180	7	26
Peanut Butter	190	10	22
Sandwich Cremes:			
Peanut Butter (4)	170	8	22
Vanilla (4)	170	7	23
Great American Cookies: *Per Cookie*			
Chewy Choc. Supreme	200	9	29
Chewy Pecan Supreme	230	12	31
Double Fudge with Reese's	230	11	33
Original with Reese's or M&M's	240	12	31
Peanut Butter with M&M's	250	14	29
White Chunk Macadamia	250	14	30

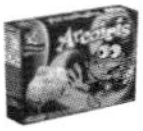

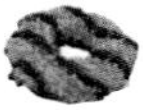

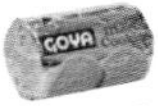

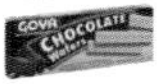

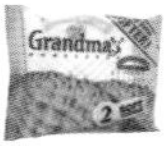

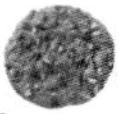

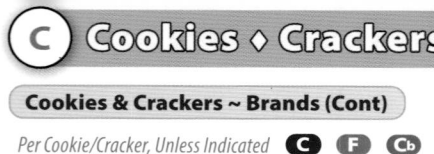

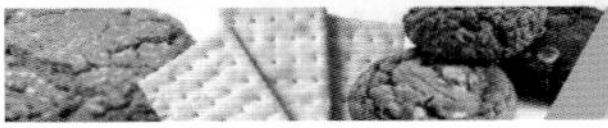

Cookies & Crackers ~ Brands (Cont)

Per Cookie/Cracker, Unless Indicated	C	F	Cb
Great American Cookies (Cont): *Per Cookie*			
Double Doozies:			
Original, 5.3 oz	690	34	94
M&M Big Bite, 2.5 oz	340	17	46
Cookie Cakes:			
16", 3.5 oz	460	22	67
16" M&M, 4 oz	500	24	73
Heart Shaped, 3.5 oz	440	21	64

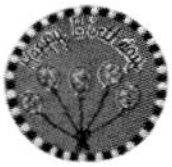

Great Value *(Walmart):*			
Caramel Coconut & Fudge, (2)	130	6	18
Chocolate Chip Chippers, Mini:			
Original, 1 Pack, 1 oz	130	6	18
Orange, 1 pack, 1 oz	140	7	21
Fudge: Grahams, (1)	110	5	16
Covered Peanut Butter Filled (2)	160	9	17
Striped Shortbread (3)	170	7	25
Iced Apple Oatmeal, Minis, 1 pack	140	6	21
Pecan Shortbread, (2)	160	9	19
Sandwich: Chocolate Cremes (3)	160	7	24
Vanilla (3)	170	7	26
Twist & Shout, Dble Choc Filled (2)	140	7	20
Snickerdoodle, (1)	110	5	15
Strawberry Filled Wafers, (4)	160	8	22
White Melting Wafers, (9)	80	4.5	10
Crackers:			
Buttery Smooth, (4), 0.5 oz	70	3	9
Cheddar Cheese, (28), 1 oz	150	8	18

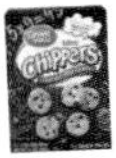

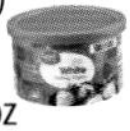

Keebler:			
Animals, Frosted (8)	160	8	22
Chips Deluxe: Original (2)	160	8	19
With Peanut Butter (2)	170	9	20
Chocolate Lovers (2)	170	9	20
Chunk (2)	170	9	21
Coconut (2)	160	9	19
Deluxe Triple Choc (2)	150	8	20
Simply Made (2)	140	7	17
Soft Batch (2)	150	7	21
Soft 'n Chewy (2)	150	6	21
Rainbow, Choc. Chip wih M&M's (2)	160	8	21

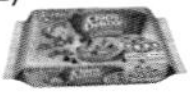

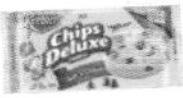

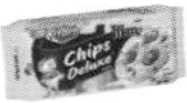

Per Cookie/Cracker, Unless Indicated	C	F	Cb
Keebler (Cont):			
Danish Wedding, (5)	160	8	22
E.L. Fudge: Original (2)	170	7	25
Chocolate (2)	170	7	26
Double Stuffed (2)	180	9	24
Vanilla (2)	180	7	26
Fudge:			
Caramel Nut Dreams, (2)	190	11	20
Coconut Dreams Fudge Covered (2)	170	9	20
Deluxe Grahams (2)	140	7	18
El Fudge: Original Elfwich (2)	170	7	25
Double Stuffed (2)	180	9	24
Fudge Sticks:			
Original (3)	150	8	20
Fudge Stripes: Original (2)	140	7	19
Birthday (2)	140	6	19
Coconut Dreams (2)	140	8	17
Dark Chocolate (2)	130	6	20
Whoopsy!: (2)	170	8	23
Cookies & Cream (2)	170	8	23
Mint (2)	170	9	23
Grasshopper (4)	150	7	20
Peanut Butter Dreams (2)	170	11	16
Gripz, Chips Deluxe, 0.9 oz pouch	120	5	18
Oatmeal, Country Style (2)	130	6	19
Pitter Patter, P'nt Butter Creme (2)	140	6	19
Sandies Shortbread Cookies:			
Cashew (2)	170	9	19
Classic (2)	160	9	19
Pecan(2)	170	10	19
Simply Made Cookies:			
Butter (2)	140	7	18
Chocolate Chip (2)	140	7	17
Chocolate S'wich (2)	140	6	20
PB Chocolate Chip (2)	140	8	15
Vienna Fingers,			
Creme Filled (2)	150	6	22
Wafers, Vanilla Filled (4)	150	7	22

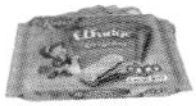

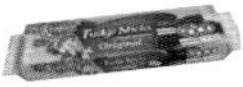

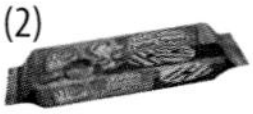

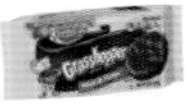

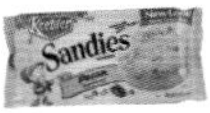

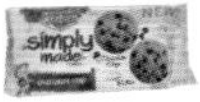

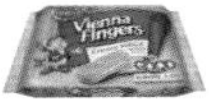

continued next page...

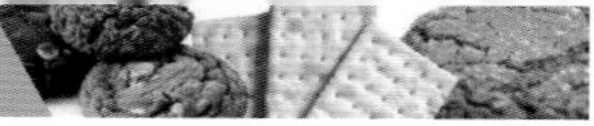

Cookies & Crackers ~ Brands (Cont)

Per Cookie/Cracker, Unless Indicated	C	F	Cb
Keebler (Cont):			
Crackers:			
Town House: Original (5)	80	5	9
Dippers, Original, (3)	70	3.5	8
Flatbread Crisps, all flavors (8)	70	2	11
Flip Side: Original (5)	70	3.5	10
Thins: Sea Salt (6)	70	3.5	10
Focaccia:			
Rosemary & Olive Oil (3)	70	3.5	9
Tuscan Cheese (3)	80	4	9
Pita:			
Mediterranean Herb (6)	70	2.5	12
Parmesan Cheese (6)	70	2.5	11
Kroger:			
Chip Mates: Original Choc. Chip (3)	130	6	17
Chewy Chocolate Chip (2)	150	7	20
Chunky Chocolate Chip (2)	140	7	18
Peanut Butter Chocolate Chunk (2)	130	7	15
White Chip Chocolate Chunk (2)	140	7	18
Sandwich Cookies:			
Kaleido: Original Chocolate (3)	160	6	25
Coconut Lime (3)	150	7	22
Salted Caramel (3)	140	6	21
Maple Creme, (2)	140	5	22
Olde Southern Pecan Shortbread, (2)	150	9	16
Vanilla Wafers, (8)	130	4	23
Crackers:			
Grahams, Orig.; Honey, (4)	130	3	24
Saltines, Original (5), 0.5oz	60	1.5	10
Lance: *Per Pack of 6 Cookies/Crackers*			
Nekot Cookies:			
Choc-O-Lunch/Van-O-Lunch, av.	220	8	34
Lemon Creme; Peanut Butter, av.	240	10	34
Crackers:			
Captain's Wafers:			
Cream Cheese & Chives	200	10	23
Grilled Cheese	190	9	25
PB & Honey	200	9	23
Cracker Sandwiches:			
Malt, with Peanut Butter Filling	180	8	20
Nip Chee, Cheddar Cheese	200	9	24
Toastchee, Peanut Butter	220	11	25
Toasty, Peanut Butter	190	9	21
Wholegrain: Cheddar Cheese	200	10	26
Peanut Butter	210	9	25

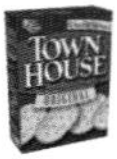

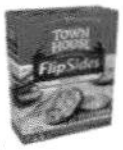

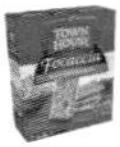

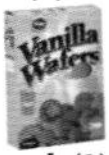

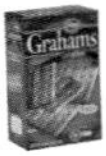

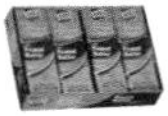

Little Debbie:	C	F	Cb
Choc. Chip Cream Pie, (1), 3 oz	380	16	58
Fudge Rounds, (1)	150	6	23
Marshmallow Pies, (1)	190	6	31
Nutty Buddy, (1)	120	7	12
Oatmeal Creme Pie, (1)	170	7	26
Big Size (1), 2.65 oz	330	12	52
Peanut Butter Cream Pies, (1)	170	7	25
Big Size (1), 3.1 oz	410	19	54
Star Crunch, (1)	150	6	22
Lu:			
Petit Ecolier: Dark Chocolate, (2)	130	7	15
Petit Ecolier, Milk Chocolate (2)	130	6	17
Pim's, Orange (2), 0.9 oz	100	3	17
Manischewitz:			
Crackers:			
Tam Tams: Original (10)	110	4	16
Everything; Garlic (10)	140	5	19
Mary's Gone Crackers:			
Chocolate Chip Cookies, (2)	130	6	19
Crackers:			
All Flavors, (13)	140	5	21
Super Seed:			
Rosemary; Lemon Dill (12)	140	6	17
Other Varieties (12)	150	7	16
Miss Meringue:			
Meringue Classiques:			
Cappuccino (4), 1 oz	110	0	26
Mint Choc. Chip (4), 1 oz	120	1.5	25
Triple Chocolate (4), 1 oz	120	1.5	25
Vanilla Rainbow/Van. (4), 1 oz	110	0	27
Meringue Minis, Low Fat:			
Mini: Chocolate Chip (12), 1 oz	130	1.5	27
Mint Chocolate Chip (12), 1 oz	120	1.5	26
Meringue Minis, Fat Free:			
Peppermint Crush (9), 1 oz	110	0	25
Rainbw Vanilla; Vanilla (13), 1 oz	110	0	27
Meringue Petites: Cafe au Lait (7)	100	0	25
Toasted Coconut (6)	120	2.5	23
Mother's:			
Circus Animal, (4), 1 oz	150	8	20
Chocolate Chips, (4), 1 oz	150	7	20
Coconut Cocadas, (4), 1 oz	140	7	17
Double Fudge, (1), 0.7 oz	100	4.5	14
English Tea, (2)	190	8	28
Oatmeal/Iced Oatmeal, (4), 1.2 oz	150	6	23
Peanut Butter Gauchos, (2), 1 oz	150	6	20
Taffy Dulce de Leche, (1), 0.7 oz	100	4.5	15

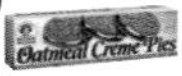

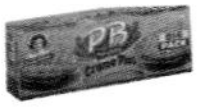

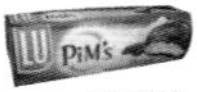

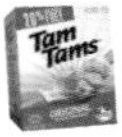

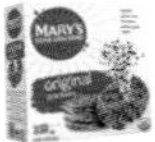

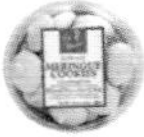

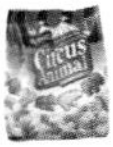

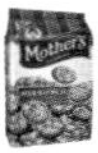

Mrs Fields Cookies ~ *See Page 219*

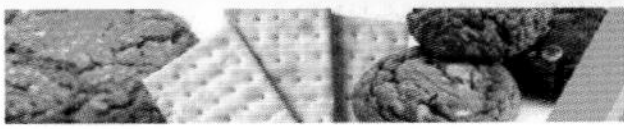

Cookies & Crackers ~ Brands (Cont)

Per Cookie/Cracker, Unless Indicated	C	F	Cb
Nabisco Cookies:			
Chips Ahoy!, Chocolate Chip:			
Original: 3 cookies, 1.2 oz	**160**	8	22
Single Serve, 2 oz	**280**	14	38
Reduced Fat (3), 1.2 oz	**150**	6	24
Mini Choc. Chips:			
Big Bag (5), 1oz	**150**	7	19
Chewy (4), 1.15 oz	**140**	5	22
Go Pak (14), 1 oz	**150**	7	20
Snak Sak, Lunch Box (5), 1.1 oz	**160**	7	21
Chewy: Regular (2), 1.1 oz	**140**	6	21
Brownie Filled (1), 0.65 oz	**80**	3.5	12
Chunky: Choc. Chunk (2), 1.2 oz	**160**	8	20
Choco Chunky; White Fudge Choc. (1)	**80**	4	11
Hot Cocoa (2), 1.1 oz	**150**	7	22
Oreo Creme, (2), 1.1 oz	**150**	7	21
Peanut Butter, (1), 0.7 oz	**90**	4	13
Lorna Doone: 100 Calorie Pack,			
Shortbread Cookie Crisps (6), 0.7 oz	**100**	3	16
Shorbreads: 1 oz pack	**140**	7	20
1.5 oz pack	**210**	10	29
Mallomars (1), 1 oz	**120**	5	18
Newtons: 100% Whole Grain:			
Blueberry (2), 1 oz	**110**	1.5	22
Fig (2), 1 oz	**110**	0	22
Strawberry (2), 1 oz	**100**	2	21
Original Fig: 1 cookie, 1 oz	**100**	2	21
Fat-Free, 1 cookie, 1 oz	**100**	0	24
Nilla Wafers: 8 Wafers, 1 oz	**140**	6	21
Reduced-Fat (8), 1 oz	**120**	1.5	24
Vanilla, 1 oz pkg	**120**	3	22
Nutter Butter:			
16 oz package, 2 cookies, 1 oz	**140**	6	19
4.8 oz package, 2 cookies, 0.8 oz	**120**	5	16
Bites, 1 package, 10 cookies, 1 oz	**150**	6	21
Snak Sak Lunch Box, 10 cookies	**150**	6	21
Wafer, 5 patties, 1.2 oz	**160**	9	19
Oreo Chocolate:			
Regular; King Size (3), 1.2 oz	**160**	7	25
Mini, 1 oz pack	**130**	5	20
Snak Sak Mini Lunchbox (9), 1 oz	**140**	6	21
Apple Pie; Chocolate Mint (2), 1 oz	**140**	7	21
Blueberry Pie; Choco Chip (2), 1 oz	**140**	7	21
Coconut (4), 1 oz	**140**	6	21
Cookie Creme Filled S'wich, 3 oz pack	**360**	16	52
Double Stuff (2), 1 oz	**140**	7	21
Thins, Choc. Creme (4), 1 oz	**140**	6	21
White Fudge Choc. Covered (1), 0.7 oz	**100**	5	13

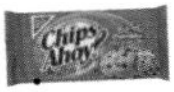

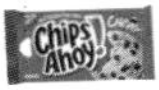

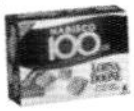
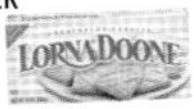

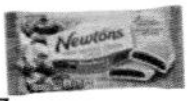

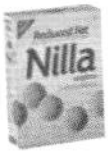

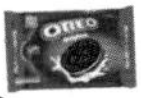

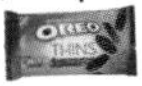

Per Cookie/Cracker, Unless Indicated	C	F	Cb
Nabisco (Cont):			
Oreo Golden: Original (1)	**55**	2.5	8
(3), 1.2 oz	**170**	7	25
Reduced Fat (3), 1.2 oz	**150**	5	27
Mini (9), 1 oz Pack	**140**	6	21
15 oz Pack	**200**	8	30
Double Stuf (2), 1 oz	**150**	7	21
Fruity Crisps (2), 1 oz	**140**	7	21
Limeade (2), 1 oz	**140**	7	20
Lemon (2), 1 oz	**150**	7	21
Mega Stuff (2), 1.3 oz	**180**	9	25
Thins, all flavors (4), 1 oz	**150**	6	21
Teddy Grahams: Cinnamon, 0.74 oz pkt	**90**	3	16
Single Serve, Honey (24), 1 oz	**120**	4	21
Nabisco Crackers:			
Barnum's Animals:			
1 oz Pack	**130**	4	21
Snack Saks (17), 1.2 oz Pack	**140**	4	24
Zoo Animals, 2 oz Pack	**250**	7	43
Cheese Nips:			
Cheddar: 29 pieces, 1 oz	**150**	6	19
Mini, Despicable Me, 1 oz Pack	**130**	4	19
Honey Maid: Chocolate 1 oz Pack	**140**	4.5	18
Grahams (8) average all varieties,	**130**	3	24
Bites, Snickerdoodle (24), 1 oz	**140**	4	18
Premium:			
Original: 5 crackers, 0.5 oz	**70**	1.5	12
Minis (17), 0.5 oz	**70**	2	11
Unsalted Tops(5), 0.5 oz	**70**	1.5	13
Rounds: Original (6), 0.5 oz	**60**	1.5	12
Wholegrain (6), 0.5 oz	**60**	1.5	11
Soup & Oyster (22), 0.5 oz	**60**	1.5	11
Triscuit: Original (6), 1 oz	**120**	3.5	20
Av. other flav. (6), 1 oz	**120**	4	20
Reduced Fat (6), 1 oz	**110**	2.5	21
Brown Rice & Wheat (6), average all varieties	**130**	3	22
Thin Crisps, Original (7)	**130**	4.5	21
Wheat Thins:			
Original (16); Big (11), 1.1 oz	**140**	5	22
Reduced Fat (16), 1 oz	**120**	3.5	22
Averae other flavors (14), 1.1 oz	**140**	5	21
Multigrain: Original (14), 1.1 oz	**130**	4	22
Toasted (13), 1 oz	**130**	5	19

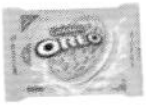

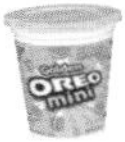

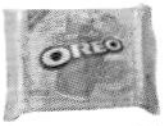

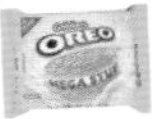

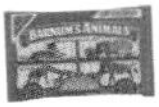
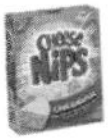

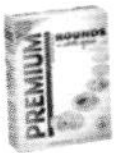

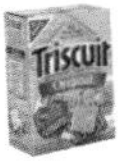

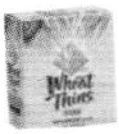

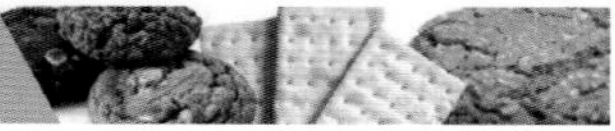

Per Cookie/Cracker, Unless Indicated	C	F	Cb
Nana's: *Per Cookie*			
Choc. Chip Walnut; Dble Choc, av.	360	13	58
Oatmeal Raisin	360	12	58
Peanut Butter	360	18	46
Gluten Free: Chocolate	340	14	50
Ginger	340	10	62
Bags:			
Cacao Nib (2)	130	7	17
Coconut; Snickerdoodle (2)	130	6	19
Lemon (2)	120	5	19
Cookie Bars, average	150	6	23

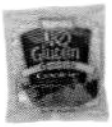
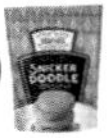

Per Cookie/Cracker, Unless Indicated	C	F	Cb
Newman's Own Organics:			
Alphabet, all flavors (10)	110	3	20
Chocolate Chip: Original (5)	150	7	20
Double Choc Chip (5)	150	7	19
Oatmeal Chocolate Chip (2)	140	6	22
Orange Chocolate Chip (2)	150	7	20
Fig Newman's:			
Fat-Free (2)	90	0	21
Low Fat & Wheat/Dairy-Free (2)	100	1.5	20
Strawberry (2)	110	1.5	21
Wheat Free Non Dairy (2)	110	1	21
Newman-O's: Orig.; Hint O Mint (2)	130	5	19
Chocolate	120	5	18
Peanut Butter (2)	120	5	17
Wheat Free Non Dairy (2)	130	5	19

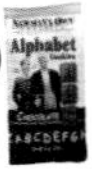
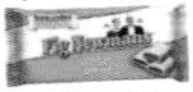
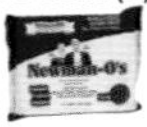

Per Cookie/Cracker, Unless Indicated	C	F	Cb
Nonni's:			
Biscotti:			
Original, 1 piece, 0.8 oz	90	3	14
Av. other varieties, 1 piece, 0.8 oz	110	4	17
Cookie Bites, all flavors (5), average	150	10	17
THINaddictives: Cranb. Alm., 1 oz	130	4.5	20
Lemon Blueberry Almond, 1 oz	130	2.5	22
Pistachio Almond, 1 oz	140	6	18
O Organics *(Signature Select)*			
Animal Cookies, Chocolate (5)	120	4.5	20
Coconut Bites (1)	100	6	11
Koala Bites, 1 piece, 0.9 oz	130	7	16
Mini Chocolate Chip, 1oz Bag	140	7	19
Crackers:			
Mini Peanut Butter S'wich (12)	140	7	17
Rosemary Flatbread Crackers, with Sea Salt (3)	120	2	23
Water Crackers (8)	60	1.5	10

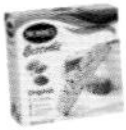
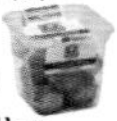

Oreo Cookies ~ *See Nabisco, Page 85*

Per Cookie/Cracker, Unless Indicated	C	F	Cb
Payaso:			
Animalitos (19)	120	1.5	23
Esponjitas (4)	95	2	18
Marias (8)	120	2.5	22
Orejitas Finas (4)	100	5	13

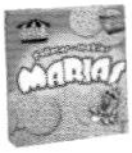

Per Cookie/Cracker, Unless Indicated	C	F	Cb
Pepperidge Farm:			
Chunk: *Per Cookie*			
Chesapeake, Dark Chocolate Pecan	140	8	16
Lexington, Milk Chocolate, Toffee Almond	130	7	16
Monauk, Milk Chocolate	140	6	22
Nantucket, Dark Chocolate	130	7	17
Sausalito, Milk Choc. Macadamia	130	7	17
Tahoe, White Chocolate Macadamia	130	7	17
Disctinctive:			
Brussels; Geneva, av. (3)	150	8	20
Chessmen, Butter (3)	120	5	18
Gingerman (4)	130	3.5	22
Milano:			
Caramel Macchiato (2)	130	7	16
Dark Chocolate (2)	180	9	22
Double Milk Chocolate (2)	130	7	17
Irish Cream; Mint; Tstd M'shmallow (2)	130	7	16
Orange; Raspberry (2)	130	7	15
Salted Caramel (2)	120	6	15
Crackers:			
Cracker Trio (3)	60	2	9
Golden Butter (4)	70	2.5	11
Harvest Wheat (3)	80	3.5	11
Goldfish Crackers (Baked):			
Cheddar; Colors (55), 1 oz	140	5	20
1.5 oz Pack	200	7	28
Flavor Blasted, Sour Cream & Onion (57)	140	5	19
Parmesan (60)	140	5	20
Pizza (55)	140	5	20
Pretzel (43)	130	2.5	24
Veggie, Sweet Carrot (56), 1 oz	140	5	21
Whole Whole Grains, Cheddar (55)	140	5	19

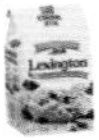

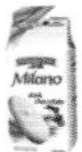
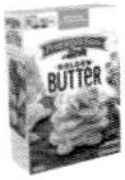
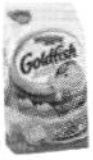

Per Cookie/Cracker, Unless Indicated	C	F	Cb
Ritz:			
Originals: Orig.;Bacon (5)	80	4.5	10
Roasted Vegetable (5)	80	3.5	10
Whole Wheat (5)	70	2.5	10
Bits: Cheese (13)	160	9	19
Peanut Butter (12)	150	8	18
Crisp & Thins, all varieties (21)	130	4.5	21
Toasted Chips: Original (13)	130	4	20
Cheddar; Sour Crm & Onion (12)	130	6	19
Multigrain (13)	130	5	19
Vegetable (13)	120	4.5	20
Sedano's:			
Cinnamon (5)	160	6	24
Maria (5)	120	3	22

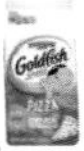
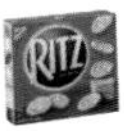
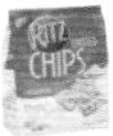
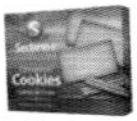

Shar Gluten Free ~ *See CalorieKing.com*

Cookies & Crackers ~ Brands (Cont)

Per Cookie/Cracker, Unless Indicated	C	F	Cb
Snackwell's Cookies:			
Choc. Creme S/wich, 1 pack (4)	210	6	38
Devil's Food Cake, 2 cookies, 32g	120	3	24
Vanilla Creme S/wich, 2 cookies, 24g	100	3	19
Special K:			
Cracker Chips, Sea Salt, 1 cup, 2 oz	190	1	46
Popcorn Chips, White Cheddar (25)	120	3	22
Stella D'Oro:			
Almond Delight (1)	140	7	18
Almond Toast (2)	110	1	24
Breakfast Treats (1), av. all varieties	90	2.5	15
Lady Stella Assorted (3)	120	4	19
Margherite: Chocolate (2)	130	6	19
Vanilla (2)	120	4	20
Original (1)	90	2	15
Swiss Fudge (3)	180	9	23
Trinkets (4)	150	7	19
Crackers:			
Breadsticks: Original (1)	40	1	7
Sesame (1)	50	2	6
Streit's:			
Flavored Wafers:			
Chocolate (3)	160	9	19
Vanilla (3)	170	11	18
Sunshine:			
Cheez-It Crackers:			
Original (27)	150	8	17
Reduced Fat (27)	140	6	19
Duos: C'rml Popcorn & Cheddar, 1 oz	130	6	18
Average other flavors (25), 1 oz	150	7	18
Extra BIG (14)	150	8	17
Four Cheese; White Cheddar (20)	150	7	18
Whole Grain (12)	150	8	17
Grooves: Orig. Cheddar (9)	140	6	19
Zesty Cheddar Ranch (9)	140	6	19
Snack Mix, Classic, ½ cup, 1 oz	130	4.5	20
Trader Joe's:			
100 Calorie Packs, av.	100	2.5	18
Almond Windmill (2)	140	6	18
Charmingly Chewy Choc Chip (2)	130	5	20
Cherry Granola (2)	110	4	18
Chocolate Chip: Small (4)	140	7	18
Large, singles, 1.7 oz	280	14	35
Deep Dish: 1/10 cookie, 1.6 oz	200	9	28
¼ Cookie, 4 oz	500	23	70
Vegan (1)	130	6	18
Caramel Cashew (3)	140	7	16
Crispy Crunchy Choc. Chip (12)	150	9	19
Crispy Oatmeal Choc. Chip (12)	150	7	19
Dark Choc Chunks w/ Almonds (3)	140	7	17
Dunkers: Chocolate Chip (2)	160	7	21
Choc. Coated Choc. Chip (2)	190	9	25

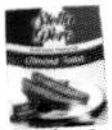
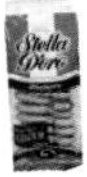

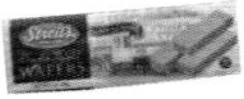
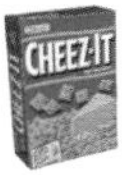
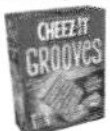
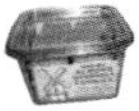
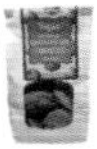

Per Cookie/Cracker, Unless Indicated	C	F	Cb
Trader Joe's (Cont):			
Ginger Snaps, Gluten Free (5)	140	6	21
Highbrow Chocolate (2)	140	7	17
Joe Joe's S'wich Cremes,			
Chocolate/ Vanilla (2)	130	6	19
Macarons A La Parisienne (2)	90	3	10
Meringues, Vanilla (4)	110	0	27
Oatmeal Raisin, 1.8 oz	270	12	35
Pecan Southern Style (4)	150	9	15
Thins: Meyer Lemon (9)	130	4.5	22
Toasted Coconut (8)	130	4.5	22
Triple Choc Chunk, 1 oz	140	7	20
Ultimate Vanilla Wafers (5)	120	6	15
Way More Chocolate Chip (3)	160	11	14
Crackers:			
Multigrain (14)	150	6	22
Savory Thin Edaname (38)	120	2	21
Water (4)	60	1	12
Triscuits ~ *See Page 85*			
Voortman: *Per Cookie Unless Indicated*			
Almond Crunch (2)	140	5	21
Chocolate Chip (1)	90	4	13
Coconut (1)	100	5	9
Fudge Striped Oatmeal (1)	110	6	14
Oatmeal Cranberry Flaxseed (1)	90	4	12
Wafers, average all flavors (3)	150	7	22
Sugar Free:			
Wafers (3), average all flavors	140	8	18
Note: Carbohydrate Figure Contains 7 g Sorbitol			
Whole Foods (365 Organic):			
Butter Shortbread (2)	150	8	17
Chocolate Chip: Bites, 1 oz pkg	150	8	19
Two Bite(3)	130	6	18
Double Chocolate Chip (2)	150	8	19
Oatmeal Raisin (2)	140	6	20

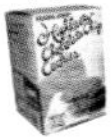
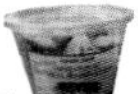
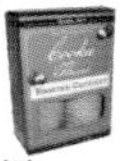

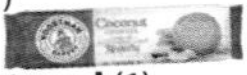
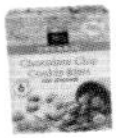

Cookie ~ Mixes

As Packaged	C	F	Cb
Betty Crocker: *Per 3 Tbsp (1 oz) Mix, Unless Indicated*			
Chocolate Chip	110	2.5	22
Double Chocolate Chunk	110	2.5	21
Snickerdoodle	110	1.5	24
Walnut Chocolate Chip	110	1.5	22
Limited Edition, Gingerbread	100	1.5	20
Snack Size, Sugar Cookie, 4 tbsp, 1 oz	120	2	23
Whole Foods (365 Organic): *Per 2 Tbsp Mix*			
Chocolate Chip, 2 tbsp	110	2.5	22
Gluten Free, ¼ cup, 0.74 oz	80	1.5	17

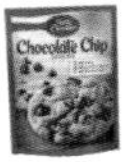

Thaw, Bake & Serve

Per Cookie/Cracker Unless Indicated

	C	F	Cb
Eat Pastry Vegan (Whole Food): *Per Cookie*			
Chocoholic Cookie Dough	50	2.5	8
Choc. Chip Cookie Dough	60	2.5	8
Gluten Free	60	2.5	8
Peanut Butter Choc. Chip	60	2.5	7
Pillsbury Cookies:			
Refrigerated Cookie Dough: *Per Cookie*			
Chocolate Chip Cookie, 1 oz	130	6	17
Peanut Butter, 1.1 oz	130	6	19
Sugar, 1 oz	120	5	18
Ready To Bake CookieDough: *Per 2 Cookies*			
Choc. Chunk & Chip Cookies, 1.34 oz	170	7	24
Chocolate Chip, 1.34 oz	170	7	24
Oreo Pieces, 1.34 oz	170	8	22
Rees'es PB, 1.34 oz	130	6	19
Shapes: Chick, 0.9 oz	110	4.5	16
Bunny; Hearts 0.9 oz	120	6	15
Sugar Cookies, 1.34 oz	160	7	23

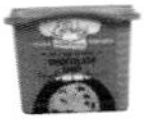
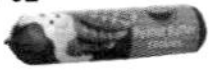
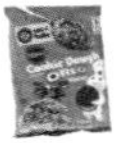
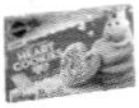

Refrigerated Sweet Buns/Rolls~ *See Page 67*

	C	F	Cb
Toll House (Nestle):			
Edible Batter, Fudge Brownie, 2 Tbsp	140	4.5	25
Edible Cookie Dough: Choc Chip, 2 T.	140	4.5	25
Funfetti, 2 Tbsp	140	4	25
PB Choc. Chip Monster, 2 Tbsp, 1.23 oz	140	5	21
Refrigerated Cookie Dough: *Per Cookie*			
Bars:			
P'B Chocolate Chip	80	4	11
Oatmeal Raisin	80	3	11
White Chip Macadamia	90	2	11
Chocolate Chip (1)	120	6	17
Chocolate Chip Lovers (1)	170	8	24
Peanut Butter (1)	130	7	15

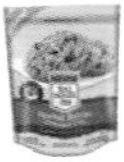
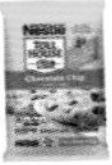

Toll House (Nestle) Cont:	C	F	Cb
Refrigerated Coookie Dough (Cont): *Per Cookie*			
Peanut Butter Chip, 1 oz	90	4.5	11
Pecan Turtle Delight (1)	180	10	21
Triple Chip, 1 oz	90	4.5	11

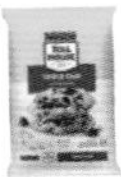

Crispbreads

Per Crispbread Unless Indicated

	C	F	Cb
Finn Crisp:			
Round: Multigrain	50	0	7.5
Original	40	0.5	8
Snacks, average all flavors, 1 oz	115	3.5	15
Thins, average all flavors	20	0.2	4
New York Flatbread Crisps,			
Everything, 3 pieces 1.1 oz	140	4	22
Ry-Krisp: Natural (2)	50	0	11
Seasoned (2)	50	0	11
Sesame (2)	50	0	9
Ryvita:			
Crispbreads: Original (4)	120	0	26
Sesame (4)	160	3	24
Thins: Caramelised Onion Flatbread (4)	120	2	21
Sweet Chilli Flatbreads (4)	110	1.5	21
WASA:			
Crispbread: Multigrain; Thin Rye (1)	35	0	8
Sourdough (1)	30	0	7
crisp'n light,			
7 Grains (3)	60	0	13
Thins: Rosemary & Sea Salt (2)	60	1.5	11
Sesame & Sea Salt (2)	60	2	10

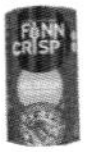

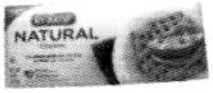

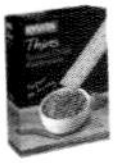
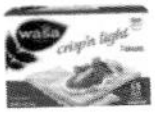 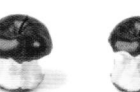
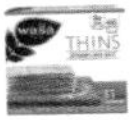

Matzos

	C	F	Cb
Manischewitz:			
Matzo: Original (1), 1 oz	110	0	24
Egg & Onion (1), 1 oz	80	0.5	17
Everything (1)	110	0.5	22
Thin Salted/Tea, average, 0.9 oz	95	0	20
Crackers:			
Tam Tams: Original (9), 1 oz	110	4	16
Unsalted (10)	120	4.5	17
Streit's:			
Matzos: Lightly Salted, (1)	110	0.5	23
Unsalted (1)	100	0	23
Moonstrips, Onion Poppy (1)	100	0.5	22

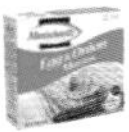
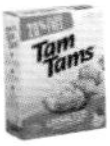

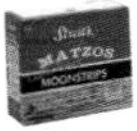

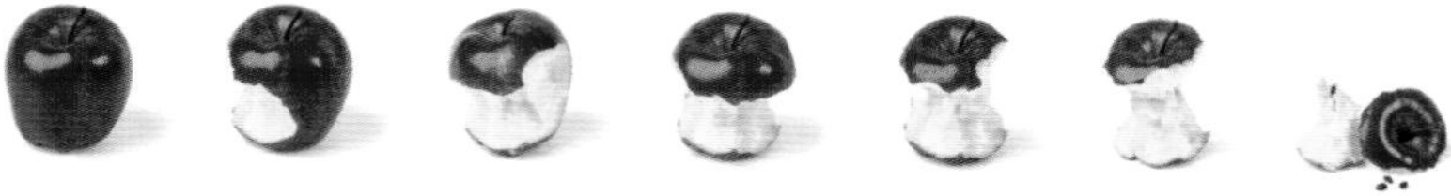

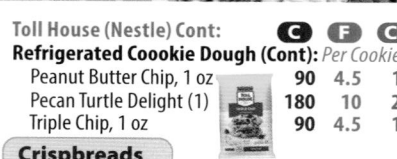

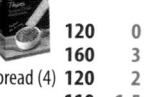

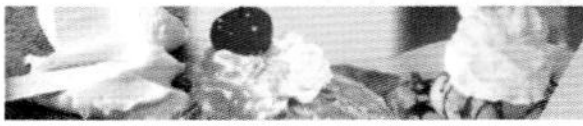

Quick Guide

Cream	C	F	Cb
Average All Brands			
Half & Half Cream:			
1 Tbsp, 0.5 oz	20	1.5	0.5
2 Tbsp, 1 oz	40	3	1
¼ cup, 2 oz	80	6	2
Light: Coffee/table (20% fat): 1 Tbsp	30	3	0.5
2 Tbsp, 1 oz	60	6	0.5
Sour Cream:			
Regular: 1 Tbsp, 0.5 oz	25	2.5	1
1 cup, 8 oz	445	45	7
Low-Fat/Light: 1 Tbsp, 0.5 oz	20	1.5	1
2 Tbsp, 1 oz	40	3	2
Fat-Free: Av., 2 Tbsp, 1 oz	20	0	3
Knudsen, 2 Tbsp, 1 oz	30	0	2
Kroger, 2 Tbsp, 1 oz	20	0	3
Sour Cream Substitute:			
Albertson's, 2 Tbsp, 1 oz	60	5	2
Tofutti, Sour Supreme, 2 Tbsp, 1 oz	85	5	9
Whipping Cream:			
Heavy, (37% fat):			
1 Tbsp fluid/2 Tbsp whipped	50	5.5	0.5
½ cup whipped	105	11	1
1 cup whipped	410	44	3.5
Light, (30% fat):			
1 Tbsp fluid/2 Tbsp whipped	45	4.5	0.5
½ cup fluid/1 cup whipped	350	37	3.5

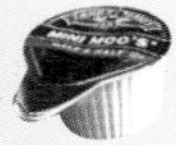
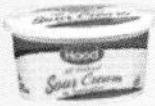
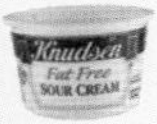
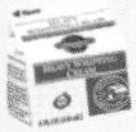

Coconut Cream/Milk

	C	F	Cb
Coconut Cream, (Canned):			
Plain/unsweetened: 2 Tbsp, 1 oz	75	6.5	3
½ cup, 4 oz	285	26	12
Sweetened:			
Coco Lopez: 1 oz	130	5	21
½ cup, 4 oz	520	20	84
Coconut Milk: (Canned):			
Thai Kitchen: Lite, ⅓ cup, 2 fl.oz	50	4.5	1
Premium/Organic, 2 fl.oz	115	10	4
Unsweetened, ⅓ cup	140	14	3
Coconut Water, (Center), 1 cup	45	0.5	9

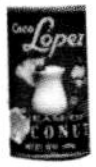
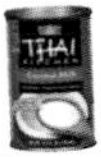

Whipped Toppings

	C	F	Cb
Average All Brands			
Cream (Pressurized): 2 Tbsp	20	1.5	1
¼ cup	40	3.5	2
Cream Topping, Lite, 2 Tbsp	20	1	3
Kraft: *Per 2 Tablespoons*			
Cool Whip: Original, 0.9 oz	25	1.5	3
Extra Creamy, 0.9 oz	25	2	2
Free, 2 Tbsp, 0.9 oz	15	0	3
Sugar Free, 0.9 oz	20	1	3

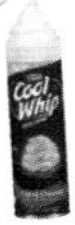
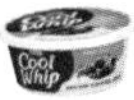

Whipped Toppings (Cont)

	C	F	Cb
Dream Whip Mix, 1/16 envolope,			
Reddi-wip:			
Original, 2 Tbsp, 0.18 oz	15	1	1
Extra Creamy, 2 Tbsp, 0.18 oz	15	1	1
Fat-Free, 2 Tbsp, 0.18 oz	5	0	1
Chocolate, 2 Tbsp, 0.18oz	15	1	1
Non Dairy: Almond, 0.18 oz	10	0.5	2
Coconut, 0.18 oz	10	0.5	2

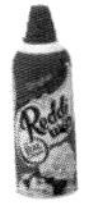

Creamers (Dairy)

	C	F	Cb
Natural Bliss: *Per Tbsp, 15 ml*			
Toasted Coconut	30	1	5
Other Flavors	35	1.5	5

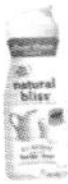

Creamers (Non-Dairy)

	C	F	Cb
Powder:			
Coffee-Mate/Cremora/N-Rich:			
Original: 1 tsp	10	0.5	1
Fat Free, 1 tsp	10	0	2
Flavors: All flavors, 0.10 oz	15	1	2
Sugar Free, all flavors, 0.07 oz	15	1	1
Liquid/Refrigerated:			
Per Tablespoon			
Baileys, Coffee Creamer,			
all flavors, 1 Tbsp, 15ml	35	1	6
Califia Farms, all flavors, 1 Tbsp	15	0	4
Coffee-Mate: *Per Tbsp, 15 ml Unless Indicated*			
Flavors: All flavors	35	1.5	5
Fat-Free, all flavors	25	0	5
Sugar free, all flavors	15	1	1
Shelf Stable, all flavors	35	1.5	5
Unflavored: Original	20	1	2
Fat-Free	10	0	1
Natural Bliss, all flavors	30	1	5
Hood, Country Creamer, 1 Tbsp	15	1	1
International Delight: *Per Tbsp*			
Regular, all flavors	35	1.5	5
Fat-Free, all flavors	30	0	7
Sugar-Free, all flavors	20	2	1
Singles, all flavors, 0.4 fl.oz	30	1	5
Kroger: *Per Tbsp*			
Coffee Creamers: Original	15	1	1
Hazelnut; White Choc Mocha	30	1	5
Fat-free, French Vanilla	25	0	5
Silk: Almond/Oat/ all flavors	25	1	4
Soy: Original	20	1.5	2
Vanilla	30	1.5	4

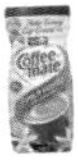
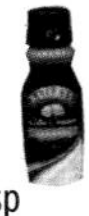
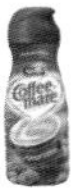
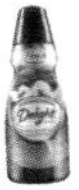
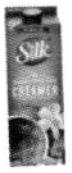

D Desserts ~ Puddings ♦ Gelatin

Ready-To-Serve

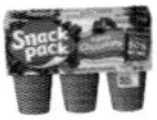
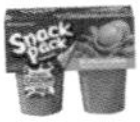
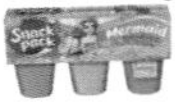
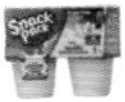
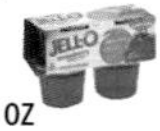

	C	F	Cb
Hunt's:			
Snack Pack Puddings:			
5.5 oz Container:			
Butterscotch	170	4	33
Chocolate	180	3.5	34
Vanilla	170	4.5	32
3.25 oz Container:			
Butterscotch	90	2.5	17
Choc.; M'maid Splashes; Unicorn Magic	100	2.5	19
Dragon Treasure	100	2	20
Tapioca	110	3	19
Vanilla	100	3	17
Sugar Free: Chocolate	70	3.5	14
Vanilla	60	3	11
Juicy Gels: All flav., 5.5 oz	160	0	39
All flavors, 3.25	90	0	21
Sugar Free, Cherry, 3.25 oz	5	0	1
Jell-O *(Kraft)*:			
Gelatin: Orig., av. all flav., 3.4 oz	70	0	17
Sugar Free, 3.2 oz	10	0	0
Puddings: *4 Packs*			
Choc. Vanilla Swirls, 3.5 oz	110	1.5	24
Strawberry Cheesecake, 3.5 oz	130	2	26
Sugar Free Puddings: *4 Packs*			
Chocolate Vanilla Swirls, 3.6 oz	60	1.5	10
Creme Brule Rice Pudding, 3.6 oz	70	2	12
Temptations: Lem. Meringue Pie, 3.4 oz	80	1.5	17
Strawberry Cheesecake, 3.5 oz	130	2.5	25
Kozy Shack:			
Flan, Creme Caramel, 1 cup, 4 oz	150	3	27
Original Puddings: *Per ½ Cup Unless Indicated*			
Chocolate, 4.6 oz	140	2.5	27
Cinn. Raisin Rice, 4.6 oz	140	2.5	26
French Vanilla Rice, 4.6 oz	140	2.5	24
Original Rice, 4.6 oz	130	2.5	24
Tapioca, 4.6 oz	130	2	25
Simply Well Puddings, average all flavors, 4 oz cup	90	1.5	14
Kroger:			
4 Pack Pudding Snacks: *Per 3.25 oz Cup*			
Butterscotch	90	2.5	17
Chocolate	100	2.5	19
Swiss Miss:			
Puddings: *Per 4 oz Cup*			
Butterscotch	130	3.5	22
Chocolate Vanilla Swirl	150	3.5	26
Creamy Milk Choc.	150	3.5	27
Tapioca; Vanilla	140	3.5	24
Triple Chocolate	160	4	27

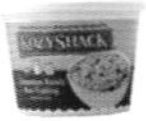
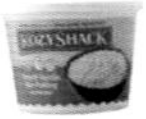
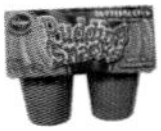
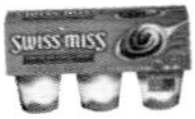

Homemade Puddings

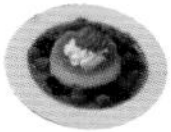
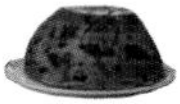

	C	F	Cb
Apple Tapioca, ½ cup	150	0	32
Bread Pudding, ½ cup	250	8	40
Blancmange, ½ cup	140	5	19
Chocolate, ½ cup	190	6	30
Crème Brulée, ½ cup	400	35	16
Plum Pudding, 2 oz	170	3	32
Rice, with Raisins, ½ cup	200	4	38
Sponge Pudding, 3.5 oz	340	16	45
Tapioca Cream, ½ cup	110	4	15
Trifle, ½ cup	180	7	26

Custards

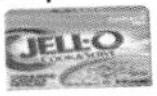

	C	F	Cb
Custard Mix *(Jello/Royal Flan)*, average:			
Dry, ¼ of 2.9 oz package, 0.7 oz	80	0	19
Prepared: whole milk, ½ cup	155	4	25
2% milk, ½ cup	140	2.5	25
Non-Fat milk, ½ cup	125	0	25
Home Made Egg Custard:			
With Whole Milk, ½ cup	170	8	18
With 2% Milk, ½ cup	155	6.5	18

Gelatin • Parfait • Jell-O

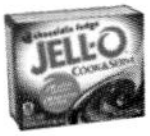
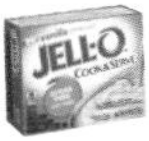
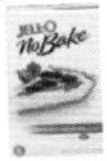

	C	F	Cb
Jell-O:			
Gelatin Dessert Mix: *Dry Mix Only*			
All flavors, 0.8 oz	80	0	19
Sugar free, all flavors, 0.3 oz	10	0	0
Cook & Serve Pudding & Pie Filling: *Dry Mix Only*			
Banana Cream, 0.77 oz	80	0	20
Butterscotch, 0.85 oz	90	0	22
Chocolate Fudge, 1 oz	100	0	25
Coconut Cream, 0.77 oz	90	2.5	17
White Chocolate, 0.8 oz	100	0	23
Sugar free, Fat-Free:			
Chocolate var., 0.3 oz	30	0	8
Vanilla, 0.2 oz	20	0	5
Instant: Banana Cream, ½ pkt, 0.85 oz	90	0	22
Butterscotch, 0.88 oz	90	0	22
No Bake Dessert Mix: *Dry Mix Only*			
Cheesecake: Classic, 1.83 oz	210	5	42
Cherry, 2.2 oz	210	4	42
Home Style, 1.87 oz	220	4.5	43
Oreo, 2 oz	260	8	47
Ida Mae, Strawberry Parfait	90	2	18
Reser's, Parfaits, Rainb.;Rasp. 3.9 oz, av.	105	2	19

Meringues

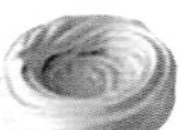

	C	F	Cb
Meringue Swirl, ½ oz	50	0	8
Meringue Shell, 1 oz	100	0	16

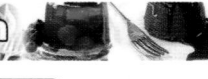

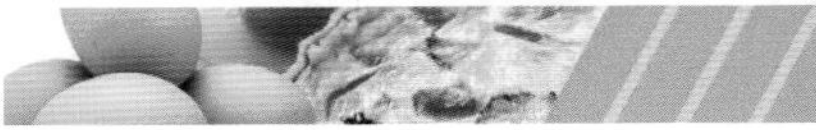

Chicken Eggs

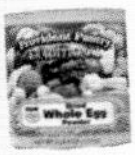

	C	F	Cb
Fresh Eggs:			
Raw:			
Small	55	4	0
Medium	65	4	0
Large	70	5	0
Extra Large	80	5.5	0
Jumbo	90	6	0
Egg Yolk, 1 extra large	55	4.5	0
Egg White, 1 extra large	17	0	0
Dried Egg Powder:			
Whole Egg: ¼ cup, 1 oz	170	12	0
1 Tbsp	30	2	0
Egg White, ¼ cup, 1 oz	105	0	0
Egg Yolk, ¼ cup, 1 oz	195	18	0

Egg Substitutes

¼ Cup (Equivalent to 1 Egg) ~ Zero Cholesterol

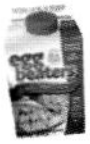

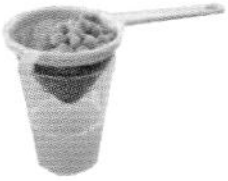

	C	F	Cb
All Whites *(Crystal Farms)*, 1.6 oz	25	0	0
Better 'n Eggs *(Crystal Farms):*			
Regular, 3 Tbsp	25	0	0
Egg Beaters *(ConAgra):*			
100% Egg White 3 Tbsp	25	0	0
Original, 3 Tbsp, 1.6 oz	25	0	0.5
Single Serve, 4 oz cup	50	0	1
Southwestern Style, 3 Tbsp, 1.6 oz	20	0	0.5
Egg Replacer *(Ener-g)*, 1.5 tsp	15	0	4
Naturegg *(Burnbrae Farms)*,			
Simply Egg White, ¼ cup, 2 oz	30	0	0
O-Organics *(Albertson's)*, Egg Whites	25	0	0
Vegan Egg Substitute:			
Aquafaba, ¼ cup, 2 oz	10	0	2

Liquid from cooked/canned beans or chickpeas. Replaces eggs and egg whites in recipes.
Extra Info: www.aquafaba.com

Other Eggs

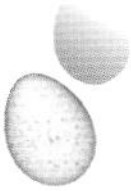

	C	F	Cb
Duck, 1 large, 2.5 oz	130	9.5	0
Goose, 1 large, 5 oz	280	19	0
Quail, 3 eggs, 1 oz	42	3	0
Turkey, 1 large, 3 oz	135	9.5	0
Turtle, 1 egg, 1.75 oz	75	5	0

Omega-3 Fat Enriched

	C	F	Cb
Egg•Land's Best, 1 large	60	4	0
Horizon Organic, 1 large	70	5	0

Note: Cholesterol content is the same as regular eggs.

Cooked Eggs

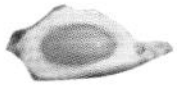

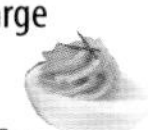

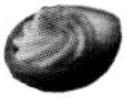

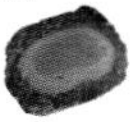

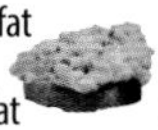

	C	F	Cb
Boiled Egg: *Same as Raw Egg*			
Hard-Cooked, Small, peeled	65	4	0
Fried Egg:			
With fat: 1 large egg	105	9	0.5
2 small eggs	175	13	1
No fat/nonstick pan, 1 large	75	5	0.5
Deviled Egg, 2 halves	145	13	0.5
Eggs Benedict, (2),			
on Toast or English Muffin	860	56	25
Eggs Florentine, (2),			
on Toast or English Muffin	890	59	25
Pickled Egg, 1 large	80	5.5	0
Poached Egg, 1 large	65	4	0
Quiche *(Homemade):*			
Egg & Bacon, 1 slice, 5.3 oz	580	43	27
Ham & Cheese, 1 slice, 5.3 oz	475	33	29
Scotch Egg, 1 egg	300	21	16
Scrambled Eggs:			
1 large egg:			
With 1 Tbsp milk + 1 tsp fat	120	9	1
With 1 Tbsp skim milk/no fat	85	5.5	1
2 large eggs:			
With 2 Tbsp milk + 2 tsp fat	260	20	2
With 2 Tbsp skim milk, w/o fat	180	11	2

Omelets

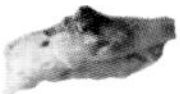

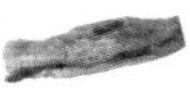

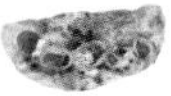

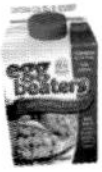

	C	F	Cb
1 Egg:			
Plain (with 1 tsp fat)	125	10	0.5
With: ½ oz cheese	175	15	0.5
½ oz cheese + ½ oz ham	200	16	0.5
2 Eggs:			
Plain (with 2 tsp fat)	250	20	1
With: 1 oz cheese	360	29	2
1 oz cheese +1 oz ham	410	32	2
3 Eggs:			
Plain (with 1 Tbsp fat)	360	29	1.5
With: 2 oz cheese	580	47	2.5
2 oz cheese+2 oz ham	680	53	2.5
Extras, Tomato/Onion/Veggies, 2 oz	20	0	4.5
Egg Substitute *(EggBeaters):*			
2 eggs (½ cup) + 1 tsp fat	100	4	2
3 eggs (¾ cup) + 2 tsp fat	160	8	3
Extras: 1 oz Cheese	110	9	1
1 oz Ham	50	3	1

Egg Nog

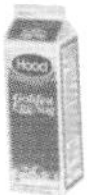

	C	F	Cb
Average all Brands,			
½ cup, 4 oz	170	8	18
Borden, Regular, 4 fl.oz	160	8	18
Hood, Golden, ½ cup, 4 fl.oz	180	9	22
Horizon, Low-Fat, 4 fl.oz	140	3	23

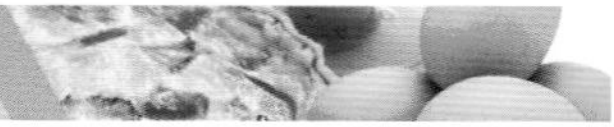

Breakfast Sides

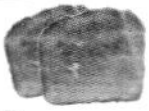
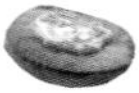
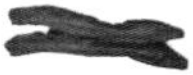
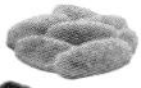
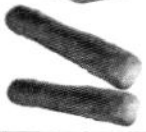

	C	F	Cb
Toast:			
Plain, 1 thick slice	85	1	13
With: 2 tsp butter/marg.	155	9	13
3 tsp/1 Tbsp fat	190	13	13
English Muffin:			
Plain, 2 oz	130	1	26
With 3 tsp fat	230	12	26
Bacon, 2 strips	70	5	0
Ham, lean, 2 oz	100	3	0
Hash Brown:			
½ cup, 3 oz	125	6.5	14
1 cup serving, 6 oz	250	13	28
Sausages, 2 oz link	180	16	1.5

Frozen Egg Breakfasts

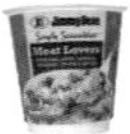
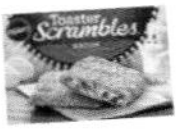
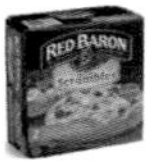

	C	F	Cb
Jimmy Dean:			
Breakfast Sandwich: *Per Sandwich*			
Biscuit, Sausage, Egg & Cheese	410	28	27
Croissant, Sausage, Egg & Cheese	400	26	29
Muffin, Meat Lovers	480	32	30
Simple Scrambles:			
Bacon, 5.32 oz pkg	290	23	4
Meat Lovers, 5.32 oz pkg	290	22	2
MorningStar Farms,			
Breakfast Muffin Sandwich,			
Veggie Sausage, Egg & Cheese	200	8	20
Pillsbury: *Per Pastry*			
Toaster Scrambles:			
Bacon, 1.8 oz	180	10	19
Bacon & Sausage	180	10	19
Sausage	180	10	19
Red Baron:			
Biscuit Scrambles:			
Bacon (1), 5.85 oz	440	21	45
Sausage (1), 5.85 oz	410	19	46

Frozen Pancake/Waffles ~ *See Page 132*
Toaster Pastries ~ *See Page 64*

Frozen Egg Rolls

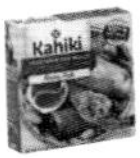
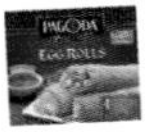

	C	F	Cb
Kahiki: *Each*			
Chicken; Vegetable, av., 2.65 oz	150	3.5	24
Pork, 2.65 oz	150	4.5	23
Teriyaki Steak, 2.5 oz	170	6	23
Lotus Restaurant:			
Imperial, Chkn/Pork (1)	160	6.5	24
Vegetarian (1)	120	5	20
Pagoda Express: *Each*			
Chicken, 2.75 oz	160	4	24
Pork, 2.75 oz	180	8	20
Vegetable, 2.75 oz	130	4	21

Fast-Foods/Restaurants

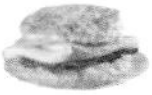
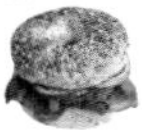
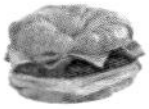
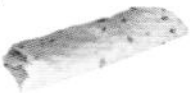
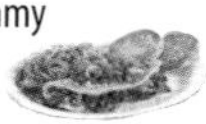
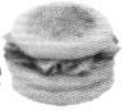
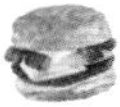
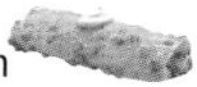
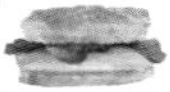

	C	F	Cb
Arby's, Bacon, Egg & Cheese Croissant	440	27	29
Au Bon Pain, 2 Egg on Plain Bagel	390	11	51
Bob Evans:			
Omelets, Low Calorie: *Without Sides*			
Three Meat & Cheese	1210	94	21
Western	650	50	11
Bojangles: Cajum Filet Biscuit	570	27	57
Bacon, Egg & Cheese Biscuit	470	27	39
Bruegger's:			
Bagel: Egg & Cheese, 6.8 oz	450	14	62
Western, 9.2 oz	560	25	64
Burger King:			
Burrito, Breakfast	375	23	27
Croissan'wich:			
Bacon, Egg & Cheese	335	18	30
Dble Ssg., Egg & Cheese	710	52	31
Ham, Egg & Cheese	335	16	31
Carl's Jr:			
Biscuit, Beyond Sausage Egg & Cheese	660	42	46
Burrito: Bacon & Egg & Cheese	580	35	32
Big Country	660	40	55
Loaded Breakfast	760	48	46
Steak & Egg	600	33	37
Chick-fil-A, Chicken, Egg & Cheese, on Sunflower Multigrain Bagel	500	20	50
Del Taco, Bacon Breakfast Burrito	640	36	38
Denny's:			
Omelettes: MyHammy	600	42	4
Ultimate	710	60	5
Dunkin Donuts:			
Bagel, Bacon, Egg & Cheese	520	18	67
Croissant, Saus., Egg & Cheese	720	52	42
Eat 'N Park:			
Omelettes: Ham & Cheese	660	47	6
Meat Lovers	750	58	6
Hardee's:			
Biscuit: Loaded Omelet	630	41	46
Southwest Omelet	660	45	42
IHOP:			
Omelette: Country	880	69	14
Spinach & Mushroom	910	71	22
Jack in the Box:			
Burritos: Grand Sausage	1070	72	70
Meat Lovers	810	51	50
McDonald's:			
Biscuit, Bacon, Egg & Cheese, reg.	460	25	39
McMuffin, Egg	300	12	30
Whataburger, Breakfast Platter, with Bacon	615	39	36

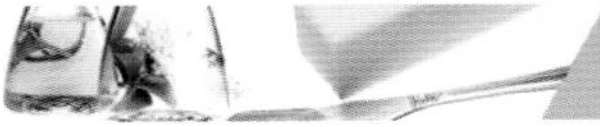

Quick Guide

Butter

Average All Brands

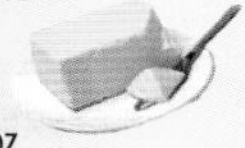
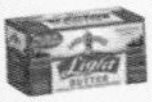
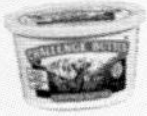
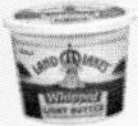

	C	F	Cb
Regular: 1 tsp, 0.2 oz	35	4	0
1 Tbsp, 0.5 oz	100	11	0
2 Tbsp, 1 oz	205	23	0
1 Stick, ½ cup, 4 oz	810	92	0
1 Pound, 2 cups, 16 oz	3255	368	0
Light: Regular, 40% Fat			
1 tsp, 0.2 oz	30	3	0
1 Tbsp, 0.5 oz	70	7.5	0
2 Tbsp, 1 oz	140	15	0
Whipped Butter: Regular			
1 tsp, 0.1 oz	20	2.5	0
1 Tbsp, 0.3 oz	65	7.5	0
1 Stick, 2 .7 oz	545	62	0
Whipped Light Butter *(Land O Lakes):*			
1 tsp, 0.15 oz	15	1.5	0
1 Tbsp, 0.4 oz	45	5	0
2 Tbsp, 0.8 oz	90	10	0

Unsalted ~ *Same as Salted*

Flavored Butter/Spreads

Average All Brands

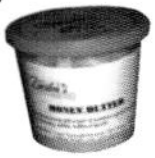
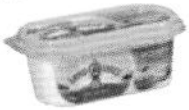

	C	F	Cb
Honey Butter, (60% Fat):			
1 Tbsp, 0.5 oz	90	8	4
Downey's, 2% Fat, 1 Tbsp, 0.5 oz	60	1	11
Garlic Butter, (80% Fat):			
1 Tbsp, 0.5 oz	100	11	0
Sweet Cream Butter:			
Land O Lakes: Reguar, 1 Tbsp	100	11	0
Honey Butter Spread, 1 Tbsp	70	6	4

Butter & Butter Blends

Per 1 Tablespoon

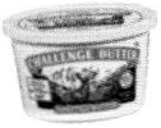
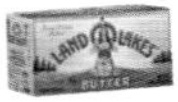

	C	F	Cb
Challenge: Stick, 0.5 oz	100	11	0
Tub, Whipped, 0.3 oz	70	7	0
Brummel & Brown,			
Spread Made with Yogurt, 0.5oz	45	5	0.5
Land O'Lakes:			
Sticks, Original, 0.5oz	100	11	0
Tubs, Butter With Olive Oil, 0.5 oz	90	10	0

Ghee (Clarified Butter)

(Example ~ *Purity Farms*)
Note: Ghee is 100% fat compared to regular butter (80% fat + 20% water)

	C	F	Cb
1 tsp, 0.2 oz	45	5	0
1 Tbsp, 0.5 oz	120	14	0

Light & Reduced Fat Spreads

Per Tablespoon

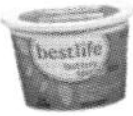
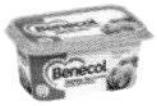
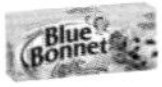

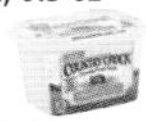
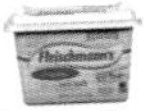
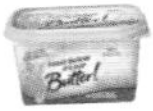
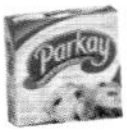
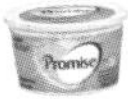
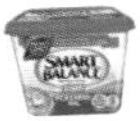

	C	F	Cb
Bestlife, Buttery Spread,			
1 Tbsp, 0.5 oz	50	5	0
Benecol: Regular, 0.5 oz	70	8	0
Light, 0.5 oz	50	5	0
Blue Bonnet:			
Stick, Lactose Free, 0.5 oz	70	7	0
Tub, Orig. Soft Spread, 0.5 oz	50	6	0
Butter Buds:			
Butter Flavored: Mix, 1 tsp	5	0	2
Sprinkles, 1 tsp	10	0	2
Country Crock *(Shedd's)*: Stick, 0.5 oz	80	8	0
Tubs: Orig; Churn Spread, 0.5 oz	50	6	0
Light Spread, 0.5 oz	35	4	0
Plant Based,			
Almond/Avocado/Ol. Oil, 0.5 oz	100	11	0
Earth Balance, Original, 1 Tbsp	100	11	0
Fleischmann's,			
Olive Oil Spread, 0.4 oz	60	6	0.5
I Can't Believe It's Not Butter!:			
Tubs: Original Spread, 0.5 oz	60	6	0
Light, 0.5 oz	40	4	0
Olive Oil Spread, 1 Tbsp	60	6	0
Molly McButter, 1 tsp	5	0	1
Parkay:			
Spread: Original, 0.4 oz	60	6	0
Light, 0.5 oz	50	6	0
Stick, Original, 0.5 oz	70	8	0.5
Promise: Activ, Spread, 0.5 oz	45	5	0
Light Spread, 0.5 oz	45	5	0
Smart Balance:			
Tubs, Buttery Spread: Original, 0.5 oz	80	9	0
EVOO, 0.4 oz	60	7	0
Light EVOO, 0.4 oz	50	5	0
Light,			
with Flaxseed Oil, 0.5 oz	50	5	0
Omega 3, Light, 0.5 oz	50	5	0

Animal Fats/Lards

Average All Types

Beef Tallow/Drippings, Lard (Pork), Chicken, Duck, Goose, Turkey:

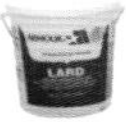

	C	F	Cb
1 Tbsp, 0.5 oz	115	13	0
2¼ Tbsp, 1 oz	255	28	0
1 cup, 7.3 oz	1850	205	0
½ pound, 8 oz	2040	227	0

Ghee/Butter/ Oil ~ *See Page 93*

Vegetable Shortening

Average All Types

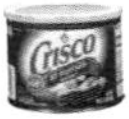

	C	F	Cb
1 Tbsp, 0.5 oz	115	13	0
2¼ Tbsp, 1 oz	250	28	0
1 cup, 7.3 oz	1810	205	0

Vegetable Oils

Includes almond, avocado, canola, corn, coconut, flaxseed, grapeseed, linseed, mustard, olive, palm, peanut, rice bran, safflower, sesame, sunflower, soybean, wheat germ. Note: Oil is 100% fat.

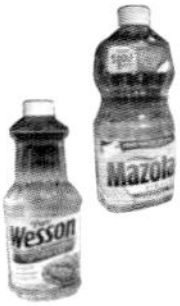

	C	F	Cb
1 tsp, 0.2 oz	45	5	0
1 Tbsp, 0.5 oz	120	14	0
2 Tbsp, 1 oz	240	28	0
1 cup, 7.3 oz	1930	205	0

Fish Oils

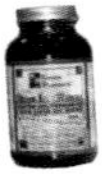

Average All Types

	C	F	Cb
(Includes Cod Liver, Herring, Salmon, Sardines): 1 Tbsp, 0.5 oz	125	14	0

Cooking Sprays/Squeezes

Cooking Sprays: (PAM, Mazola, I Can't Believe It's Not Butter, Weight Watchers, Wesson):

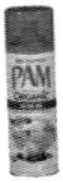

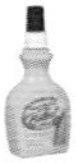

	C	F	Cb
Pam: ¼ second spray	2	0	0
1-3 second spray	6	1	0
I Can't Believe It's Not Butter, Original Spray	0	0	0
Parkay, Buttery Spray	0	0	0

Olestra (Olean)

	C	F	Cb
Olestra *(Olean)*	0	0	0

Note: Olean is Proctor & Gamble's brand name for Olestra – a no-calorie cooking oil that gives snacks (like potato chips, tortilla chips and crackers) taste and texture without adding fat or calories.

Examples:

- *Frito-Lay,* Light Products (*Lays, Ruffles, Tostitos, Doritos*)
- *Pringles,* Fat-Free Potato Crisps

Quick Guide

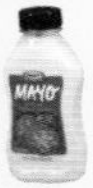

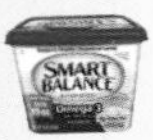

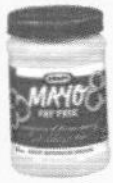

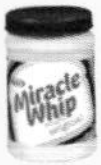

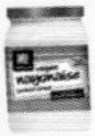

Mayonnaise:	C	F	Cb
Regular: *Per 1 Tbsp, 0.5 oz Unless Indicated*			
Average All Brands	90	10	0
Best Foods; Hellman's; Kraft:			
Original/Real	90	10	0
½ cup, 4 oz	720	80	0
Hain, Safflower Mayonnaise	100	11	0
Spectrum, Canola Mayo	100	11	0
Light/Reduced Fat: *Per 1 Tbsp, 0.5 oz*			
Best Foods/Hellman's	35	3.5	1
Kraft, Light/Olive Oil	35	3	1
Smart Balance, Omega	50	5	0
Spectrum, Light Canola Mayo, Eggless	35	3.5	0.5
Fat Free:			
Kraft: Original, 1 Tbsp	10	0	2
½ cup, 4 oz	80	0	16
Sugar Free:			
Dukes Mayo, 1 Tbsp	100	12	0
Mayonnaise Style Dressing:			
Per 1 Tbsp, 0.5 oz			
Best Foods, Sandwich Spread	60	5	2
Kraft:			
Miracle Whip Dressing:			
Original	50	5	2
Light	20	1.5	2
Fat Free	15	0	3
Mayo:			
Homestyle Rich & Creamy; Real	90	10	0
Light	35	3	2
Horseradish	50	1	2
Nasoya, Egg & Dairy Free:			
Nayonaise: Regular/Whipped	40	3.5	1
Light	20	1.5	1
Sir Kensington's, Egg/Dairy Free			
Fabanaise (Vegan Mayo)	90	10	0

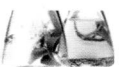

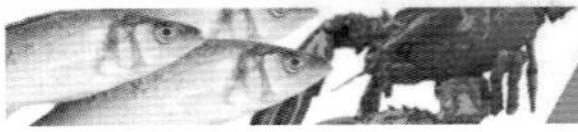

Quick Guide

Fresh Fish

Low Oil: *Less than 2.5% fat)*

White/Lightly-colored flesh. Examples:
Cod, Flounder, Haddock, Halibut, Mahi Mahi, Perch, Pike, Pollock, Snapper, Sole, Whiting.

	C	F	Cb
Raw, without bones, 4 oz	100	1	0
Steamed, broiled, baked, 4 oz	140	1.5	0
Fried: Lightly floured, 4 oz	210	8	3.5
Breaded, 4 oz	260	12	8
In Batter, 4 oz	320	16	27

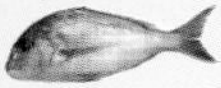

Medium Oil: *2.5-5% fat*

Lightly-colored flesh. Examples:
Bluefin Tuna, Catfish, Kingfish, Orange Roughy, Salmon (Pink), Swordfish, Rainbow Trout, Yellowtail.

	C	F	Cb
Raw, without bones, 4 oz	145	7	0
Baked/Broiled, 4 oz	195	8	0
Fried, 4 oz	230	11	8

High Oil: *Over 5% fat*

Darker-colored flesh. Examples:
Albacore Tuna, Mackerel,
Salmon (Atlantic/Chinook/Sockeye), Sardines, Trout.

	C	F	Cb
Raw, without bones, 4 oz	220	14	0
Baked/Broiled, 4 oz	275	17	0
Fried, 4 oz	340	23	12

Cooking Yields (Fin Fish):

4 oz Raw wt. = 3.5 oz Cooked weight
4 oz Cooked wt. = 5 oz Raw weight

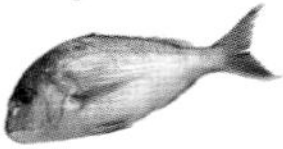

Calorie & Fat Variations:

The amount of fat/oil in fish varies with the species, season and locality. Within the same fish, fat/oil content is generally higher towards the head.

Fish & Shellfish

Edible Weights: (no bones/shell)

	C	F	Cb
Abalone: Raw, 3 oz	90	0.5	5
Fried, 3 oz	160	6	10
Ahi Tuna, grilled, 6 oz fillet (w/o fat)	235	2	0
Anchovy: Paste, 1 Tbsp, 0.5 oz	45	3	0
Canned in oil, drained, (5), 0.7 oz	40	2	0
Barracuda (Pacific), raw, 4 oz	130	3	0
Basa/Swai, raw, 4 oz fillet	70	2	0
Bass:			
Sea: Raw, 4.6 oz fillet	125	2.5	0
Baked, 3 oz	105	2	0
Striped: Raw, 1 fillet, 5.5 oz	150	3.5	0
Baked, 3 oz	105	3	0
Freshwater: Raw, 3 oz	95	3	0
Baked, 3 oz	125	4	0

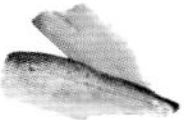

Fish & Shellfish (Cont)

Edible Weights: (no bones/shell)

	C	F	Cb
Calamari/Squid:			
Raw, 4 oz	100	1.5	3.5
Baked, 1 cup	190	6.5	5.5
Fried, 3 oz	150	6	7
Catfish:			
Farmed: Raw, 1 fillet 5.6 oz	190	9.5	0
Baked, 1 fillet 5 oz	205	10	0
Wild: Raw, 1 fillet, 5.6 oz	150	4.5	0
Baked, 1 fillet, 5 oz	150	4	0
Breaded, fried, 1 fillet, 3 oz	200	12	7
Caviar, black/red, 1 Tbsp, 16g	40	3	0.5
Clams: Raw (4 large/9 small), 3 oz	70	1	3
Breaded, fried (20 small), 6.6 oz	380	21	20
Canned, drained, ½ cup, 2.8 oz	115	1	0
Steamed (10 small), 3.3 oz	140	2	5
Cod:			
Atlantic: Raw, 4 oz	95	1	0
Baked, 3 oz	90	1	0
Canned, solids & liquid	90	0.5	0
Pacific: Raw, 4 oz	80	0.5	0
Baked, 3 oz	70	0.5	0
Crab:			
Alaska King, 1 leg, cooked, 4.7 oz	130	2	0
Blue: Raw, 1 crab, 6 oz	150	1	0
Steamed, 3 oz	70	0.5	0
Canned, drained, 6.5 oz can	105	0.5	0
Dungeness: Raw, 1 crab, 5.8 oz	140	1.5	0
Steamed, 4.45 oz	140	1.5	0
Crab Cakes *(Capt. D's)*, (1), 2.8 oz	250	16	16
Crayfish:			
Farmed: Raw, 3 oz	60	1	0
Steamed, 3 oz	75	1	0
Wild: Raw 3 oz	65	1	0
Steamed, 3 oz	70	1	0
Cuttlefish, raw, 3 oz	70	1	1
Dolphinfish ~ *See Mahi-Mahi*			
Eel: Raw, 3 oz	155	10	0
Baked, 3 oz	200	13	0
Fish & Chips *(Red Lobster)*, battered, without condiments	700	33	61
Fish Sandwich *(Burger King)*, without Tartar Sauce	340	9	49
Fish Oil, 1 Tbsp, 0.5 oz	125	14	0
Flounder/Sole:			
Raw, 4 oz	80	2	0
Baked, 3 oz	75	2	0

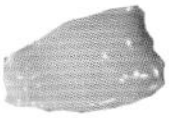
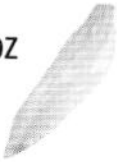
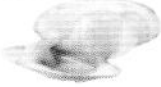
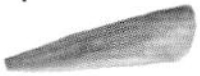
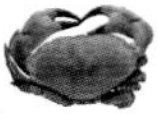
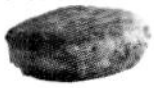
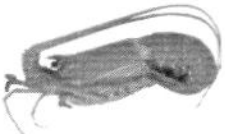
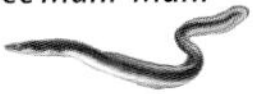
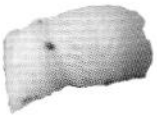

Frozen Fish ~ *See Pages 114-122*

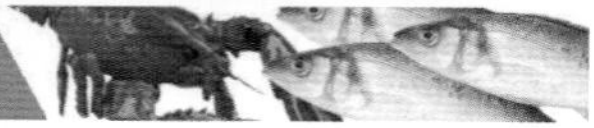

Fish & Shellfish (Cont)	C	F	Cb
Edible Weights: Without Bones or Shell			
Haddock: Raw, 4 oz	85	0.5	0
Baked, 3 oz	75	0.5	0
Smoked, 3 oz	100	1	0
Halibut:			
Atlantic: Raw, 4 oz	105	1.5	0
Baked, ½ fillet, 5.6 oz	175	2.5	0
Herring:			
Atlantic, raw, 4 oz	180	10	0
Canned: Plain, drained, 3 oz	130	8	0
In Tomato Sauce, 3.5 oz	140	8	2
Pickled, 2 pieces, 1 oz	75	5	3
Smoked, kippered, 4 oz	245	14	0
Jellyfish: Raw, 4 oz	30	0	0
Dried, Salted, 1 cup, 2 oz	20	1	0
Ling, raw, 4 oz	100	0.5	0
Lobster, Northern:			
1.5 lb Whole Lobster, edible portion:			
Raw, 6.3 oz	140	1.5	0
Boiled, 5 oz	140	1	0
Lobster Salads, average, ½ cup	220	13	5
Lobster Newberg, average, ¾ cup	360	20	9
Lobster Thermidor, av., 1 serving	370	22	15
Lobster Tail (Rock),			
Red Lobster, grilled/roasted	230	6	2
Lox, Regular/Nova, 2 oz	65	2.5	0
Mackerel, Atlantic: Raw, 4 oz	230	16	0
Baked, 3 oz fillet	225	15	0
Pacific/Jack: Raw, 4 oz	180	9	0
Baked, 3 oz	170	9	0
Spanish: Raw, 4 oz	160	7	0
Baked, 3 oz	135	5.5	0
Mahi-Mahi/Dolphinfish:			
Raw, 4 oz	95	1	0
Baked, 4 oz	125	1	0
Monkfish: Raw, 4 oz	85	1.5	0
Baked, 3 oz	80	2	0
Mullet, Striped: Raw, 4 oz	135	4.5	0
Baked, 3 oz	130	4	0
Mussels:			
Raw: 4 oz (edible wt)	100	2.5	4
1 cup, 5.3 oz (edible weight)	130	3.5	5
Cooked, moist heat, 3 oz	150	4	6
Ocean Perch:			
Atlantic: Raw, 4 oz	90	2	0
Baked, 3 oz	80	1.5	0
Octopus:			
Common: Raw, 4 oz	95	1	3
Boiled, 3 oz	140	2	4
Orange Roughy:			
Raw, 4 oz	85	1	0
Baked, 3 oz	90	1	0

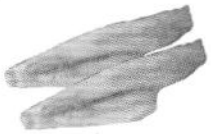
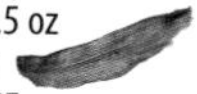
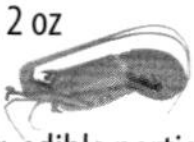
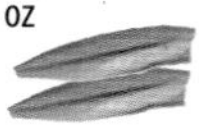
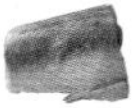
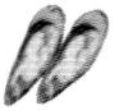
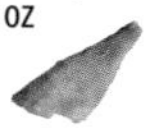
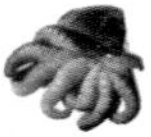
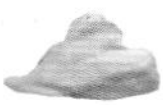

Fish & Shellfish (Cont)	C	F	Cb
Edible Weights: Without Bones or Shell			
Oysters, Common, Raw, 3 oz	70	2	4
Eastern:			
Farmed: Raw, 6 medium, 3 oz	50	1.5	5
Cooked, dry heat, 6 med., 2 oz	45	1.5	5
Wild: Raw, 6 medium, 3 oz	45	1.5	3
Cooked, dry heat, 6 med., 2 oz	45	1.5	3
Breaded & Fried, 6 med., 3 oz	175	11	10
Pacific: Raw, 1 medium, 1.8 oz	40	1	3
Steamed, 1 medium, 0.8 oz	40	1	3
Perch ~ *See Ocean Perch*			
Pike: Northern: Raw, 4 oz	100	1	0
Baked, 3 oz	95	1	0
Walleye: Raw, 4 oz	105	1.5	0
Baked, 3 oz	100	1.5	0
Pollock, Atlantic: Raw, 4 oz	105	1	0
Baked, 3 oz	100	1	0
Pompano, Florida, raw, 4 oz	185	11	0
Red Snapper ~ *See Snapper*			
Roe, raw, 2 Tbsp, 1 oz	40	2	0.5
Sablefish: Raw, 4 oz	220	17	0
Smoked, 3 oz	220	17	0
Salmon:			
Atlantic, Farmed: Raw, 4 oz	235	15	0
Baked, 3 oz	175	10	0
Steaks: Raw, 7 oz	410	27	0
Baked, 6 oz	365	22	0
Atlantic, Wild: Raw, 4 oz	160	7	0
Baked, 3 oz	155	7	0
Steaks: Raw, 7 oz	280	13	0
Baked, 6 oz	310	14	0
Chinook: Raw, 4 oz	205	12	0
Baked, 3 oz	195	11	0
Smoked, 3 oz	100	3.5	0
King: Raw, 3.5 oz	185	12	0
Kippered, 3.5 oz piece	265	16	0
Smoked & canned, 3.5 oz	150	6	0
Coho:			
Farmed: Raw, 4 oz	180	8.5	0
Baked, 3 oz	150	7	0
Wild: Raw, 4 oz	165	6.5	0
Steamed, 3 oz	155	6.5	0
Pink/Chum: Raw, 4 oz	145	5	0
Baked, 3.5 oz	155	5.5	0
Canned: Drained solids, 11 oz	435	16	0
Without skin & bones, 8.5 oz	330	10	0
Sockeye: Raw, 4 oz	160	6.5	0
Baked, 3 oz	145	5.5	0
Canned, Drained solids, 3 oz	140	6.5	0
Smoked, 3.5 oz	205	7.5	0
Salmon Cake (1), 3 oz	240	15	6

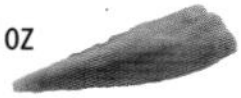
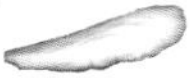
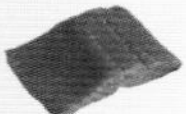
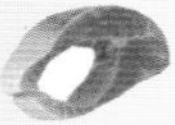
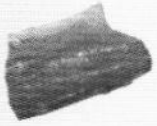
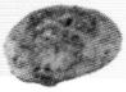

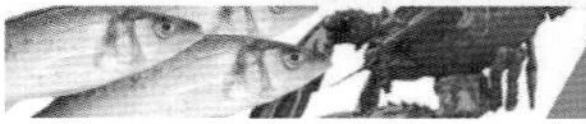

Fish & Shellfish (Cont)

	C	F	Cb
Sardines: *Canned, Average all Brands*			
Drained of Oil:			
¼ cup drained, 2.2 *oz*	**130**	9	0
3.75 oz can, drained, 3.3 oz	**190**	11	0
1 large/2 medium, ⅗", 0.8 oz	**50**	3	0
in Tomato Sauce, 3.8 oz	**150**	8	3
Sashimi ~ *See Japanese Foods, Page 171*			
Scallops: Raw, 6 lge/15 small, 3 oz	**65**	0.5	3
Breaded, Fried (6), 5 oz	**385**	20	39
Steamed, 3 oz	**95**	0.5	0
Sea Bass ~ *See Bass*			
Seafood Salad, Deli Style, ½ cup, 3.5 oz	**250**	21	11
Shark: Raw, 4 oz	**145**	5	0
Baked, 4 oz	**185**	7	0
Batter-dipped, fried, 4 oz	**260**	16	7
Shrimp:			
Raw: Small/Medium (4), 0.8 oz	**15**	0	0
Large (4), 1 oz	**20**	0	0
Breaded & Fried, 4.8 oz	**395**	24	27
Steamed, in shell, 3 oz	**100**	1.5	0
Canned, 1 can, 4.5 oz	**130**	2	0
Snapper: Raw, 4 oz	**115**	1.5	0
Baked: 3 oz	**110**	1.5	0
6 oz fillet	**220**	3	0
Sole: Raw, 4 oz	**80**	2	0
Baked, 3 oz	**75**	2	0
Squid ~ *see Calamari*			
Surimi, (Imitation Crab), 4 oz	**110**	0.5	17
Swai/Basa, raw, 4 oz	**70**	2	0
Swordfish: Raw, 4 oz	**165**	7.5	0
Medium Steak, 6 oz	**250**	11	0
Baked: Small Steak, 4 oz	**205**	7	0
Medium Steak, 6 oz	**290**	13	0
Tilapia: Raw, 4 oz	**110**	2	0
Baked: 3 oz	**110**	2.5	0
Trout, Rainbow:			
Farmed: Raw, 4 oz	**160**	7	0
Baked, 3 oz	**145**	6.5	0
Wild: Raw, 4 oz	**135**	4	0
Baked, 3 oz	**130**	5	0
Tuna:			
Raw: Bluefin, 4 oz	**165**	5.5	0
Skipjack, Yellowfin, av., 4 oz	**120**	1	0
Baked: Bluefin, 3 oz	**155**	5.5	0
Skipjack, Yellowfin, av., 3 oz	**110**	1	0
Canned: *in Water, drained*			
Chunk Light: 2 oz	**50**	1	0
3 oz can	**75**	1.5	1
5 oz can	**125**	2.5	1.5
Tuna (Cont): *in Water, drained (Cont)*			
Solid White: 2 oz	**60**	0.5	0
5 oz can	**150**	1.5	0
7 oz can	**210**	2	0
in Oil, drained:			
Chunk Light: 2 oz can	**80**	4	0
5 oz can	**200**	10	0
Solid White: 2 oz can	**90**	4	0
6 oz can	**270**	12	0
Whitefish: Raw, 4 oz	**150**	6.5	0
Baked, 3 oz	**145**	6.5	1
Smoked, 3 oz	**90**	1	0
Whiting: Raw, 4 oz	**100**	1.5	0
Baked, 3 oz	**100**	1.5	0
Yellowtail: Raw, 4 oz	**165**	6	0
Grilled, 3 oz	**160**	6	0

Other Canned/Packaged Fish

	C	F	Cb
Bumble Bee: *Skinless, Boneless*			
Mackerel, in oil, drained, 1.9 oz	**160**	15	0
Pink/Red Salmon, av., 3 oz	**115**	4.5	0.5
Sardines, in oil, drained, 2.6 oz	**160**	12	0
Tuna: *Drained*			
Chunk, Light, in water, 3 oz	**60**	0.5	0.5
Prime Fillets: Solid White, 4 oz	**140**	1.5	0
with Chipotle & Olive Oil, 2 oz	**140**	9	1
Pouch, in water, 5 oz	**190**	6	0
Solid White, in oil, drained, 4 oz	**160**	5	0
Snack Kits, per 2.5 oz Pouches:			
Cracked Pepper	**60**	0.5	0.5
Jalapeno Seasoned	**70**	0	2
Spicy Thai Chili	**90**	1	8
Sun-Dried Tomato & Basil	**60**	0	2
Chicken of the Sea: *Drained*			
Pink Salmon: Skinless/boneless: 3 oz	**80**	2	0
Traditional, 14.75 oz can, 2.1 oz serve	**90**	5	0
Sardines, in oil, smoked, 3.75 oz can	**150**	10	0
Tuna: Chunk In Water, 5 oz can, 2 oz sv.	**50**	1	0
Solid in Water, 5 oz can, 2 oz serving	**60**	1	0
Starkist:			
Lunch To Go Kit, Tuna Salad, 4.1 oz	**260**	9	25
Pouch: *Per 2.6 oz Pouch*			
Albacore White Tuna in water	**80**	1.5	0
Pink Salmon in Water	**70**	1	1
Ready To Eat Kit:			
Ranch Tuna Salad, 3.28 oz	**130**	3.5	13
Sweet & Spicy Tuna Salad, 2.75 oz	**70**	0.5	7
Salmon Creations:			
Lemom Dill, 2.6 oz	**70**	1	0.5
Mango Chipotle, 2.6 oz	**90**	1	5
Tuna Creations:			
Bold Thai Chili Style, 2.6 oz	**90**	1	7
Herb & Garlic, 2.6 oz	**110**	4	2

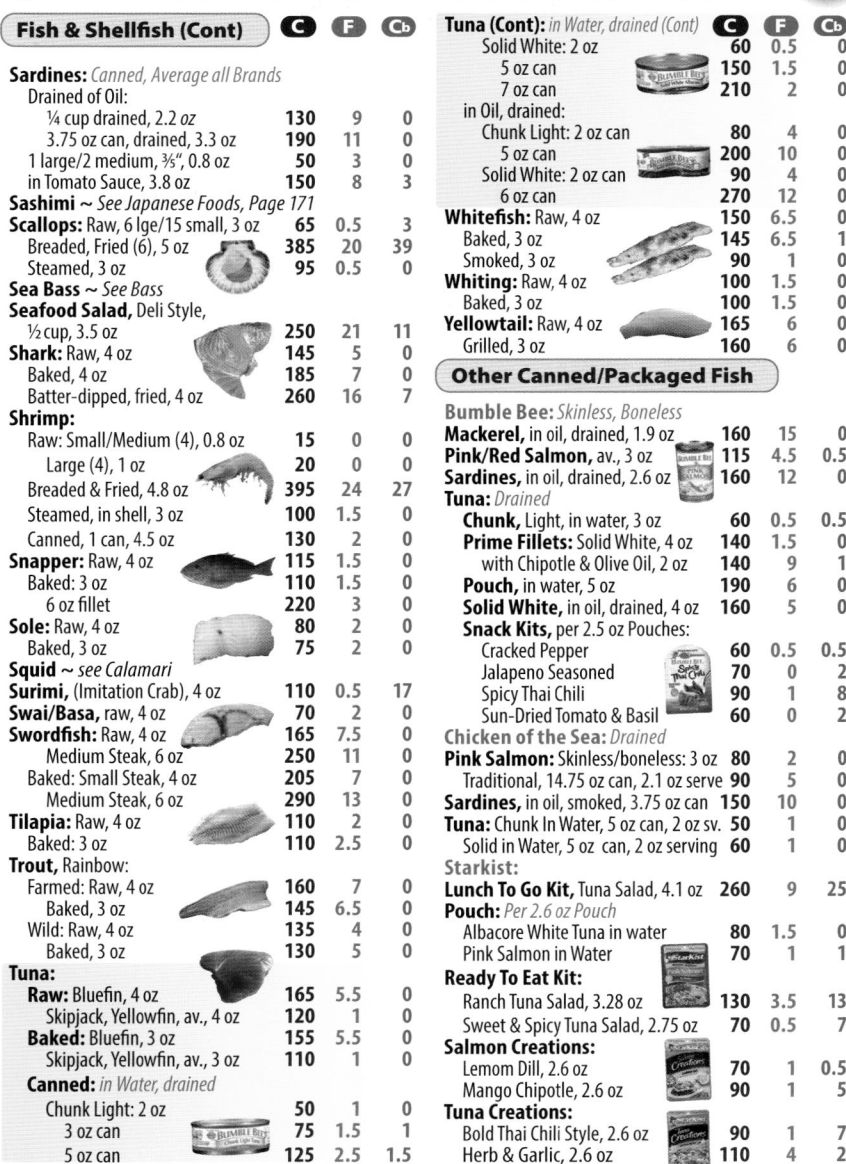

F Flours & Grains

Flours & Grains	C	F	Cb
Amaranth Flour *(Bob's Red Mill)*,			
½ cup, 2.2 oz	220	4	40
Arrowroot Flour, ½ cup, 2.3 oz	230	0	56
Barley: Grain, regular, ½ cup, 2.6 oz	255	1	55
Pearled, raw, 3.5 oz	350	1	78
Buckwheat: Grain, ½ cup, 3 oz	290	3	61
Flour, whole-groat, ½ cup, 2 oz	200	2	42
Groats: Roasted, dry, ½ cup, 3 oz	285	2	62
Roasted, cooked, 3.5 oz	80	0.5	17
Bulgur: Dry, ½ cup, 2.5 oz	240	1	53
Cooked, ½ cup, 3.2 oz	75	0.5	17
Carob Flour, ½ cup, 1.8 oz	115	0.5	46
Coconut Flour, 2 Tbsp, 0.6 oz	60	3.5	10
Corn Kernels, cooked, av., ½ cup	80	0.5	18
Corn Bran, ½ cup, 1.3 oz	85	0.5	33
Corn Flour/Masa, ½ cup, 2 oz	215	2.5	43
Corn Grits:			
Dry, ½ cup, 2.8oz	290	1	62
Cooked, ½ cup, 4.3 oz	70	0.5	15
Corn Germ, toasted, ½ cup, 4 oz	100	1.5	22
Cornmeal, average all varieties:			
3 Tbsp, 1 oz	105	0.5	22
½ cup, 2.5 oz	255	1	54
Mixes, same as above	230	1	48
Cornstarch: 1 Tbsp, 0.3 oz	30	0	8
½ cup, 2.3oz	245	0	58
Couscous: Dry, 1 oz	110	0	22
Cooked, 1 cup, 5.5 oz	175	0.5	37
Farina: Dry, ½ cup, 3 oz	325	0.5	69
Cooked, ½ cup, 4 oz	55	0	12
Flaxseed: Whole, 1 T., 0.3 oz	45	3.5	2
Ground, 2 Tbsp, 0.3 oz	60	4.5	4
Garbanzo, (Chick Pea), ½ cup, 1.6 oz	180	3	27
Gluten Free Flour, 3 Tbsp	100	0	24
Hemp Flour, Wholemeal, ½ cup, 3.5 oz	300	10	5
Matzo Meal, ½ cup, 2.2 oz	230	0.5	48
Millet: Raw, ½ cup, 3.5 oz	380	4	73
Cooked, ½ cup, 3 oz	105	1	21
Oat Bran: Raw, ⅓ cup, 1 oz	75	2	21
Cooked, ½ cup, 3.8 oz	45	1	13
Oats, Rolled/Oatmeal:			
Dry/Groats, ½ cup, 1.5 oz	160	3	28
Cooked, ½ cup, 4.2 oz	75	1	13
Polenta ~ *See Cornmeal*			
Potato Flour, ½ cup, 2.8 oz	285	0.5	66
Psyllium Husks, 1 Tbsp, 0.2 oz	10	0	4
Quinoa: Dry, ½ cup, 3 oz	320	5	59
Cooked, ½ cup, 3.8 oz	130	2	24
Rice Bran, ½ cup, 2 oz	180	12	28
Rice Flour, ½ cup, 2.8 oz	290	1	63

Flours & Grains (Cont)	C	F	Cb
Rice Polish, ½ cup, 3.5 oz	360	0.5	80
Rye Flour:			
Dark, ½ cup, 2.3 oz	210	2	44
Light, ½ cup, 1.8 oz	190	1	41
Medium, ½ cup, 1.8 oz	180	1	40
Rye Grain: ½ cup, 3 oz	280	2	59
Flakes, ¼ cup, 1 oz	100	0.5	21
Semolina Flour, ½ cup, 3 oz	300	1	61
Sorghum, ½ cup, 3.4 oz	325	3	72
Soy Flour:			
Defatted, 1 cup, 3.5 oz	330	1	38
Low-Fat, 1 cup, 3 oz	325	6	33
Full-Fat, 1 cup, 3 oz	365	17	29
Soy Meal, defatted, 1 cup, 4.3 oz	415	3	49
Spelt Flour, ½ cup, 2 oz	190	1	41
Tapioca Pearl:			
Dry, ½ cup, 2.7 oz	270	0	67
3 Tbsp, 1 oz	100	0	25
Teff Seed Flour, 2 oz	215	2	42
Tortilla Flour Mix,			
½ cup, 2 oz	220	6	37
Triticale:			
½ cup, 3.4 oz	325	2	70
Flour, wholegrain, ½ cup, 2.3 oz	220	1	48
Wheat Bran, unprocessed, ½ cup, 1 oz	65	1	19
Wheat Flakes, ½ cup, 1.5 oz	160	1	35
Wheat Germ:			
Raw, ¼ cup, 1 oz	105	3	15
Toasted, ¼ cup, 1 oz	110	3	14
Wheat Flour:			
White, All Purpose/Self-Rising:			
1 level Tbsp, 0.3 oz	30	0	6
½ cup, 2.2 oz	230	0.5	48
1 cup, 4.4 oz	455	1.5	95
Whole Wheat, 1 cup, 4.2 oz	405	2	87

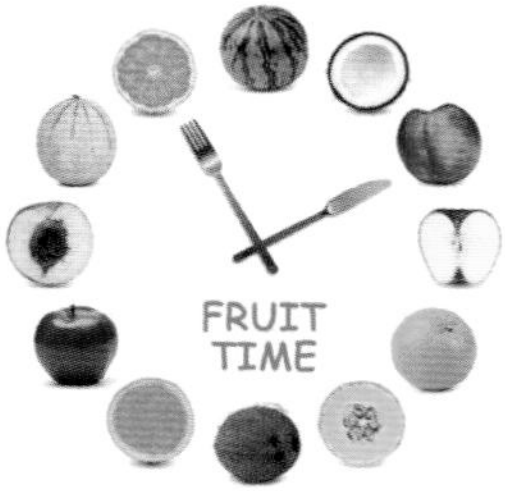

Fruit ~ Fresh

Weights As Purchased

	C	F	Cb
Apples, all varieties, average:			
Whole, with skin:			
1 small, 4 oz	55	0	14
1 medium, 5.5 oz	75	0	19
1 large, 8 oz	110	0	28
1 extra large, 11 oz	145	0	36
Flesh only, no skin or core: 1 oz	15	0	3.5
Slices, 1 cup, 4 oz	55	0	14
Candy/Caramel Apple, 1 med., 6.5 oz	245	4	54
Chiquita, Apple Bites, 14 slices, 5 oz	80	0	20
Apricots: 1 small, 1.5oz	20	0	4
1 medium, 2 oz	25	0	6
1 large, 3 oz	40	0	10
1 extra large, 4 oz	50	0	12
Asian Pear, (Nashi Fruit), 1 med., 7 oz	85	0	21
Avocado:			
Fuerte (Florida) variety:			
¼ medium, 2.7 oz pulp	90	7.5	6
½ medium, 5.4 oz pulp	180	15	12
Mashed, 2 Tbsp, 1 oz	35	3	2
Hass variety (Californian/Mexican):			
Cubes, ½ cup, 2.5 oz	120	11	6
Mashed: 2 Tbsp, 1 oz	50	4	2
¼ cup, 2 oz	95	8	5
Pulp: ¼ medium, 1.5 oz	70	6.5	3
½ medium, 3 oz	140	13	7
1 medium (8.5 oz whole), 6 oz	280	26	14
Salad slices (3), 1 oz	50	4	2

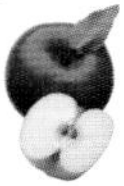
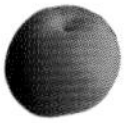
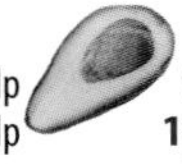
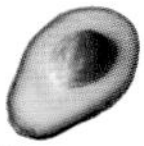

Note: The fat of avocados is heart-healthy. Avocados are very low in carbs ~ most is fiber. This benefits blood sugar and cholesterol levels. Use in place of butter and other high-fat spreads.

	C	F	Cb
Banana:			
Weight with skin:			
1 baby, 3 oz	50	0	12
1 small (5"), 4 oz	65	0	16
1 medium (7"), 5 oz	80	0	20
1 large (8"), 8 oz	120	0	30
1 extra large (9"), 9 oz	135	0	34
Flesh only, weight without skin:			
Mashed, ½ cup, 4 oz	100	0	25
Slices, ½ cup, 2.5 oz	65	0	16
Green Bananas, weight with skin:			
1 medium (7"), 5 oz	75	0	18
1 large (8"), 7 oz	110	0	27
Blackberries, 1 cup, 5 oz	60	0.5	14
Blueberries: ¼ cup, 1 oz	15	0	4
1 cup or ½ pint ctn, 5 oz	80	0	20
1 pint container, 10 oz	160	0	40

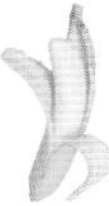
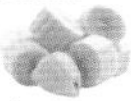
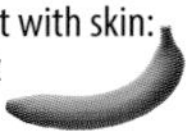
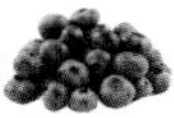

Weights As Purchased

	C	F	Cb
Boysenberries, 1 cup, 4.5 oz	60	4.5	14
Breadfruit, ½ cup, 4 oz	115	0	30
Cactus Fruit:			
1 small, 2 oz	15	0	4
1 medium, 5 oz	40	0	9
1 large, 7 oz	55	0	13
Pulp, no skin, 1 cup, 5.3 oz	60	0	14
Cantaloupe: Flesh, without skin, 1 oz	10	0	2
Pieces/Balls, 1 cup, 5.5 oz	55	0	13
Slices, ½ circle, without rind:			
1 thin (buffet), ⅛"), 0.5 oz	5	0	1
1 medium (¼"), 1 oz	10	0	2
1 thick (½"), 2 oz	20	0	5
Wedges, length cut, without skin:			
1 thin, 1/16 medium, 2 oz	20	0	5
1 thick, ⅛ medium, 4 oz	40	0	9
Whole, weight with seeds and skin:			
½ small, 20 oz	195	1	46
½ medium, 28 oz	270	1.5	65
½ large, 2.5 lb	370	2	90
Cape Gooseberries, 1 cup, 5 oz	70	1	15
Cherimoya: Pulp, ½ cup, 3 oz	60	0	14
1 Fruit (11 oz), 8 oz edible	170	1	40
Cherries, (Red/White), sweet, raw:			
6 medium or 4 large, 2 oz	30	0	7
1 cup, 4.5 oz	75	0	18
½ lb quantity	130	0	32
Sour, red, raw, 1 cup, 4 oz	50	0	12
Clementine, 1 medium, 2.6 oz	35	0	9
Coconut, raw:			
Young, sweet,			
Pieces: 1 piece (2" x 2"), 1.5 oz	35	2	4
½ cup, 3.5 oz	80	5	9
Mature, hard, 1 piece (2"x 2"), 1.5 oz	160	15	6
Crabapples, slices, ½ cup, 2 oz	40	0	11
Cranberries,			
fresh, ¼ cup, 1 oz	25	0	6.5
Custard Apple ~ *See Cherimoya*			
Dates: Medium (1), 0.3 oz	20	0	5
Large Medjool (1), 0.5 oz	40	0	10
Extra Large Medjool (1), 0.9 oz	65	0	16
Chopped, ½ cup, 3 oz	240	0	58
Dragon Fruit, (Pitahaya):			
1 medium, 4" long, 12 oz	60	0	12
1 large, 5"long, 16 oz	80	0	18
Durian, pulp, 4 oz	165	6	31
Elderberries, ½ cup, 2.5 oz	55	0.5	13

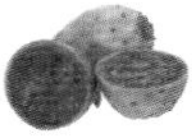
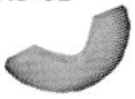
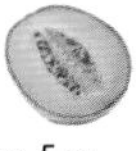
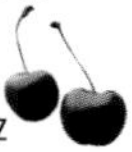
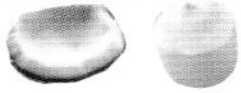
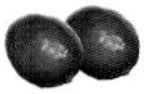
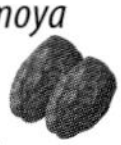
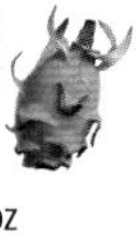

F Fruit ~ Fresh 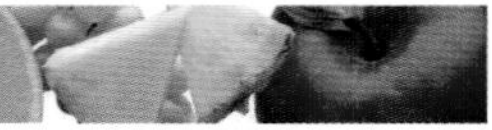

Weights As Purchased	C	F	Cb
Feijoa, (Pineapple Guava), 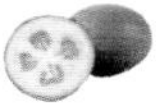			
1 medium, 2 oz	**30**	0.5	5.5
Figs, green/black: 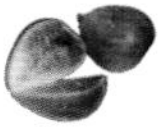			
1 medium, 2 oz	**40**	0	10
1 large, 3 oz	**60**	0	15
Gooseberries, raw, 1 cup, 5 oz	**65**	1	15
Grapefruit, all varieties, average: 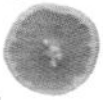			
½ fruit, 10 oz (6 oz flesh)	**55**	0	13
1 cup sections w/ juice, 8 oz	**75**	0	18
Grapes: Average, 1 cup, 5.5 oz 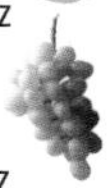	**105**	0	28
1 small bunch, 4 oz	**80**	0	20
1 medium bunch, 7 oz	**140**	0	36
1 large bunch, 16 oz	**315**	0	82
Granadilla, pulp, ½ cup, 4 oz	**110**	0	27
Guanabana, pulp, ½ cup, 4 oz	**75**	0	19
Guava, 1 medium, 4 oz 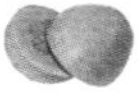	**80**	1	16
Honeydew: 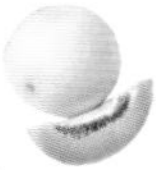			
1 slice, ¾" thick, 3 oz	**30**	0	7
1 wedge (⅛ of 7" diameter), 12 oz (with rind)	**80**	0	20
Cubes/Balls, 1 cup, 6 oz	**60**	0	14
½ small (4½ lb whole)	**180**	0.5	42
½ medium (6 lb whole)	**230**	1	56
Honey Murcots, 1 only, 5 oz	**45**	0	11
Jaboticaba, 1 cup, 5.5 oz	**55**	0	14
Jackfruit, flesh, ⅛, 4 oz 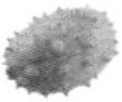	**105**	0	27
Kiwano, ½ medium, 5 oz	**35**	0	8
Kiwifruit: 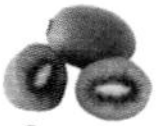			
1 Medium, 2.7 oz	**45**	0	11
1 Large, 3.2 oz	**55**	0	13
Langsat, Duku, 1 medium, 2 oz	**25**	0	5
Lemons: 1 medium, 5oz 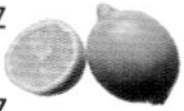	**20**	0	4
1 wedge, 1 oz	**5**	0	1
Limes, 1 medium, 2.4 oz	**20**	0	7
Loganberries, frozen, ½ cup, 2.5 oz	**40**	0	9
Longans, 5 fruit, 0.5oz 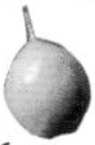	**10**	0	2.5
Loquats, 4 fruit, 2.3 oz	**30**	0	8
Lychees, 4 fruit, 2.3 oz	**30**	0	7
Mamey Apple, cubes, 1 cup, 6 oz	**85**	1	20
Mandarin Orange: 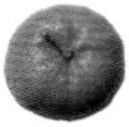			
1 small, 3 oz	**35**	0	9
1 medium, 4 oz	**45**	0	11
1 large, 6 oz	**50**	0	13
Mango: 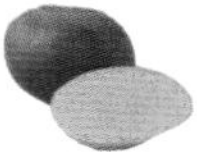			
Slices, ½ cup, 3 oz	**55**	0	14
1 small mango, 7 oz	**90**	0.5	24
1 medium: 10 oz	**130**	0.5	34
Side cheek, 4 oz	**60**	0	14
1 large, 17 oz	**220**	1	58
1 extra large, 24 oz	**310**	1.5	82
Marionberries, 1 cup, 5 oz 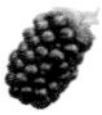	**75**	1	15

Weights As Purchased	C	F	Cb
Melons, all varieties, average, 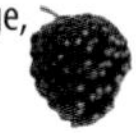			
cubes/balls, 1 cup, 6 oz	**60**	0	14
Mulberries, 20 fruit, 1 oz	**15**	0	3
Nashi Fruit/Asian Pear, 1 med. 7 oz	**85**	0	21
Nectarines: 1 medium, 5oz 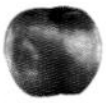	**60**	0	14
1 large, 7 oz	**80**	0	18
Oheloberries, ½ cup, 2.5 oz	**20**	0	5
Olives, Pickled: Green, 10 lge, 1.5 oz	**60**	6.5	1.5
Ripe, Greek Style, 10 medium, 1 oz	**70**	6	4
Ripe (Black) Californian:  			
1 small/medium	**5**	0	0.2
1 large/extra large	**6**	0.5	0.5
1 jumbo	**7**	0.5	0.5
1 colossal	**11**	1	0.5
Oranges, all varieties, average, weights with skin: 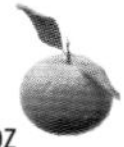			
1 small, (2.5" diam.), 5 oz	**45**	0	11
1 medium (3") 7 oz	**75**	0	18
1 large, (3.5") 10 oz	**105**	0	25
1 extra large, (4"), 14 oz	**130**	0	30
Flesh/Pulp only, 1 cup, 6 oz	**85**	0	21
Peel, 1 Tbsp	**0**	0	0
California Navel (3"), 7 oz	**70**	0	17
California Valencia, 1 medium (2¾" diam.) 6 oz	**60**	0	14
Florida Orange, 1 med., 7 oz 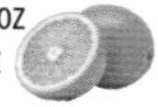	**70**	0	17
Sunkist Navel, large, 14 oz	**130**	0	30
Papaya: 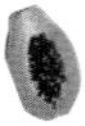			
1" pieces, 1 cup, 5 oz	**60**	0	15
1 medium, 16 oz	**120**	0	30
Green (unripe), ½ cup, 3.5 oz	**20**	0	5
Passionfruit: 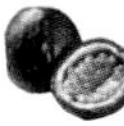			
1 small, 1.5 oz	**15**	0	3
1 large, 2.7 oz	**30**	0	6
Pulp, ½ cup, 4 oz	**110**	0	27
Peaches: 1 baby/donut, 3 oz 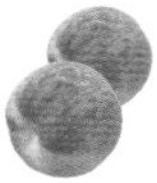	**30**	0	7
1 small, 5 oz	**50**	0	12
1 medium, 6 oz	**60**	0	14
1 large, 7 oz	**70**	0	16
1 extra large, 9 oz	**90**	0	21
Pears, all varieties, average: 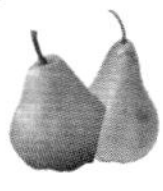			
1 mini, 2.5 oz	**35**	0	8
1 small, 5 oz	**75**	0	18
1 medium, 7 oz	**100**	0	25
1 large, 9 oz	**130**	0	33
1 extra large, 12 oz	**170**	0	42
Pepino, ½ medium, 4 oz 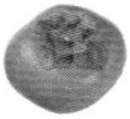	**20**	0	4
Persimmons: Native, 1 oz	**35**	0	9
Japanese (2½"d. x 2½"h), 7 oz	**120**	0	30
Maui, seedless, 1 medium, 5 oz	**100**	0	25

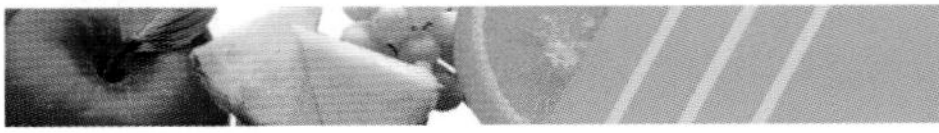

Weights As Purchased	C	F	Cb
Pineapple, average all varieties:			
Weights without skin: 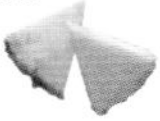			
1 thin slice (½"), 2 oz	30	0	7
1 thick slice (¾"), 3 oz	40	0	10
1 cup, chunks, 6 oz 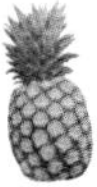	80	0	20
Whole fruit, wt with skin:			
Baby/Mini, 16 oz	150	0	39
Medium size, 3 lbs	450	1	118
Canned ~ *See Page 102*			
Pitanga, (Surinam-Cherry) (5), 1.2 oz	10	0	2
Plaintain:			
Fresh/Raw, weight with skin: 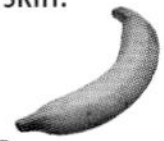			
1 medium, 10 oz	220	0	55
Slices, 1 cup, 5 oz	180	0	44
Cooked:			
Mashed, ½ cup, 3.5 oz	115	0	30
Slices, 1 cup, 5.5 oz	180	0	47
Fried in oil: 10 slices (¼"), 2 oz	160	6	26
1 cup, 4.2 oz	360	14	58
Plums, all varieties, average:			
1 mini/Damson, (1" diam), 0.5 oz	10	0	1.5
1 small (2"), 2.3oz 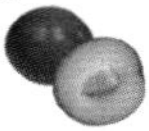	30	0	7
1 medium (2½"), 3.5 oz	45	0	10
1 large (3"), 5 oz	60	0	14
Plumcot, 1 medium, 6 oz	75	0	18
Pomegranate: 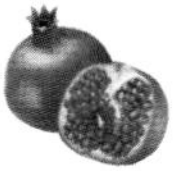			
1 small (3"), 5.5 oz	70	1	15
1 medium (3½"), 10 oz	125	2	27
1 large (4"), 16 oz	230	3	50
Seeds/Arils, ¼ cup, 2 oz	40	1	10
Pomelo, flesh, ½ cup, 3.5 oz	35	0	9
Prickly Pear ~ *See Cactus Fruit*			
Quince, 1 medium, 3.5 oz 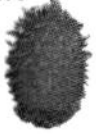	55	0	14
Rambutan/Rambotang,			
Red/Yellow, 1 medium, 2 oz	15	0	4
Raspberries: ½ cup, 2 oz	30	0	7
10 raspberries, 0.8 oz 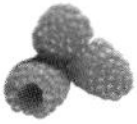	10	0	2
1 cup, 4.3 oz	65	1	15
1 pint, 11 oz	160	2	37
Sapodilla: 1 medium, 6 oz	140	2	34
Pulp, 1 cup, 8.5 oz	200	2.5	45
Sapote: 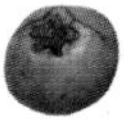			
Black: 1 medium, 4.5 oz	60	0	14
Pulp only, ½ cup, 4 oz	100	1	22
Mamey, piece, 1 cup, 6 oz	220	1	50
Satsuma Tangerine, 1 medium, 3 oz	45	0	11
Soursop, pulp, 1 cup, 8 oz	150	0.5	38
Starfruit, (Carambola): 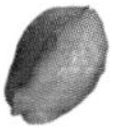			
1 medium, (3½" long), 3 oz	30	0	6
1 large (4½"), 4.5 oz	40	0	8
Strawberries: 1 cup, 5.5 oz 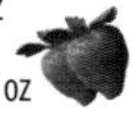	50	0.5	12
6 medium/3 large, 2 oz	20	0	4
1 pint container, heaping, 16 oz	130	1	32
Chocolate dipped, 1 large	45	2.5	6

Weights As Purchased	C	F	Cb
Sugar-Apple (Sweetsop), 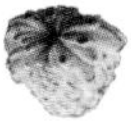			
pulp, ½ cup, 4 oz	120	0	28
Sugar Cane:			
Unpeeled, 1 baton (7" long), 4 oz	30	0	7
Peeled, 1 small stick (3"), 2 oz	35	0	8
Tamarillo, 1 medium, 3 oz 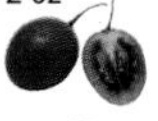	20	0	3
Tamarind: 1 fruit (3"x1")	5	0	1.5
Pulp, ½ cup, 2 oz 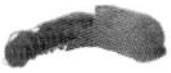	140	0.5	37
Tangelo: 1 small, 4 oz	55	0	13
1 medium, 5 oz 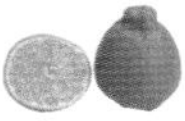	70	0	17
1 large, 7 oz	95	0	23
Tangerine, 1 med., (2½" diam.), 4 oz	50	0	13
Tangor, 1 medium, 4 oz	35	0	7
Tomatillos: 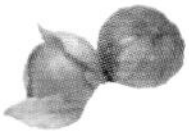			
3 medium, 3.5 oz	35	0.5	6
1lb (16 oz) quantity	160	2	27
Tomatoes:			
1 small (2¼" diameter), 3 oz 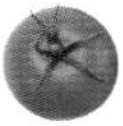	15	0	3
1 medium (2¾"), 5 oz	25	0	5
Sliced: 2 thin slices, 1 oz	5	0	1
2 thick (⅜"), 2 oz 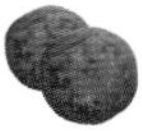	10	0	2
Wedge, ¼, 1.3 oz	6	0	1
1 large (3½"), 8 oz	40	0.5	9
1 extra large (4"), 12 oz	60	0.5	14
Cherry: 4 medium, 2 oz	10	0	2
1 cup, 5 oz 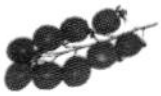	25	0	6
Grape, 5 medium, 2 oz	10	0	2
Yellow Tear Drop, 3 medium, 1 oz	5	0	2
Canned Tomatoes/Products ~ *See Page 144*			
Tree Tomato/Tamarillo, 3 oz	20	0	5
Ugli Fruit, Tangelo type, 5 oz 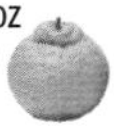	40	0	8
Watermelon:			
Flesh only, weights without skin:			
1 thin slice (½"), ¼ circle, 3 oz	25	0	6
1 thick slice (1"): ¼ circle, 6 oz	50	0	12
½ circle, 12 oz 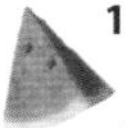	100	1	24
Buffet Slice, small, thin, 1 oz	8	0	2
Cubes or Balls, 1 cup, 5.5 oz	45	0	11
Round Seedless Melon, weight with skin:			
Medium size, 13 lb, (8" diam.):			
whole melon, 13 lb	1160	5	280
wedge, ⅛ whole, 26 oz	145	1	35
Mini size, 6 lb, (6.5" diam.): 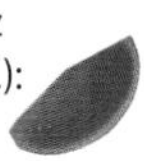			
whole melon, 6 lb	480	2.5	110
wedge, ⅛ whole, 12 oz	60	0	14

Dried Fruit

	C	F	Cb
Apples, 5 rings, 1 oz	80	0	19
Apricots, 8 halves, 1 oz	65	0	16
Banana Chips, ⅓ cup, 1 oz	180	9	16
Banana Flakes, 4 Tbsp, 1 oz	80	0	20
Cranberries *(Craisins):*			
Original, ¼ cup	130	0	33
Reduced Sugar, ¼ cup	100	0	31
Chocolate Covered, ¼ cup, 2 oz	180	8	28
Dates ~ *See Dates in Fresh Fruit*			
Figs, 3 medium figs, 1 oz	90	0	23
Goji Berries, 3 Tbsp, 1 oz	100	0	21
Mango Slices, 5 pieces, 1.4 oz	25	0	6
Papaya Spears, 2 pieces, 1.4 oz	120	0	30
Peaches, 2 halves, 1 oz	60	0	15
Pears, 3 halves, 2 oz	140	0.5	34
Plums *(Sunsweet)*, (5), 1.4 oz	100	0	24
Prunes/Dried Plums:			
with pits, 3 medium, 1 oz	70	0	17
without pits, 4 medium, 1 oz	70	0	17
Cooked: with sugar, ½ cup, 5 oz	155	0	38
without sugar, ½ cup, 4.5 oz	135	0	33
Raisins: 2 Tbsp, 1 oz pack	85	0	22
½ cup, (unpacked), 2.5 oz	215	0	56
White Mulberries, 1 oz	90	0.5	22

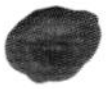
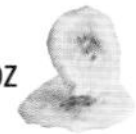
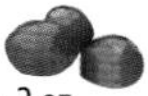
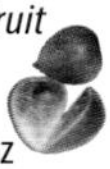
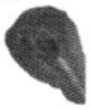
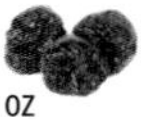
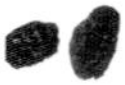

Candied/Glazed Fruit

	C	F	Cb
Apricot, 1 medium, 1 oz	70	0	17
Cherry, Maraschino (1)	8	0	2
Citron/Fruit Peel, 1 oz	85	0	20
Ginger, 1 oz	90	0	21
Pineapple, 1 slice, 1.3 oz	120	0	29
Tamarind, dried, sweetened, 1 oz	70	0	17

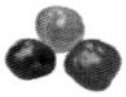
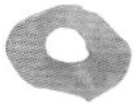

Fruit Leather Rolls

	C	F	Cb
Betty Crocker: Fruit By The Foot, 1 roll, 0.8 oz	80	0	17
Fruit Gushers, 1 oz	90	1	20
Fruit Roll-Ups, 1 roll	50	1	12
Stretch Island, Leathers, 1 pouch, 0.5 oz	45	0	12

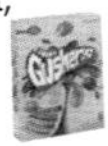

Canned/Bottled Fruit

Solids & Liquids:
Per ½ Cup, 4½ oz Unless indicated

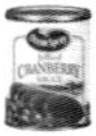

	C	F	Cb
Apricots/Peaches/Pears:			
in juice, light	60	0	15
in heavy syrup	105	0	28
in water/diet	35	0	8
Black/Blueberries:			
in heavy syrup	120	0	30
in light syrup	110	0	26

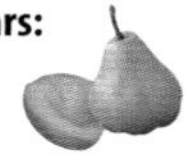
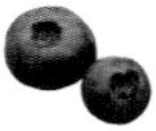

Canned/Bottled Fruit (Cont)

	C	F	Cb
Cherries, pitted:			
in heavy syrup	105	0	27
in light syrup	85	0	22
in water	55	0	15
Maraschino, 1 oz	50	0	12
Fruit Cocktail/Salad:			
in heavy syrup	95	0	25
in juice, light	60	0	16
in water/diet	35	0	10
Gooseberries, light syrup	90	0	24
Grapefruit, in light syrup	75	0	20
Lychees, ½ cup, 4.5 oz	105	0	26
Mixed Fruit: in fruit juices/light syrup	70	0	18
in heavy syrup	90	0	24
in water/diet	40	0	10
Pineapple: in heavy syrup, 4.3 oz	110	0	26
in own juice, 4 oz	60	0	15
Prunes: with syrup, 3 oz	90	0	23
Stewed in water, ½ cup	135	0	35

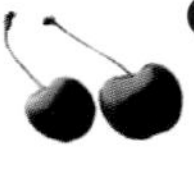
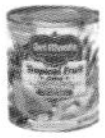
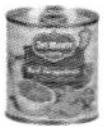
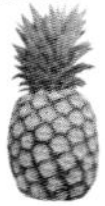

Fruit Snack Cups

	C	F	Cb
Deli/Take-Out: Small, 6 oz	70	0	16
Large, 12 oz	140	0	32
Yogurt and Fruit Cup, 15 oz	380	4.5	75
Del Monte:			
Bubble Fruit, all flavors, 4 oz cup,	60	0	14
Fruit & Oats, average, 7 oz	185	2.5	36
Fruit Refreshers, average, 7 oz cup	95	0	23
Fruit Snack Cups: Average, 4 oz	70	0	17
No Sugar Added, average, 4 oz	50	0	14
Parfaits: Pineapple Coconut	180	7	31
Average other varieties, 6.25 oz	200	8	31
Dole:			
Fruit Bowls In 100% Juice:			
Diced Pears, 4 oz cup	90	0	22
Mixed Fruit, 4 oz cup	70	0	15
Fridge Packs In Juice: *Per 4.3 oz Container*			
Peach Slices	80	0	21
Pineapple Chunks	70	0	16
Other Fruits	90	0	21

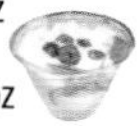
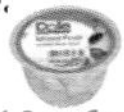

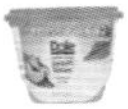

Apple & Fruit Sauces

	C	F	Cb
Apple Sauce:			
Regular/sweetened, 2 Tbsp, 1 oz	20	0	6
Cranberry, Jellied, ¼ cup	110	0	25
Fruit Sauces & Purees:			
All fruit types, average: 2 Tbsp, 1 oz	25	0	6
½ cup, 4 oz	100	0	24
Mott's:			
Apple Sauce: Original, 4 oz	60	0	14
Unsweetened Mango Pineapple, 3.9 oz	50	0	13
Ocean Spray, Jellied Cranb. Sce, 2.5 oz	110	0	28

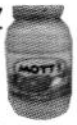

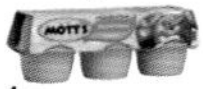

Quick Guide

Ice Cream

Average all Flavors:

Regular (10% fat):

Examples: Dreyer's Grand, Hood, Friendly's

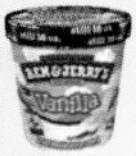

	C	F	Cb
½ cup, 4 fl.oz	140	7	16
1 cup, 8 fl.oz	280	14	32
1 pint, 16 fl.oz	560	28	64

Rich/Premium (16-17% fat):

Examples: Baskin Robbins, Ben & Jerry's, Haagen-Dazs

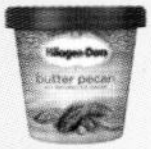

	C	F	Cb
½ cup, 4 fl.oz	250	16	24
1 cup, 8 fl.oz	500	32	48
1 pint, 16 fl.oz	1000	64	96

Reduced-Fat/Light (5% fat):

Examples: Breyers ½ The Fat, Friendly's Light, Hood Light

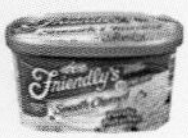

	C	F	Cb
½ cup, 4 fl.oz	140	5	21
1 cup, 8 fl.oz	280	10	42
1 pint, 16 fl.oz	560	20	84

Fat-Free:

Example: Breyers

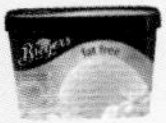

	C	F	Cb
½ cup, 4 fl.oz	90	0	21
1 cup, 8 fl.oz	180	0	42
1 pint, 16 fl.oz	360	0	84

Scoop Shops:

Average all Brands

Add extra for cone (see next column)

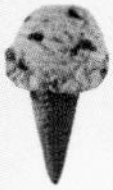

	C	F	Cb
Kids, 3 fl.oz	125	8	12
Regular, 6 fl.oz	250	16	24
Large, 9 fl.oz	375	24	36

Soft Serve:

Average all Brands

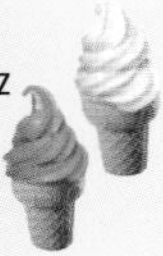

	C	F	Cb
Regular: ½ cup, 4 fl.oz	255	15	25
1 cup, 8 fl.oz	510	30	50
Light: ½ cup, 4 fl.oz	145	3	25
1 cup, 8 fl.oz	290	6	50

Quick Guide

Frozen Yogurt

Average all Brands

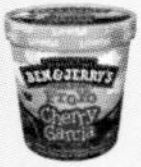

	C	F	Cb
Hard: Low-Fat, ½ cup	110	3	19
Non-Fat, ½ cup	110	0	24
Soft: Low-Fat, ½ cup	120	4	17
Non-Fat, ½ cup	100	0	30

Brands ~ *See Ice Cream & Novelties Section*

Quick Guide

Gelato/Ices/Frozen Custard

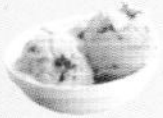

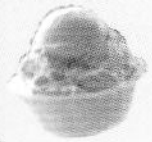

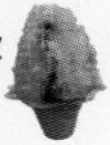

	C	F	Cb
Gelato: *Per ½ Cup*			
Milk base: Vanilla	160	6	25
Chocolate Hazelnut	230	15	21
Water base, ½ cup	100	0	26
Frozen Custard, Choc./Vanilla, av:			
½ cup	210	11	23
Single Scoop, 5 oz wt	300	15	38
Double Scoop, 10 oz wt	600	30	76
Ice (Milk base): *Average all flavors*			
Hard (4% fat), ½ cup	100	3	15
Soft Serve (3% fat), ½ cup	110	2	19
Shaved Ice, average, 12 fl.oz	160	0	40
Sherbet, average, ½ cup	110	1.5	22
Sorbet, Fruit, fat free, ½ cup	70	0	19
Fruit Ice Pops	80	0	20

Sundaes

Baskin Robbins:

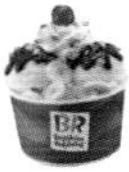

	C	F	Cb
Classic: Banana Royale	690	28	103
Choc. Chip Cookie Dough	1130	48	164
Made with Snickers	1110	43	165

Toppings ~ *See Page 195*

McDonald's:

Sundaes:

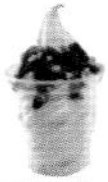

	C	F	Cb
Hot Caramel	340	8	60
Hot Fudge	330	10	52

Ice Cream Cones & Cups

Average all Brands

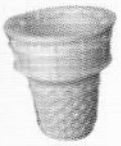

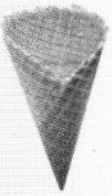

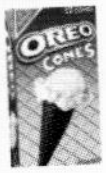

	C	F	Cb
Wafer Cone/Cup, average	20	0	4
Sugar Cone, average	50	0	14
Waffle Cone:			
Small	50	1	10
Large	90	0.5	19
Brands:			
Comet, Sugar Cone	50	0	11
Keebler, Sugar Cone	50	0	10
Oreo, Chocolate Cone	50	1	10

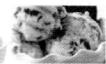

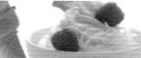

Ice Cream ~ Brands

Baskin-Robbins ~ *See Fast-Foods Section*

Ben & Jerry's:

Scoop Shop Ice Cream: *Hand Scooped, 3 oz Serving*

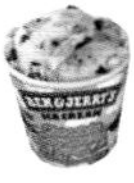
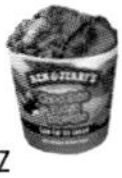
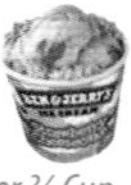

	C	F	Cb
Americone Dream	240	13	26
Boots on the Moooo'n	250	16	25
Butter Pecan	250	19	17
Cannoli	230	14	24
Chip Happens	240	14	24
Choc. Chip Cookie Dough	230	13	26
Chocolate Fudge Brownie	220	11	26
Chunky Monkey	240	15	24
Coconut Seven Layer Bar	250	16	24
Coffee, Coffee, BuzzBuzzBuzz	220	13	23
Mint Chocolate Chunk	220	14	22
Netflix & Chilll'd	250	15	25
New York Super Fudge Chunk	260	17	24
Salted Caramel Blondie	220	11	26
Strawberry Cheesecake	200	12	22
Sweet Cream & Cookies	210	12	23
Triple Caramel Chunk	220	12	26

Ice Cream, 1 Pint Tubs: *Per ⅔ Cup*

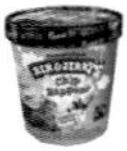
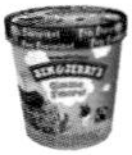
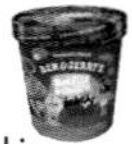

	C	F	Cb
Berry Sweet Mascarpone	350	22	32
Cannoli	360	21	38
Cherry Garcia	340	20	36
Chip Happens	390	24	40
Chocolate Therapy	330	18	38
Everything But The	420	26	40
Gimme S'more!	410	24	45
Netflix & Chilll'd	390	24	38
Peanut Butter Half Baked	370	20	43
Salted Caramel Almond	380	23	38
Strawberry Cheesecake	340	20	37
Triple Caramel Chunk	370	20	42
Vanilla Caramel Fudge	390	21	44
Core: Born Choclatta! Cookie	380	24	36
Peanut Butter Fudge	420	26	40
Salted Caramel	360	19	41

Light Ice Cream, 1 Pint Tubs: *Per ⅔ Cup*

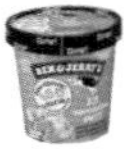

	C	F	Cb
Chocolate Mint	190	6	30
Chocolate Cookie EnlightenMint	190	6	30
Mocha Fudge Brownie	200	4.5	36
P.B. Marshmallow Swirl	230	7	34

Non Dairy: *Per ⅔ Cup*

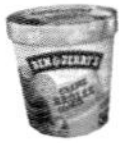

	C	F	Cb
Coffee Caramel Fudge	340	17	44
Creme Brulee Cookie	310	14	46
Choc. Salted 'n Swirled	320	15	44
Mint Chocolate Cookie	300	14	40
PB & Cookies	380	22	41

Fro Yo Frozen Yogurt: *Per ⅔ Cup*

	C	F	Cb
Cherry Garcia	230	4	44
Half Baked	230	3.5	45

Blue Bunny:

Premium Ice Cream, 1 Pint Cont: *Per ⅔ Cup*

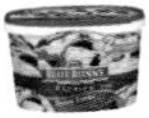

	C	F	Cb
Banana Split, 3.5 oz	220	9	30
Bunny Tracks, 3.35 oz	260	14	29
Chocolate, 3.1 oz	180	8	23
Cookies 'n Cream, 3.1 oz	200	10	26
Peanut Butter Party, 3.6 oz	280	16	29

Sweet Freedom: *Per ⅔ Cup*

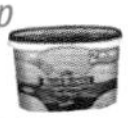

	C	F	Cb
Bunny Tracks, 3.35 oz	180	9	30
Butter Pecan, 3.38 oz	140	6	25
Double Strawberry Swirl, 3.38 oz	120	3	26

Note: Carbohydrate figures include 5-10 g sugar alcohols

Frozen Yogurt: *Per ⅔ Cup*

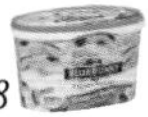

	C	F	Cb
Vanilla Bean, 3.17 oz	140	3	25

Bars/Pops ~ *See Page 108*

Breyers:

Classics: *Per ⅔ Cup*

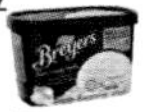

	C	F	Cb
Chocolate Chip/Mint, av., 3.1 oz	200	11	24
Other Choc. varieties, av., 3.1 oz	175	9	21
Natural Strawberry, 3.2 oz	150	7	20
Vanilla:			
Extra Creamy, 2.85 oz	140	4.5	24
Other Varieties, av., 3.1 oz	175	9	20
Carb Smart: Chocolate; Vanilla, 2.75 oz	110	6	17
Peanut Butter, 2.85 oz	150	9	17

Note: Carbohydrate figures include 7-8g sugar alcohol and 4g fiber

Cookies & Candy: *Per ⅔ Cup*

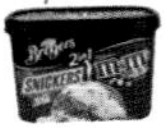

	C	F	Cb
Oreo, 2.9 oz	170	6	27
Reeses, 3.1 oz	200	8	30
Snickers, 3.3 oz	210	8	32
2 in 1, Snickers & M&M's, 3.2 oz	200	7	30

Delights: *Per ⅔ Cup*

	C	F	Cb
Cookies & Cream, 3.3 oz	110	3	24
Creamy Chocolate, 3.2 oz	90	2.5	22

Note: Carbohydrate figures include 6g sugar alcohol

No Sugar Added: *Per ⅔ Cup*

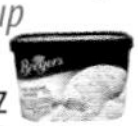

	C	F	Cb
Butter Pecan, 2.7 oz	130	7	17
Salted Carармel Swirl, 2.7 oz	120	5	21
Vanilla Choc. Strawberry, 2.6 oz	110	4	17

Note: Carbohydrate figures include 8-12g sugar alcohol and 0-2g fiber

Non Dairy: *Per ⅔ cup*

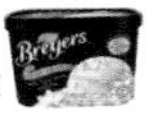

	C	F	Cb
Oreo Cookies & Crm, 2.9 oz	190	9	26
Van. P'nut Butter, 2.96 oz	190	11	21

Gelato: *Per ⅔ Cup*

	C	F	Cb
Raspberry Cheesecake, 3.7 oz	200	6	34
Vanilla Caramel, 3.7 oz	220	8	34

Bruster's: *Per Small Dish*

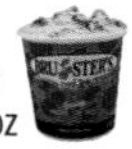

	C	F	Cb
Ice Cream: Banana, 4.93 oz	280	14	36
Butterscotch Ripple, 4.93 oz	310	15	40
Chocolate Mudslide, 4.93 oz	340	14	49
Non Dairy:			
Graham Central Station, 4.93 oz	260	5	52
Mint Chocolate Chip, 4.93 oz	230	7	40
Vanilla, 4.93 oz	160	2	36

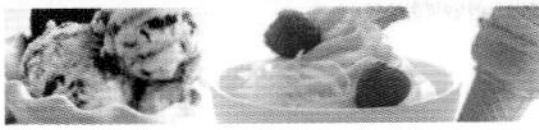

Ice Cream ~ Brands (Cont)

	C	F	Cb
Carvel Ice Cream ~ *See Fast-Foods Section*			
Coldstone Creamery ~ *See Fast-Foods Section*			
Dairy Queen/Brazier ~ *See Fast-Foods Section*			
Dannon: *Per ⅔ Cup, 3.88 oz*			
Premium Frozen Yogurt,			
Average all flavors	155	4	25
Low Fat Frozen Yogurt:			
Chocolate Caramel Turtle	160	2	33
Cake Batter; Dulce De Leche	140	2	28
Fancy French Vanilla	130	0.5	27
Fudge Brownie Batter	150	0.5	33
No Sugar Added Nonfat Frozen Yogurt:			
Cheesecake	110	0	24
Praline	110	0	25
Raspberry	110	0	23
Strawberry Banana	110	0	24
Note: Carbohydrate figure includes 5-6g sugar alcohol			
Dairy Free Sorbet: Choc Fudge 2.9 oz	140	1	34
Average other flavors, 2.9 oz	110	0	20
Gelato, average all flavors, 3.88 oz	185	7	26
Dippin' Dots: *Per ⅔ Cup*			
Original Dots:			
Banana Split, 3.88 oz	180	9	22
Chocolate, 3.88 oz	190	9	25
Choc. Chip Cookie Dough, 3.5 oz	230	10	31
Cookies 'n Cream, 3.25 oz	210	10	26
Cotton Candy, 3.25 oz	170	9	20
YoDots: *Per 2.53 oz Package*			
Cookies 'n Cream	110	2	20
Cookie Dough	110	2	22
Cotton Candy	80	1	20
Dreyer's/Edy's:			
Classic Ice Cream: *Per ⅔ Cup, 3 oz*			
Butter Pecan	200	11	20
Chocolate; Coffee, av.	175	9	21
Choc. Peanut Butter Cup	240	14	23
Mint Choc. Chip; Mocha Alm. Fudge	205	11	23
Rocky Road	210	11	24
Slow Churned Light Classics: *Per ⅔ Cup*			
Butter Pecan, 2.85 oz	170	7	22
Caramel Delight, 2.9 oz	160	4.5	26
Chocolate; Coffee, 2.8 oz	140	4.5	20
Double Fudge Brownie, 2.8 oz	160	4	26
Mint Cookie Crunch, 2.8 oz	150	3.5	26

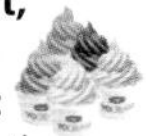
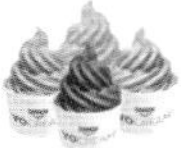
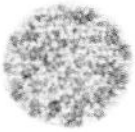
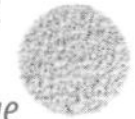
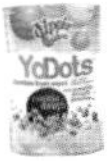
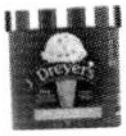
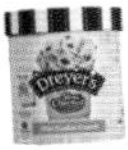

Dreyers/Eddys (Cont):	C	F	Cb
Slow Churned No Sugar Added: *Per ⅔ Cup*			
Butter Pecan, 2.9 oz	150	6	21
Triple Chocolate, 2.9 oz	150	5	23
Vanilla Bean	130	4	19
Slow Churned Triple Filled: *Per ⅔ Cup*			
Choc. Fudge Cores, 3 oz	170	4	29
Crmy Chocolatey Cores, 3.1 oz	140	3	26
Rich Caramel Cores, 3.25 oz	200	6	33
Salted Caramel Cores, 3 oz	150	3.5	27
Gelati-da:			
Gelato: *Per ½ Cup, 4 oz*			
Amaretto Chocolate	150	4.5	23
Choc Mint Milano	120	2.5	22
Coffee Fudge Latte	130	2	22
Limoncello; Vanilla Marsala, average	120	2.5	21
Red Raspberry	130	1.5	25
Great Value *(Walmart): Per ⅔ Cup*			
Ice Cream: Butter Pecan, 3.5 oz	240	15	23
Cherry Chocolate, 5.4 fl.oz	190	10	22
Chocolate, 3.14 oz	180	8	23
Circus Cookie, 3.14 oz	200	11	24
Cookies & Cream, 3.14 oz	210	10	27
Mint Choc. Chip	140	8	17
Unicorn Sparkle, 3.2 oz	190	8	25
Vanilla Bean, 3.14 oz	170	9	21
Sherbet, av. all flav., ½ cup	110	0	26
Haagen-Dazs:: *Per ⅔ Cup*			
Ice Cream, 14 fl.oz Tubs:			
Bourbon Praline Pecan	380	21	42
Caramel Cone	400	25	38
Cherry Vanilla	290	18	29
Chocolate Peanut Butter	450	29	36
Coffee Chip	340	22	30
White Chocolate Raspberry Truffle	360	20	41
Crispy Trio Layers:			
Coconut Caramel Chocolate	370	24	34
Belgian Choc. Van. & Blackberry	360	24	30
Decadent:			
Banana Peanut Butter Chip	440	30	33
Honey Salted Caramel Almond	350	22	33
Heaven: Choc Caramel Sea Salt	230	8	30
Cold Brew Espresso Chip	220	9	27
Non Dairy:			
Coconut Caramel	240	11	34
Raspberry Sorbet	170	0	42

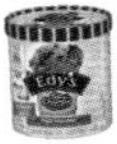
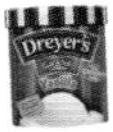
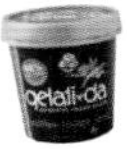
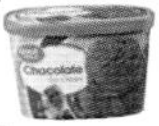
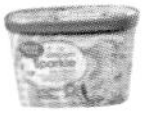
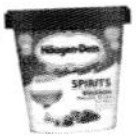
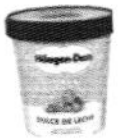
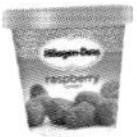

Bars ~ *See Page 109*

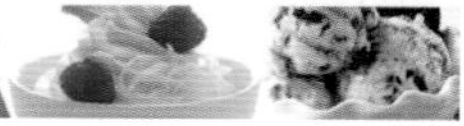

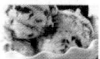

Ice Cream ~ Brands (Cont)

Hood:	C	F	Cb
Classic: *Per ⅔ Cup*			
Chocolate	190	9	25
Classic Trio	180	9	23
Coffee Cookies 'N Crm	200	10	26
Cookie Dough	210	10	28
Creamy Coffee	180	10	22
Fudge Twister	190	8	27
Golden Vanilla; Patchwork, av.	190	10	22
Maple Walnut Flavored	200	11	22
Churned, Light: *Per ⅔ Cup*			
Chocolate Chip	170	6	26
Coffee	140	4	24
Under The Stars	210	10	25
Vanilla	140	4	24
Frozen Fat-Free Yogurt: *Per ⅔ Cup*			
Chocolate; Strawberry, av.	125	0	26
Mocha Fudge	130	0	29
Salted Caramel Espresso	150	1.5	29

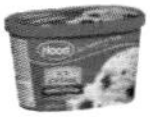
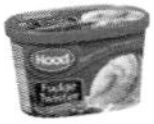
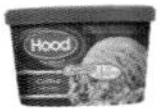
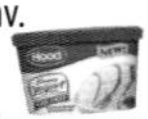

New England Creamery ~ *www.CalorieKing.com*

Lucerne *(Vons): Per ⅔ Cup*	C	F	Cb
Frozen Dairy Dessert: Chocolate	130	4	22
Cookies & Cream	160	5	26
Neapolitan	130	4	22
Orange Vanilla Swirl	150	3	30
Vanilla	130	3.5	21

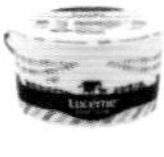

Oberweis:	C	F	Cb
Super Premium Ice Cream: *Per ⅔ Cup*			
Black Cherry, 3.8 oz	280	17	28
Chocolate Chip, 3.8 oz	340	22	33
Cookies & Cream, 3.8 oz	300	19	28
Cookie Dough P'nut Butter, 3.9 oz	320	19	35
Espresso Caramel Chip, 3.9 oz	310	18	36
Vanilla, 3.77 oz	280	19	24

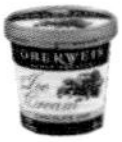
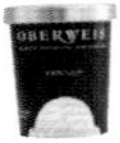

Oikos ~ *see Dannon*

Pinkberry:	C	F	Cb
Frozen Yogurt: *Without Toppings*			
Original: Mini, 3.2 oz wt	90	0	19
Small, 4.9 oz wt	150	0	31
Medium, 8 oz wt	240	0	50
Large, 13 oz wt	390	1	81
Chocolate Hazelnut, 8 oz	360	9	59
Cookies & Cream, 8 oz	320	4.5	59
Passionfruit, 8 oz	240	0	50
Peanut Butter, 8 oz	390	16	49
Vanilla Latte, 8 oz	240	0	47

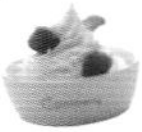
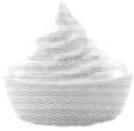

Red Mango (Stores):	C	F	Cb
Frozen Yogurt: *1 Cup, 8 oz, Without Toppings*			
Original	200	0	46
Banana	220	0	50
Blueberry	220	0	48
Caribbean Coconut; Vanilla Bean	260	0	58
Dark Chocolate	260	1	60
Mango	260	0	58
Milk Chocolate; Raspberry, average	260	0	61
Peanut Butter	300	10	44
Pomegranate	240	0	54
Pomegranate Dark Chocolate	240	0	54
Fro-Yo Mashups: *Per ½ Cup, 4 oz*			
Brownie Brittle; Cookie Butter, av.	140	3	25
Cake Batter; Coffee	120	1	25
NY Cheesecake; Pistachio Mustachio	130	1.5	26
Vanilla Latte	120	1	25
White Chocolate	140	1	29

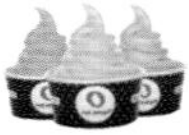
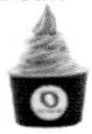

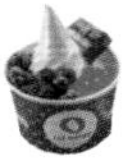

Bars ~ *See Page 110*

So Delicious: *Per ⅔ Cup*	C	F	Cb
Frozen Dessert:			
Cashew Milk:			
Bananas Foster, 4 oz	240	13	29
Chocolate Cookies & Cream, 4 oz	250	13	25
Creamy Chocolate, 3.88 oz	220	13	25
Dark Chocolate Truffle, 4.1 oz	250	15	30
Salted Caramel Cluster, 4 oz	250	13	32
Snickerdoodle, 4 oz	240	11	34
Very Vanilla, 3.67 oz	240	11	34
Coconut Milk: Chocolate, 3.8 oz	200	11	25
Choc. P'Nut Butter Swirl, 4.1 oz	300	20	29
Mocha Almond Fudge, 3.8 oz	250	15	28
No Sugar Added:			
Mint Chip, 3.84 oz	160	11	25
Vanilla Bean, 4 oz	130	9	24

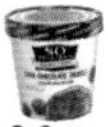
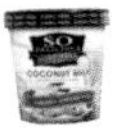

Note: Carbohydrate Figure Includes 4-5g Sugar Alcohol

	C	F	Cb
Mousse: Mint Chip, 2.2 oz	110	4.5	22
Peanut Butter Swirl, 2.2 oz	110	5	20
Salted Caramel Swirl, 2.2 oz	110	4	23
Oatmilk: C'rmel Apple Crumble, 4.16 oz	230	10	36
P'nut Butter & Rasp., 4 oz	250	14	30
Soy Milk,			
Creamy Vanilla, 3.66 oz	160	4	31

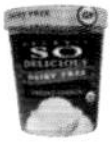

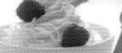

Ice Cream ~ Brands (Cont)

	C	F	Cb
Stonyfield Organic:			
Organic Frozen Yogurt: *Per ⅔ Cup*			
Chocolate	170	4.5	28
Creme Caramel	210	5	35
Vanilla	170	4	27
Vanilla Fudge Swirl	190	3.5	33
Stop & Shop *(Ahold):*			
Churn Style Ice Cream: *Per ⅔ Cup*			
Chocolate	135	4	23
Choc. Chip Cookie Dough	160	5	25
Cookies & Cream	160	5	27
Moose Tracks	200	8	28
Real Ice Cream: *Per ⅔ Cup*			
Black Raspberry	180	10	22
Cafe Au Lait	130	6	16
Cherry Vanilla	140	7	18
Chocolate	200	11	23
Chocolate Moose Tracks	260	15	29
Cookies & Cream	200	10	26
Espresso Chip	210	11	26
Neapolitan	190	10	24
Salted Caramel Toffee	220	11	29
Tasti D-Lite:			
Soft Serve: *Per 3 oz Wt*			
Vanilla: Banana	70	1.5	14
Birthday Cake	80	1.5	14
Black Cherry	90	1.5	16
Brownie Batter	90	2	16
Butter Pecan	80	1.5	16
Cappuccino	80	1.5	15
Chocolate Mousse	80	1.5	16
Cinnamon Crunch	140	3	26
Creme Brulee; New York Chsecake	90	1.5	17
Mango	80	1.5	16
Mud Pie	100	2	19
Nutella Fusion	110	4	17
Oreo Mint	130	3	22
Peanut Butter	100	4	15
Tofutti *(Milk Free):*			
Premium Pints: *Per ⅔ Cup*			
Better Pecan	320	20	36
Chocolate	280	18	27
Vanilla	280	18	28
Vanilla Almond Bark	320	20	32
Van. Fudge; Wild Berry Supreme, av.	260	12	34

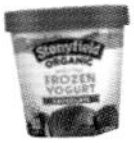
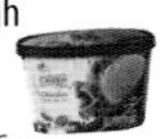
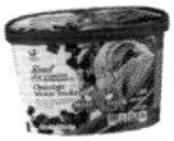
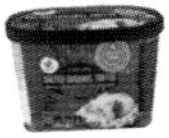
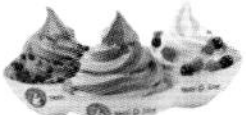
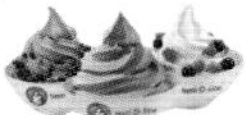
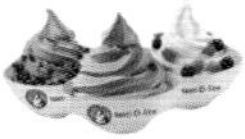 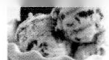
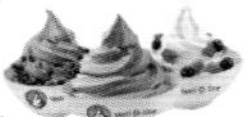
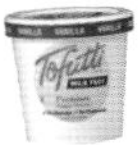

TCBY ~ *See Page 250*

	C	F	Cb
Turkey Hill:			
All Natural: *Per ⅔ Cup, 3.3 oz Unless Indicated*			
Belgian Style Choc.	220	11	27
Butter Almond & Choc.	230	13	23
Raspberry Chocolate Chip	210	11	24
Salted Caramel	210	10	27
Vanilla Peanut Butter	250	16	21
Red. Fat, Moose Tracks, 2.9 oz	190	8	26
No Sugar Added,			
Vanilla Bean, 3.2 oz	100	0	26
Premium Ice Cream: *Per ⅔ Cup, 3 oz*			
Black Raspberry	170	8	23
Choco Mint Chip	200	11	23
Chocolate Peanut Butter Cup	230	13	24
Cookies 'n Cream; Tin Roof Sundae	200	10	25
Raspberry Cream Swirl	170	6	28
Vanilla Bean	170	9	21
Vanilla Chocolate Crunch	210	12	25
Stuff'd, average all flavors, ⅔ cup	195	8	29
Frozen Dairy Desserts: *Per ⅔ Cup, 3.2 oz*			
Butter Pecan	170	6	24
Pistachio Almond	160	5	25
Rocky Road	180	4.5	32
Sherbet, Fruit Rainbow, 4 oz	160	1.5	36
Wawa:			
Premium Ice Cream: *Per ½ Cup*			
Butter Pecan; Mint Choc. Chip, av.	180	10	20
Chocolate; Vanilla Bean, average	160	8	20
Cookies & Cream	180	9	21
Strawberry Shortcake	160	7	22
Wegmans: *Per ⅔ Cup Unless Indicated*			
Ice Cream: Choc. Peanut Butter Swirl	200	12	20
Coconut Almond Fudge	250	14	29
French Vanilla	200	9	26
Mint Chip	200	10	26
Neapolitan	180	9	23
Peanut Choc. Stampede	260	15	29
Vanilla & Chocolate	180	9	22
White Chocolate Raspberry	220	11	30
Light: *Per ⅔ Cup*			
Mint Chip	170	4	29
Pecan Praline	170	3.5	32

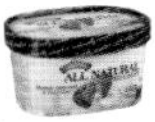
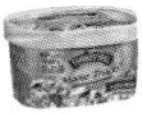
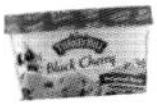
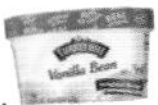
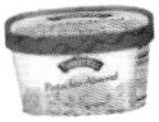
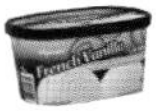
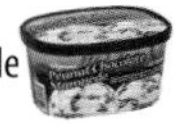
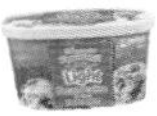

Ice Cream Bars & Pops ~ Brands

Per Bar/Serving Unless indicated	C	F	Cb
Ben & Jerry's:			
Pint Slices:			
Amer. Dream; Choc Chip Cookie Dough	280	18	30
Cherry Garcia	250	15	27
Choc Fudge Brownie	250	16	26
The Tonight Dough	290	18	31
Vanilla P'nut Butter Cup	300	22	24
Big Bear ~ *See Klondike*			
Blue Bunny:			
Big Alaska Bar	250	15	27
Sandwich Bars:			
Big: Bopper	400	16	61
Double Strawberry	230	6	42
Mississippi Mud	260	7	47
Single Bars: Chocolate Eclair	210	10	29
Cookies 'n Cream	250	12	32
Fudge Bar	40	0	9
Heath Bar	270	18	26
Nutt'n Better Bar	270	18	24
Strawberry Shortcake	200	10	26
Turtle Bar	360	23	33
Snacks, CMint Choc. Chip	150	5	24
Cones, 6 Pack:			
Caramel Lovers	310	16	38
Chocolate Lovers	270	12	36
Cookies 'n Cream	270	13	37
Big Dipper: Chocolate Lovers	260	12	36
Cookies 'n Cream	260	12	35
Breyers:			
Carb Smart, 6 Pack:			
Almond Bar, 2 oz	150	12	11
Caramel Swirl, 2 oz	60	2.5	11
Fudge Bar, 1.7 oz	60	3	10
Vanilla Ice Cream Bar, 2 oz	140	11	11

Note: Carbohydrate figure includes 4-5g sugar alcohol

Butterfinger Bar ~ *See Nestle Page 110*			
Diana's Bananas:			
Banana Babies:			
Milk/Dark Chocolate (1)	130	6	18
Milk Choc. & Peanuts (1)	215	13	21
Banana Bites, (4), 1.5 oz	100	6	13

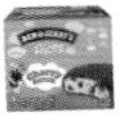
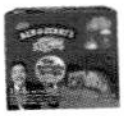
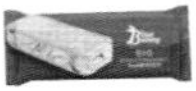
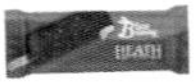
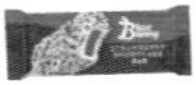
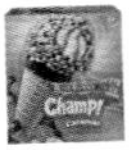

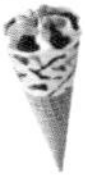
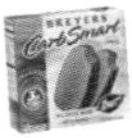
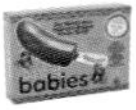

Per Bar/Serving Unless indicated	C	F	Cb
Dove:			
Single Bars: *Per 2.6 oz Bar*			
Milk Chocolate, Vanilla	250	16	24
Dark Chocolate, Choc.	250	16	26
Miniatures, Variety Pack, w/ Milk/Dark Choc.,1 piece	60	4	6
Sorbet Bars: Dark Chocolate Raspb.	150	8	19
Milk Chocolate Strawberry	150	7	20
Drumstick *(Nestlé)*:			
Classic Sundae Cones: Banana	290	15	34
Banana with Fudge	300	15	38
Dulce de Leche	290	13	41
Strawberry with Fudge	300	15	38
Vanilla; Vanilla Fudge, average	300	5	37
Vanilla Caramel	310	15	39
Dipped: Choc. Cookie	280	13	38
Vanilla Caramel	290	14	32
Super Nugget: Strawberry	300	16	35
Vanilla	310	17	35
Vanilla Fudge	320	17	39
King Size: Triple Chocolate	340	14	50
Vanilla with Choc. Swirls	350	14	52
Lil' Drums: Choc. w/ Choc. Swirls	110	5	16
Vanilla with Choc. Swirls	120	5	17
Simply Dipped: Mint	260	12	37
Vanilla	270	12	38
Edy's ~ *See Dreyer's*			
Eskimo Pie ~ *See Nestle*			
Fudge Bar ~ *See Nestle*			
Fat Boy:			
Cones: Chocolate Fudge Brownie	300	15	40
Sundae Best	310	17	34
Other Flavors	310	15	40
Freeze Pops, Orange Cream	110	3	21
Sandwiches: Chocolate, 3 oz	210	8	32
Cookies 'n Cream, 3 oz	220	9	34
Mint Chocolate Chip, 3 oz	230	10	33
Premium Vanilla	210	8	32
S'mores, 3 oz	230	9	35
Strawberry, 3 oz	180	7	29
Sundae On A Stick: Caramel Pretzel	230	9	35
Cherry Cordial	230	16	20
Toffee Crunch	290	21	25
Vanilla Nut	270	18	25
Fudgsicle *(Breyers)*:			
Fudge Bar: Original	80	3	14
Low Fat	60	1.5	11
No Sugar Added	80	2	18

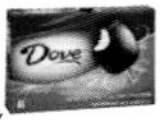

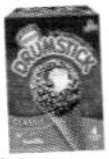
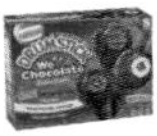
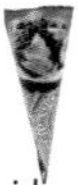
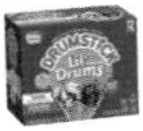
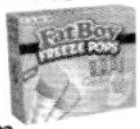
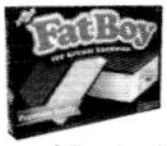

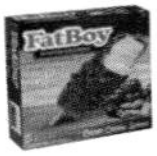
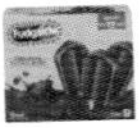

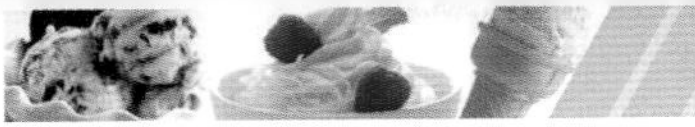

Ice Cream Bars/Pops ~ Brands (Cont)

Per Bar/Serving	C	F	Cb
Good Humor:			
Cones:			
Single: Giant King Cone, Choc. & Vanilla, 5 oz	390	22	44
King Cone, Vanilla, 2.7 oz	230	14	25
4-Packs: Oreo Cone, 2.65 oz	200	9	29
King Cones, Vanilla, 3 oz	240	12	31
Dessert Bars, Singles:			
Original Vanilla, 2.8 oz	240	15	23
Birthday Cake, 2.6 oz	200	10	25
Chocolate Eclair, 2 oz	150	7	21
Creamsicle, 3 oz	100	2	20
Oreo, 1.8 oz	150	8	19
Reese's, 1.8 oz	180	11	20
Toasted Almond, 2 oz	160	9	18
Sandwiches:			
Single: Giant Neapolitan;Van., 3.6 oz	220	5	39
Choc. Chip Cookie, 2.7 oz	250	10	40
Stickless: *4 or 6-Pack*			
Reese's PB Dessert Cup, 2.43 oz	260	17	25
Haagen-Dazs:			
Dark Chocolate Bar, Chocolate	280	20	22
Milk Chocolate Bars:			
Coffee & Almond Crunch	290	21	22
Vanilla & Almonds	290	21	21
Vanilla	270	19	22
Snack Size:			
Coffee & Almond Crunch	190	14	15
Vanilla & Almonds	195	15	13
Gelato, Vanilla Caramel Pizzelle	290	19	25
Healthy Choice: Fudge Bar	80	0.5	15
Smoothie Bars: Mango Peach	70	0.5	14
Raspberry	80	0.5	15
Strawberry	70	0.5	13
Hershey's:			
Bars, Gluten Free: Banjo	170	11	17
Fudjo	120	0	24
Orange Blossom	80	3	13
Cones: Incredible	290	14	38
Moose Tracks	480	28	52
P-Nutty	260	15	30
Low fat, Cookies & Cream; Crazy, av.	120	2	25

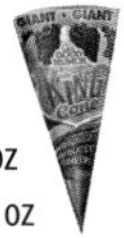
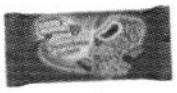
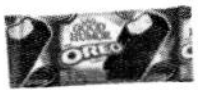
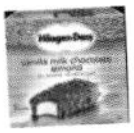
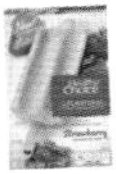
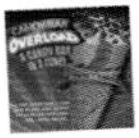

Per Bar/Serving	C	F	Cb
Hershey's (Cont):			
Ice Pops, all flavors	35	0	10
Sandwiches:			
Vanilla Ice Cream, 4 oz	210	9	30
Giant:			
Andes Creme de Menthe, 6 oz	350	16	48
Neapolitan, 6 oz	280	12	40
Vanilla, 6 oz	300	12	43
Signature Bars: Chocolate Eclair	220	10	30
Salty Caramel Brownie	240	12	30
Strawb. Shortcake	240	11	32
Hood:			
Bars: Ice Cream Bar	130	7	14
Red Sox Sports Bar	250	16	26
Hoodsie:			
Cups, Chocolate; Vanilla, 3 oz	100	5	12
Sundae Cups, 3 oz	120	5	19
Sandwich: Av., 2.2 oz	175	6	29
Mini's, 1.2 oz	90	3.5	14
Klondike:			
Bars:			
Single, Orig. Vanilla, 5.5 oz	300	17	34
4-Pack:			
Mint Choc. Chip, 2.8 oz	230	14	26
6 Pack: Cookies & Cream, 2.15 oz	200	10	24
Double Chocolate, 3 oz	240	14	27
Oreo, Cookies & Cream, 37 oz	250	15	27
Reeses, PB Cup , 2.75 oz	250	15	28
8-Count Snack Size: Orig., 1.4 oz	120	7	13
English Toffee, 2.6 oz	230	14	24
Choco Taco, Original, 4 oz	250	12	34
Kandy, Caramel & Peanuts, 2.7 oz	250	14	28
Sandwiches:			
Single: Mrs Fields, 3.9 oz	340	12	55
Oreo, 4.5 oz	220	7	37
4-Pack: Mrs Fields, 2.3 oz	210	8	34
Oreo, 2.4 oz	210	7	35
6-Pack, Vanilla, 2.7 oz	180	5	31
Kroger: *Per Bar*			
Arctic Blasters:			
Fudge Bar	100	1	21
Ice Cream Bar	150	11	13
Orange Cream	100	3	18
Strawberry Shortcake	140	8	16
Toffee Bar	160	11	14
Mighty Pops, Grape Cherry, Orange (3)	140	0	33
Luigi's: *Per 6 fl.oz cup*			
Real Italian Ice: Blue Rasp. Lemon	130	0	27
Cherry; Lemon; Strawb.	100	0	26
Cherry & Lemon Swirl	120	0	30

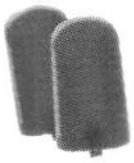
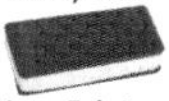
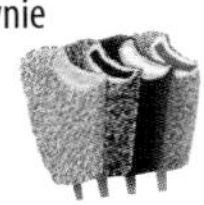
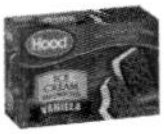
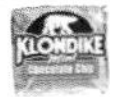
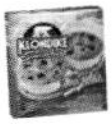
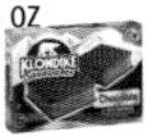
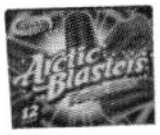

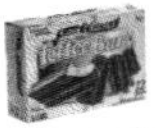
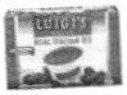

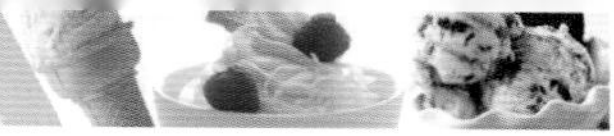

Ice Cream Bars/Pops ~ Brands (Cont)

Per Bar/Serving	C	F	Cb
M&M's:			
Cone, Single, 2.6 oz	250	12	32
Sandwiches: Choc. Ice Cream, 2.9 oz	240	10	36
Vanilla Ice Cream, 2.9 oz	240	10	37
Magnum:			
Singles: Almond 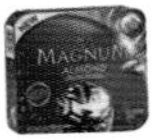	270	18	25
Dark Chocolate	240	16	23
Double Caramel	270	17	29
White	240	15	24
Double: Cookies & Cream	280	17	30
Raspberry 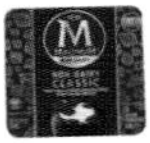	260	16	28
Minis, Almond	170	11	15
Non Dairy: Classic	230	14	26
Almond	250	16	25
Minute Maid, Juice Bars, 2.25 fl.oz	40	0	10
Nestlé:			
Bars: Butterfinger 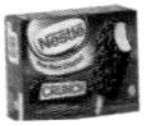	290	17	30
Cookies N' Cream	180	11	19
Crunch	150	9	15
Crushed It: Cookies N' Cream	170	9	21
Vanilla Fudge	180	9	22
Eskimp Pie 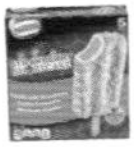	150	5	15
Fudge Bar	110	2	20
Strawberry Shortcake	140	6	20
Dibs, Crunch, 3.3 oz container	320	21	31
Drumsticks ~ See Page 108			
Push-Up Pops, all flavors	70	1	16
Sandwiches, Vanilla 	160	3	30
Popsicle:			
Fruit Pops: Strawberry	150	0	34
Average Other Fruit Flavors	165	0	40
Fruit Stacker, Banana, Orange, Strawb.	160	0	38
Fudgsicle, Low Fat	60	2	11
Scribblers, 2 Pops	60	0	14
Reeses Dessert Bar~*See Good Humor*			
Skinny Cow: *Per Item*			
Bars: Fudge; Chocolate Truffle, av.	120	3	19
Vanilla Almond Crunch 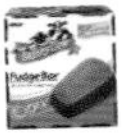	190	11	19
Cones, all flavors	170	5	28
Minis, Salted C'rmel Pretzel	90	6	9
Sandwiches, all flavors	160	3.5	29
Snickers:			
Bars: Milk/Dark Choc. 1.7 oz 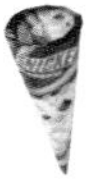	180	11	18
2.8 oz bar	250	15	25
Cone, 2.7 oz	250	13	31
Snow Cone *(Wonder)*, av. all, 7 fl.oz	60	0	15

Per Bar/Serving	C	F	Cb
So Delicious *(Turtle Mountain):*			
Almond Based:			
Bars, Mocha Alm. Fudge 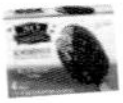	180	13	16
Sandwich, Vanilla, 1.3 oz	100	4	14
Cashewmilk:			
Dipped Bars: Dble Choc Delight, 2 oz	170	13	16
Salted Caramel Bar, 2 oz	180	13	17
Coconut Milk:			
Dipped Bar: Coconut Alm., 1.85 oz	190	14	15
Vanilla Bean, 1.8 oz	170	12	14
Fudge Bar, 2 oz 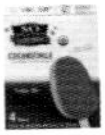	100	6	13
Sandwiches:			
Coconut, 1.3 oz	100	4	14
Vanilla Bean, 1.3 oz	100	4	14
Tampico, Freezer Pops, all var., 1.4 oz	30	0	7
Tofutti: *Per Item*			
Bars: Chocolate Fudge, 1.4 oz	30	0	6
Hooray Hooray, 1.4 oz 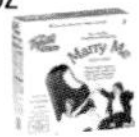	120	8	8
Marry Me, 1.4 oz	170	8	22
Totally Fudge Pops	95	2	19
Note: Carb figures include 0-7g sugar alcohols			
Cone, Yours Truly Sundae 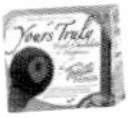	170	8	22
Cuties, average all flavors	130	6	18
Toll House *(Nestle)*:			
Sandwiches:			
Chocolate Choc. Chip Cookie, 4 oz	380	16	54
Vanilla Choc. Chip Cookie, 2.1 oz	210	8	32
Mini, Vanilla 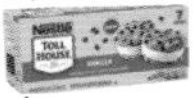	105	4	16
Turkey Hill:			
Sandwiches: Double Decker	200	8	31
Vanilla Bean 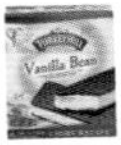	190	7	30
Reduced Fat	170	3	33
Sundae Cone, Van. Fudge	360	22	35
Twix:			
Cookies & Cream, 2.4 oz	250	14	29
Vanilla Ice Cream Bar: 3 fl.oz	250	14	28
1.6 fl.oz Bar	160	9	18
Wegmans: 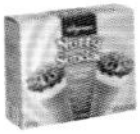			
Bars: Organic Fudge	190	12	16
Chocolate Sundae Crunch	180	10	22
Strawberry Sundae Crunch	180	9	22
Sandwiches: Vanilla, 3.5 fl.oz	160	5	27
Light Vanilla, 3.5 fl.oz	160	3	29
Weight Watchers: *Per Item*			
Bars: Dark Choc. Raspberry 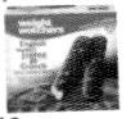	70	2	11
English Toffee	80	3.5	11
Giant Bar, Chocolate Fudge	90	1	21
Snack Bars: Cookies & Cream	90	3	15
Divine Triple Chocolate	90	3	14
Salted Caramel	90	3	14

Canned & Packaged Meals ~ Brands

	C	F	Cb
Amy's:			
Frozen:			
Bowls: *Per Package*			
Asian Dumplings	370	13	47
Broccoli & Cheedar Bake, 9.5 oz	460	21	50
Cheese Ravioli, 9.5 oz	340	11	48
General TSO's, 8 oz	270	11	36
Meatless Pepperoni Mac & Cheese, 9 oz	490	21	52
Pesto Tortellini, 9.5 oz	530	22	63
Vegan: Baked Ziti, with Cheeze, 9.5 oz	380	13	54
Tortilla Casserole, w/ Cheeze, 9.4 oz	360	15	48
Burrito, Org. Vegan Bean & Cheeze	340	10	51
Entrees: Cheese Enchilada, 9 oz	360	16	39
Greek Red Rice & Veggies, 8.65 oz	500	29	50
Indian Mattar Paneer, 10 oz	370	13	49
Macaroni & Cheese, 9 oz	450	18	55
Sweet & Sour Asian Noodle, Light, 8 oz	260	4	47
Tofu Scramble, 9 oz	420	27	24
Vegan Brocc. & Cheeze Bake, 9.5 oz	400	18	54
Pot Pie, Vegetable, 7.5 oz	440	24	46
Snacks: Chse & Bean Nachos, 5-6 pcs	230	9	28
Pizza: Cheese, 6 pieces	220	9	25
Meatless Pepperoni Pizza, 6 pcs	220	10	22
Wraps:			
Indian Samosa, 5 oz	270	12	32
Teriyaki, gluten free, 5.5 oz	250	6	38
Armour-Star:			
Beef Stew, 9 oz	230	12	21
Chili, Orig., with Beans, 7 oz	380	19	31
Corned Beef, 2 oz	120	7	1
Corned Beef Hash, 7 oz	420	26	22
Potted Meat, Chicken/Pork, 2.1 oz	170	16	0
Roast Beef with Gravy, 5.3 oz	140	3.5	7
Atkins: *Per 9 oz Tray/Bowl*			
Frozen:			
Beef Merlot; Chsy Chkn Risotto, av.	305	20	9
Chicken & Broccoli Alfredo	290	18	10
Chili Con Carne	340	23	11
Crustless Chkn Pot Pie	300	19	9
Meatloaf, with Portobello Mshrm Gravy	340	21	13
Mongolian-Style Beef	270	18	10
Pork Verde	300	20	10
Shrimp Scampi	290	19	19

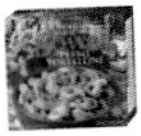
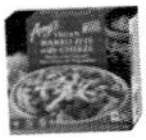
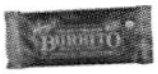
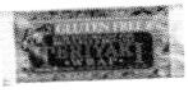
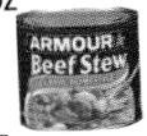

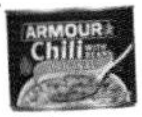

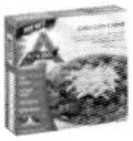
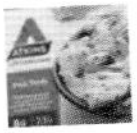

	C	F	Cb
Bagel Bites: *Per 4 Pieces*			
Frozen:			
Bagel Dogs	200	10	19
Pizza Snacks:			
Cheese & Pepperoni	210	6	33
Cheese, Sausage & Pepperoni	190	5	27
Cheesy Garlic Bread	220	8	27
Extreme Beef Nacho, Mini	190	5	27
Mozzarella Cheese	170	4	27
Three Cheese	200	5	32
B&M:			
Baked Beans: *Per ½ cup, 4.6 oz*			
Original; Maple Flavor, av.	160	1	32
Bacon & Onion; Boston's Best, av.	185	1	36
Country Style	170	1	35
Homestyle	190	2	39
Vegetarian	160	0.5	32
Brown Bread, Orig., 1 slice (1/2"), 2 oz	130	0.5	28
Banquet:			
Bowls: Dynamite Penne & M'balls	640	34	56
Kung Pao Chicken	550	20	77
Nashville Hot Fried Chicken	470	22	48
Sesame Chicken Lo Mein	570	11	97
Homestyle Bakes: *1 Cup, Prepared*			
Creamy Cheesy Chicken Alfredo	380	19	39
Creamy Chicken & Biscuits	420	21	48
Frozen Meals ~ *Per Package*			
Backyard BBQ & Mshd Potato	290	11	35
Chicken:			
Fettuccine Chicken Alfredo	330	12	42
Cheesy Rice Chicken	260	6	40
Parmesan	340	10	48
Strip Meal	430	17	49
Homestyle Patty	340	17	32
Lasagna with Meat Sauce	250	9	31
Mac & Cheese	240	9	32
Pepper Steak,	320	13	39
Rigatoni & Italian Sausage, with Meatballs	300	12	35
Salisbury Steak w/ Mshd Potatoes	350	16	39
Spaghetti & Meatballs	320	14	34
Swedish Meaballs	370	17	39
Turkey	270	10	29
Family: *Per ⅙ Package*			
Gravy & Meat Loaf, 4 oz	120	6	9
Salisbury Steak & Gravy, 4.5 oz	170	12	8
Zesty Marinara Sauce & M'balls, 6 oz	170	10	11
Pot Pie: Beef	410	26	35
Chicken	350	18	35
Chicken & Broccoli	330	18	31
Salisbury Steak Deep Dish	410	22	45
Turkey	320	18	31

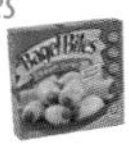
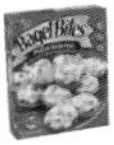
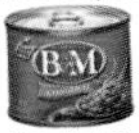

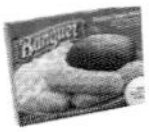
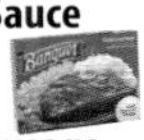
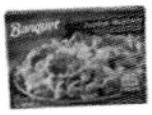
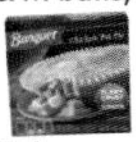

	C	F	Cb
Barilla:			
Entrees: *Per Container*			
Chicken Alfredo, 8.5 oz	**310**	18	22
Marinara/Tom. & Basil Penne, av., 9 oz	**305**	4	60
Meat Sauce Gemelli, 9 oz	**350**	6	61
Betty Crocker: *Dry Mix Only*			
Chicken Helper:			
Chicken Fettuccine Alfredo, 1.38 oz	**140**	2	28
Chicken Fried Rice, 1.15 oz	**110**	0	24
Hamburger Helper:			
Bacon Chsebgr; Beef Pasta, av., 1 oz	**100**	0.5	21
Cheddar Cheese Melt, 1 oz	**100**	0.5	20
Cheeseburger Macaroni, 1.2 oz	**120**	1	25
Cheesy: Enchilada, 1.4 oz	**140**	2	30
Fajita, 1.1 oz	**110**	0.5	24
Hashbrowns, 1.1 oz	**120**	0	27
Ranch Burger, 1.23 oz	**120**	1	26
Del. Beef Strog.; Four Chse Lasag 1. oz	**110**	1	23
Potato Stroganoff, 0.9 oz	**80**	0	19
Tuna Helper:			
Creamy Broccoli, 1.4 oz	**140**	1	28
Fettuccine Alfredo, 1.3 oz	**130**	1	27
Tetrazzini, 1.4 oz	**150**	1	30
Birds Eye:			
Frozen:			
Casseroles:			
Chicken Alfredo Pasta, 8.6 oz	**310**	13	27
Lasagna with Meat Sauce, 8.7 oz	**270**	9	36
Three Cheese Ziti, 7.9 oz	**310**	11	41
Meals For One: Five Cheese Las.	**330**	10	38
Meatless Be'f Lasagna	**330**	9	43
Sheet Pan Meals:			
Chicken:			
Balsamic Flav. Sweet Pot., 4.86 oz	**150**	6	14
Rosemary Brown Butter Pot., 4.2 oz	**140**	5	14
Ital. Sausage with Peppers, 5.3 oz	**220**	14	16
Voila!: Alfredo Chicken, 7.6 oz	**210**	7	27
Cheesy Ranch Chicken, 6.8 oz	**210**	5	30
Chicken Florentine, 7.5 oz	**220**	6	28
Garlic Chicken, 6.2 oz	**210**	7	29
Garlic Shrimp, 6.7 oz	**220**	7	31
Meatless Alfredo Chick'n, 5.9 oz	**170**	5	20
Shrimp Scampi, 9 oz	**230**	4	36

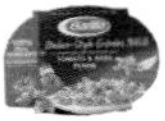
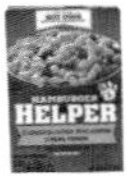

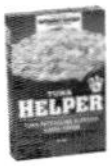

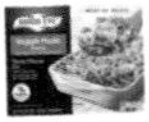
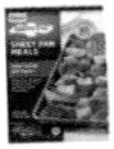
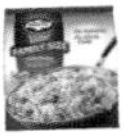

	C	F	Cb
Boca:			
Burger Patties: *Per Patty*			
Original: Original Chik'n	**130**	4	13
Original Vegan Veggie	**70**	1	6
Chik'n Veggie	**130**	4	13
Crumbles, Original Veggie, 2 oz	**60**	0	5
Falafel Bites, average all flavors (4)	**150**	6	23
Boston Market: *Per Package*			
Frozen:			
Bowls: Fr. Chkn w/ Loaded Mshd Pot.	**350**	14	38
Philly Cheese Steak with Rice & Veg.	**390**	17	42
Slow Cooked Beef with Red Potatoes	**320**	16	28
Carver's Cut:			
Herb Seasoned Grilled Chicken	**350**	13	22
Roadhouse Beef Meatloaf	**520**	28	44
Slow Cooked Pulled Pork	**480**	17	55
Entrees:			
Boneless Pork Rib Shaped Patty	**580**	29	60
Chicken Fettuccine Alfredo	**390**	14	42
Salisbury Steak	**530**	32	38
Smothered Turkey	**430**	11	57
Pot Pie, Chicken	**470**	34	35
Buitoni:			
Refrigerated:			
Ravioli, Four Cheese, 3.7oz	**330**	12	42
Tortellini: Herb Chkn, 3.9 oz	**330**	8	52
Mixed Cheese, 3.7 oz	**330**	8	47
Tortelloni, Sweet Italian Ssg., 4 oz	**350**	10	51
Dry Pasta ~ *See Page 133*			
Bush's Best: *Per ½ cup, 4.6 oz*			
Baked Beans: Original	**150**	1	30
Honey Sweet	**160**	1	33
Vegetarian	**150**	0	30
Black Beans	**110**	0	20
Chili, Pinto, mild sauce	**120**	1	21
Dark Red Kidney Beans	**130**	0	24
Garbanzo Beans (Chick Peas)	**120**	2	20
Grillin' Beans: Honey Chipotle	**170**	0.5	36
Smokehouse; Bourbon & Br. Sugar	**165**	0	34
Pinto Beans	**90**	0	17
Refried Beans, Traditional, 4.4 oz	**140**	3	21
Campbell's:			
Pork & Beans, 11 oz can, ½ cup, 4.6 oz serving	**130**	0.5	27
Spaghetti O's: *Per 1 Cup*			
Original, 8.9 oz	**170**	1	33
With Franks, 8.9 oz	**220**	7	29
With Meatballs, 8.9 oz	**230**	7	31

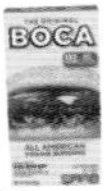

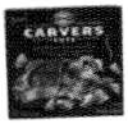

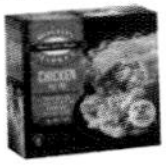
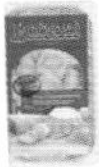
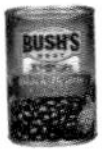

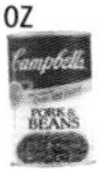
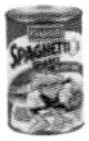

Chef Boyardee:	C	F	Cb
Boxed Pizza Maker Kits: *Single Kits*			
Pepperoni, ⅛ package, 4 oz	260	6	43
Traditional, ⅛ package, 4 oz	240	4	46
Canned: *Per Cup*			
Beefaroni, 8.8 oz	200	7	27
Ravioli:			
Beef in Pasta Sauce	180	5	30
Cheese, in Tomato Sauce	200	2	39
Overstuffed Italian Sausage	240	6	38
Spaghetti: with Meatballs	250	10	30
Mini Rings & Meatballs, 8.6 oz	250	11	29
Cauliflower Pasta: *Per Microwaveable Bowl*			
Rings & Meatballs	200	9	23
Rings & Veggies in Sauce	130	3	22
Microwaveable: *Per 7.5 oz Bowl*			
Beefaroni; Lasagna, average	215	8	28
Ravioli: Beef In Tom. & Meat Sce	200	7	28
Cheese in Tomato & Meat Sauce	190	5	28
Mini Micro Beef	180	5	30
Pizza Sauce, w/ Cheese, ¼ c., 2 oz	35	2	4

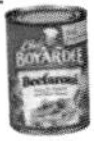
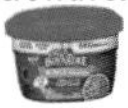

Dennison's Chili: *Per 15 oz Can*	C	F	Cb
Chili Con Carne:			
Original: with Beans	550	23	56
without Beans	440	24	30
Chunky, with Beans	510	22	51
Hot, with Beans	540	21	57
Turkey with Beans	380	6	57
Vegetarian, 99% fat free	280	2	52

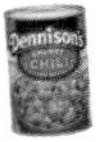
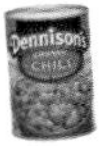

Devour ~ *See Heinz Page 114*

Dinty Moore (Hormel):	C	F	Cb
Big Bowl (Microwave): *Approx. ½ of 15 oz Bowl*			
Beef Stew, 8.3 oz	200	10	17
Chicken & Dumplings, 8.5 oz	210	6	29
Can, Chicken & Dunplings, 8.5 oz	200	7	24
Microwave:			
Cup, Scalloped Pot, with Ham, 7.5 oz	260	16	19
Tray, Beef Stew, XL, 13 oz	330	17	29
Dr. McDougall's:			
Asian Noodles:			
Pad Thai, 2 oz	200	2	43
Spicy Kung Pao, 2 oz	200	2	38
Eden Foods (Organic):			
Black Beans & Quinoa Chili, 8.8 oz	190	2	35
Kidney Beans & Kamut Chili, 8.8 oz	220	2	41
Pinto Beans & Spelt Chili, 8.8 oz	200	2	40
Spanish Rice & Pinto Beans, 8.46 oz	200	2	40

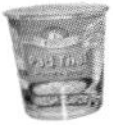

Farmhouse: *Per 1 Cup Prepared*	C	F	Cb
Pasta: Fettuccine Alfredo	460	22	51
White Cheddar	380	14	51
Rice: Long Gr., & Wild Herbs & Butter	250	7	44
Mexican	230	5	42
Roasted Chicken Flavor	230	5	44
French's:			
French Crispy Fried Onions:			
Original; White Cheddar:2 Tbsp	45	4	3
4 tablespoons	90	7	6
8 tablesooons	180	14	12
GardenBurger:			
Veggie Burger: *Per 3 oz Burger*			
Original	110	4	17
Black Bean Chipotle	90	3	16
Portabella	90	2	16

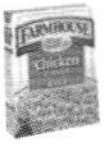
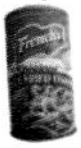
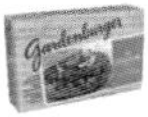

Garden Lites: *Per Package*	C	F	Cb
Bakes: Broccoli Cheddar Bake	190	6	25
Butternut Squash Souffle	180	1	38
Roasted Vegetable Bake	150	3	24
Spinach	140	3	22
Zucchini	150	3	25
Cakes: Broccoli Cheddar (1)	90	6	5
Superfood Veggie (1)	80	4	8
Frittata: Mushroom & 3 Cheese, 2 oz	80	4	6
Roasted Cauliflower (1)	60	2	7
Spinach Egg White, 2 oz	70	4	5
Veggie, Bacon & Potato, 2 oz	80	5	6

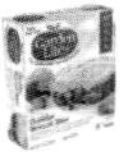

Gorton's:	C	F	Cb
Frozen:			
Delicious Classics:			
Clams, Crunchy Breaded, 15 pieces	210	10	22
Flounder, Crispy Batt. Fillets (2)	250	13	25
Pollock: Beer Battered Fillets (2)	230	12	23
Crispy Battered Fillets (2)	230	11	23
Crunchy Breaded Fish Sticks (4)	230	10	26
Potato Crunch Fillets (2)	230	11	24
Popcorn Shrimp, 3.5 oz	370	15	23
Everyday Gourmet:			
New England Cod: Pub Style (1)	380	24	29
Fish Sticks, Crunchy Panko (4)	270	13	26
Simply Bake:			
Roasted Garlic Butter Salmon (1)	140	3	8
Shrimp Scampi (9)	180	7	5
Tilapia, with Seasoning (1)	130	3	6

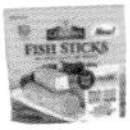

continued nex page...

Gorton's (Cont):	C	F	Cb
Frozen:			
Smart Solutions: *Per Fillet*			
Haddock, Grilled	70	1	0
Pollock: Grilled Lemon Butter	70	0.5	0
Italian Herb Grilled	80	2	2
Tilapia: Grilled	100	4	1
Grilled Rosted Garlic Butter	100	3	1
Great Value *(Walmart)*:			
Frozen:			
Breakfast Bowls: Meat Lovers, 7 oz	430	30	14
Sausage & Gravy, 7 oz	340	25	14
Meals: Beef Shepherd's Pie, 6.4 oz	190	10	15
Rstd Turkey Breast & Mshd Pot, 10 oz	230	6	25
Spaghetti with Meat Sauce, 10 oz	360	12	48
Spinach Pesto Chkn & Veggie, 10 oz	240	10	21
Sweet & Sour Chicken, 10 oz	380	5	76
Turkey & Dressing Bake, 9.5 oz	370	18	35
Steam Meal, Lem. Herb Chicken, 12 oz	350	6	51
Healthy Choice:			
Frozen:			
Cafe Steamers:			
Beef Teriyaki, 9.5 oz	270	4	43
Chicken & Noodles, 10 oz	260	7	31
Chicken Fajita, 9.5 oz	200	5	23
Crustless Chicken Pot Pie, 9.6 oz	300	6	40
General Tso's Spicy Chicken, 10.3 oz	290	4	47
Grilled Chkn Pesto with Veg., 9.6 oz	290	7	36
Sweet & Sour Chicken, 10 oz	390	9	63
Gluten Free: Beef Merlot, 9.5 oz	180	4	24
Cajun Style Chkn & Shrimp, 9.6 oz	220	3	35
Classics: Chicken Parmigiana, 11.6 oz	320	9	44
Lemon Pepper Fish, 10.7 oz	280	4	48
Power Bowls: *Per Bowl*			
Adobo Chicken	330	8	38
Chicken Feta & Farro	310	9	34
Cuban-Style Pork	340	8	46
Italian Chicken Sausage & Peppers	290	9	36
Vegetatian/Vegan:			
Cauliflower Curry, 10 oz	290	4	50
Falafel & Tahini, 9.6 oz	360	13	49
Simply Steamers: *Per Package*			
Beef & Broccoli, 10 oz	270	5	39
Beef Chimichurri, 9 oz	220	6	24
Chicken & Vegetable Stir Fry, 9.2 oz	200	5	16
Gr. Chicken & Broc. Alfredo, 9.15 oz	190	5	8
Meatball Marinara, 10 oz	280	6	36

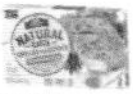
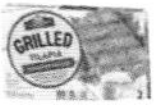
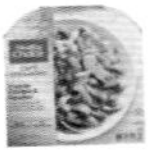
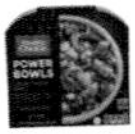
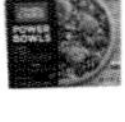

Heinz:	C	F	Cb
Beans, Baked in Tom. Sauce, 4.6 oz	100	0	17
Frozen:			
Devour Meals: *Per Package*			
Buffalo Chicken Mac & Cheese	640	33	58
Cajun Syle Alfredo w/ Ssg & Chkn	410	19	34
Loaded Potato w/ Beef & Bacon	330	14	31
Pesto Ravioli w/Spicy Italian Ssg	670	37	55
Pulled Chicken Burrito Bowl	440	15	45
Smokehouse Meat & Potatoes	430	13	57
Bowls: Creamy Alfredo Mac & Chse	390	14	51
Sharp Chedd. Mac & Chse w/ Bacon	380	13	51
Sandwiches:			
Buffalo Chicken Grilled Cheese	500	18	59
Philly Cheesesteak Grilled Cheese	460	15	59
Hormel:			
Frozen:			
Chili with Beans: *Per 8.7 oz Cup*			
Regular; Hot; Chunky, av.	265	9	32
Turkey, 98% Fat-Free	220	3	29
Vegetarian, 99% Fat Free	200	2	35
Chili No Beans: *Per 8.3 oz Cup*			
Angus Beef	330	23	14
Hot; Chunky, average	255	13	18
Turkey, 98% Fat-Free	190	3	16
Compleats, Comfort Classics: *Per 7.5 oz Pkg*			
Beefy Mac	240	5	37
Chicken & Noodles,	180	6	20
Dumplings & Chicken	190	4	32
Noodles & Beef	170	2	28
Spaghetti & Meat Sauce	220	6	31
Compleats, Homesyle: *Per Package*			
Beef Pot Roast	200	6	20
Chicken Alfredo	350	18	30
Chkn Brst, Gravy & Mashed Potatoes	220	5	28
Meatloaf, Gravy & Mashed Potates	300	14	28
Salisbury Steak	300	16	27
Swedish Meatballs	280	13	26
Refrigerated Entrees: *Per Package*			
H'style Meat Loaf & Tom. Sce, 5 oz	220	9	14
Sliced Rstd Turkey Brst & Gravy, 5 oz	110	3	3
Slow Simm. Beef Tips w/ Gravy, 4.3 oz	170	10	3
Side Dishes: Bacon Mac & Chse, 8.2 oz	340	11	45
Chipotle Chedd. Mac & Chse, 8.2 oz	340	14	41
Tamales: Beef in Chile Sauce, 7.5 oz	190	9	22
Beef, Hot & Spicy in Chile Sce, 7.5 oz	180	8	22

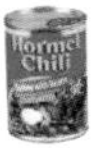
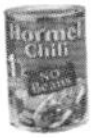
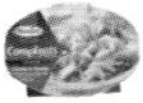
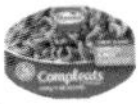
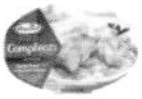
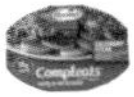

Hot Pockets:	C	F	Cb
Sandwiches: *Per Pocket*			
Big & Bold: Chicken Bacon Ranch	450	17	58
Sriracha Steak	440	18	56
Crispy Buttery Crust:			
Hickory Ham & Cheddar	270	9	39
White Meat Chkn, Brocc. & Chedd.	270	9	38
Crispy Crust:			
Five Cheese Pizza	290	12	36
Pepperoni Pizza	320	15	36
Croissant Crust,			
Hickory Ham & Cheddar	280	10	38
Garlic Buttery Crust: Four Chse	280	11	36
Four Meat & Four Cheese Pizza	300	13	35
Pepperoni	310	14	35
High Protein:			
Crispy Butter Crust,			
Steak & Cheddar	310	13	33
Garlic Buttery Crust,			
Four Meat & Four Cheese Pizza	300	14	32
Breakfast: Bacon, Egg & Cheese	290	10	41
Ham. Egg & Cheese	270	9	38
Sausage, Egg & Cheese	280	12	35
Hungry Jacks:			
Casserole Potatoes: *Per 1 oz dry mix, prepared*			
Au Gratin	160	5	25
Cheddar & Bacon	160	5	25
Cheesy Scalloped	160	5	26
Hashbrowns: *Per ½ oz dry mix, prepared*			
Original, ⅓ cup, 0.5 oz	90	4	13
Mashed Potatoes: *Per ⅓ cup dry mix, prepared*			
Original, ½ cup prepared	150	6	19
Four Cheese, ½ cup prep.	100	2	19
Roasted Garlic, ⅔ cup prep.	110	2	20
Supreme Baked, 1/2 cup prepared	100	2	19
Hungry Man: *Per Package*			
Frozen:			
Bowls: Double Chicken Bacon Ranch	570	29	30
Double Meat Angus Meatloaf	580	35	37
Dinners: Backyard BBQ	690	24	91
Country Fried Chicken	530	27	54
Roasted Carved White Meat Turkey	400	10	61
Smokin' Backyard Barbeque	710	27	96

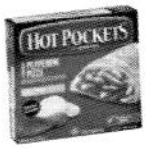

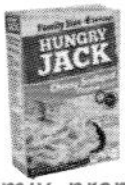

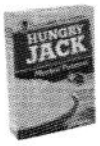

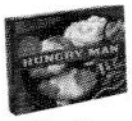

Hungry-Man (Cont):	C	F	Cb
Selects: *Per Package*			
Classic Fried Chicken: Classic	970	59	59
Mesquite Flavored	1050	72	60
Spicy	940	63	51
Fried Chicken & Ham	630	23	78
Mexican Style Fiesta Enchiladas	640	19	103
José Olé:			
Breakfast Burritos: *Per 4 oz Burrito*			
Egg, Cheese & Bacon	260	10	30
Egg, Sausage & Cheese	240	9	28
Burritos: *Per Burrito*			
Beef & Cheese	350	15	41
Beef & Jalapeno	320	12	40
Chimichangas: *Per Chimichanga*			
Beef & Cheese	390	20	40
Chicken & Cheese	330	13	42
Loaded Beef Nacho	420	25	36
Queso Chicken Nacho	330	16	33
Minis & Bites:			
Beef & Cheese (5)	230	11	24
Queso Chicken Nacho (5)	220	10	24
Taquitos: Beef, Corn Tortillas (3)	230	12	26
Beef & Cheese, Flour Tortillas, (2)	250	13	25
Chicken, Corn Tortillas, (3)	220	9	26
Chicken & Cheese, Flour Tortillas, (3)	220	10	25
Kashi:			
Bowls: *Per Package*			
Chimichurri Quinoa	240	7	41
Creamy Cashew Noodle	360	14	46
Mayan Harvest Bake	330	8	56
Sweet Potato Quinoa	270	6	48
Kid Cuisine: *Per Meal*			
All American Chkn Breast Nuggets	420	16	53
All Star Chicken Breast Nuggets	440	16	56
Carnival Mini Corn Dogs	470	16	68
Catch A Wave Mac & Cheese	410	13	62
Popstar Popcorn Chicken	470	18	65

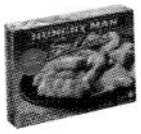
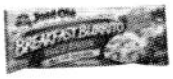
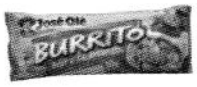

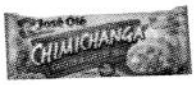

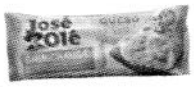
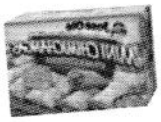
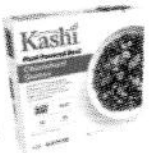

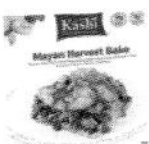

Kraft:	C	F	Cb
Macaroni & Cheese:			
Original (7.25 oz Box), 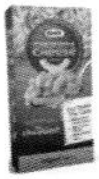			
2.5 oz (makes 1 cup)	**250**	2	42
Thick & Creamy:			
2.5 oz (makes 1 cup)	**250**	2	49
Whole Grain (6oz Box),			
2.5 oz (makes 1 cup)	**250**	2	45
Deluxe:			
Original; 4 Cheese, average:			
¼ box, 3.5 oz (makes 1 cup)	**315**	10	42
White Cheddar, Galic & Herbs,			
¼ box, 3.5 oz (makes 1 cup	**280**	9	38
Microwave Cups: 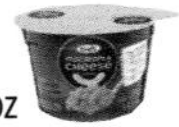			
Avg all flavors, 2 oz	**215**	4	39
Orig. Cheddar, 2.4 oz	**210**	8	30
Big Cup, Triple Cheese, 4 oz	**440**	7	79
Velveeta: *Per Container*			
Cheesy Bowls: Bacon Mac & Chse	**340**	14	48
Chicken Alfredo 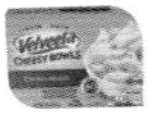	**300**	9	35
Lasagna with Meat	**350**	17	36
Ultimate Cheeseburger Mac	**370**	17	39
Shells & Cheese Cups:			
Original, 5 oz 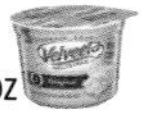	**460**	16	65
2% Milk Cheese, 2.2 oz	**180**	3	31
Queso Blanco, 2.4 oz	**220**	8	30
Kroger:			
Frozen:			
Bacon & Cheddar Meatloaf, 4 oz	**270**	19	5
Beef Ravioli, 5 oz 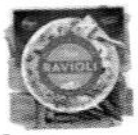	**280**	7	44
Cheese Ravioli, 5.1 oz	**280**	6	43
Chicken Fried Rice, 4.23 oz	**220**	5	32
Vegetable Fried Rice, 4.23 oz	**220**	6	37
Meatballs: 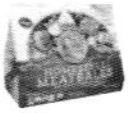			
Homestyle, 3 oz	**240**	19	6
Italian Style, Beef & Pork, 3 oz	**240**	19	6
Reduced Fat Turkey (6), 3 oz	**160**	9	6
Meat Lasagna, Party Size, 1 cup	**280**	10	34
Heat & Serve: 			
Beef Barbacoa, 5 oz	**200**	10	2
Mac. & Cheese, 110 oz	**350**	13	44
Pork Burnt Ends in BBQ Sauce, 5 oz	**190**	4	21

Lean Cuisine:	C	F	Cb
Bowls: *Per Bowl* 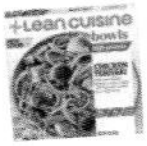			
Chicken Pad Thai	**390**	5	65
Chicken Teriyaki	**310**	5	45
Four Cheese Tortelloni w/ Pesto Sce	**320**	9	43
Garlic parmesan Alf 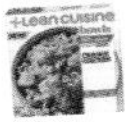			
Glazed chicken	**320**	7	41
Mango Chicken w/ Coconut Rice	**360**	6	55
Orange Chicken	**350**	6	59
Oven Fried Chicken w/ Mshd Pot.	**290**	9	36
Oven Fried Chicken w/ Buffalo			
Style Mac & Cheese 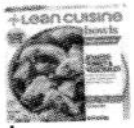	**340**	8	45
Peanut Chicken Stir Fry	**400**	10	56
Roasted Turkey & Vegetables	**230**	5	29
Savory Sesame Chicken & Veggies	**390**	9	61
Sesame Stir-Fry with Chicken	**350**	7	46
Shrimp Alfredo 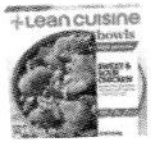	**320**	9	41
Sticky Ginger Chicken	**320**	5	51
Sweet & Sour Chicken	**400**	8	67
Unwrapped Chicken Burrito	**340**	7	44
Cauli Bowls: *Per Bowl* 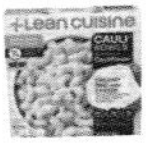			
Creamy Mac & Cheese	**260**	6	37
Crmy Tom. Vodka Pasta	**240**	7	36
Fettuccini with Meat Sauce	**260**	7	36
Garlic Parm Alfredo w/ Broccoli	**250**	8	34
Favorites: *Per Package*			
Alfredo Pasta with Chkn & Brocc.	**280**	5	39
Baked Chicken with Pot. & Stuffing	**240**	7	30
Broccoli Cheddar Rotini 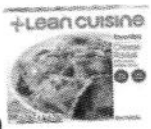	**300**	8	42
Cheese Ravioli	**250**	6	39
Chicken Enchilada Suiza	**300**	5	53
Chicken Fried Rice	**300**	6	44
Chicken Fettuccini 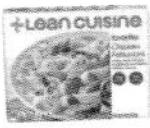	**310**	7	42
Classic Mac. & Beef	**270**	6	39
Fettuccini Alfredo	**290**	5	49
Glazed Turkey Tenderloins	**300**	6	47
Grilled Chicken Caesar 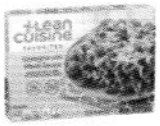	**270**	9	27
Lasagna w/ Meat Sce	**310**	7	44
Macaroni & Cheese	**270**	5	44
Spaghetti with Meat Sauce	**310**	4	53
Spaghetti with Meatballs	**280**	5	43
Swedish Meatballs	**300**	6	44

Lean Cuisine (Cont):

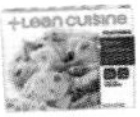
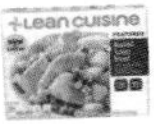
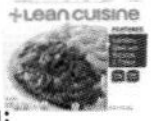
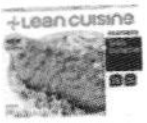

	C	F	Cb
Features: *Per Package*			
Apple Cranb. Chicken	320	4	56
Buffalo Style Chicken	200	6	20
Butternut Squash Ravioli	290	6	49
Chicken Club Panini	340	7	45
Chicken Marsala	200	7	21
Chicken Parmesan	340	9	44
Chicken in Sweet BBQ Sauce	230	5	33
Roasted Turkey Breast	300	5	50
Salisbury Steak w/ Mac & Cheese	250	5	28
Sesame Chicken	330	9	51
Shrimp Scampi	350	9	50
Spinach, Artichoke Ravioli	340	10	44
Steak Portabella	160	5	10
Tortilla Crusted Fish	310	8	45

Pizzas ~ *See Page 137*

Extra Product Listings ~ *www.CalorieKing.com*

Lightlife (Meatless):

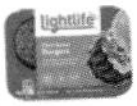
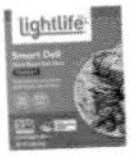
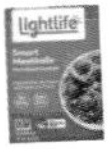
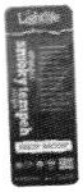

	C	F	Cb
Burger Patty, 4 oz	250	17	6
Italian Sausage, 3 oz cooked	210	15	5
Smart Deli: Bologna, 4 slices	90	3	3
Ham, 4 slices	90	3	3
Turkey, 4 slices	100	3	3
Smart Dogs (1)	50	3	2
Smart Ground: Original, 1.94 oz	70	2	4
Meatballs (3)	150	6	10
Mexican, 1.94 oz	70	2	5
Smart Tenders, 3 oz	150	5	10
Tempeh: Original, 3 oz	160	5	12
Buffalo Strips (2), 3.5 oz	190	7	13
Smoky Strips, 4 strips	140	5	10

Lunchables: *Per Package*

	C	F	Cb
Without Drink:			
Ham & Cheddar with Crackers	260	13	22
Nachos, Chse Dip & Salsa	370	20	42
Pepperoni & Mozzarella	250	15	19
Turkey & Cheddar with Crackers	260	13	22

Lunchmakers (Armour): *Per Pkg*

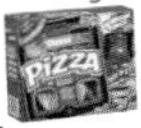

	C	F	Cb
Chkn Cracker Crunchers	200	9	21
Nachos Meal Kit	200	9	29
Pepperoni Cracker Crunchers	230	14	19
Pepperoni Pizza with Crunch	220	10	25
Turkey Cracker Crunchers	210	10	22

Marie Callender's:

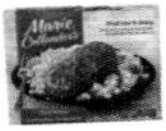
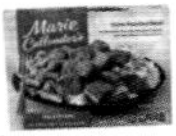
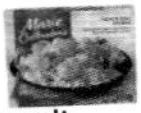
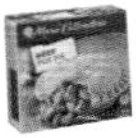
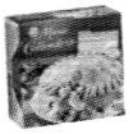
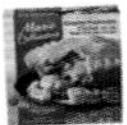
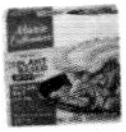
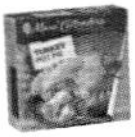

	C	F	Cb
Frozen:			
Beef: *Per Container*			
Beef Pot Roast	200	5	26
Meat Loaf & Gravy	370	15	37
Salisbury Steak	510	23	53
Slow Roasted Beef	240	7	28
Steak & Roasted Potatoes	240	5	32
Bowls: *Per Bowl*			
Aged Cheddar Cheesy Chkn & Rice	380	13	46
Creamy Chicken & Dumplings	370	14	39
Four Cheese Fettuccini Alfredo	460	22	47
Garden Tomnato Four Cheese Rav.	320	13	39
Grilled Chicken Alfredo Bake	390	16	37
Grilled Chicken Pesto Cavatelli	370	9	45
Red Chili Grilled Chicken Burrito	360	10	44
Savory Swedish Meatballs	460	21	47
Slow Roasted Beef Pot Roast	220	6	26
Spicy Buffalo Style Chkn Mac & Chse	590	26	64
Sweet & Spicy Chicken & Noodle	330	7	48
Chicken/Turkey: *Per Container*			
Country Fried Chicken & Gravy	390	17	44
Fettuccini with Chicken & Broccoli	440	18	43
Honey Roasted Turkey Breast	260	6	31
Sweet & Sour Chicken	550	15	88
Pasta: *Per Container*			
Fettuccini, Chicken & Broccoli	440	18	43
Italian Lasagna	350	16	33
Pot Pies: *Per 1 Cup, 7 oz*			
Beef	400	21	40
Brocc. & Cheddar Potato	680	40	69
Cheesy Chicken & Bacon	510	32	41
Chicken Corn Chowder	460	28	38
Creamy:			
Mushroom Chicken	430	25	39
Parmesan Chicken	430	26	36
Layered: Beef Shepherd's	350	18	28
Chicken & Bacon Shepherd's	380	19	32
Kansas City BBq Sce Chkn & Crnbrd	550	23	64
Turkey & Stuffing Thanksgiving	280	9	33
Plant Based: Meatless Be'f	450	25	44
Meatless Chick'n	440	25	41
Pub Style:			
Herb Roasted Chicken	760	45	69
Steak & Ale	790	51	62
Turkey	480	28	46

Maruchan:	C	F	Cb
Bowls, all var., 3.3 oz 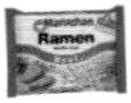	380	16	50
Ramen Noodle Soup,			
average all, 3 oz pkg	380	15	52
Instant Lunch, 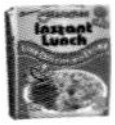			
average, 1 container	290	11	39
Yakisoba: *Per 4 oz Pkg*			
Chicken/Teriyaki Beef Flavor, av.	500	19	69
Cheddar Chse Flavor 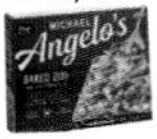	540	24	68
Michael Angelo's:			
Frozen:			
Signature: Baked Ziti w/ M'balls, 11 oz	480	20	51
Chicken Parmigianan, 10 oz	400	15	44
Creamy Chicken Florentine, 8.1 oz	280	7	41
Eggplant Parmigiana, 11 oz	460	32	29
Lasagna with Meat Sauce, 8.1 oz	230	8	29
Manicoti w/ Sauce, 11 oz 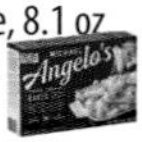	440	19	41
Shrimp Scampi, 10 oz	580	28	61
Three Chse Baked Ziti, 11 oz	530	20	63
Vegetable Lasagna, 11 oz	350	13	40
Minute Rice:			
Ready To Serve: *Per 4.4 oz Container, Prepared*			
Brown/Chicken Rice	220	3	43
Fried/Yellow Rice Mix, average	220	3	45
Quinoa, Red & White	160	2	34
Morningstar Farms (Meatless):			
Burgers: Grillers Original (1)	130	5	8
Mediterranean Chickpea (1)	120	5	13
Spicy Black Bean (1) 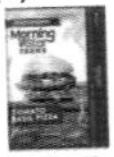	110	5	13
Tomato & Basil Pizza (1)	120	6	8
Chik'n:			
Nuggets: BBQ (3) 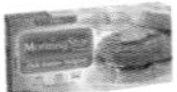	200	8	20
Sweet Mustard (3)	200	7	23
Incogmeato Plant Based):			
Beef Pattie	280	18	14
Chik'n Tenders 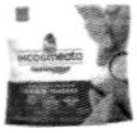	230	9	22
Ital. Based Sausage (1)	170	9	9
Veggitizers:			
Chk'n & Chse Taquito Bites (3)	200	9	21
Chorizo Nacho Bites (3) 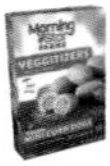	220	10	27
Wings: Buffalo (5)	200	8	21
Parmesan Garlic (5)	190	8	19
Nissin:			
Chow Mein: *Per 4 oz Package*			
Chicken	490	22	65
Shrimp Flavor	560	30	63
Teriyaki Beef Flavor 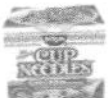	510	24	63
Cup Noodles:			
All flavors, 1 cup	290	11	41

Nissin (Cont):	C	F	Cb
Cup Noodle Stir Fry, av. all flav.	370	13	55
Top Ramen: *Per Package With Soy Sauce*			
Beef; Chicken, average	390	14	57
Shrimp 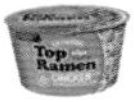	450	22	54
Old El Paso:			
Dinner Kits: *Per 2 Tortillas, Sauce & Seasoning Only*			
Caribbean Inspired Jerk; Fajita, av	185	5	32
Fiesta Taco 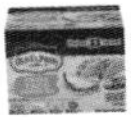	160	6	18
Taco	190	5	32
Rice & Beans:			
Cheesy Mex. Rice, 2.6 oz dry mix	270	0.5	59
Spanish Rice, 2.6 oz dry mix	260	0.5	58
Traditional Refried Beans, 4.23 oz	110	3	14
Ortega: *Per ½ cup, 4.6 oz*			
Black Beans	110	0	20
w. Diced Jalapeños 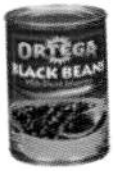	130	2	23
Refried Beans:			
Traditional	130	3	21
w. Diced Green Chiles	140	3	22
Fat Free Refried Beans	120	0	21
Vegetarian Refried Beans	120	0	21
Meal Kits: *Per Serving*			
Bakeable Tortilla Bowl 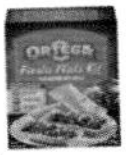	120	2	22
Fiesta Flats Taco	160	6	22
Hard & Soft Grande Taco	230	4	41
Soft Taco	230	4	42
Taco Dinner 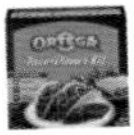	140	6	21
Taco Pizza	200	4.5	35
Pasta Roni: *Per Cup, Prepared*			
Angel Hair with Herbs	310	12	42
Butter & Herb Italiano; Chkn Flav., av.	300	12	40
Chicken & Broccoli 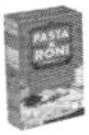	360	15	47
Fettuccine Alfredo	440	24	48
White Cheddar & Broccoli	310	13	39
P.F. Chang's: *Per ½ Package, 11 oz*			
Frozen:			
Entrees: Beef with Broccoli, 9.47 oz	270	10	25
General Chang's Chicken, 10.8 oz	370	11	50
Mongolian Style Beef, 8.57 oz	230	5	31
Sesame Chicken, 10.2 oz	230	10	17
Sweet & Sour Chicken, 9.2 oz	280	6	44
Ramen: Chicken Tonkotsu, 9.5 oz	450	23	37
Veggie Shoyu, 9.5 oz	270	5	48
Sides, Chang's Signature Rice, 8 oz	290	2	61

Prego:	C	F	Cb
Ready Meals: *Per Pouch*			
Creamy Three Cheese Alfedo Rotini	**370**	19	37
Creamy Tomato Penne	**400**	15	57
Marinara & Italian Sausage Rotini	**350**	9	55
Roasted Tomato & Vegetables Penne	**300**	4	55
Rice-A-Roni:			
Classic Favorites: *Per Cup, Prepared*			
Beef	**310**	9	51
Chicken & Broccoli	**230**	4	41
Chicken & Garlic	**250**	8	41
Mexican Style	**250**	8	41
Rice Pilaf	**310**	8	52
Single Serve Cups:			
Cheddar Broccoli	**230**	5	41
Chicken Flavor	**190**	1	41
Creamy Four Cheese	**240**	6	43
Rosarita:			
Black Beans, 4.5 oz	**110**	0.5	19
Pinto Beans, 4.5 oz	**120**	0	22
Refried Beans:			
Traditional, 4.5 oz	**120**	3	18
No Fat, 4.5 oz	**100**	0	18
Restaurant Style, 4.4 oz	**90**	3	13
Vegetarian, 4.5 oz	**120**	2	19
Safeway Select *(Albertsons):*			
Frozen:			
Signature Select:			
Lasagna Five Cheese, 1 cup	**290**	9	40
Lasagna with Meat Sauce, 8 oz	**270**	7	39
Lemongrass Chkn & Jasm. Rice, 9.5 oz	**350**	9	52
Portobello Mushroom Ravioli, 9 pcs	**270**	6	43
S & W: *Per ½ Cup, 4.6 oz*			
Chili, average	**125**	1	22
Classic, average	**110**	0	21
Flavored Savory Sides:			
Indian Style Savory Sides	**150**	3.5	24
Jalapeno Black Beans	**130**	2	22
New Orleans Style Savory	**160**	4	23
Southwest Style	**110**	0	22
Tuscan Style Savory	**130**	2	21

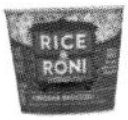

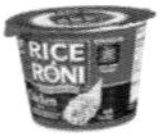

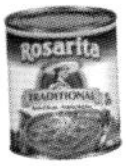

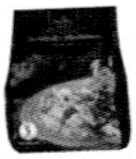

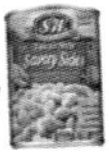

Seapak ~ *See www.calorieking.com*

Simply Asia: *Per Container*	C	F	Cb
Noodles & Broth:			
Japanese: Ramen Noodles	**200**	1	42
Ramen Soy Chicken Broth	**40**	1	2
Udon Noodles	**190**	0.5	41
Noodle Bowls: Roasted Peanut	**460**	12	75
Sesame Teriyaki	**420**	4	87
Soy Ginger	**440**	6	86
Smart Ones *(Weight Watchers):*			
Frozen:			
Smartmade: *Per Package*			
Chicken with Spinach Fettuccine	**230**	6	20
Grilled Sesame Beef & Broccoli	**220**	5	31
Mexican Style Chicken Bowl	**260**	5	33
Roasted Turkey & Veggies	**240**	3	37
Smart Ones: *Per Package*			
Angel Hair Marinara	**200**	2	38
Beef Pot Roast	**180**	4	18
Broccoli & Chicken Rigatoni	**260**	4	40
Cheese Ravioli In Mushroom Sauce	**300**	7	47
Cheese Scramble with Hash Brown	**190**	7	16
Chicken Enchilada Suiza	**290**	5	49
Chicken Fettuccini	**300**	5	44
Chicken Parmesan	**280**	6	35
Crustless Chicken Pot Pie	**190**	4	20
Florentine Lasagna	**300**	10	41
Florentine Ravioli	**280**	5	48
Meat Sauce Lasagna	**330**	12	41
Meat Sauce Lasagna Bake	**300**	5	51
Stagg:			
Chili with Beans, 15 oz Can: *Per Cup*			
Classic, 8.7 oz	**290**	13	26
Dynamite Hot, 8.7 oz	**340**	16	33
Laredo, 8.7 oz	**300**	17	23
Silverado Beef, 8.7 oz	**250**	9	25
Turkey Ranchero	**260**	6	32
Vegetarian Garden 4-Bean Chili	**200**	2	37
Starkist Creations Microwavables: *Per 4.5 oz Pouch*			
Latin Citrus	**160**	4	19
Spicy Rice & Beans	**160**	3	22
Thai Green Curry	**160**	5	18
Tomato Basil	**170**	5	18

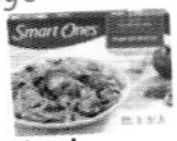

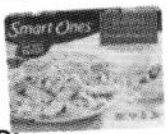

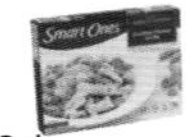

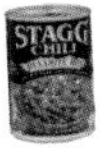

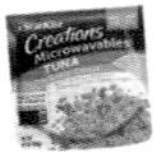

Stouffer's:

Frozen:

Bowl-FULLS: *For One*

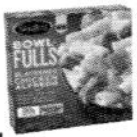

	C	F	Cb
Blackened Chicken Alfredo	**580**	25	59
Cheesy Chicken Parmesan	**520**	16	66
Chicken Bacon Ranch Pasta	**610**	26	58
Classic Pub Meatballs & Potatoes	**470**	20	42
Fried Chicken & Mashed Potatoes	**450**	17	51
Philly Cheese Steak Mac & Cheese	**560**	26	54
Slow Roasted Steak & Potatoes	**360**	14	38
Spicy Italian Sausage Pasta	**660**	35	63
Other Entrees: *For One*			
Baked Chicken	**260**	11	18
Cheddar Potato Bake	**510**	30	44
Chicken a la King	**400**	15	48
Chicken & Mushroom Marsala	**300**	7	40
Chicken Pot Pie Bites (4)	**190**	10	18
Fettuccini Alfredo	**640**	37	58
Fish Fillet with Mac & Cheese	**490**	21	49
Fried Chicken	**380**	18	32
Four Cheese Mac with Bacon	**440**	19	47
Fried Chicken	**340**	16	28
Green Pepper Steak	**290**	9	34
Pub Classics: BBQ Burger & Bacon	**390**	14	40
Ranch Fried Chicken	**480**	19	48
Rigatoni with Chicken & Pesto	**410**	17	40
Romano Crusted Chicken	**470**	19	51
Salisbury Steak	**340**	16	26
Spaghetti w/ Meatballs	**450**	13	60
Spaghetti w/ Meat Sauce	**410**	13	54
Swedish Meatballs	**500**	23	48
Three Cheese Ravioli	**370**	13	43
Tuna Noodle Casserole	**420**	19	40
Turkey Tetrazzini	**470**	24	42
White Meat Chicken Pot Pie, large	**630**	37	55

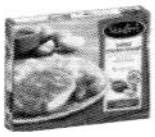

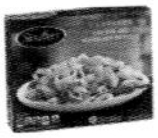

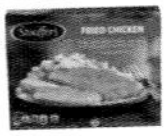

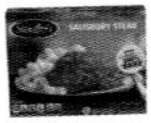

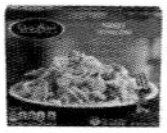

Swanson:

Frozen:

Dinners: *Per Package*

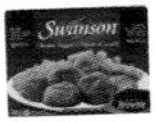

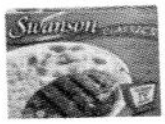

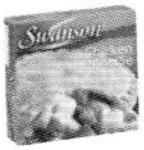

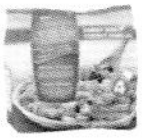

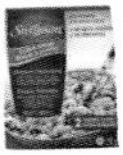

	C	F	Cb
Chicken Nuggets	**590**	25	71
Chicken Parmigiana	**450**	23	45
Chicken Strips	**480**	19	61
Fried Chicken	**520**	26	54
Meatloaf	**450**	23	45
Rib Style Boneless Pork	**540**	23	71
Salisbury Steak	**450**	22	44
Turkey	**330**	9	45
Meat Pies: Beef	**430**	26	37
Chicken	**370**	20	37
Turkey	**400**	23	38
Skillets: *For Two*			
Alfredo Chicken	**370**	12	42
Beef Lo Mein	**360**	6	55
Chicken Florentine	**310**	7	40
Chicken Parmesan	**430**	14	60
Creamy Cheddar Chicken	**360**	8	52
Garlic Chicken	**420**	15	51
Garlic Shrimp	**390**	14	49
Teriyaki Chicken	**290**	3	51
Tasty Bite:			
Mains: *Per ⅔ Cup*			
Bombay Potatoes, 4.9 oz	**130**	5	18
Channa Masala	**160**	6	28
Coconut Vegetables	**130**	7	13
Jaipur Vegetables	**180**	12	12
Jodhpur Lentils	**120**	4	14
Kashmir Spinach	**120**	9	6
Madras Lentils	**140**	6	17
Mushroom Masala	**100**	4.5	13
Punjab Eggplant	**110**	5	12
TGI Friday's:			
Buffalo Style Chicken Wings, with Sauce, 4.5 oz	**240**	16	10
Cheddar & Bacon Potato Skins (1)	**190**	13	15
Cheeseburger Sliders w/ BBQ Sce	**250**	13	24
Honey BBQ Chicken Wings, 3 oz	**290**	15	24
Mozzarella Sticks, with Marinara Sauce (1)	**100**	5	12
Poppers, Crm Chse Stuffed Jalapeno (3) with Raspberry Habanero Dip	**250**	14	27

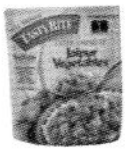

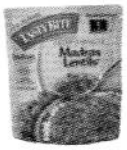

Thai Kitchen:	C	F	Cb
Curry & Noodle Kits (Gluten Free):			
Pad Thai	260	1	58
Thai Peanut	200	4	37
Noodle Carts (Gluten Free):			
Pad Thai, 9.77 oz	440	3	98
Thai Peanut, 9.77 oz	540	12	96

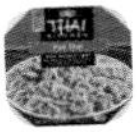

Trader Joe's:			
Baked Beans, Organic, av., ½ cup	140	0	29
Black Beans:			
Regular, ½ cup	110	0	19
Cuban Style, ½ cup	100	0.5	19

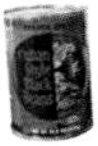

Black Bean & Jack Cheese Burrito	600	20	77
Chicken Chili with Beans, 1 cup	290	9	32
Potatoes: Garlic Mashed, ½ cup	150	7	19
Cheddar Cheese Au Gratin, ½ cup	140	5	21
Turkey Chili w/ Beans, 1 cup	240	4.5	30
Frozen:			
Black Beans & Chse Taquitos (2)	190	7	26
Butternut Squash Mac & Cheese, 8 oz	250	8	38
Chicken Quesadilla, (1), 6 oz	320	16	26
Fiery Chicken Curry, 9.5 oz	360	13	40
Mac & Cheese: Regular, 1 cup, 7 oz	360	15	42
Reduced Guilt, 7 oz	270	6	40
Pies: Chicken Pot Pie, ½ pie, 8 oz	360	22	28
Shepherd's Pie, 1 cup, 8 oz	170	3	22
Plant Based Protein Patties:			
Burger Patties (1), 4 oz	290	20	11
Turkeyless Patties (1), 4 oz	240	14	7
Spaghetti & Beef Meatballs, 1 cup, 9 oz	380	13	48
Spicy Beef & Broccoli, 1¾ cups	430	13	64
Trad. Carnitas, Mexican Style, 3 oz	200	14	1
Veggie & Sobda Noodle Stir Fry, 1 cup, 3 oz	80	2	14
Tyson:			
Any'tizers Snacks:			

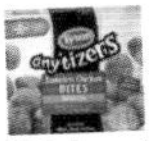

24 oz Bags Boneless Chicken Bites:			
Buffalo Style, 3 oz	180	9	12
Honey BBQ, 3 oz	210	9	20
Homestyle Chicken Fries, 3.2 oz	260	16	16
Popcorn Chicken, 3 oz	170	7	14
Wings, Tequila Lime flavored, 3 oz	170	11	3

Tyson (Cont):	C	F	Cb
Frozen:			
Beef:			
Country Fried Steak (1)	300	21	15
Steak Fingers, 3 oz	250	18	14

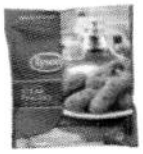

Breaded Chicken: *Per 3 oz Unless Indicated*			
Crispy Chicken Strips	210	10	17
Fun Nuggets 2.7 oz	180	11	10
Honey Batt. Breast Tender	210	13	13
Nuggets, 3.2 oz	270	17	15

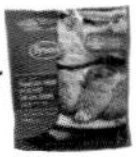

Parm. Herb Encrusted Crispy Strips	210	10	13
Southern Breast Tenderloins, 3 oz	180	9	12
Spicy Breast Patties, 2.7 oz	200	13	10
Grilled Chkn Breasts: Blackened, 3 oz	110	3	1
Breast Fillets, 3.5 oz	130	4.5	2
Fajita Strips, 3 oz	100	2	2
Oven Roasted, Diced, 3 oz	100	3	1

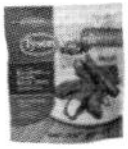

Sweet Teriyaki Chicken Fillets, 3 oz	140	6	4
Meal Kits: Chipotle Chicken, with Honey Lime Glaze, 4.5 oz	160	5	3
Instant Pot:			
Cajun Style Chicken & Rice, 7 oz	330	10	41
Teriyaki Chicken & Rice, 7.2 oz	410	8	63
Uncle Ben's:			
Flavored Grains: *Dry Mix Only*			
Average all flavors, ¼ cup	155	1	31
Long Grain Varieties, ¼ cup	200	0.5	42
Flavor Infusions, dry mix, av., 1.7 oz	155	0.5	34
Ready Rice: *Per Pouch Unless Indicated*			
Butter & Garlic Flavored	370	6	73
Creamy Four Cheese Flavored Rice, with Vermicelli, 1 cup, 5.65 oz	220	5	40
Garden Vegetable Rice, 1 c., 5.1 oz	210	3	42
Jambalaya Rice, 1 cup, 5 oz	200	2	40
Risotto: Cheese	430	10	76
Mushroom	420	8	77

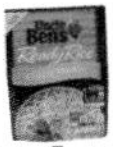

Roasted Chicken Flavored, 1 c., 5 oz	210	3	42
Spanish Style Rice, 1 cup, 5 oz	200	3	40
Van Camp's:			
Baked Beans: Orig., ½ cup, 4.8 oz	150	0.5	30
Bacon, ½ cup, 4.8 oz	160	1	30
Beanee Weenee: Original, 7.75 oz	260	8	33
Barbecue, 7.75oz	280	8	39
Smoked Hickory, 7.75 oz	320	8	48
Chili, with Beans, 9 oz	410	24	34
Pork & Beans, in Tom. Sce, 4.6 oz	120	1	23

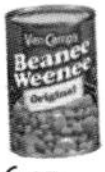

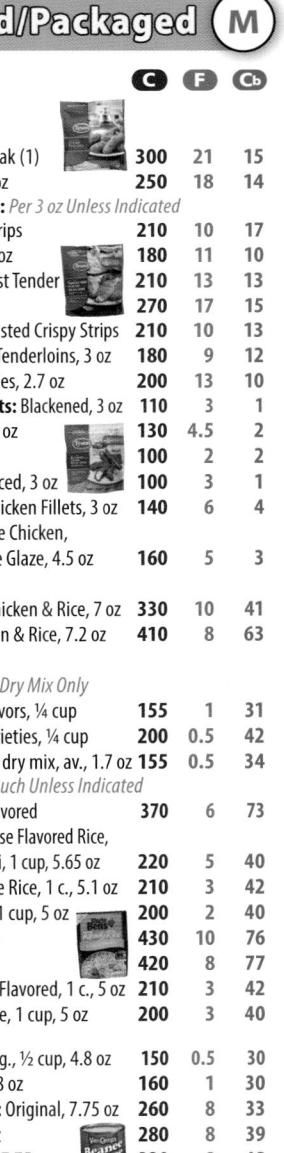

Van De Kamp's:	C	F	Cb
Frozen:			
Fillets: Beer Battered, 3.8 oz	210	10	21
Cracked Black Pepper Salmon, 4.5 oz	230	8	20
Crispy, 3.8 oz	210	10	21
Crunchy, 3.8 oz	240	12	24
Fish Sticks:			
Crunchy, 3.6 oz	220	10	20
Nacho, 3 oz	200	10	18
Ranch (4), 3 oz	200	10	18

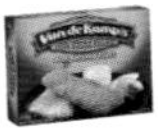
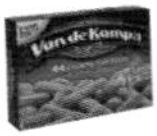

Whole Foods (365):	C	F	Cb
Macaraoni & Cheese, 1 c. prepared	400	17	50
Plant-Based:			
Chicken-Style: Breaded Patties (1)	130	5	12
Meatballs (4), 2 oz	170	11	9
Nuggets (4)	140	6	13
Tradtnl Burgers, 1 Patty	80	3	7
Pasta Rings in Tom. Sauce, 7.5 oz	140	0	30

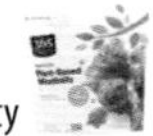

Worthington/Loma Linda *(Vegan)*:	C	F	Cb
Big Franks, 1 link, 1.8 oz	110	6	3
Burger, 1.94 oz	70	2	3
Chili, 1 cup, 8.10 oz	280	10	25
Choplets, 2 slices, 3.2 oz	90	1	4
Complete Meal Solution:			
Chipotle Bowl, 5 oz	130	0	23
Hearty Stew, 10 oz	270	2	47
Italian Bolognese, 5 oz	90	3	10
Medit. Tom. & Olive with Pasta, 5 oz	100	3	12
Pad Thai, 5 oz	130	4	18
Southwest Chunky Stew, 5 oz	125	2	19
Thai Red Curry, 5 oz	130	6	12
Thai Green Curry, 5 oz	155	5	23
Tikka Masala, 5 oz	125	3	19
Linketts (1), 1.3 oz	70	4	1
Nutolene, 2 slices, 3 oz	230	20	2
Redi-Burger, 3 oz slice	120	3	7
Saucettes (1), 1.34 oz	90	6	1
Sloppy Joe, ⅓ cup, 1.62 oz	40	0.5	6
Swiss Stake with Gravy, 3.25 oz	120	6	7
Tuno: In Spring Water, 2 oz	40	0	2
Lemon Pepper, 2 oz	55	1	5
3 oz pouch	80	2	7
Sesame Ginger, 3 oz pouch	87	1	13
Sriracha, 2 oz	70	3	6
Thai Sweet Chili, 3 oz pouch	90	0.5	13
Vege-Burger, ¼ cup, 1.9 oz	60	0.5	2
Veja-Links (1)	45	2	3

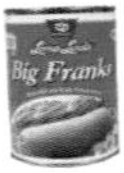

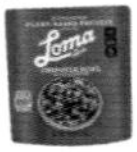

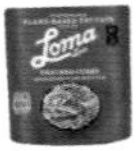

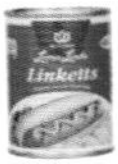

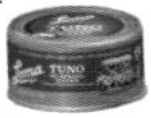
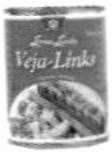

Yves Veggie Cuisine *(Meatless)*:	C	F	Cb
Appetizers:			
Balls, Falafel (3)	150	7	17
Bites: Broccoli (4)	80	3	11
Kale & Quinoa (4)	90	3	13
Sweet Potato & Chickpea (4)	100	3	17
Burger Patties:			
Gluten Free Veggie (1)	110	6	5
Kale & Root Vegetables (1)	110	6	5
Deli Veggie Slices:			
Bologna (3)	60	1	2
Ham (5)	80	1	5
Pepperoni (10)	45	1	3
Salami (5)	80	1	5
Turkey (5)	80	1	4
Veggie Dogs:			
Good Dog, 1.35 oz	45	1	2
Regular (1)	50	0.5	2
Jumbo (1), 2.7 oz	110	2	4
Tofu (1)	50	1	2
Ground Rounds:			
Original Veggie, 1.9 oz	60	0.5	5
Garden Veggie Crumble, 1.95 oz	80	2	9

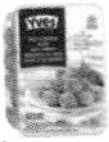

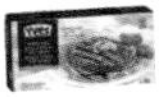
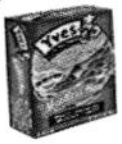

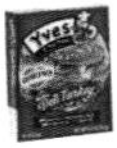

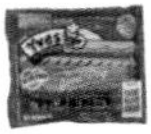

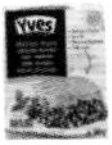

Other Vegan Plant Based Meals ~ *See Page 124*

Zatarain's:	C	F	Cb
Rice Mixes New Orleans Style: *Per Dry Mix Only*			
Creole Piiaf Mix, with Long Grain & Wild Rice, 2 oz	220	1	46
Jambalaya Mix, 1.74 oz	170	0.5	37
Red Beans & Rice, 3 oz	250	1	50
Red. Sodium: Dirty Rice, 1.74 oz	180	0.5	39
Red Beans & Rice, 3 oz	250	1	50
Frozen Entrees: *Per Single Serve*			
Blackened Chicken Alfredo, 10.5 oz	500	22	54
Blackened Chkn w/ Yellow Rice, 10.5 oz	540	17	77
Bourbon Chicken Pasta, 10.5 oz	460	18	52
Creamy Cajun Style Pasta, 10.5 oz	420	16	48
Dirty Rice with Beef & Pork, 10 oz	430	13	64
Jambalaya Flavored w/ Ssg, 12 oz	440	7	86
Red Beans & Rice with Sausage, 12 oz	480	14	78
Sausage & Chicken Gumbo with Rice, 12 oz	310	10	45
Shrimp Alfredo, 10.5 oz	490	17	62
Shrimp Scampi with Pasta, 10.5 oz	350	10	47

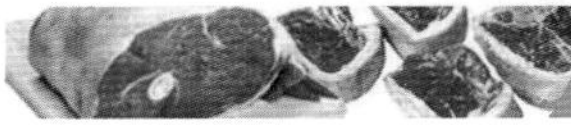

Note: Cooking reduces weight of meat by 20-45% due to water and fat losses. Average weight loss is 30%. Actual loss depends on cooking method and cooking time.

Examples:

4 oz raw weight = approx. 3 oz cooked weight

4 oz cooked weight = approx. 5½ oz raw weight

What 3 oz Cooked Meat Looks Like:

- Rectangular piece (4" x 2½" x ½" thick)
- Deck of cards (3½" x 2½" x ⅝" thick)

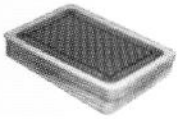

Quick Guide

Sirloin (Choice Grade):
External fat trimmed to ½"
Broiled, Edible Portion (no bone)

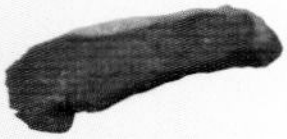

	C	F	Cb
Small/Regular Serving, 3 oz, cooked weight:			
(from 4-4½ oz raw)			
Lean + external fat (⅛"), 3 oz	**220**	13	**0**
Lean + marbling, 3 oz	**185**	9	**0**
Lean only, 3 oz	**160**	6	**0**
(No external fat or marbling)			
Medium Serving, 5 oz, cooked weight:			
(from approximately 7 oz raw)			
Lean + external fat (⅛"), 5 oz	**365**	22	**0**
Lean + marbling, 5 oz	**310**	15	**0**
Lean only, 5 oz	**265**	10	**0**
Large Serving, 8 oz, cooked weight:			
(from approximately11-12 oz raw)			
Lean + external fat (½"), 8 oz	**585**	36	**0**
Lean + marbling, 8 oz	**500**	24	**0**
Lean only, 8 oz	**425**	15	**0**
Extra Large Serving, 12 oz, cooked weight:			
(from approximately 16-17 oz raw)			
Lean + external fat (⅛"), 12 oz	**875**	54	**0**
Lean + marbling, 12 oz	**745**	36	**0**
Lean only, 12 oz	**640**	22	**0**
Pan Fried:			
Sirloin (Choice), medium serving,			
Lean + external fat (⅛"), 5 oz	**445**	30	**0**

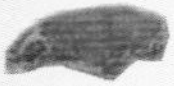

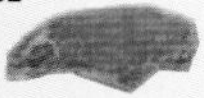

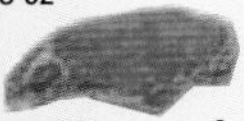

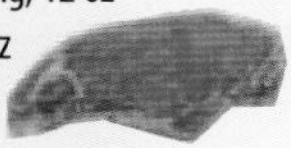

Other Steaks

	C	F	Cb
Filet Mignon (Tenderloin):			
1 Medium steak, 6 oz raw weight:			
Broiled, with ¼" fat trim:			
Lean + fat (¼"), 4 oz	**360**	27	**0**
Lean only, 3.5 oz	**230**	12	**0**
New York/Club Steak:			
Top Loin/Short Loin:			
1 steak, regular (9.25 oz raw, ¼" fat):			
Broiled: Lean + fat (¼"), 6.3 oz	**580**	43	**0**
Lean + marbling, 5.5 oz	**400**	25	**0**
Lean only, 5.25 oz	**360**	20	**0**
Porterhouse Steak:			
1 Medium, 6 oz raw weight, w/out bone, broiled:			
Lean + fat (¼"), 4.3 oz	**410**	33	**0**
Lean only, 3.5 oz	**210**	11	**0**
1 Large ,12 oz raw weight, without bone, broiled:			
Lean + fat (¼") 8.5 oz cooked	**820**	66	**0**
Lean only, 7 oz cooked	**420**	22	**0**
T-Bone Steak: *Broiled or Grilled*			
Medium Size: *8 oz raw weight, without bone*			
Approximately 6 oz cooked:			
Lean + Fat (¼"), 5 oz	**400**	28	**0**
Lean only, 4 oz	**265**	12	**0**
Large Size: *12 oz raw weight*			
Approximately 9 oz cooked:			
Lean + fat (¼"), 7 oz, without bone	**560**	39	**0**
Lean only, 6 oz, without bone	**400**	18	**0**
Extra Large Size: *20 oz raw weight*			
Approximately 16 oz cooked:			
Lean + Fat (¼"), 12 oz, without bone	**960**	66	**0**
Lean Only, 10 oz, without bone	**660**	30	**0**

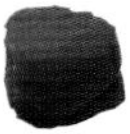

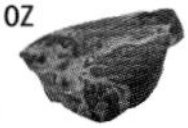

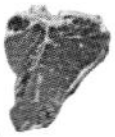

Also See Fast-Foods & Restaurants Section ~
Lone Star Steakhouse; Outback Steakhouse

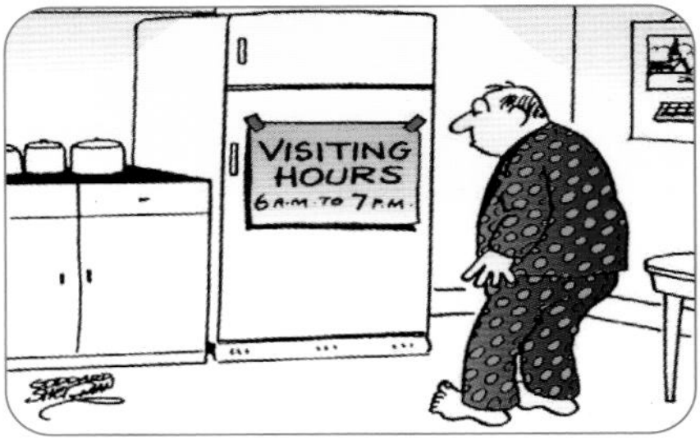

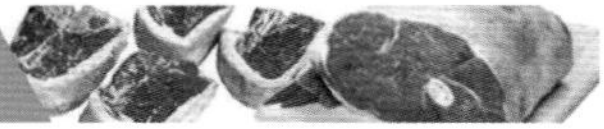

Beef – Individual Cuts

Average All Grades
Edible Weight, Without Bone

	C	F	Cb
Brisket, whole, braised:			
Lean + fat (¼" trim), 3 oz	330	27	0
Lean + marbling, 3 oz	250	17	0
Lean only, 3 oz	185	9	0
Chuck Blade, braised:			
Lean + fat (¼"), 3 oz	310	24	0
Lean + marbling, 3 oz	295	22	0
Lean only, 3 oz	245	13	0
Flank: Raw, 4 oz	175	8	0
Braised, 3 oz	225	14	0
Broiled, 3 oz	155	6	0
Round, bottom, braised:			
Lean + marbling, 3 oz	190	7.5	0
Lean only, 3 oz	185	6.5	0
Round, eye/tip, rstd:			
Lean + fat (¼"), 3 oz	205	11	0
Lean, w/ marbling, 3 oz	150	5	0
Round, top: *Per 3 oz, Cooked Weight*			
Braised, Lean + fat	210	10	0
Lean only	170	4	0
Broiled, Lean + fat	180	8	0
Lean only	160	5	0
Pan-fried, Lean + fat	235	13	0
Lean only	195	7	0

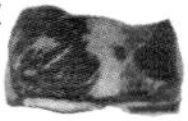
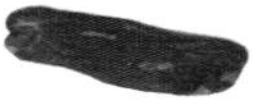
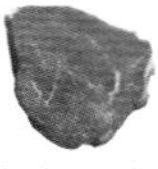
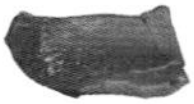

Beef Ribs

	C	F	Cb
Back Ribs: *7" long, visible fat trimmed to ¼"*			
10.3 oz raw w/ bone or 3.5 oz cooked, braised, w/o bone			
1 average rib	410	34	0
3 ribs	1230	102	0
Short Ribs: *2½" long, visible fat trimmed to ¼"*			
6 oz raw with bone or 2.52 oz cooked, braised, w/o bone			
1 average rib	320	28	0
3 ribs	960	85	0

Ground Beef

	C	F	Cb
Ground Beef, Raw: *Per 4 oz*			
70% lean (30% fat)	380	34	0
75% lean (25% fat)	335	29	0
80% lean (20% fat)	290	23	0
85% lean (15% fat)	245	17	0
90% lean (10% fat)	200	12	0
95% lean (5% fat)	155	6	0
Baked/Broiled: Regular (70%), 3 oz	230	16	0
Lean (80%), 3 oz	215	14	0
Extra lean (90%), 3 oz	185	10	0
Pan-Broiled:			
Regular (70%), 3 oz	230	15	0
Lean (80%), 3 oz	210	14	0
Extra lean (90%), 3 oz	195	10	0
Ground Beef Patties: *Average, 23% Fat*			
Raw, 4 oz	330	25	0
Broiled, 3 oz (from 4 oz raw)	250	19	0

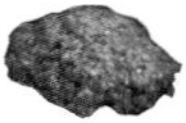
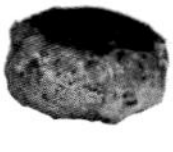

Quick Guide

	C	F	Cb
Roast Beef			
Round (Eye/Tip, average): *Average All Cuts*			
Small/Regular Serving: *3 oz*			
(2 thin slices/1 thick slice)			
Lean + fat (⅛" fat trim)	180	9	0
Lean only	145	4	0
Medium Serving: *5 oz*			
(3-4 thin slices)			
Lean + fat (⅛" fat trim)	300	15	0
Lean only	245	6.5	0
Large Serving, 8 oz: *3 thick slices*			
Lean + fat (⅛" fat trim)	480	24	0
Lean only	385	11	0
Beef Kebab: Cooked			
Beef & Veggies, 2 oz	160	10	4
If very lean meat	100	4	4

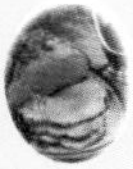
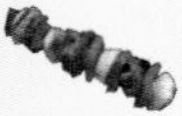

Meat Alternatives (Vegan)

	C	F	Cb
Beyond Meat:			
Beyond: Burger Patty, 4 oz	260	18	5
Cookout Classic, Burger Patties	290	22	4
Crumbles: Beefy, 1.94 oz	90	3	2
Fiesty Crumbles, 1.94 oz	90	2.5	2
Ground Beef, 4 oz	260	18	5
Sausage: Original Brat, 2.9 oz	190	12	5
Hot/Swseet Italian (1), cooked, 2.7 oz	190	12	5
Gardein:			
Beefless: Burger Patty, 3 oz	130	4.5	7
Sliders (1) with Bun, 2.5 oz	130	2.5	20
Tips, ¾ cup, 3.5 oz	170	7	8
Chick'n: BBQ Wings, w/o Sce, 2.5 oz	120	5	5
Crispy Patty (1), 3.1 oz	160	7	12
Mandarin Crispy, w/out Sce, 2.68 oz	150	7	6
Fishless: Golden Filet (2), 3.38 oz	180	10	14
Mini Crabless Cakes (3), 2.65 oz	130	6	11
Meatless Meatballs, (3), 3.17 oz	150	7	9
Porkless, Sweet & Sour Bites, 2.47 oz	120	3	9
Quorn:			
Meatless: Buffalo Dippes, 3.7 oz	230	10	21
Chipotle Cutlets (1), 3.5 oz	205	9	24
Fillets (1), 2.2 oz	70	1	7
Fishless Sticks, 3.5 oz	200	8	30
Pieces, 3.9 oz	120	3	11
Spicy Patties, 2.3 oz	130	5	14
Tofurky:			
Burger Patty, (1), 4 oz	250	16	7
Crumbles: Beef Style, 1.94 oz	100	5	4
Chorizo, 1.94 oz	130	9	5
Ham Style Roast, 3.2 oz	170	6	8
Roast w/ Wild Rice Stuffing, 5.2 oz	290	10	17

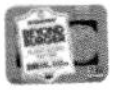
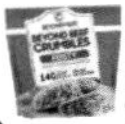
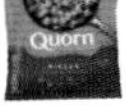

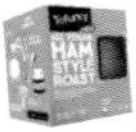

Yves Veggie Cuisine/Loma Linda ~ *See page 122*

Lamb

	C	F	Cb
Choice Grade:			
Leg (Whole), roasted:			
Lean + fat, 3 oz	**220**	14	0
Lean only, 3 oz	**160**	7	0
Leg (Sirloin Half), roasted:			
Lean + fat, 3 oz	**250**	18	0
Lean only, 3 oz	**175**	8	0
Leg (Shank Half), roasted:			
Lean + fat, 3 oz	**190**	11	0
Lean only, 3 oz	**155**	6	0
Loin Chop, broiled:			
1 chop (raw weight,4.25 oz):			
Lean + fat (2.25 oz edible)	**180**	12	0
Lean only (1.6 oz edible)	**85**	3.5	0
Rib Chop, broiled:			
1 chop (raw wt., 3.5 oz):			
Lean + fat (2.5 oz edible)	**255**	21	0
Lean only (1.75 oz edible)	**105**	6	0
Shoulder (Arm/Blade):			
Braised: Lean + fat, 3 oz	**295**	21	0
Lean only, 3 oz	**240**	12	0
Broiled: Lean + fat, 3 oz	**240**	17	0
Lean only, 3 oz	**170**	8	0
Roasted: Similar to Broiled			
Cubed Lamb (Leg/Shoulder):			
For stew or kebab:			
Braised, lean only, 3 oz	**190**	8	0
Broiled, lean only, 3 oz	**160**	6	0

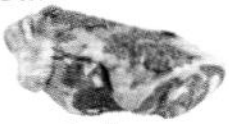
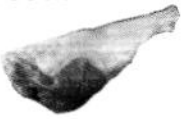
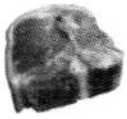
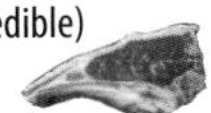
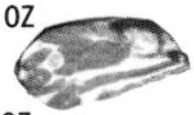
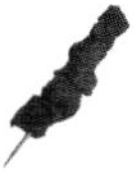

Veal

	C	F	Cb
Edible Weights:			
Leg (Top Round):			
Braised: Lean + fat, 3 oz	**180**	6	0
Lean only, 3 oz	**175**	5	0
Pan-fried, breaded:			
Lean + fat, 3 oz	**195**	8	9
Lean only, 3 oz	**185**	6	9
Pan-fried, not breaded:			
Lean + fat, 3 oz	**180**	7	0
Lean only, 3 oz	**155**	4	0
Roasted: Lean + fat, 3 oz	**135**	4	0
Lean only, 3 oz	**130**	3	0

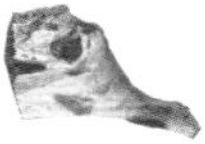
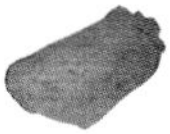
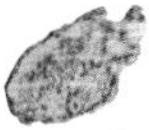
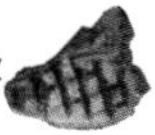

Veal (Cont)

	C	F	Cb
Loin Chop: *1 chop, 7 oz raw weight*			
Braised: Lean + fat, 3 oz	**240**	15	0
Lean only, 3 oz	**190**	8	0
Roasted: Lean + fat, 3 oz	**185**	11	0
Lean only, 3 oz	**150**	6	0
Rib, roasted: *Lean + fat, 3 oz*	**195**	12	0
Lean only, 3 oz	**150**	7	0
Shoulder, Arm/Blade, roasted:			
Lean + fat, 3 oz	**155**	7	0
Lean only, 3 oz	**140**	5	0
Sirloin, roasted:			
Lean + fat, 3 oz	**170**	9	0
Lean only, 3 oz	**145**	6	0
Cubed for Stew, braised:			
Leg/Shoulder, lean only, 3 oz	**160**	4	0
(1 lb raw yields approximately 9.25 oz cooked)			

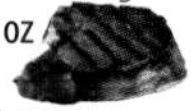
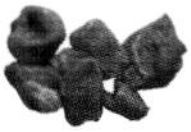

Pork

	C	F	Cb
Fresh Pork: *Cooked Weight, without bone): 4 oz raw weight = approx. 3 oz cooked weight*			
BBQ, Pulled:			
2 oz	**90**	2.5	10
4 oz	**180**	5	20
8oz	**360**	10	40
Blade Steak, broiled:			
Lean + fat, 3 oz	**220**	15	0
Lean only, 3 oz	**190**	11	0
Country Style Ribs, broiled/roasted:			
Lean + fat, 3 oz	**280**	22	0
Lean only, 3 oz	**210**	13	0
Spareribs, braised: *Lean & fat, 6 oz*			
(from 1 lb raw weight)	**675**	52	0
Leg (Ham), whole, roasted:			
Lean + fat, 3 oz	**230**	15	0
Lean only, 3 oz	**180**	8	0
Loin Chops, broiled: *Average* (From 1 chop: 5 oz raw weight with bone or 4 oz raw weight, without bone)			
Lean + fat, 3 oz	**200**	11	0
Lean only, 3 oz	**165**	7	0
Loin Roast, roasted:			
Lean + fat, 3 oz	**210**	13	0
Lean only, 3 oz	**180**	8	0
Rib Chops, (Boneless), broiled:			
Lean + fat, 3 oz	**220**	14	0
Lean only, 3 oz	**185**	9	0
Rib Roast:			
Lean + fat, 3 oz	**215**	13	0
Lean only, 3 oz	**180**	9	0

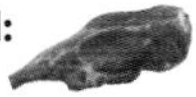
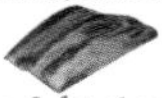
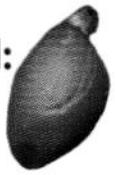
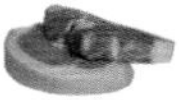
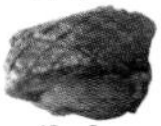
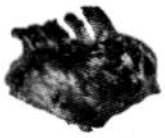

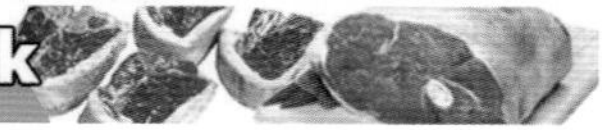

Pork (Cont)

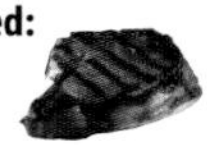
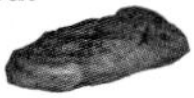
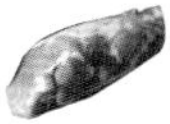
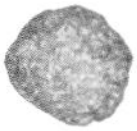

	C	F	Cb
Sirloin Chop, broiled:			
Lean + fat, 3 oz	180	8	0
Lean only, 3 oz	165	6	0
Sirloin Roast, roasted:			
Lean + fat, 3 oz	175	8	0
Lean only, 3 oz	170	7	0
Tenderloin (Boneless), roasted:			
Lean + fat, 3 oz	125	4	0
Lean only, 3 oz	120	3	0
Ground Pork:			
Raw, average, 1/4 lb, 4 oz	300	24	0
Broiled, 3 oz	250	18	0
Pan-fried, drained, 3 oz	260	19	0

Bacon

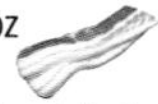
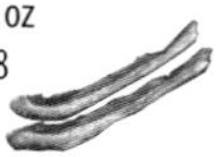
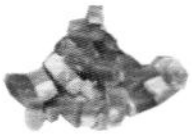

	C	F	Cb
Raw: 1 med. slice, 0.75 oz	95	9	0
1 thick slice, 1.3 oz	175	17	0
(1 lb raw yields approximately 5 oz cooked)			
Broiled/Pan-Fried:			
1 medium slice, 0.3 oz	40	3	0
3 medium slices, 0.8	125	10	0
2 thin slices, 0.5 oz	75	6	0
1 thick slice, 0.9 oz	65	5	0
Canadian Bacon:			
Cooked: 1 slice, 1 oz	45	2	0.5
2 slices, 2 oz	90	4	1
Bacon Bits, 1 Tbsp, 0.3 oz	35	2	0
Breakfast Strips, Broiled, 1 sl., 0.4 oz	50	4	0

Ham

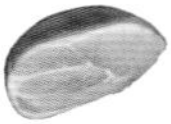
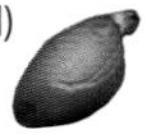

	C	F	Cb
Boneless Ham, cooked:			
Regular, (approximately 13% fat):			
Roasted, 3 oz	150	8	0
Extra Lean (5% fat),			
Roasted, 3 oz	125	5	0
Whole Ham, cooked:			
Lean + fat (as purchased)			
Roasted, 3 oz	210	15	0
Lean only, Roasted, 3 oz	135	5	0
Canned Ham: *Similar to boneless ham*			
Chopped, canned, 3 oz	200	16	0
Ham Patties, cooked, (1), 2.3 oz	220	20	1
Ham Steak, extra lean, 2 oz	70	2.5	0

Lunch Slices ~ *See Deli Meats, Page 128*

Game & Other Meats

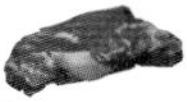
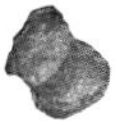
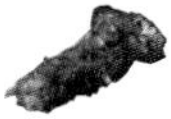
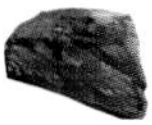
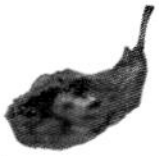

	C	F	Cb
Bison Steak,			
lean, 6 oz (raw)	205	4	0
Boar (wild), roasted, 3 oz	140	4	0
Buffalo Steak,			
New West Foods, 4 oz	70	3	0
Caribou, roasted, 3 oz	140	4	0
Deer/Venison, roasted 3 oz	135	3	0
Goat (Capretto):			
Raw, 3 oz	95	2	0
Roasted, 3 oz	120	2.5	0
Ostrich:			
Blackwing Ostrich Meats:			
Sausage Patties, 4 oz	110	1.5	0
Strip Filet, 6 oz	160	1.5	0
New West Foods:			
Ground Ostrich, 4 oz	165	7	0
Ostrich Steak, 4 oz steak	130	2.5	0
Rabbit: Roasted, 3 oz	165	7	0
Stewed, 1 cup, diced, 5 oz	290	12	0

Variety & Organ Meats

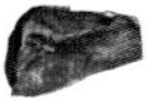
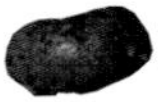
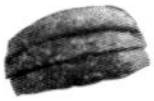
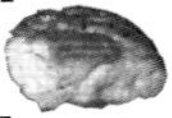
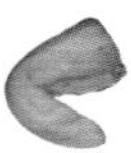

	C	F	Cb
Brain (Lamb): Braised, 3 oz	125	9	0
Pan-fried, 3 oz	230	19	0
Chitterlings, pork, simmered, 3 oz	260	25	0
Ears, pork, simmered, 1 ear, 4 oz	185	12	0
Feet, Pork: Simmered, 3 oz	200	14	0
Cured, pickled, 3 oz	170	14	0
Hormel, 2 oz	80	6	0
Head Cheese (Pork Snouts/Ears/Vinegar/Spices),			
1 oz slice	50	4	0
Heart, Beef, braised, 3 oz	140	4	0
Jowl, pork, raw, 4 oz	750	80	0
Kidneys, braised, 3 oz	140	5	0
Liver (beef): Raw, 4 oz	150	4	4
Braised, 3 oz	140	4	3
Pan-fried, 3 oz	185	7	7
Pancreas, pork, braised, 3 oz	185	8	0
Pork Cracklins, 0.5 oz	80	6	0
Pork Hocks, 1 piece, 6 oz	340	23	0
Scrapple, pork, 2 oz	120	8	8
Spleen, pork, braised, 3 oz	130	3	0
Stomach, pork, raw, 4 oz	185	12	0
Sweetbreads:			
Beef,/Lamb, cooked, 3 oz	125	9	0
Tail, pork, simmered, 3 oz	340	31	0
Tongue: Raised Veal, 3 oz	170	9	0
Beef/Lamb/Pork, av., 3 oz	235	17	0
Tripe, beef, raw, 3 oz	85	3.5	0

Quick Guide

	C	F	Cb
Franks & Weiners			
Average All Brands			
Regular (Pork Mix): *Per Frank*			
Regular, 1.5 oz	140	13	1
Bun Length/Jumbo, 2 oz	185	17	2
Extra Long, 2.75 oz	255	24	2
Small/Cocktail, each	30	3	0.5
Beef Franks: *Per Frank*			
Regular, 1.5 oz	140	13	2
Bun Length/Jumbo, 2 oz	175	17	2.5
1/4 lb Dog, 4 oz	375	33	5

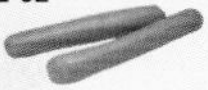

Franks & Weiners

	C	F	Cb
Ball Park: *Per 2 oz Frank Unless Indicated*			
Angus Beef:			
Orig.; Bun Size, 1.76 oz	160	15	2
Bun Size, 1.76 oz	70	5	2
Beef: Original; Bun Size, 1.8 oz	180	15	4
Deli Style, Regular, 1.76 oz	160	15	2
Grillmaster, Hearty, 2.9 oz	260	24	3
Lean, 1.76 oz	80	5	2
Classic: Cheese (1), 1.76 oz	120	10	2
Chicken & Pork(1); Bun Size, 1.9 oz	130	11	2
Turkey, (1), 1.76 oz	110	7	6
Foster Farms, Chicken; Turkey, 1.5 oz	110	9	1
Hebrew National: *Per Frank*			
Beef: Regular, 1.7 oz	150	13	2
All Natural, 1.7oz	140	12	2
Bun Length, 2 oz	170	15	2
Jumbo, 3 oz	260	23	3
97% Fat-Free, 1.6 oz	45	1	2
Reduced Fat, 1.6 oz	100	8	2
Jennie-O: *Per Frank*			
Turkey Franks:			
1.2 oz	70	6	1
Jumbo, 2 oz	120	9	2
Turkey Bratwurst, 3.85 oz	150	8	0
Uncured Breast Frank, 1.83 oz	90	6	0
Oscar Mayer: *Per Frank*			
Angus Beef:			
Bun Length; Jumbo, 1.76 oz	170	15	0
Beef, Classic, 1.48 oz	130	12	0
Cheese, 1.48 oz	120	10	0
Weiners, Classic, 1.48 oz	110	10	0
Shelton's: *Per Frank*			
Chicken, uncured, 1.2 oz	80	7	0
Turkey, 1.2 oz	60	4.5	1
Zacky Farms, Chkn; Turkey, av, 2 oz	115	10	4

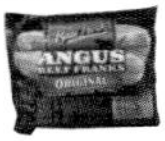

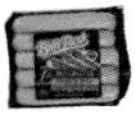

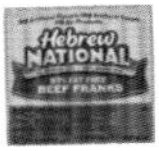

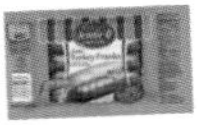

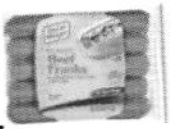

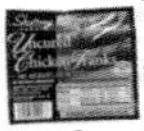

Quick Guide

	C	F	Cb
Fresh Sausages			
Pork/Beef: *Average All Types*			
Small: Raw, 4" link, 1 oz	85	7.5	0
Broiled/Pan-fried	80	7	0
Medium: Raw, 2 oz	170	15	0
Broiled/Pan-fried	165	14	0
Large: Raw, 3 oz	255	22	0
Broiled/Pan-fried	245	21	0
Italian: Raw, 3.2 oz	315	28	1
Cooked, 2.4 oz	230	18	3
Chorizo: Beef Chorizo, 2.5 oz piece	250	23	5
Pork Chorizo, 2 oz piece	250	23	5

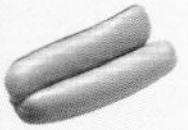

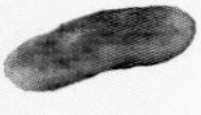

Note: Fat is lost in broiling/pan frying.
Cooked weight = approx. 60-70% raw weight

Smoked Sausages

	C	F	Cb
Per Link:			
Butterball, Turkey, 2 oz	100	5	5
Eckrich:			
Original, Natural Casing, (1)	180	15	4
Skinless Rope: Beef (1), 2 oz	180	15	5
Cheddar (1), 2 oz	180	16	3
Turkey (1), 2 oz	110	7	5
Hillshire Farm:			
Basil Pesto Chicken, 2 oz	110	7	3
Beef, 2 oz	170	14	3
Cheddarwurst, 2 oz	180	16	2
Chicken, Roasted Garlic, 2 oz	100	6	3
Hot Smoked, 2 oz	180	16	3

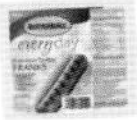

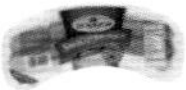

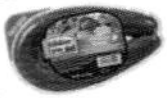

Johnsonville ~ *See CalorieKing.Com*

Breakfast Sausages/Patties

	C	F	Cb
Butterball: *Fully Cooked*			
Turkey: B'fast Sausage Links (3), 2 oz	90	5.5	0
Patties (2), 2 oz	90	5.5	0
Jimmy Dean: *Fully Cooked*			
Heat 'N Serve Sausage Links:			
Pork, Regular (3), 1.9 oz	210	19	2
Turkey (3), 2 oz	130	8	2
Heat 'N Serve Sausage Patties:			
Pork, Original (2), 1.8 oz	200	17	2
Turkey (2), 1.8 oz	120	8	1
Maple Pork Sausages,(3), 2.4 oz	280	26	4
Pork Patties, (2), 2.4 oz	280	27	1

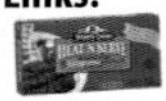

Breakfast Sandwiches ~ *See Page 92*

	C	F	Cb
Jones Dairy Farm:			
Golden Brown Sausages: *Fully Cooked*			
Mild/Maple Pork (3), average, 2 oz	250	24	2

Vegetarian Patties:

Boca ~ *See Page 112*
GardenBurer ~ *See Page 113*

Bagel, Corn & Hot Dogs

	C	F	Cb
Hot Dogs, Ready-To-Go:			
Includes Ketchup/Relish			
Regular, 1.5 oz frank, 1.5 oz bun	260	15	22
Bun Length, 2 oz frank, 1.5 oz bun	290	18	21
Jumbo Dog, 2 oz frank, 2 oz bun	360	20	36
¼ lb Beef Dog, 2 oz bun	480	15	36
Mile Long Dog, 2.6 oz dog, 1.5 oz bun	360	24	23
Corn Dogs:			
Beef/Pork Frank, average, 2.6 oz	170	10	16
Foster Farms:			
Corn Dogs:			
Cheese & Jalapeno (1)	180	8	20
Honey Crunchy:			
Regular (1), 2.7 oz	180	9	18
Mini (4), 2.7 oz	220	13	19
Gluten Free, 2.7 oz	180	9	20
State Fair: *Per Dog*			
Beef Corn Dog, 2.7 oz	240	13	26
Classic Corn Dog: Regular (2), 4 oz	330	11	34
Mini (5), 3.3 oz	270	14	29
Bagel Dogs:			
Hebrew National:			
Beef Bagel Dogs, 4 pieces, 2.75 oz	240	13	22
Schwanns: Classic Corn Dog (1), 2.7 oz	230	11	25
Mini Corn Dogs (4), 2.7 oz	220	13	21
Vienna Beef,			
Mini Bagel Dogs,(5), 4.6 oz	310	18	31

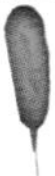
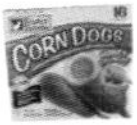
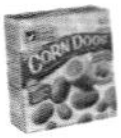
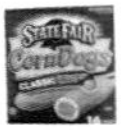
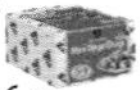

Hot Dog Toppings/Extras:

	C	F	Cb
American Cheese, 1 slice, 1 oz	110	9	1
Chili Con Carne, ¼ cup	50	2	5.5
Ketchup, 1 Tbsp	15	0	4
Mustard, 1 Tbsp	20	0	1
Onions, chopped, 1 Tbsp	5	0	1
Pickle Relish, 1 Tbsp	20	0	5
Sauerkraut, ½ cup	20	0	5

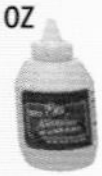
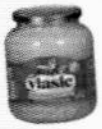

Deli/Lunch Meats & Sausage

	C	F	Cb
Beef Jerky/Meat Snacks,			
Berliner (pork/beef), 1 oz	65	5	1
Beerwurst (Beef):			
Small (2¾"diam), 1/16" slice	20	2	0
Large (4" diam), ⅛" slice	75	7	0.5
Beerwurst (Pork):			
Small (2.75"diameter), 1/16" slice	15	1	0
Large (4"diameter), ⅛" Slice	55	4	0.5
Blood Sausage, 1 oz	100	9	0.5

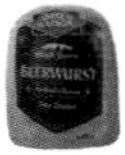
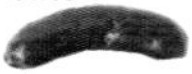

Deli/Lunch Meats & Sausages (Cont)

Bologna:	C	F	Cb
Beef Bologna: 1 slice, 1 oz	90	8	0
Light, 1 slice, 1 oz	60	4	2
Oscar Mayer: Regular, 1 oz	90	8	0
Light, 1 slice, 1 oz	60	4	1
Chicken & Pork Bologna,			
Oscar Mayer, with added Beef, 1 oz	80	7	0
Pork Bologna: 1 Slice, 1 oz	65	6	1
Fat-Free, 1 slice, 1 oz	20	0	2
Pork & Beef,			
Boar's Head, 2 oz	150	13	1
Turkey Bologna, av., 1 oz	60	5	0.5
Oscar Mayer, 1 oz	50	4	0
Bratwurst, average, 1 oz	80	7	1
Braunschweiger, (Pork/Liver/Sausage),			
Oscar Mayer, Liver, 2 oz	190	14	0
Chicken, average:			
1 thick or 2 thin slices, 1 oz	30	1	1
2 oz slice	60	2	2
Hillshire Farm,			
Rotisserie S'snd Chicken Breast, 2 oz	60	1	3
Corned Beef, average, full fat, 1 oz	60	5	0.5
Ham, Sliced: *Per 1 oz Slice*			
Baked/Broiled	35	1	1
Honey/Brown Sugar, average	35	1	1
Oscar Mayer, Honey Ham	60	1.5	1
Prosciutto, average	70	5	0
Ham & Cheese Loaf, average, 1 oz	70	5	1
Oscar Mayer, 1 oz	70	4.5	1
Italian Sausage, 2.6 oz	250	20	3
Kielbasa: Polish Sausage, 2 oz	65	5	1
Beef, 2 oz link	190	17	1
Knockwurst, av., 1 oz	90	8	0.5
Linguica *(Gaspar's),* 2 oz	130	9	1
Liverwurst, 1 oz	65	5	2
Liver Pate, fresh, average, 1 oz	90	8	1
Mortadella: 1 oz	105	9	0
Boar's Head, 6 slices	160	14	0
Olive Loaf: Average, 1 oz	70	5	3
Oscar Mayer, 1 oz	80	6	1
Pancetta, *Boars Head, 0. 5 oz slice*	50	4.5	0

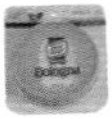
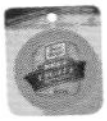
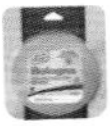
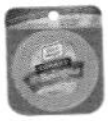
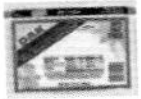
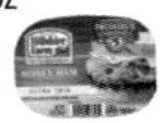
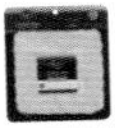
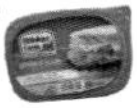
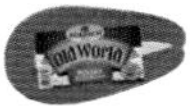
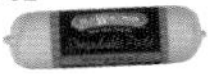
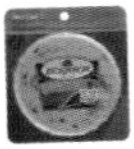

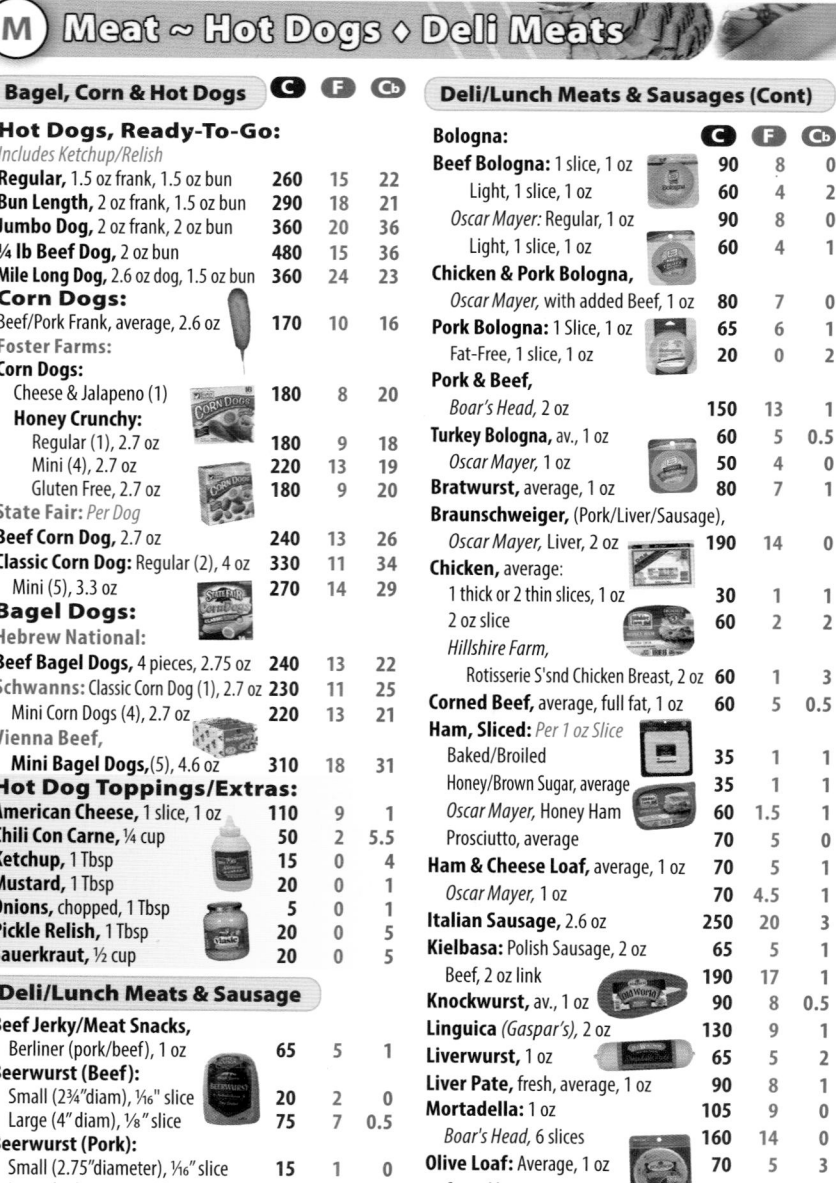

Deli/Lunch Meats & Sausages (Cont)

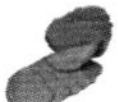
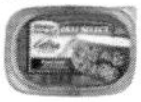
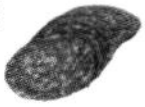
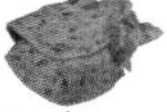
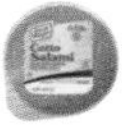
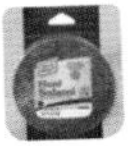

	C	F	Cb
Pastrami (Beef):			
Boar's Head:			
1st cut Pastrami Brisket, 2 oz	90	4	2
Top Round Pastrami, 2 oz	80	3	0.5
Hillshire, Deli Select,			
Ultra Thin. 2 oz	60	1.5	0.5
Peppered Beef, 1 oz slice	40	2	1
Pepperoni, 5 slices, 1 oz	140	13	0
Pickle Loaf, average, 1 oz	70	5	5
Pickle & Pepper Loaf,			
Boars Head, 2 oz	150	13	2
Proscuitto/Proscuitti, av., 1 oz	70	5	1
Roast Beef, Lean, 1 oz	40	2	0
Salami:			
Beef, average, 1 oz	80	7	1
Beef Chicken Pork,			
Oscar Mayer: Cotto, 1 slice, 1 oz	50	4	0
Beer Salami, average, 1 oz	50	4	0.5
Pork: Genoa, sliced, average, 1 oz	100	8	1
Boarshead, 2 oz	190	15	1
Fortuna's Stick, 1 oz	110	8	1
Pork & Beef:			
Dry, Hard, av., 1 oz	100	8	1
Boar's Head, 5 slices	110	9	1
Oscar Mayer: Hard: 1 slice, 1.8 oz	100	8	0.5
Cracked Black Pepper, 1 oz	110	9	0
White Cheddar Cheese, 3.45 oz	400	27	7

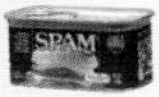
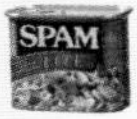
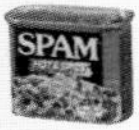
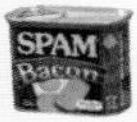
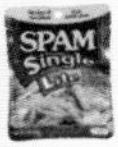

	C	F	Cb
SPAM (Hormel): *Per 2 oz*			
Classic: 2 oz serving	180	16	1
7 oz can	630	56	3.5
12 oz can	1080	96	6
Spam Lite: 2 oz	110	8	1
12 oz can	660	48	6
Other Spam Products: *Per 2 oz Unless Indicated*			
Hickory Smoke Flavor	180	16	1
Hot & Spicy	160	14	2
Oven Roasted Turkey	80	4.5	1
Spam Fries, 3 oz	300	23	14
Spam Spread	160	12	5
Spam with Bacon	180	16	1
Spam with Cheese	170	15	1
25% Less Sodium	180	16	1
Spam Singles: *Per 3 oz*			
Classic, 2.5 oz package	210	18	2
Lite, 2.5 oz package	130	9	2

Deli/Lunch Meats & Sausages (Cont)

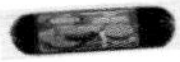
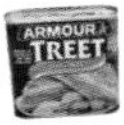
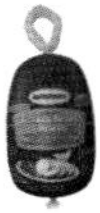
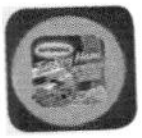

	C	F	Cb
Summer Sausage:			
Armour, Beef, 2 oz	190	17	2
Hillshire Farm, 2 oz	190	16	1
Treet *(Armour),* Luncheon Loaf,			
Original, 2 oz	140	11	4
Turkey, average: 1 oz slice	30	1	0.5
0.8 oz slice	22	0.5	0.5
Turkey Breast:			
Butterball, Oven Roasted:			
1 slice 1 oz	30	0.5	1
Deli Inspirations,			
Extra Thin Slices, 4 slices, 2 oz	50	1	3
Hillshire, Deli Select,			
Oven Roasted, 6 slices, 2 oz	50	0.5	2
Turkey Ham, 1 slice, 1 oz	35	1.5	0.5
Turkey Loaf, 1 oz	30	1	0.5
Turkey Pastrami, 1 oz	35	1.5	1
Turkey Roll, 1 oz	40	2	0.5

Vegetarian Deli ~ *See Page 118*

Meat Spread

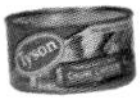
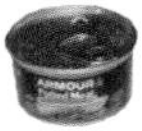
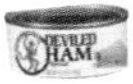
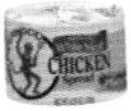

	C	F	Cb
Average All Brands:			
Chicken, white meat, 2oz	140	11	2
Corned Beef, 2 oz	140	11	1
Ham, Deviled, 2 oz	180	15	1
Liverwurst, 2 oz	160	13	4
Roast Beef, 2 oz	130	10	2
Turkey, 2 oz	110	7	2
Underwood: *Per 2 oz*			
Deviled Ham	180	15	1
Liverwurst	160	13	4
Roast Beef	140	10	2
White Meat Chicken	130	8	3

Paté

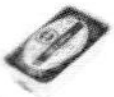
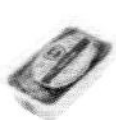
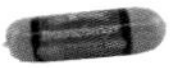

	C	F	Cb
Les Trois Petit Cochons: *Per 8 oz Package*			
Pate: au Poivre Noir, 2 oz	210	19	2
de Campagne 2 oz	240	22	2
de Canard a l'Orange, 2 oz	210	18	3
Paysan, 2 oz	160	13	2
Rustique, 2 oz	240	22	2
Wild Boar, 2 oz	180	15	4
Old Wisconsin Pate,			
Braunschweiger, 2 oz	210	18	3

N Nuts

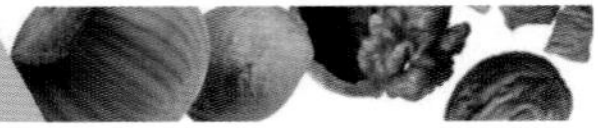

Nuts

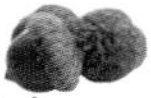
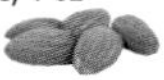
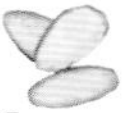
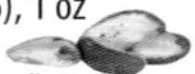
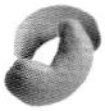

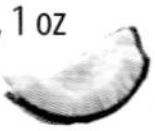
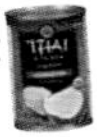

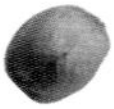
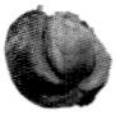
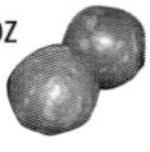
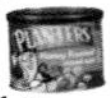

Per 1 oz Unless Indicated	C	F	Cb
Acorns, raw 1 oz	110	7	12
Almonds: Dried/Dry Roasted:			
Whole: 12 medium size, 0.5 oz	85	7.5	3
23-25 medium size, 1 oz	170	15	6
½ cup, 2.5 oz	420	37	13
Ground, 1 cup, 3.4 oz	545	47	20
Sliced, ½ cup, 1.6 oz	260	22	10
Slivered, ½ cup, 2 oz	310	27	12
Chocolate Coated (5-6), 1 oz	150	10	15
Honey Roasted, 1 oz	170	14	8
Oil Roasted (*Blue Diamond*), 1 oz	170	16	5
Brazil Nuts, 8 medium, 1 oz	185	19	3
Cashews, dry or oil roasted:			
14 large/18 med./26 small: 1 oz	165	14	9
½ cup, 2.4 oz	375	31	20
Honey Roasted, 1 oz	165	13	10
Chestnuts:			
Average, dried, 1 oz	105	1	22
Raw/Fresh, 5-6 nuts, 1 oz	60	0	13
Canned, water chestnuts, sliced/whole/drained, 1 oz	30	0	7
Coconut, Fresh:			
1 piece, 2"x2"x ½ ", 1 oz	185	18	7
Shredded, fresh, ½ cup, 1.4 oz	140	13	6
Dried (Desiccated):			
Sweetened: Shredded, 1 oz	145	10	14
Grated, ½ cup, 1.3 oz	185	13	18
Unsweetened, 1 oz	185	18	7
Cream (canned), ½ cup, 5.2 oz	285	26	12
Milk (canned), unsweetened, ¼ cup, 2 fl.oz	100	10	3
Water (center liquid), ½ cup, 4.3 oz	25	0	4.5
Filberts or Hazelnuts:			
Shelled, 18-20 nuts	180	17	4.5
Chopped, ¼ cup, 1 oz	180	18	5
Ground, ¼ cup, 0.6 oz	120	12	3
Ginkgo Nuts, canned, 14 med., 1 oz	32	0.5	6.5
Hickory, 30 small nuts, 1 oz	200	18	5
Macadamia Nuts, Shelled:			
Raw or Dry Roasted, avg:			
12 small or 8 med., 1 oz	200	21	4
6-7 large, 1 oz	200	21	4
½ cup, 2.3 oz	480	51	10
Mixed Nuts: Raw, 18-22 nuts, 1 oz	170	15	7
Oil Roasted, all types	170	16	6
Sweet Roasts, 26 pieces, 1 oz	160	12	10
Planters, Dry Roasted/Honey, 1 oz	150	11	11
Nut Toppings, chopped, 1 Tbsp, 0.3 oz	40	4	1.5

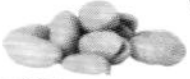
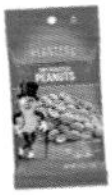
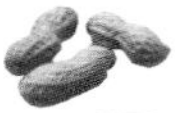
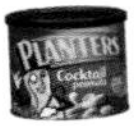

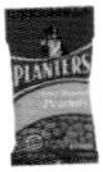

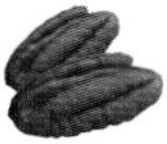
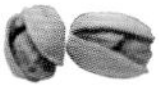
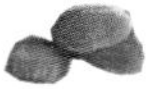
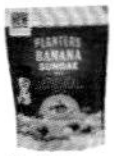

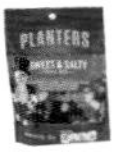

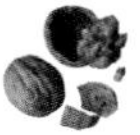

Per 1 oz Unless Indicated	C	F	Cb
Peanuts:			
Dry or oil roasted, average:			
Small handful, ¾ oz	125	10	4
⅕ cup, 1 oz	165	14	6
½ cup, 2.5 oz	415	35	15
3 oz bag	500	42	18
7 oz bag	1160	98	42
Raw: Shelled, 1 oz	160	14	4.5
In shell, 1 oz	115	110	3
Planters:			
Cocktail, all varieties	170	14	5
Honey Roasted	160	13	7
Spanish Redskins	170	15	4
Sweet N' Crunchy	140	8	15
Japanese Style Peanuts, Coated in Crunchy Shell	150	8	13
Pecans, roasted:			
10 halves, 0.5 oz	95	10	2
20 Halves, 1 oz	195	20	4
1 cup, halves, 3.5 oz	680	71	14
Pilinuts, dried, 1 oz	215	24	1
Pine Nuts, dried, 1 Tbsp, 0.3 oz	70	7	1.5
Pistachios, raw:			
Shelled, 45 nuts, 1 oz	160	13	8
Unshelled, 2 oz	165	14	7
Lance, Roasted, 1.5 oz	120	9	6
Sesame Nut Mix, 1 oz	160	13	9
Soy Nuts: Dry Roasted	130	6	9
½ cup, 3 oz	390	18	28
Revival, Chocolate Covered, 2 oz	200	12	20
Trail Mix *(Planters):*			
Dessert Mixes: Banana Sundae, 1 oz	150	10	13
Oatmeal Raisin Cookie,1 oz	140	7	17
Turtle Sundae, 1 oz	160	11	13
Energy Mix, 1.4 oz	240	19	14
Peanut Butter Chocolate, 1.15 oz	180	12	13
Spicy Nuts & Cajun Sticks, 1 oz	150	11	11
Sweet & Salty, 1.1 oz	150	9	15
Tropical Fruit, 1.1 oz	150	9	15
Walnuts, average all types:			
7-10 halves, 0.5 oz	90	9	2
15-20 halves, 1 oz	175	17	3
Chopped, ½ cup, 2.2 oz	380	36	6
Ground, ¼ cup, 0.7 oz	130	13	3

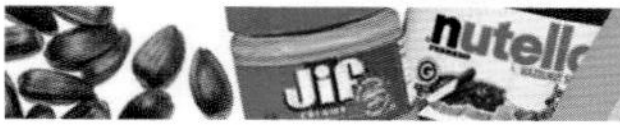

Quick Guide

	C	F	Cb
Peanut Butter: *Average All Brands*			
1 level tsp, 0.2 oz	35	3	1
1 level Tbsp, 0.6 oz	100	8.5	3.5
1 oz Quantity	165	14	6
½ cup, 5 oz	835	72	29

Peanut Butter ~ Brands

	C	F	Cb
Jif: Regular, all varieties, 2 Tbsp	190	16	8
Honey Varieties, 2 Tbsp	190	15	10
No Added Sugar, 2 Tbsp	200	17	7
Reduced Fat, all varieties, 2 Tbsp	190	12	15
Laura Scudder's:			
Natural: Smooth; Nutty, 2 Tbsp	190	16	7
Smooth, Unsalted, 2 Tbsp	190	16	7
Organic, Smooth; Nutty, 2 Tbsp	180	16	5
Peter Pan:			
Just Peanuts: Creamy/Crunchy, 2 T.	210	17	6
Honey Roast Creamy, 2 Tbsp	200	16	6
Natural, Creamy/Crunchy, 2 Tbsp	210	17	6
Planters, Creamy/Crunchy, 2 Tbsp	180	15	8
Smucker's, Goober,			
Grape/Srawberry, av., 3 Tbsp. 2 oz	220	11	30
Skippy: *Per 2 Tbsp*			
Blended with Plant Protein, all var.	210	16	6
Creamy; Super Chunky	190	16	6
Reduced Fat, Creamy/Crunchy	190	12	14
Roasted Honey Nut, Creamy	200	16	6

Peanut Butter & Jelly Sandwich

	C	F	Cb
1 sandwich: *With 2 oz Bread*			
Thin Spread, 1 Tbsp Peanut Butter + 1 Tbsp Jelly	310	10	48
Thick Spread, 2 Tbsp Peanut Butter + 2 Tbsp Jelly	480	19	67

Nut & Chocolate Spread

	C	F	Cb
Nutella:			
1 Tbsp, 0.7 oz	110	6	11
2 Tbsp, 1.3 oz	200	11	22

Note: Nutella contains approx. 50% sugar & 13% hazelnuts

Other Nut & Seed Butters

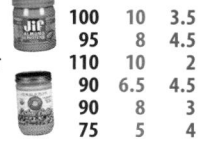

	C	F	Cb
Per 1 Tbsp, 0.5 oz			
Almond Butter	100	10	3.5
Cashew Butter	95	8	4.5
Hazelnut Butter; Pecan Butter	110	10	2
Pistachio Butter	90	6.5	4.5
Sesame Butter (Tahini)	90	8	3
Soy Nut Butter	75	5	4

Seeds

	C	F	Cb
Alfalfa Seeds, sprouted, ½ cup, 0.5 oz	5	0	1
Caraway/Fennel, 1 tsp	7	0.5	1
Chia Seeds: 1 Tbsp, 0.4 oz	45	3	4
3 Tbsp, 1 oz	140	8.5	12
Cottonseed Kernels, roasted, 1 Tbsp	50	3.5	2
Flaxseeds, 3 Tbsp, 1 oz	140	9	9
Hemp Seeds, 3 Tbsp, 1 oz	160	14	3
Lotus Seeds, dried, ½ cup, 0.5 oz	55	0.5	10
Poppy Seeds, 1 tsp	15	1	1
Pumpkin/Pepita Seeds, whole:			
Roasted/Tamari: 1 oz	150	12	4
½ cup, 4 oz	590	48	15
Dried (hulled), ¼ cup, 1 oz	155	13	5
Safflower Kernels, dried, 1 oz	150	11	10
Sesame Seeds:			
Dried, 1 Tbsp, 0.3 oz	50	4.5	2
Roasted/Toasted, 1 oz	160	14	7.5
Sunflower Kernels/Seeds:			
Dried, ¼ cup w/out hulls, 0.3 oz	200	18	7
Dry Roasted: 1 Tbsp, 0.3 oz	45	4	2
¼ cup, 1 oz	165	14	7
Oil Roasted, ⅕ cup, 1 oz	170	14	6.5
Watermelon Seeds, dried, ¼ cup, 1 oz	150	13	4

Nut eaters are healthier and live longer, say scientists.

Nuts are a nutritious source of protein, vitamins, minerals, fiber, healthy fats, and antioxidants.

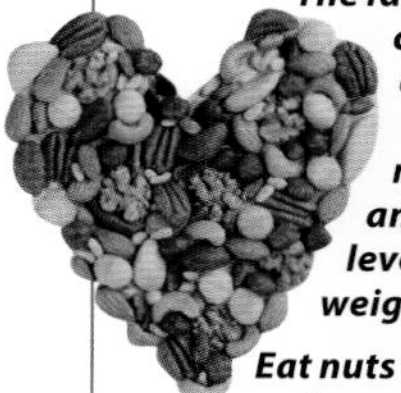

The fat and fiber of nuts can help reduce blood cholesterol. Their protein and fiber also promotes meal satiety (fullness) and reduces hunger levels – of benefit in weight control.

Eat nuts instead of high-sugar snacks, candy and soft drinks. Add chopped nuts to breakfast cereals.

P Pancakes & Waffles

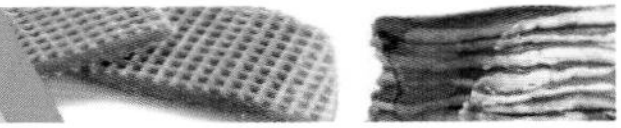

Quick Guide

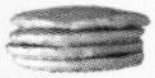
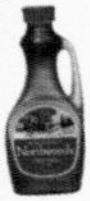
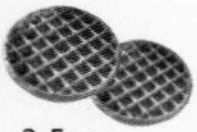

	C	F	Cb
Pancakes:			
Plain: *Average All Types*			
Small (3″ diameter), 0.8 oz	50	2	6
Medium (4″ diameter), 1.3 oz	85	3.5	11
Large (6″ diameter), 2.5 oz	175	7.5	22
Add Extra for Syrups/Butter			
Pancake Syrup: Regular, 1 Tbsp	50	0	12
¼ cup, 4 Tbsp	185	0	49
Lite, 1 Tbsp	25	0	6.5
¼ cup, 4 Tbsp	100	0	27
Butter/Margarine:			
Regular, 1 Tbsp	100	11	0
Whipped, 1 Tbsp	65	7.5	0
Waffles:			
Homemade, 7″ waffle, 2.5 oz	220	11	25
Frozen + Toasted, (4″ diam.), 1 oz	105	3	16

Pancake Brands

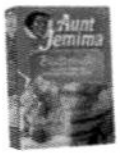

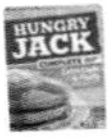

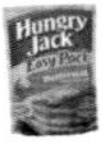

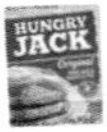

	C	F	Cb
Prepared as Directed			
Aunt Jemima: *Prepared*			
Mixes: *Makes 4″ Pancakes*			
Original (2)	190	5	30
Buttermilk (2)	180	5	30
Whole Wheat Blend (3)	200	5	30
On The Go, average, 2 oz mix	225	4.5	42
Bisquick: *Prepared with Water*			
Pancake/Waffle Mix: *Makes 3 Pancakes*			
Complete Whole Grain, ½ cup, 2 oz	210	3	40
Hungry Jack: *Just Add Water*			
Pancake & Waffle Mixes: *Makes 3 4″ Pancakes*			
Complete Mixes:			
Buttermilk, 1.9 oz	190	1	39
Chocolate Chip, 1.9 oz	190	2.5	39
Extra Light & Fluffy, 1.8 oz	180	1	38
Easy Packs:			
Buttermilk, 1.9 oz	190	1	39
Chocolate Chip, 1.9 oz	190	2.5	39
Traditional:			
Original, 1.7 oz	160	1	34
Buttermilk, 1.7 oz	160	1	34
Extra Light & Fluffy, 1.6 oz	150	1	32
Northern Pines, Just Add Water,			
Premium Mix (3), prepared	200	3.5	38

Frozen Breakfasts

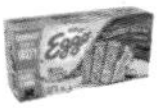
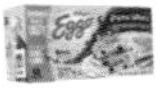
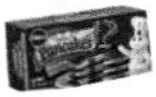

	C	F	Cb
Eggo *(Kellogg's):*			
Cinna-Toasts, Cinnamon Roll			
1 slice (set of 4), 1.4 oz	110	4	18
French Toast, Thick & Fluffy:			
Blueberry (1)	160	6	24
Classic (1)	120	2.5	21
French Toaster Sticks:			
Original (2)	210	6	35
Cinnamon (2)	220	6	38
Pancakes:			
Blueberry (3)	250	7	42
Chocolatey Chip (3)	260	8	42
Bites, Chocolatey Chip, 1.7 oz pouch	130	3.5	24
Minis, Buttermilk Pancakes, (11)	270	9	44
Pillsbury:			
Pancakes,			
Buttermilk; Homestlye, (3)	230	4	45

Frozen Waffles

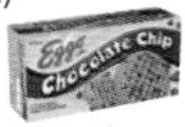
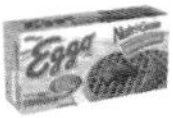
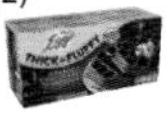
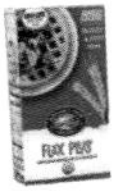
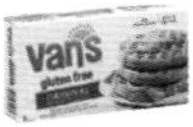

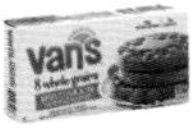

	C	F	Cb
Eggo *(Kellogg's):*			
Blueberry; Strawberry (2)	180	6	29
Buttermilk (2)	180	6	28
Chocolatey Chip (2)	200	7	32
Homestystyle (2)	180	5	30
Nutri-Grain:			
Blueberry (2)	180	6	30
Whole Wheat , low fat (2)	140	2.5	27
Thick & Fluffy:			
Original (1)	160	7	22
Cinnamon Brown Sugar (1)	170	7	25
Double Chocolately (1)	160	6	25
Nature's Path:			
Ancient Grains (2)	180	6	30
Buckwheat Wildberry (2)	190	7	33
Chia Plus; Homestyle (2)	210	7	34
Dark Chocolate Chip (2)	220	7	34
Flax Plus (2)	200	8	30
Maple Cinnamon (2)	180	6	28
Van's:			
Original, (2)	160	6	26
Blueberry, (2)	210	7	27
Gluten Free: Original (2)	210	7	34
Apple Cinnamon (2)	200	6	35
Blueberry (2)	210	7	34
Homestyle, (2)	190	8	29
Mini Chocolate Chip, (12)	210	6	35
Multigrain, (2)	160	5	29

Spaghetti/Pasta

- Pasta includes all shapes and sizes; (e.g. spaghetti, fettuccini, elbows, shells, twists, sheets, cannelloni, linguini, tubes, ziti).
- All regular pasta products have the same cals/fat/carbs on a weight basis.
- 1 oz Dry = approximately 2.5 -3 oz cooked.

Dry Spaghetti/Pasta

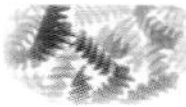
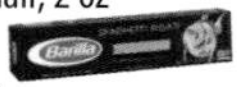
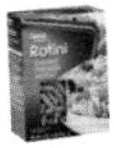

	C	F	Cb
1 oz quantity	105	0.5	21
1lb box/pkg, 16 oz	1685	7	339
Elbows, 1 cup, 4 oz	380	2	80
Shells, small, 1 cup, 3.3 oz	330	1.5	69
Spirals, 1 cup, 3 oz	305	1.5	64
Barilla:			
Blue Box: Angel Hair, 2 oz	200	1	42
Fettuccini, 2 oz	200	1	42
Other varieties, 2 oz	200	1	42
Great Value:			
Angel Hair, 2 oz	200	1	41
Penne Rigate, 2 oz	200	1	42
Rigatoni, 2 oz	200	1	41

Cooked Spaghetti/Pasta

	C	F	Cb
Plain, All Types (no added fat):			
Firm/Al Dente (8-10 minutes), 1 oz	42	0.5	8.5
Medium (11-13 minutes), 1 oz	37	0.5	7.5
Tender (14-20 minutes), 1 oz	32	0.5	7
Longer cooking increases water absorbed			
Spaghetti: ½ cup, 2.5 oz	90	0.5	18
Medium serving, 1 cup, 5 oz	225	1.5	44
Large serving, 2 cups, 10 oz	450	3	88
Extra large, 3 cups, 15 oz	675	5	132
Elbows/Spirals, 1 cup, 5 oz	220	1.5	43
Small Shells, 1 cup, 4 oz	180	1	36
Protein-fortified:			
Dry, 1 c., 3.4 oz	350	2	63
Cooked, 1 cup, 5 oz	230	0.5	45
Spinach/Vegetable:			
Dry, 1 cup, 3 oz	310	1	61
Cooked, 1 cup, 5 oz	180	0.5	38
Whole-wheat:			
Dry, 1 cup, 3.8 oz	365	1.5	79
Cooked, 1 cup, 5 oz	175	1	37

Fresh Pasta (Refrigerated)

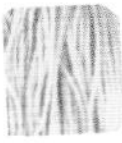
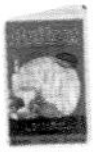
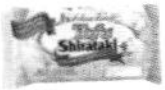
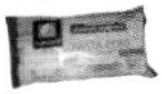

	C	F	Cb
Average All Brands:			
Plain/Spinach/Tomato:			
As purchased, 4.5 oz	370	3	70
Cooked, 1 cup, 5 oz	185	1.5	35
Home-made, w/o egg, cooked, 1 c. 5 oz	175	1	35
Buitoni:			
Cut Pasta:			
Angel Hair, 2.8 oz	220	1.5	45
Fettuccine/Linguine, av., 3 oz	235	1.5	46
House Foods:			
Tofu Shirataki Noodles:			
Angel Hair/Fettuccini, Macaroni/Spaghetti, 4 oz	20	1	6
Nasoya,			
Shirataki Spaghetti, Pasta Zero, ⅔ cup, 4 oz	15	0	4

Macaroni & Cheese

Packaged (Kraft) ~ *See Page 116*

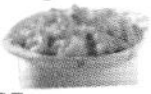

	C	F	Cb
Restaurant: *Average*			
Side Serve, 6 oz	265	13	26
Medium serve, 1 cup, 9 oz	350	17	34
Large serve, 2 cups, 18 oz	700	34	68

Noodles

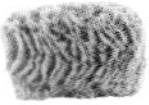
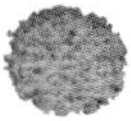
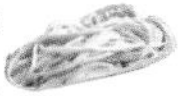
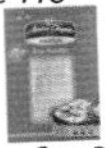

	C	F	Cb
Plain/Egg: Dry, 1 oz	110	1.5	20
1 cup, 1.4 oz	145	1.5	27
Cooked: ½ cup, 2.8 oz	110	1.5	20
1 cup, 5.5 oz	220	3.5	40
Stir-Fried: 1 cup, 5.5 oz	270	9	40
2 cup serving, 11 oz	540	18	80
Low Carb Noodles, (Konjac/Shiritaki), 4 oz	5	0	2
Note: Carbs are from glucomannan fiber			
Yolk Free (Cooked):			
Manischewitz, Yolk Free, 2 oz	200	1	41
Chinese: Cellophane/Rice, dry, 1 oz	100	0	25
Chow Mein/hard, dry, 1 oz	150	9	16
Japanese: Soba: Dry, 1 oz	95	0.5	21
Cooked, 1 cup, 4 oz	115	0.5	24
Somen: Dry, 1 oz	100	0.5	21
Cooked, 1 cup, 6 oz	230	0.5	49
Japanese Style Pan Fried,			
Yaki-Soba (*Maruchan's*), av., 5.6 oz	260	3	50
Ramen Noodles ~ *See Page 118*			
Rice Noodles: Dry, 3.5 oz	365	0.5	83
Cooked, 1 cup, 6.2 oz	190	0.5	44
Annie Chun's, 2 oz	190	0	43

Simply Asia/Thai Kitchen ~ *See Pages 119 & 121*

Egg Roll/Won Ton Wrappers

	C	F	Cb
Egg/Spring Roll (1), 0.8 oz	65	0	15
Won Ton Wrapper (1), 0.3 oz	20	0	4

Quick Guide

	C	F	Cb
Fruit Pies: *Average All Brands, 9" Pie*			
Apple; Blueberry; Cherry:			
Small Serving, ⅛ pie, 4.8 oz	350	16	49
Medium Serving, ⅙ pie, 6.5 oz	465	22	65
Large Serving ¼ pie, 9.5 oz	700	33	98
Whole Pie (9"), 38 oz	2800	131	392
Other Pies: *Per Serving, 1/6 of 9" Pie*			
Chocolate Cream Pie	345	22	38
Custard: Egg Pie	220	12	22
Coconut Pie	330	18	35
Lemon Meringue Pie	305	10	53
Peach Pie	260	12	39
Pecan Pie	440	23	57
Pumpkin Pie	315	14	41
Shoo-Fly Pie	400	13	70

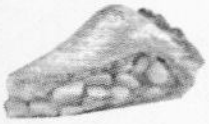
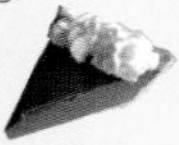
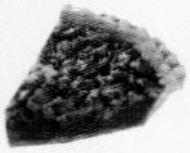

Dessert/Fruit Pies ~ Brands

	C	F	Cb
Hostess:			
Apple, 4.5 oz	450	19	65
Cherry Pie, 4.5 oz	480	20	69
Marie Callender's:			
Key Lime Pie, 4.5 oz	490	19	72
Lattice Cherry Pie, 4.5 oz	380	16	56
Peach Cobbler Pie, 4 oz	330	16	43
Peanut Butter Pie, 4.7 oz	620	46	43
Southern Pecan Pie, 4 oz	530	30	60
Turtle, 4.7 oz	560	36	55
Mrs Smith's:			
Cobblers: Blackberry, 4 oz	240	8	38
Peach, 4 oz	240	8	39
Flaky Crust: *Per 1/8 Pie*			
Apple, 4.6 oz	330	18	41
Cherry, 4.4 oz	340	17	43
Peach, 4.6 oz	330	18	41
Sara Lee: *Per Slice*			
Creme Pies:			
Chocolate, ⅕ pie, 3.9 oz	440	27	46
Coconut, ⅙ pie, 4.5 oz	370	20	44
Key Lime, ⅕ pie, 4.8 oz	410	17	59
Fruit Pies: Apple, 4.27 oz	320	13	44
Cherry, 4.27 oz	310	14	44
Peach, 4.27 oz	300	13	42
Raspberry, 4.27 oz	320	13	48
Seasonal Pies: Pumpkin, 4.27 oz	260	11	38
Sweet Potato, 4.27 oz	260	9	43
Tastykake: Baked Apple Pie (1)	300	12	45
Orange Kream-Cicle Pie (1)	320	15	42

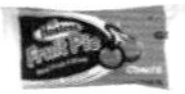
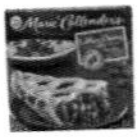
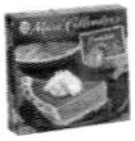
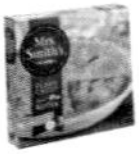
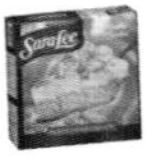

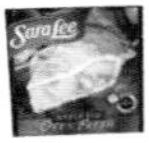

Croissants

	C	F	Cb
Average all Brands			
Plain/Butter/Cheese: Mini, 1 oz	115	6	13
Small, 1.5 oz	170	9	19
Medium, 2 oz	230	12	26
Large, 2.5 oz	290	15	32
Sweet Croissants:			
Almond Filled, 3 oz	330	18	39
Chocolate Filled, 3 oz	360	19	43
Dunkin' Donuts, Plain Croissant	340	19	37

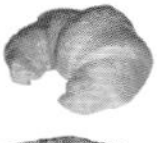
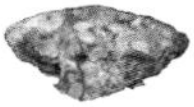

Croissant Sandwiches ~ *See Page 165*

Pastry & Pie Crust

	C	F	Cb
Pie Crust, Baked, 9" diameter shell:			
1 Pie Shell, 6.5 oz	970	64	87
2-crust Pie, 9", 11.3 oz	1660	109	150
Filo Pastry: 4 sheets, 2.5 oz	210	2.5	40
Athens, Phyllo Dough, 5 sheets, 2 oz	180	1	36
Puff:			
Pepperidge Farms: Sheets, 1.5 oz	160	10	16
Bake & Fill Shells, 1.7 oz	180	11	18
Arrowhead Mills,			
Graham Cracker Pie Crust, ⅛ of 9"	110	4.5	15
Keebler:			
Ready Crust: *Per ⅛ of 9" Crust*			
Chocolate	100	4.5	14
Graham	100	4.5	13
Low Fat	100	3.5	15
Shortbread Crust	100	5	14
Marie Callenders,			
Pastry Pie Shell, ⅛, 1 oz	130	8	13
Mrs Smith's,			
Deep Dish Pie Crust, ⅛ pie, 1 oz	130	8	14
Nabisco:			
Honey Maid,			
Graham Cracker Crust, ⅛ pie, ¾ oz	110	5	14
Nilla, Pie Crust,			
⅛ of Pie, 0.75	100	3	16
Pillsbury, Pie Crusts,			
Refrigerated, ⅛ pie, 0.9 oz	100	6	12
Trader Joe's, Pie Crust, ⅛ pie, 1.37oz	190	13	17

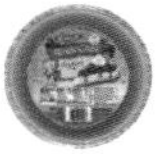
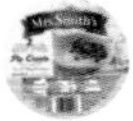
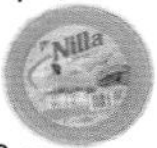

Pie Fillings ~ Canned

	C	F	Cb
Apple/Blueb./Cherry/Strawb., average:			
Sweetened: ⅓ cup, 3.2oz	90	0	22
1 cup, 9.5 oz	270	0	66
1 can, 21 oz	600	0	150
Light/Lite, ⅓ cup, 3.2 oz	60	0	15
Unsweetened, ⅓ cup, 3.2 oz	35	0	8
Lemon Crm/Creme, ⅓ cup, 3.2 oz	130	1.5	28

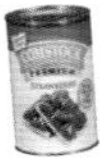

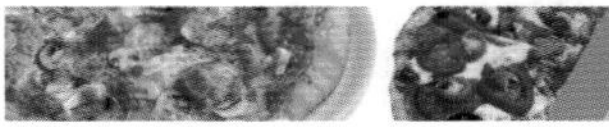

Pizzas ~ Ready to Eat

Figures Based On Pizza Hut

Cheese

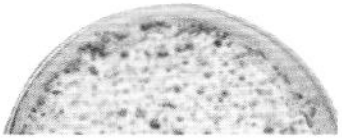

	C	F	Cb
Medium Size (12"):			
Hand Tossed Crust:			
⅛ Pizza (1 slice)	210	8	26
½ Pizza (4 slices)	840	32	104
Whole Pizza (8 slices)	1680	64	208
Original Pan: ⅛ Pizza (1 slice)	240	10	28
½ Pizza (4 slices)	960	40	112
Whole Pizza (8 slices)	1920	80	224
Thin 'N Crispy Crust:			
⅛ Pizza (1 slice)	190	7	22
½ Pizza (4 slices)	760	28	88
Whole Pizza (8 slices)	1520	56	176

Ham & Pineapple

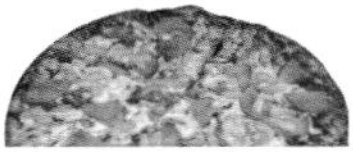

	C	F	Cb
Figures Based On Domino's			
Medium Size (12"):			
Hand Tossed Crust:			
⅛ Pizza (1 slice)	190	7	23
½ Pizza (4 slices)	760	28	92
Whole Pizza (8 slices)	1520	56	184
Handmade Pan: ⅛ Pizza (1 slice)	290	14	29
½ Pizza (4 slices)	1160	56	116
Whole Pizza (8 slices)	2320	112	232
Thin Crust:			
⅛ Pizza (1 slice)	140	7	13
½ Pizza (4 slices)	560	28	52
Whole Pizza (8 slices)	1120	56	104

MeatZZA

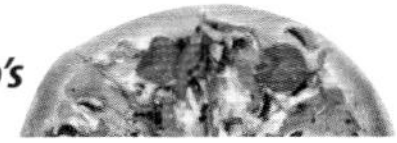

	C	F	Cb
Figures Based On Domino's			
Medium Size (12"):			
Hand Tossed Crust:			
⅛ Pizza (1 slice)	270	13	24
½ Pizza (4 slices)	1080	52	96
Whole Pizza (8 slices)	2160	104	192
Handmade Pan: ⅛ Pizza (1 slice)	360	20	29
½ Pizza (4 slices)	1440	80	116
Whole Pizza (8 slices)	2880	160	232
Thin Crust: ⅛ Pizza (1 slice)	220	14	14
½ Pizza (4 slices)	880	56	56
Whole Pizza (8 slices)	1760	112	112

Pepperoni

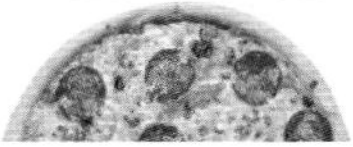

	C	F	Cb
Figures Based On Pizza Hut			
Medium Size (12"):			
Hand Tossed Crust:			
⅛ Pizza (1 slice)	220	9	25
½ Pizza (4 slices)	880	36	100
Whole Pizza (8 slices)	1760	72	200
Original Pan: ⅛ Pizza (1 slice)	250	11	28
½ Pizza (4 slices)	1000	44	112
Whole Pizza (8 slices)	2000	88	224
Thin 'N Crispy: ⅛ Pizza (1 slice)	210	9	22
½ Pizza (4 slices)	840	36	88
Whole Pizza (8 slices)	1680	72	176

Large Pizzas

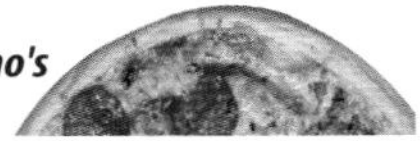

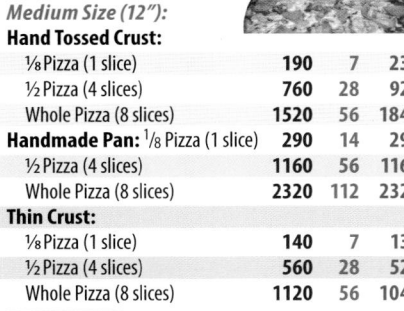

	C	F	Cb
Figures Based On Domino's			
Large (14")			
Hand Tossed Crust:			
ExtravaganZZa: ⅛ Pizza (1 slice)	390	19	36
½ Pizza (4 slices)	1560	76	144
MeatZZA: ⅛ Pizza (1 slice)	370	18	34
½ Pizza (4 slices)	1480	72	136
Pepperoni: ⅛ Pizza (1 slice)	280	12	31
½ Pizza (4 slices)	1120	48	124

Extra Large NY, Single Slice

	C	F	Cb
Figures Based On Sbarro			
Cheese	430	15	51
Classic Hawaiian	470	15	57
Sausage	520	24	50
Spinach & Tomato	370	15	42

Individual Personal Pan Pizzas

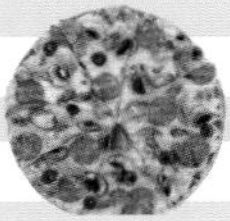

	C	F	Cb
Pan (6"): Figures Based On Pizza Hut			
Buffalo Chicken	640	20	88
Cheese	600	24	68
Pepperoni	600	28	68
Supreme	680	32	72
Veggie Lovers	560	20	72
Chicago-Style Deep Dish: Per Individual, 6 slices			
Figures Based On Uno Pizzeria			
Cheese & Tomato	1680	78	108
Chicago Classic	2160	156	114
Prima Pepperoni	1680	190	108

Frozen Pizzas

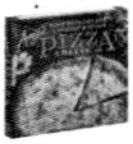
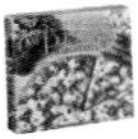

	C	F	Cb
Amy's: Per ⅓ Pizza			
Cheese	290	12	33
Margherita	270	12	31
Meatless Pepperoni	340	16	34
Mushroom & Olive	260	11	31
Pesto & Artichoke	300	16	34
Gluten-Free, Roasted Vegetable	320	11	51
Spinach	300	12	36
Vegan: Meatless Pepperoni, gluten free	320	15	40
Pesto & Rstd Artichoke, ½ pizza	370	20	45
Supreme, ⅓ pizza	290	12	37

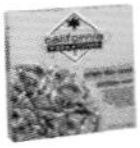

	C	F	Cb
California Pizza Kitchen: Per ⅓ Pizza			
Cauliflower: Artisanal Style Cheese	270	12	29
Pepperoni, Mushroom & Sausage	300	15	28
Crispy Thin Crust: BBQ Recipe Chkn	290	11	33
Four Cheese; Margherita, average	320	16	29
Sicilian Recipe	350	17	31
Signature Pepperoni	330	17	29
White Recipe	280	11	31
Gluten-Free:			
BBQ Recipe Chicken, **½** pizza	290	9	37
Margherita, ⅓ pizza	190	8	21
Single Serve: BBQ Recipe Chicken	300	11	31
Five Cheese & Tomato	280	12	29

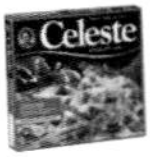

	C	F	Cb
Celeste: Per Pizza			
Pizza For One: Original 4 Cheese	380	16	48
Deluxe	360	15	47
Pepperoni	370	16	46
Sausage	370	16	47
Daiya (Vegan):			
Cheese Lovers, ⅓ pizza, 5,22 oz	400	15	60
Meatless: Meat Lover's, ¼ pizza, 4.8 oz	340	14	48
Pepperoni, ⅓ pizza, 5.53 oz	410	17	61
M'shrm & Rstd Garlic, ¼ pizza, 4.27 oz	290	11	45
Supreme, gluten free, ¼ pizza	310	11	45
DiGiorno:			
Bacon & Cheese Stuffed Crust:			
Bacon Me Crazy, ¼ pizza	410	21	34
Better with Bacon ⅕ pizza	330	17	28
Cheese Stuffed Crust:			
Bacon Cheeseburger, ⅕ pizza	330	17	29
Buffalo Style Chkn, ¼ pizza	380	16	40
Five Cheese; Pepperoni, av., ⅕ pizza	315	15	29
Three Meat; Supreme, av., ⅕ pizza	355	18	31

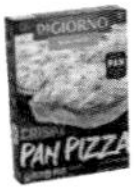
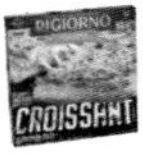
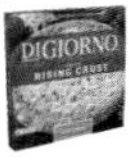
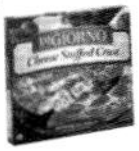
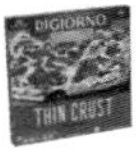
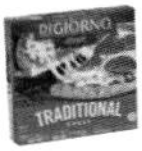

	C	F	Cb
DiGiorno (Cont):			
Crispy Pan: *Per ⅕ Pizza*			
Cheesy Garlic	410	20	40
Four Cheese	430	22	40
Pepperoni	430	22	39
Croissant Crust: *Per ⅕ Pizza*			
Four Cheese	370	18	36
Pepperoni	380	20	35
Three Meat	410	22	36
Rising Crust: *Per ⅙ Pizza*			
Four Cheese; Spicy Chkn Supreme, av	300	10	38
Hawaiian Style	280	8	39
Italian Sausage	340	13	48
Small Pizzas: *Per Pizza*			
Cheese Stuffed Crust:			
Four Cheese	650	29	67
Pepperoni; Supreme	660	31	66
Thin Crispy Crust:			
Pepperoni	580	25	68
Supreme	580	23	68
Traditional Crust:			
Four Cheese	690	29	83
Pepperoni	750	34	83

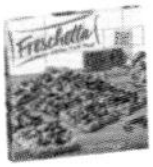
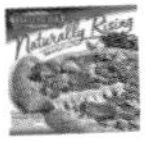

	C	F	Cb
Freschetta:			
Brick Oven: *Per ⅕ Pizza Unless Indicated*			
5 Cheese, ¼ Pizza, 5.2 oz	370	17	39
Pepperoni, 4.55 oz	330	17	32
Spinach & Roasted M'shrms, 4.5 oz	270	10	34
Three Meat, 4.6 oz	340	18	32
Supreme, 4.6 oz	310	14	33
Naturally Rising:			
4 Cheese, 5 oz	370	14	48
Canada Style Bacon P'apple, 4.5 oz	290	9	41
Pepperoni, 4.55 oz	330	13	40
Supreme, 5.2 oz	350	15	41

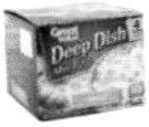
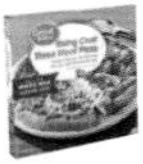

	C	F	Cb
Great Value (Walmart):			
Deep Dish Minis: Cheese (1)	400	16	48
Supreme (1)	410	19	47
Three Meat (1)	400	17	47
Rising Crust:			
Cheese, 4.6 oz	300	10	41
Supreme, 5.11 oz	330	12	42
Three Meat, 4.6 oz	320	11	41
Thin Crust: Four Cheese, 5.15 oz	370	18	33
Pepperoni, 5.43 oz	410	22	34

Frozen Pizzas (Cont)

	C	F	Cb
Kroger:			
3 Minute Microwave: *Per 7.2 oz Pizza*			
Cheese	480	18	62
Pepperoni	540	25	63
Three Meat	510	21	64
Self Rising Crust: *Per ⅙ pizza*			
Double Bacon	300	9	43
Four Cheese	300	8	43
Supreme	330	12	42
Three Meat	340	13	44
White Chicken	310	11	41
Lean Cuisine:			
Favorites: *Per Package*			
French Bread Pepperoni	300	7	44
Features: *Per Package*			
Farmer's Market	340	9	50
Four Cheese	360	7	55
Margherita	330	8	51
Pepperoni; Supreme. av	395	8	60
Deep Dish: Spinach & Mushroom	360	8	54
Three Meat	390	9	56
Thick Crust, BBQ Recipe Chicken	340	5	54
Red Baron:			
Brick Oven: *Per ¼ Pizza*			
Cheese Trio, 4.4 oz	320	15	34
Meat-Trio, 4.6 oz	320	15	35
Pepperoni, 4.5 oz	330	17	33
Classic Crust: *Per ¼ Pizza*			
Four Cheese, 5.25 oz	380	17	40
Sausage & Pepp.,4.4 oz	320	16	32
Supreme, 4.7 oz	310	15	33
Deep Dish Minis:			
Cheese, 4 pieces, 5.4 oz	380	15	48
Pepperoni, 4 pieces, 5.6 oz	430	20	48
Deep Dish Singles: *Per Pizza*			
Hawaiian Style, 5.6 oz	370	14	48
Meat-Trio, 5.6 oz	400	18	47
Sausage, 5.8 oz	440	20	49
Scrambles: Bacon, 5.85 oz	440	21	45
Sausage, 5.85 oz	410	19	46
Thin & Crispy Crust: *Per ⅓ Pizza*			
Five Cheese, 5 oz	350	16	38
Pepperoni, 5.3 oz	390	20	38
Supreme, 4.4 oz	300	15	31

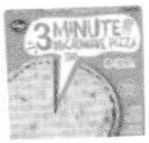

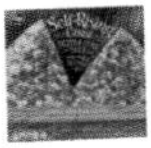
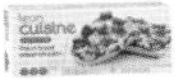

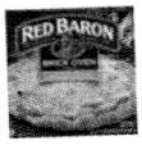

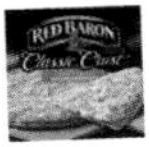

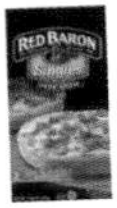

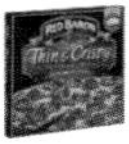

	C	F	Cb
Signature Select *(Albertsons):*			
Rising Crust: *Per ⅙ Pizza*			
Five Cheese	330	12	41
Pepperoni	380	17	41
Supreme	360	15	41
Ultra Thin Crust: *Per ⅓ Pizza*			
Italian Sausage; Sausage, average	345	19	27
Smart Ones *(Weight Watchers):*			
Thin Crust: Cheese	290	6	42
Pepperoni Pizza, 4.37 oz	310	10	39
Stouffer's:			
French Bread Pizzas:			
Two Per Box:			
Cheese (1)	360	15	43
Deluxe (1)	430	21	44
Three Meat (1)	470	25	43
Nine Per Box, Pepperoni (1)	430	21	44:
Tombstone:			
Original: *Per ¼ Pizza*			
Canadian Bacon, 4.9 oz	300	12	33
Deluxe; Supreme, av.	345	16	35
Five Chees; Hamburger	340	15	34
Pepperoni;Pepperoni & Sausage, av.	350	17	34
Pepperoni & Sausage	340	16	34
Sausage; Sausage & Mushroom	350	16	35
Veggie	300	12	35
Half & Half: *Per ¼ Pizza*			
Pepperoni & Sausage/Cheese	350	17	34
Garlic Bread Crust,			
Pepperoni; Supreme, av., ⅙ pizza	340	14	37
Tony's:			
Pizzeria Style Crust: *Per ¼ Pizza*			
Cheese, 4.7 oz	330	13	41
Meat Trio, 5 oz	360	16	41
Pepperoni, 4.7 oz	330	14	40
Sausage & Pepperoni, 4.83 oz	350	15	41
Supreme, 5.1 oz	350	15	41
Totino's:			
Crisp Crust Party Pizza: *Per ½ Pizza*			
Canadian Bacon	330	16	37
Cheese	320	16	37
Hamburger	360	19	38
Pepperoni & Bacon	340	17	37
Trader Joe's:			
Cauliflower Crust Cheese, ⅓ pizza	250	12	24
Org. Six Cheese & Tomato, ¼ pizza	340	16	35

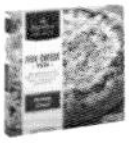
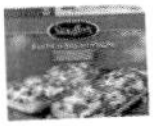
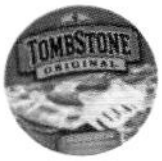

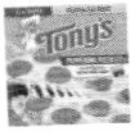

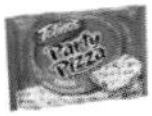

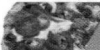

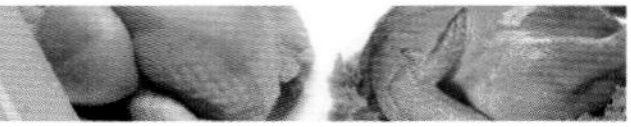

Quick Guide

Chicken

From 3lb ready-to-cook chicken

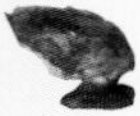

Breast/Wing Quarter:	C	F	Cb
Roasted: with skin	300	15	0
without skin	185	5	0
Fried, batter dipped	530	30	17

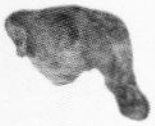

Leg Quarter:	C	F	Cb
Thigh & Drumstick:			
Roasted: with skin	270	16	0
without skin	185	8	0
Fried, batter dipped	435	25	15

KFC ~ *See Fast-Foods Section*

Per 4 oz Edible Portion

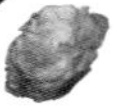

Average of Light Meat: *Per 4 oz without Bone*	C	F	Cb
Roasted: with skin	250	12	0
without skin	175	4.5	0
Stewed: with skin	230	12	0
without skin	180	4.5	0
Fried: Batter-dipped, with skin, 4 oz	315	17	11
Flour-coated, with skin, 4 oz	280	14	2

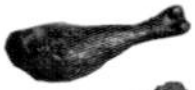

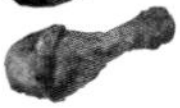

Average of Dark Meat: *Per 4 oz without Bone*	C	F	Cb
Roasted: with skin	290	18	0
without skin	235	11	0
Stewed: with skin	265	17	0
without skin	220	10	0
Fried: Batter-dipped, with skin, 4 oz	340	21	11
Flour-coated, with skin, 4 oz	325	19	5

Chicken Parts

Broilers or Fryers: *Edible Weights (no bone)*

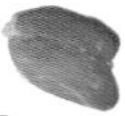

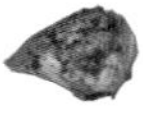

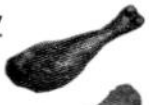

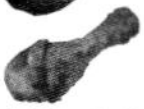

	C	F	Cb
Breast: *Per ½ Breast*			
Raw: with skin, 5 oz	250	14	0
without skin, 4.25 oz	140	3	0
Roasted: with skin, 3.5 oz	195	8	0
without skin, 3 oz	140	3	0
Stewed: with skin, 4 oz	200	8	0
without skin, 3.3 oz	145	3	0
Fried: Batter-dipped, w/ skin, 5 oz	365	19	13
Flour-coated, with skin, 3.5 oz	220	9	2
Drumstick: *Per Drumstick*			
Roasted: with skin, 2 oz	115	6	0
without skin, 1.5 oz	75	2.5	0
Stewed: with skin, 2 oz	115	6	0
without skin, 1.5 oz	80	3	0
Fried: Batter-dipped, w/ skin, 2.5 oz	195	11	6
Flour-coated, with skin, 1.8 oz	120	7	1

Chicken Parts (Cont)

Broilers or Fryers (Cont): *Edible Weights (no bone)*

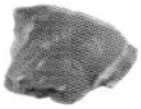

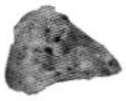

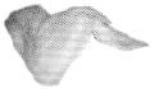

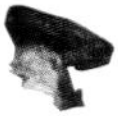

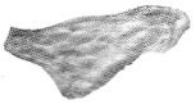

	C	F	Cb
Thigh Portion:			
Raw: with skin, 3.3 oz (4¼ oz with bone)	200	14	0
without skin, 2.4 oz	80	3	0
Roasted: with skin, 2.3 oz	155	10	0
without skin, 2 oz	110	6	0
Stewed: with skin, 2.5 oz	160	10	0
without skin, 2 oz	105	5	0
Fried: Batter-dipped, with skin 3 oz	240	14	8
Flour-coated, with skin, 2.3 oz	165	9	2
Wing: *Per Wing, Bone In*			
Raw Weight, 3.2 oz			
Raw: with skin	110	8	0
without skin	35	1	0
Roasted: with skin	100	7	0
without skin	45	2	0
Fried: Batter-dipped, with skin	160	11	5
Flour-coated, with skin	105	7	1
Stewed, with skin, 4 oz	100	7	0
Buffalo Wings ~ *See Fast-Foods Section*			
Neck: Simmered, with skin	95	7	0
without skin	30	2	0
Skin Only: *Skin from ½ Chicken*			
Raw skin, 3 oz	275	26	0
Roasted skin, 2 oz	255	23	0
Stewed skin, 2.5 oz	260	24	0
Fried, flour-coated, 2 oz	280	24	5
Fried, batter-dipped, 6.8 oz	750	55	44

Roasters: *Average of Light & Dark Meat*	C	F	Cb
Roasted: with skin, 4 oz	250	15	0
without skin, 4 oz	190	8	0
Dark Meat, without skin	200	10	0
Light Meat, without skin	175	5	0

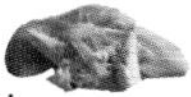

Stewing Chicken: *Per 4 oz, average of Light & Dark Meat*	C	F	Cb
Stewed: with skin	325	22	0
without skin	270	14	0
Dark Meat, without skin	290	17	0
Light Meat, without skin	240	9	0

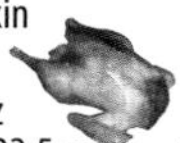

Capon Chicken:	C	F	Cb
Roasted: with skin, 4 oz	260	13	0
½ Chicken, with skin, 22.5 oz	1460	74	0

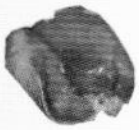

Chicken Offal & Stuffing:	C	F	Cb
Giblets: Simmered, 1 Cup	230	7	0.5
Fried, flour-coated, 1 Cup	400	20	6
Gizzard, simmered, 1 Cup	210	4	0
Heart, simmered, 1 Cup	270	12	0.2
Liver: Raw, 4 oz	130	5.5	0
Simmered, 1 Cup	215	8.5	1
Liver Pate, fresh, 1 Tbsp, 0.5 oz	30	2	1
Stuffing, average, ½ Cup	180	9	22

Chicken Products

	C	F	Cb
Bumble Bee:			
Chicken In Water: *Per 2 oz Drained*			
Premium White	70	1.5	0
Premium Breast	70	1	1
Foster Farms:			
Chicken Breast Strips, grilled, 3 oz	100	2	1
Wings: Chipotle, 3 wings, 3 oz	190	13	4
Honey BBQ Glazed, 3 wings, 3 oz	190	11	7
Hot 'n' Spicy, 3 wings, 3 oz	190	14	1
Tyson:			
Anytizers, Frozen:			
Wings:			
Hot Wings, Buffalo Style (3)	190	13	1
Honey BBQ Seasoned (3)	190	12	8
Wyngz, Boneless:			
Buffalo Style, 3 pieces, 3 oz	150	7	8
Sweet Garlic Glazed, 3 pcs, 2.8 oz	130	5	10

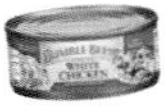

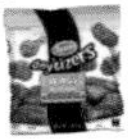

Duck, Goose, Quail

	C	F	Cb
Duck, Roasted:			
with skin, 3 oz	290	24	0
without skin, 3 oz	170	10	0
½ duck, with skin, 13.5 oz	1290	108	0
Goose: Roasted with skin, 3 oz	260	19	0
without skin, 3 oz	200	11	0
Pheasant, cooked, 3 oz	210	10	0
Quail, cooked, 1 whole, 6 oz	385	24	0

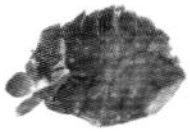

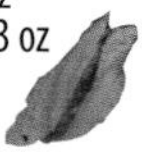

Turkey

	C	F	Cb
Fryer-Roasters: *Per 3 oz Serving*			
Roasted:			
Light Meat: with skin	140	4	0
without skin	120	1	0
Dark Meat: with skin	155	6	0
without skin	140	4	0
½ of Whole Turkey: (Approx. 3.3 lbs raw weight without neck and giblets; 1.8 lbs cooked weight)			
Roasted: with skin	1650	74	0
without skin	1125	31	0
Ground Turkey, raw: (4 oz raw wt. = 3 oz cooked wt.)			
85% lean, regular, 4 oz	170	10	0
93% lean: Average, 4 oz	160	8	0
Jennie-O, 4 oz	170	8	0
Trader Joe's, 4 oz	150	8	0
94% lean,			
Foster Farms, 4 oz	150	7	0
Breast, no skin, 4 oz	115	1	0
Patties: Small, 3 oz	130	7	0
Medium, 4 oz	170	10	0

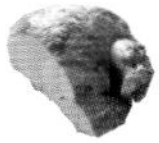

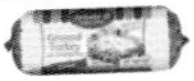

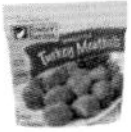

Turkey Parts

	C	F	Cb
Roasted, Edible Weights, without bone:			
Breast, (½), (from 17.3 oz raw weight with bone):			
with skin, 12 oz (no bone)	525	11	0
without skin, 10.8 oz	415	2	0
Back (½): with skin, 4.5 oz	265	13	0
without skin, 3.5 oz	165	6	0
Leg (Thigh & Drumstick): (from 1 lb raw weight with bone)			
with skin, 8.5 oz (without bone)	410	13	0
without skin, 7.8 oz (w/out bone)	355	8.5	0
Wing: (From 7.3 oz raw weight)			
with skin, 3 oz (without bone)	185	9	0
without skin, 2 oz (w/out bone)	100	2	0
Neck: Simmered, 1 neck, 9 oz (with bone)	275	11	0
Giblets, simmered, 1 Cup, 5 oz	240	7	3

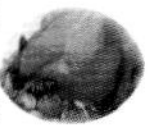

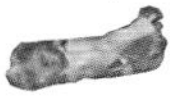

Young Hens (Roasted)

	C	F	Cb
Light Meat:			
with skin, 3 oz	175	8	0
without skin, 3 oz	135	3	0
Dark Meat: with skin, 3 oz	200	11	0
without skin, 3 oz	165	7	0
Young Toms ~ *Similar to Young Hens*			

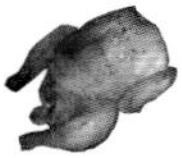

Turkey Products

	C	F	Cb
Foster Farms:			
Raw: Breast Cutlets, 4 oz	120	0.5	0
Ground Turkey, 85% lean, 4 oz	230	17	0
Tenderloins, Island Teriyaki, 4 oz	120	1	5
Hormel, Canned Turkey Breast, 97% Fat Free, in water, 2 oz	50	1	0
Jennie-O:			
Cooked: Meatballs, Italian, 3 oz	180	13	2
Home Style, 3 oz	180	13	3
Raw: Bacon, raw, 1 slice,	30	2.5	0
Bratwurst, lean, 1 link, 3.85 oz	150	8	0
Patties, 93% Lean All Natural, 4 oz	150	8	0
Spam, Oven Roasted Turkey, 2 oz	80	4.5	1
Valley Fresh, 100% Natural, Canned White Turkey Breast, in water, 2 oz	50	1	0

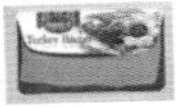

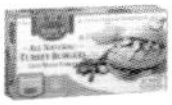

White Rice

	C	F	Cb
Raw:			
Glutinous, 1 Cup, 6.5 oz	685	1	151
Long Grain, 1 Cup, 6.5 oz	675	1	148
Short Grain, 1 Cup, 7 oz	715	1	158
Wild Rice, 1 Cup, 5.5 oz	570	2	120
Cooked Rice: *Boiled/Steamed*			
Short/Medium Grain:			
½ Cup, 3.3 oz	140	0	30
1 Cup (½ Pint), 7.2 oz	265	0.5	59
2 Cups (1 Pint), 13 oz	480	1	106
Long Grain: ½ Cup, 2.8 oz	100	0	22
1 Cup, 5.5 oz	205	0.5	44
Glutinous/Sticky, 1 Cup, 6 oz	170	0.5	37
Parboiled, ½ Cup, 3 oz	105	0.5	22
Precooked/Instant:			
Dry, ½ Cup, 3.5 oz	380	1	82
Cooked, ½ Cup, 3 oz	95	0.5	21
Wild Rice,			
Cooked, 1 Cup, 5.8 oz	165	0.5	35

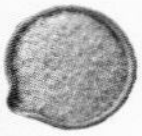
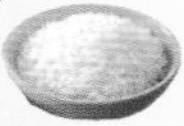
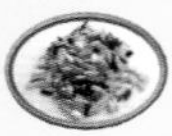

Brown Rice

	C	F	Cb
Average of Short or Long Grain			
Raw/Dry: ½ Cup, 3.3 oz	340	2.5	71
1 Cup, 6.5 oz	685	5.5	143
Cooked: ½ Cup, 3.5 oz	110	1	22
1 Cup, 7 oz	220	2	46

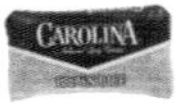

Rice Dishes

	C	F	Cb
Chinese Fried Rice:			
½ Cup, 2.5 oz	140	4.5	21
1 Cup, (½ Pint), 5 oz	280	9	42
2 Cups, (1 Pint), 10 oz	565	18	84
Mexican Style Rice:			
Taco Time, Seasoned, 4.6 oz	200	3	40
Rice-A-Roni ~ *See Page 119*			
Rice with Raisins/Pinenuts, 1 Cup	400	11	60
Rice Pilaf: Restaurant, 1 Cup	275	7.5	46
O'Charley's, side dish, 1 portion	160	4	27
Rice Pudding,			
Kozy Shack, Original, 1 pudding cup	130	2.5	24
Risotto, 1 Cup	420	12	70
Saffron Rice, 4 oz	175	7	25
Spanish Rice: 1 Cup, 5 oz	390	9	72
El Pollo Loco, Small, 4.5 oz	160	1.5	32
Sticky Rice, 1 Cup, 5 oz	155	0.5	34
Sushi Rice: 1 Tbsp	25	0	5
1 Cup, 5.2 oz	390	0	77
Other Packaged Rice Products:			
Uncle Ben's / Zatarain's ~ *See Page 121*			

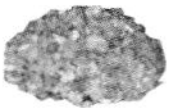
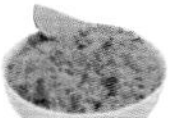
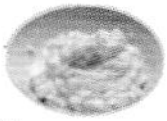
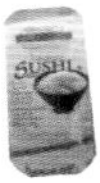

CalorieKing.com Recipes

See the CalorieKing website for a salubrious selection of healthy recipes – all analyzed for calories, fat, protein, carbohydrate, fiber and sodium.

Choose from:

- ***Starters/Appetizers***
- ***Salads***
- ***Entrees: Meat, Fish and Chicken***
- ***Vegetarian***
- ***Desserts***
- ***Cakes, Cookies***
- ***Drinks***

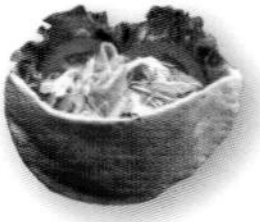

www.CalorieKing.com/recipes

HEALTHY RECIPE TIPS

- **Use non-fat milk** in place of whole or 2% milk
- **Use low-fat yogurt** in place of sour cream
- **Skim fat** from surface of soups and casseroles after cooling
- **Add extra vegetables** to soups and hot entreés
- **Cakes/cookies/muffins:** Replace most or all the fat/oil with applesauce and/or prune puree (Example, *Sunsweet Lighter Bake*)
- **Drinks:** Replace sugar with no-calorie sweeteners such as *Equal, Stevia, Splenda and Sweet 'N Low*

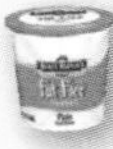
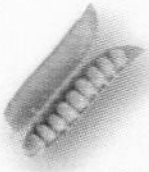
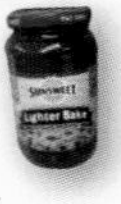
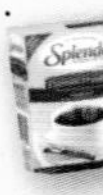

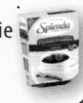

Deli Salads

	C	F	Cb
Average All Outlets			
Antipasto Salad, ½ Cup	135	8	13
3-Bean Salad, ½ Cup	90	4.5	12
Bulgur Salad, ½ Cup	70	2	12
Caesar Salad, Classic, 1 Cup	200	14	15
Side Salad, without Dressing	25	0	6
Carrot Raisin: with Dressing, ½ Cup	135	12	6
without Dressing, ½ Cup	20	0	5
Chef's Salad: Regular, w/o Dressing	620	37	8
with 2 oz Thousand Island Drssng	860	61	8
Chicken Salad, ½ Cup/scoop, 4 oz	280	21	2
Coleslaw: Traditional, ½ Cup	150	8	18
w/ Low Cal Dressing, ½ c.	50	2	8
Corn, Mexican, ½ Cup	240	12	33
Cucumber: Non-Oil Dressing, ½ Cup	60	0	14
with Oil Dressing, ½ Cup	140	12	8
Eggplant Salad, ½ Cup	75	5	7
Fettucini, with veges, ½ Cup	135	6	16
Garden Salad, without Dressing, 1 Cup	10	0	2
Greek Salad, 1 Cup	105	8	7
Greek Vegetables, 1 Cup	110	8	6
Lobster Salad, ½ Cup, 4 oz	250	21	11
Macaroni Salad, ½ Cup, 5 oz	360	26	26
Nicoise, 1 Cup	450	32	18
Pasta Salad, ½ Cup	200	11	19
Potato Salad: Dijon, 3 oz	120	7	13
with Mayonnaise, ½ Cup, 4 oz	215	15	17
Lowfat, ½ Cup	110	1.5	21
Rice Salad, ½ Cup	150	10	13
Saffron Rice, 4 oz	175	7	25
Spinach Salad, 1 Cup	180	13	13
Tabouli, ½ Cup	125	7	13
Three Bean Salad, ½ Cup	90	4.5	12
Tomato & Mozzarella, ½ Cup	180	14	10
Tortellini, with Basil Pesto, ½ Cup	150	9	15
Waldorf, with Mayo, ½ Cup	110	7	12

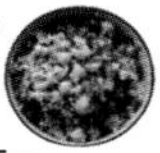
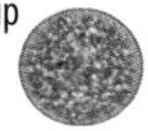
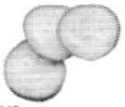
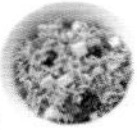
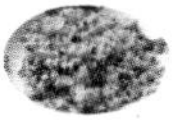
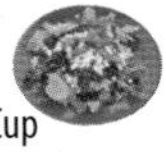

Signature Salads: *Per 6 oz Serving*
(Supplied to Deli's and Institutions)

	C	F	Cb
Antipasto Salad	510	50	4
Artichoke Salad, marinated	400	41	8
California Medley	120	7	15
Cheese Agnolotti	250	8	23
Chicken Salad	420	33	11
Crabmeat Flavored	450	38	20
Egg Salad	300	23	14
Fresh Button Mushroom	190	16	6

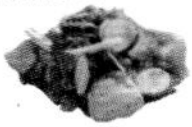
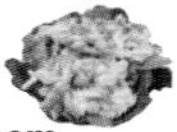

Signature Salads (Cont): *Per 6 oz*	C	F	Cb
Fresh Button Mushroom	190	16	6
Ham Salad	400	32	14
Prima Pasta Salad	360	30	18
Seafood Pasta Del Mar	170	10	21
Seafood, Crab & Shrimp	420	34	20
Shrimp Salad	360	32	8
Tuna Salad	450	36	14

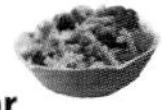
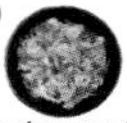

~ *Also See Fast-Foods & Restaurants Section*

Fresh Salad Packs

	C	F	Cb
Pre-Packaged (Supermarkets):			
Dole:			
Kits: *Per 3.5 oz, with Dressing*			
Blueberry Bliss	170	12	13
Caesar: Classic	150	13	8
Ultimate	170	13	10
Chopped Kits: Bacon & Bleu	150	13	6
BBQ Ranch	140	10	11
Sesame Asian	140	10	12
Salad Blends: *Per 3 oz, Without Dressing*			
American	15	0	3
Arugula; Baby Spinach	20	0	3
Field Greens; Very Veggie	20	0	4
Fresh Express:			
Chopped Salad Kits: *Per Serving*			
Twisted Asian Caesar, 3.84 oz	190	15	13
Twisted Greek Caesar, 3.72 oz	90	6	7
Gourmet Kits: *Per Container*			
Chef Salad	300	23	10
Grilled chicken Caesar	170	29	13
Saute Kits: *Per 3.9 oz Serving*			
Lemon Garlic Spinach	160	13	9
Tuscan Kale with Genovese Pesto	120	8	10
Ready Pac:			
Bistro Bowls: *Per Container*			
Apple Bleu Pecan, 4.5 oz	220	14	23
Caprese, 5 oz	210	17	12
Complete Chopped Salad Kits: *Per 3.5 oz*			
Asian,	100	6	11
Kale Cranberry Pecan	200	14	17
Mediterranean	130	10	11

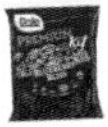
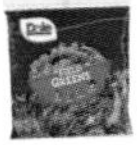
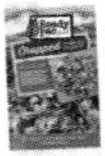

Salad Toppings

	C	F	Cb
Bac'n Pieces, *McCormick*, 1Tbsp, 0.3 oz	30	1	2
Bacon Bits *(Hormel)*, 1Tbsp	25	1.5	0
Bac-Os, Bits *(Betty Crocker)*, 1 Tbsp	30	1	2
Chow Mein Noodles, dry, ½ Cup	120	7	13
Croutons, 2 Tbsp, 0.3 oz	40	1	7
Salad Toppins, *McCormick*, 4 tsp	35	1.5	3
Sunflower Seeds, 1 Tbsp, 0.3 oz	45	4	1.5
Toasted Sliced Almonds, 2 T., 0.5 oz	85	7	3

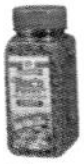
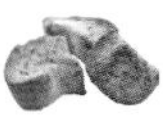

Quick Guide

Salad Dressings

Average All Brands: Per 2 Tbsp, Approx 1 fl.oz

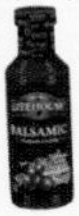
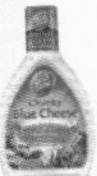
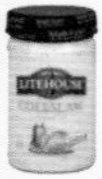
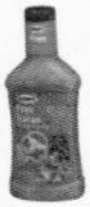
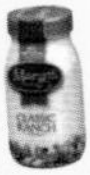
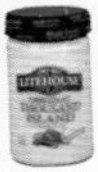

	C	F	Cb
Balsamic Vinaigrette:			
Regular	90	9	3
Light, 2 Tbsp	45	4	2
Fat Free, 2 Tbsp	25	0	6
Blue Cheese: Regular, 2 Tbsp	145	15	1.5
Regular, 1/4 cup, 2 oz	280	30	3
Light, 2 Tbsp	30	1	4
Caesar: Regular, 2 Tbsp	165	17	1
Regular, 1/4 cup, 2 oz	310	34	2
Light, 2 Tbsp	35	1.5	5.5
Coleslaw: Regular, 2 Tbsp	125	11	8
Regular, 1/4 cup, 2 oz	245	21	15
Light, 2 Tbsp	110	7	14
French: Regular	145	14	5
Regular, 1/4 cup, 2 oz	260	25	9
Light, 2 Tbsp	65	4	9
Fat/Oil-Free, 2 Tbsp	40	0	10
Italian: Regular, 2 Tbsp	85	8.5	3
Regular, 1/4 cup, 2 oz	165	16	6
Light, 2 Tbsp	55	5.5	2
Fat/Oil-Free, 2 Tbas	15	0	2.5
Ranch: Regular, 2 Tbsp	145	16	2
Regular, 1/4 cup, 2 oz	290	30	4
Light, 2 Tbsp	60	4	6.5
Fat-Free, 2 Tbsp	35	0.5	8
Thousand Island: Reg., 2 T.	115	11	4.5
Regular, 1/4 cup, 2 oz	210	20	9
Light, 2 Tbsp	60	3.5	7
Fat-Free, 2 Tbsp	40	0.5	10

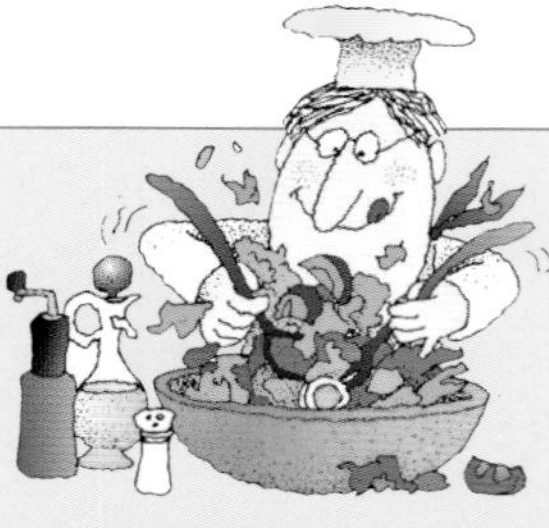

Enjoy a healthy salad but don't drown it in high-fat salad dressings.

Use 'light' dressings to halve the fat and calories.

Brands ~ Salad Dressings

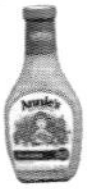
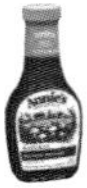
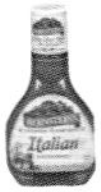
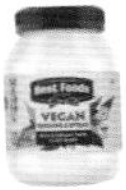
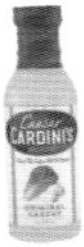
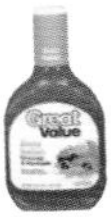
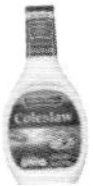

	C	F	Cb
Annie's Naturals: *Per 2 Tbsp*			
Organic: Goddess Dressing	120	12	2
French	110	10	3
Original Caesar	100	11	2
Papaya Poppy Seed	90	8	5
Vinaigrettes:			
Red Wine & Olive Oil	140	14	1
Sesame Ginger	90	8	4
Shiitake & Sesame	130	13	2
Bernstein's: *Per 2 Tbsp*			
Creamy Caesar	120	13	1
Herb Garden French	130	12	6
Italian	90	9	2
Restaurant Recipe Italian	120	12	1
Fat-Free, Cheese & Garlic Italian	10	0	2
Light Fantastic: Cheese Fantastico	30	1.5	3
Roasted Garlic Balsamic	45	3.5	3
Best Foods: *Per 1 Tbsp Unless Indicated*			
Mayonnaise: Real	100	11	0
Light	35	3.5	1
Organic	100	11	0
Olive Oil	60	6	1
Sunflower Oil	60	7	0.5
Vegan Dressing & Spread	70	8	0.5
Cardini's: *Per 2 Tbsp*			
Caesar: 80 Calorie	80	8	1
Original	140	15	0.5
Garlic Lemon	150	16	1
Red Jalapeno	140	15	0.5
Three Cheese; Vinaigrette	140	15	0.5
Vinaigrette, Balsamic:			
Regular	100	8	5
Lite Greek	50	4.5	2
Great Value *(Walmart): Per 2 Tbsp Unless Indicated*			
Creamy: Caesar	120	12	2
Thousand Island	120	12	4
Light Mayo, 1 Tbsp	35	3.5	1
Ranch: Buttermilk	110	11	2
Classic	130	14	1
Traditional Italian	80	7	5
Hidden Valley: *Per 2 Tbsp*			
Creamy: Coleslaw	150	15	4
Southwest Chipotle	100	10	2
Greek Yogurt: Cucumber Dill	60	5	3
Ranch	60	5	3
Spinach & Feta	60	5	3
Light, Butterilk Ranch; Ccumber, av.	65	5	3

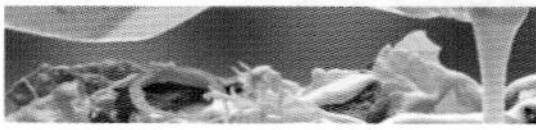

Brands ~ Salad Dressings (Cont)

Hidden Valley (Cont): *Per 2 Tbsp*

	C	F	Cb
Ranch: Bacon; Cheddar & Bacon	100	11	2
Buffalo	110	11	2
Simply Ranch: Buttermilk	110	12	2
Chili Lime	120	12	2
Classic Ranch	110	12	2

Kraft: *Per 2 Tbsp*

 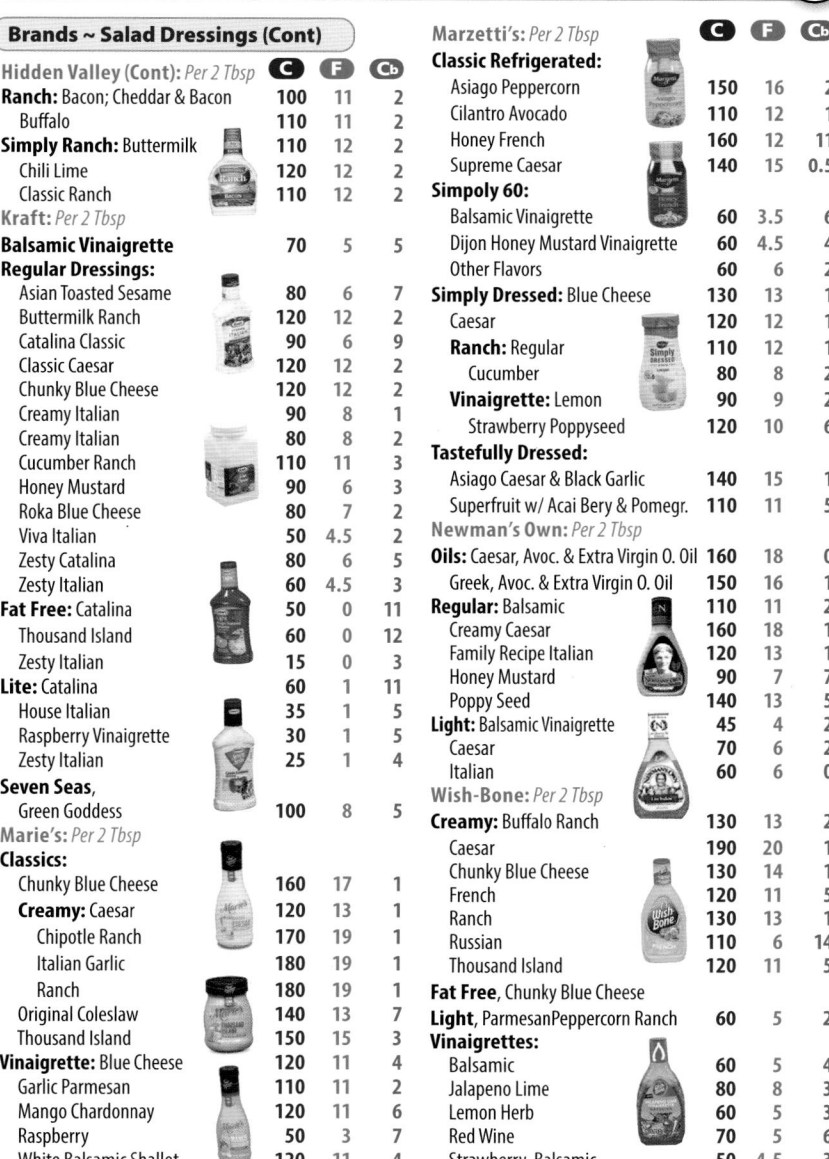

	C	F	Cb
Balsamic Vinaigrette	70	5	5
Regular Dressings:			
Asian Toasted Sesame	80	6	7
Buttermilk Ranch	120	12	2
Catalina Classic	90	6	9
Classic Caesar	120	12	2
Chunky Blue Cheese	120	12	2
Creamy Italian	90	8	1
Creamy Italian	80	8	2
Cucumber Ranch	110	11	3
Honey Mustard	90	6	3
Roka Blue Cheese	80	7	2
Viva Italian	50	4.5	2
Zesty Catalina	80	6	5
Zesty Italian	60	4.5	3
Fat Free: Catalina	50	0	11
Thousand Island	60	0	12
Zesty Italian	15	0	3
Lite: Catalina	60	1	11
House Italian	35	1	5
Raspberry Vinaigrette	30	1	5
Zesty Italian	25	1	4
Seven Seas, Green Goddess	100	8	5

Marie's: *Per 2 Tbsp*

	C	F	Cb
Classics:			
Chunky Blue Cheese	160	17	1
Creamy: Caesar	120	13	1
Chipotle Ranch	170	19	1
Italian Garlic	180	19	1
Ranch	180	19	1
Original Coleslaw	140	13	7
Thousand Island	150	15	3
Vinaigrette: Blue Cheese	120	11	4
Garlic Parmesan	110	11	2
Mango Chardonnay	120	11	6
Raspberry	50	3	7
White Balsamic Shallot	120	11	4

Marzetti's: *Per 2 Tbsp*

	C	F	Cb
Classic Refrigerated:			
Asiago Peppercorn	150	16	2
Cilantro Avocado	110	12	1
Honey French	160	12	11
Supreme Caesar	140	15	0.5
Simpoly 60:			
Balsamic Vinaigrette	60	3.5	6
Dijon Honey Mustard Vinaigrette	60	4.5	4
Other Flavors	60	6	2
Simply Dressed: Blue Cheese	130	13	1
Caesar	120	12	1
Ranch: Regular	110	12	1
Cucumber	80	8	2
Vinaigrette: Lemon	90	9	2
Strawberry Poppyseed	120	10	6
Tastefully Dressed:			
Asiago Caesar & Black Garlic	140	15	1
Superfruit w/ Acai Bery & Pomegr.	110	11	5

Newman's Own: *Per 2 Tbsp*

	C	F	Cb
Oils: Caesar, Avoc. & Extra Virgin O. Oil	160	18	0
Greek, Avoc. & Extra Virgin O. Oil	150	16	1
Regular: Balsamic	110	11	2
Creamy Caesar	160	18	1
Family Recipe Italian	120	13	1
Honey Mustard	90	7	7
Poppy Seed	140	13	5
Light: Balsamic Vinaigrette	45	4	2
Caesar	70	6	2
Italian	60	6	0

Wish-Bone: *Per 2 Tbsp*

	C	F	Cb
Creamy: Buffalo Ranch	130	13	2
Caesar	190	20	1
Chunky Blue Cheese	130	14	1
French	120	11	5
Ranch	130	13	1
Russian	110	6	14
Thousand Island	120	11	5
Fat Free, Chunky Blue Cheese			
Light, ParmesanPeppercorn Ranch	60	5	2
Vinaigrettes:			
Balsamic	60	5	4
Jalapeno Lime	80	8	3
Lemon Herb	60	5	3
Red Wine	70	5	6
Strawberry Balsamic	50	4.5	3

S Sauces & Gravy

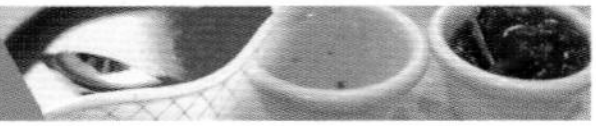

Gravy

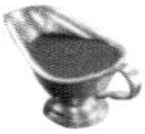
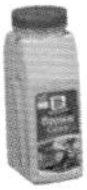

	C	F	Cb
Homemade Gravy, average:			
Thin, little fat,			
2 Tbsp, 1 oz	**20**	1	3
Thick: 2 Tbsp, 1.3 oz	**50**	2	9
¼ cup, 2.5 oz	**100**	4	18
McCormick:			
Brown, 1 Tbsp	**20**	0.5	4
Turkey, 1 Tbsp	**20**	0.5	4

Gravy-In-Jars

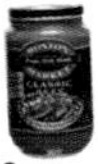
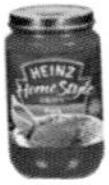

	C	F	Cb
Boston Market,			
Classic Beef, ¼ cup, 2 oz	**30**	1	4
Campbell's,			
Beef/Chicken/Turkey, ¼ cup, 2 oz	**30**	1	4
Heinz: *Per ¼ Cup, 2 oz*			
Homestyle: Bistro Au Jus	**15**	0	2
Classic Chicken	**30**	2	3
Mushroom; Pork	**20**	0.5	3
Roasted Turkey	**25**	2	3
Savory Beef	**25**	1	3
Safeway, Chicken, ¼ cup, 2 oz	**40**	2.5	3

Tomato Products

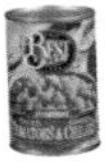
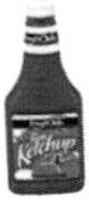
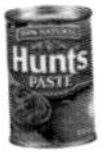
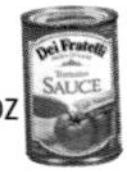
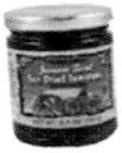

	C	F	Cb
Whole/Chopped/Crushed/Diced:			
Regular: 1 Cup, 8.5 oz	**50**	0	10
In Aspic, ½ Cup	**50**	0	12
with Green Chili, 1 c., 8.5 oz	**60**	0	16
Stewed, ½ Cup, 1.7 oz	**40**	1.5	7
Wedges in Tomato Juice, 1 Cup	**70**	0.5	18
Salsa, average, 2 Tbsp, 1 oz	**25**	0	6
Tomato Ketchup:			
Regular: 1 Tbsp, 0.5 oz	**15**	0	4
Single Serve, 1 packet	**10**	0	3
Heinz, Simply Heinz			
1 Tbsp, 0.5 oz	**15**	0	4
Tomato Paste:			
Regular: 2 Tbsp, 1 oz	**25**	0	6
¾ cup, 6 oz	**140**	1	32
Tomato Puree, ½ Cup, 4.5 oz	**50**	0	10
Tomato Sauce:			
Regular, ½ Cup, 4.4 oz	**50**	0	11
Spanish Style, ½ Cup, 4.3 oz	**40**	0	9
with Mushr., ½ Cup, 4.3 oz	**45**	0	10
with Onions, ½ Cup, 4.3 oz	**50**	0	12
Tomato Seasoning, 3 tsp	**20**	0	4
Sundried Tomatoes:			
Natural, 5-6 pieces, 0.4 oz	**20**	0	5
In Oil, drained, 6 pieces, 0.5 oz	**40**	2.5	4

Sauces ~ Brands

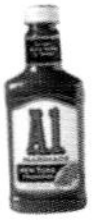
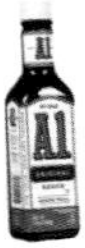
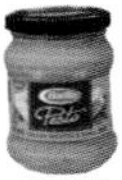
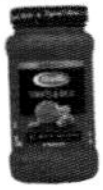
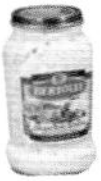
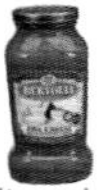
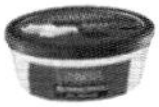
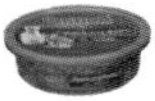
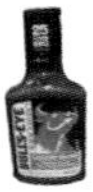
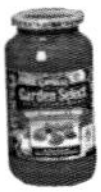

	C	F	Cb
A-1 *(Kraft):*			
Marinades: *Per Tbsp, ½ oz*			
Chicago Steakhouse	**20**	1	2
Classic	**15**	0	4
New Orleans Cajun	**25**	0	6
New York Steakhouse	**20**	0	5
Sauce: Original	**15**	0	3
Bold & Spicy	**20**	0	4
Smoky Black Pepper	**30**	0	6
Spicy Chipotle	**30**	0	7
Sweet Chili; Thick & Hearty	**25**	0	6
Sweet Hickory	**25**	0	5
Barilla:			
Pesto: *Per ¼ cup*			
Creamy: Genovese Pesto	**310**	29	8
Ricotta & Arugula	**270**	26	7
Rustic Basil	**200**	19	5
Sun-Dried Tomato	**130**	10	7
Regional: *Per ½ Cup*			
Fire Roasted Marinara	**45**	1	9
Marinara; Tomato Basil	**50**	1	11
Roasted Garlic; Savory Tomato, av.	**60**	1	11
Tomato Rosa	**80**	3	8
Bertolli:			
Alfredo Sauces: *Per ¼ Cup*			
Creamy Basil	**100**	10	2
Four Cheese Rosa	**110**	10	5
Garlic with Parmesan	**100**	10	2
Rustic Cut Marinara,			
with Traditonal Vegetables	**100**	6	10
Traditional: *Per ½ Cup*			
Five Cheese w/ Ricotta	**90**	3	12
Portobello Mushroom	**70**	2.5	9
Vodka	**140**	10	10
Buitoni: *Per ¼ Cup Unless Indicated*			
Pasta Sauces:			
Alfredo: Regular	**140**	13	3
Light	**70**	5	4
Marinara, ½ Cup	**70**	3	9
Pesto: With Basil	**290**	27	5
Reduced Fat	**230**	18	8
Bull's-Eye: Per 2 Tbsp			
BBQ Sauce: Original	**50**	0	4
Hickory Smoke	**60**	0	5
Regional, average all varieties	**50**	0	4
Catelli: *Per ½ Cup*			
Garden Select Pasta Sauce:			
Country Mushroom	**45**	1	9
Garlic & Onion	**45**	1	9
Meat Sauce	**50**	1.5	8
Pizza Sauce, all varieties	**60**	1.5	11

Sauces ~ Brands (Cont)

Cento:

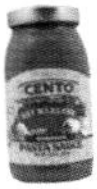

	C	F	Cb
Arrabbiata, ½ Cup	60	3.5	6
Italiano, ¼ cup	25	0	6
Marinara, ¼ cup	60	3.5	6
Porcini, ½ Cup	70	4	7
Puttanesca, ½ Cup	70	4.5	7
Vodka, ½ Cup	100	5	8

Classico:

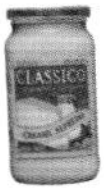

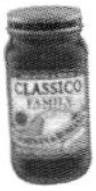

	C	F	Cb
Alfredo: *Per ¼ Cup*			
Creamy, 2 oz	50	3.5	3
Roasted Garlic, 2 oz	45	3.5	3
Family Favorites: *Per ½ Cup*			
Meat, 4.4 oz	60	1	10
Parm. & Romano, 4.4 oz	70	2	10
Traditional, 4.4 oz	80	2.5	13

Contadina: *Per ¼ Cup*

	C	F	Cb
Pizza Sauce: Four Cheese, 2.2 oz	30	0	6
Tomato, 2.2 oz	30	0	6
Tomato Sauce, average	20	0.5	4

Crosse & Blackwell:

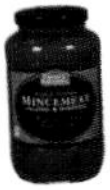

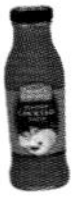

	C	F	Cb
Meat: Ham Glaze, 1 Tbsp	25	0	6
Mint Meat Sauce, 1 tsp	5	0	2
Mincemeat: *Per ¼ Cup*			
Regular	140	0	35
Rum & Brandy	140	0	36
Seafood: *Per ¼ Cup*			
Cocktail Sauce, 2.5 oz	90	0	21
Shrimp Sauce, 2.5 oz	90	0	21

Dave's Gourmet:

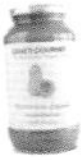

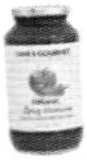

	C	F	Cb
Pasta Sauce: *Per ½ Cup*			
Butternut Squash	100	4	16
Creamy Parmesan Romano	120	8	9
Hearty Marinara	70	3.5	9
OrganicRed Heirloom	70	2.5	9
Rstd Garlic & Sweet Basil	70	4.5	8
Spicy Heirloom Marinara	45	1.5	7
Vegan Bolognese	80	4	8

Del Monte:

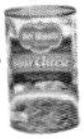

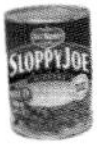

	C	F	Cb
Pasta Sauces: *Per ½ Cup*			
Four Cheese; Traditional, av.	60	1	12
Mushroom	60	1	11
Average other varieties	60	1	13
Sloppy Joe Sauce: *Per ¼ cup*			
Hickory	60	0	14
Original	60	0	13

Emeril's:

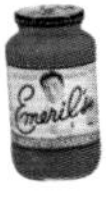

	C	F	Cb
Alfredo, Four Cheese Sauce, ¼ cup	60	5	4
Pasta Sauces: *Per ½ Cup*			
Homestyle Marinara	90	3	14
Kicked Up Tomato	80	3.5	11
Roasted Gaaahlic	80	3.5	12
Roasted Red Pepper	70	3.5	9
Vodka Sauce	110	7	12

Francesco Rinaldi:

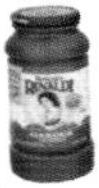

	C	F	Cb
Alfredo, all flavors, ¼ cup	90	8	2
Cheese,			
Three Cheese, ½ Cup	70	1	15
Garden, all var., ½ Cup	60	1	12
Meat: Meat Flavored, ½ Cup	70	2.5	13
Sicilian Family, Sausage, ½ Cup	70	2.5	11
Pizza, ¼ cup	20	0	4
Tomato, Marinara, ½ Cup	60	1	12

French's,

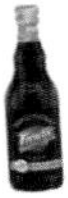

	C	F	Cb
Worcestershire Sauce, 1 tsp	0	0	1

Heinz: *Per 1 Tbsp*

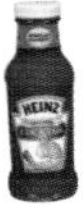

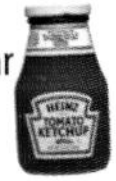

	C	F	Cb
57 Steak Sauce	20	0	4
Chili Sauce	20	0	5
Cocktail Sauce, Original, ¼ cup, 2.2 oz	70	0	18
Horseradish Sauce, tsp, 5 ml	25	2	1
Tartar Sauce, 2 tbsl	120	11	5
Tomato Ketchup: Regular	20	0	5
No Sugr Added	10	0	1
Worcestershire Sce, tsp	0	0	0

House of Tsang:

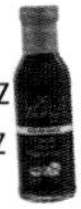

	C	F	Cb
Bangkok P'nut Sce, 1.16 oz	80	5	8
Classic Stir Fry Sauce, 0.6 oz	25	0.5	5
Ginger Sriracha Sce, 1.23 oz	15	0	4
General Tsao, 0.67 oz	45	0.5	10
Green Thai Curry Sauce, 1.1 oz	60	4	6
Korean BBQ Sauce, 0.67 oz	25	0	6
Oyster Flavored Sauce, 0.63 oz	30	0	7
Saigon Sizzle Sauce, 0.63 oz	40	1	7
Sweet & Sour Sauce, 0.63 oz	30	0	7

Hunt's:

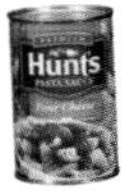

	C	F	Cb
BBQ Sauces, average, 2 Tbsp	70	0	16
Pasta Sauce: *Per ½ Cup*			
Four Cheese	60	1	11
Garlic & Herb	40	0.5	8
Mushroom	60	0.5	11
Zesty & Spicy	60	1.5	11

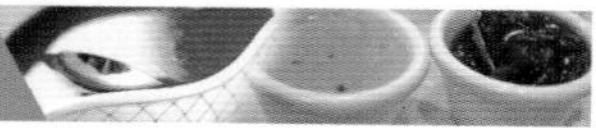

Brands (Cont)

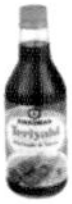
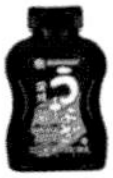

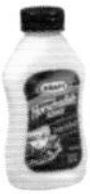
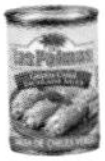
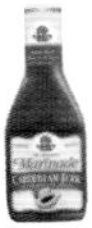
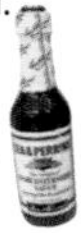

	C	F	Cb
Kikkoman: *Per Tablespoon*			
Marinade: Gourmet Teriyaki	25	0	6
Roasted Garlic & Herbs	15	0	3
Toasted Sesame	40	0.5	7
Asian Authentics: *Per Tbsp, Unless Indicated*			
Katsu	20	0	5
Kotteri Mirin	50	0	12
Plum Sauce, 2 Tbsp	90	1	21
Sukiyaki	25	0	5
Tempura	5	0	1
Unagi Sushi	40	0	10
Wasabi, 1 tsp	10	1	0.5
Knorr: *Dry Mix Only*			
Classic Sauce Mix:			
Bernaise, teaspoon	10	0	2
Creamy Pesto, 1 Tbsp	25	0	5
Four Cheese, 1 Tbsp	30	1	4
Hollandaise, teaspoon	10	0	2
Pesto, 1 tbsp	20	0	3
Kraft:			
Horseradish, 2 Tbsp	100	9	4
Mesq. Smoke BBQ Sauce, 2 T.	60	0	15
Tartar, 1 Tbsp	70	6	4
Las Palmas: *Per ¼ Cup*			
Green Enchilada Sauce, all varieties, 2 oz	25	1.5	3
Red Chili Sauce	15	0.5	3
La Victoria,			
Red/Green Enchilada Sauce, av., 2 oz	25	1.5	3
Lawry's:			
30 Minute Marinade: *Per Tbsp*			
Baja Chipotle	10	0	2
Caribbean Jerk with Papaya	20	0	4
Chipotle Molasses	30	0	7
Herb & Garlic; Lemon Pepper	10	0	2
Honey Bourbon	20	0	5
Mesquite, w/ Lime Juice	10	0	2
Sesame & Ginger	20	0	5
Steakhouse	10	0	2
Teriyaki with Pineapple Juice	15	0	4
Sweet Asian	20	0	4
Lea & Perrins:			
Marinade, Chkn; Rstd Garlic, 1 T.	15	0	4
Tradit. Steak Sauce, 1 Tbsp	20	0	5
Worcestershire Sauce:			
Original,1 tsp, 5 ml	5	0	1
Reduced Sodium, 1 tsp, 5 ml	5	0	1

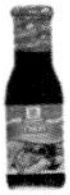
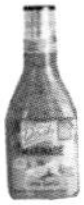
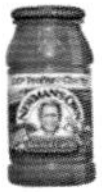
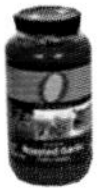
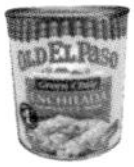
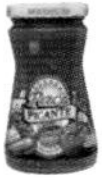
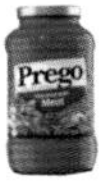

	C	F	Cb
McCormicks:			
Cooking, Tomato, Garlic & Wine, 1 T.	15	0	3
Seafood Sauces: *Per 2 Tbsp*			
Asian; Santa Fe Style, av.	50	2	7
Cajun Style	15	0	3
Lemon Butter Dill	100	9	4
Lemon Herb	80	8	0
Scampi	160	17	2
Mrs. Dash			
Marinades: *Per 1 Tbsp*			
Garlic Herb	15	0	3
Lime Garlic	15	0	3
Sweet Teriyaki	35	0	9
Newman's Own: *Per ½ Cup Inless Indicated*			
Pasta Sauce: Alfredo, 2.1 oz	50	4.5	3
Italian Sausage & Peppers	90	3.5	10
Marinara; Sockarooni	70	1	12
Roasted Garlic	60	1.5	11
Tomato & Basil Bombolina	70	2	11
Vodka	140	9	11
O Organics *(Von's): Per ½ Cup Unless Indicated*			
Enchilada, average, ¼ cup	20	0.5	4
Pasta: Arrabiata	60	1.5	10
Classic Alfredo	70	7	3
Marinara; Roasted Garlic, av.	60	1.5	11
Portobello Mushroom	45	1.5	7
Old El Paso: *Per ¼ Cup*			
Creamy: Queso, 1 Tbsp	20	1.5	2
Salsa Verde, 1 Tbsp	40	3.5	1
Enchilada Sauce:			
Green Chile, 2.15 oz	25	1.5	4
Red, all, 2.1 oz	20	0	4
Taco Sauce, all,1 Tbsp	5	0	1
Pace: *Per 2 Tbsp*			
Picante Sauce, all varieties	10	0	2
Queso,			
Salsa: Regular, all varieties	10	0	3
Salsa con Queso	40	3	3
Prego: *Per ½ Cup, Unless Indicated*			
Alfredo, all varieties, ¼ cup	70	6	3
Basil Pesto Italian	200	19	4
Classic Italian: Chnky Tom. & Greens	70	1.5	11
Italian: Chunky Zucchini	60	1.5	10
Rstd Garlic Parm.; Three Chse, av.	70	1.5	13
Spicy Sausage Meat	110	4	15
Favorite:			
Italian: Flavored with Meat	90	3	13
Fresh Mushroom	70	1.5	12
Sausage & Garlic Meat	90	3	12
Premier Japan, Hoisin;Teriyaki, 1 T.	15	0	3

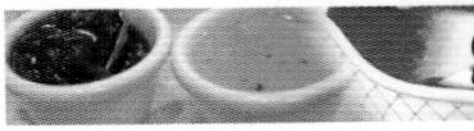

Brands (Cont)

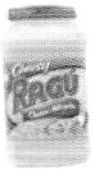
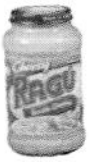
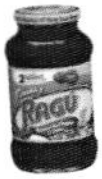
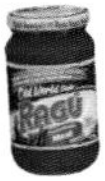
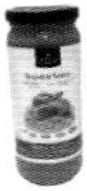
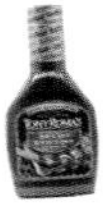

	C	F	Cb
Ragu:			
Cheese Sauce: *Per ¼ Cup*			
Butter Parmesan	60	5	2
Classic/Creamy Alfredo, av.	90	9	2.5
Double Cheddar	100	9	3
Light Parmesan Alfredo	60	4	2
Roasted Garlic Parmesan	90	8	3
Chunky Sauce: *Per ½ Cup*			
Garden Combination	90	2.5	14
Mama's Special Garden	90	2.5	15
M'shrm & Green Peppers	80	2	13
Parmesan & Romano	80	2.5	13
Six Cheese	90	2.5	14
Super Chunky Mushroom	80	2	14
Old World Style: *Per ½ Cup*			
Flavored with Meat	90	4	12
Marinara; Mushroom, av.	75	2	11
Traditional	60	1	11
Pizza: Homemade Style, ¼ Cup	30	1	5
Margherita, ¼ Cup	25	0.5	3
Snack Sauce, Traditional, ¼ Cup	45	1.5	6
Simply Pasta Sauce: *Per ½ Cup*			
Chunky Marinaraa	70	1.5	11
M'shrm; Rstd Garlic; Traditional, av.	60	1.5	11
Safeway Select: *Per ½ Cup Unless Indicated*			
BBQ, Carolina Style Gold, 2 Tbsp	60	1	13
Pasta Sauce: Marinara; Rstd Garlic, av.	60	1.5	11
Portobello Âushroom	45	1.5	7
Vodka	150	10	10
Simmer Sauce: Butter Chicken	160	13	11
Lemon Butter	190	15	13
Thai Coconut Curry	140	9	10
Tikka Masala	90	6	7
White Wine & Mushroom	100	5	8
Taco Bell, Creamy Jalapeno Sauce, 1 Tablespoon, 0.5 oz	70	7	1
Tony Roma's:			
Original, 2 Tbsp	50	0	12
Carolina Honey BBQ Sce, 2 Tbsp	70	0	18
Trader Joe's, Kansas City Style BBQ Sauce, 2 Tbsp	45	0	11
Walnut Acres,			
Organic Pasta Sauces, average all var., ½ Cup, 4.5 oz	50	1	10

Seasonings & Flavorings

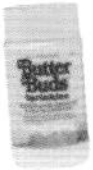
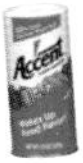
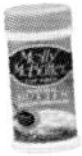
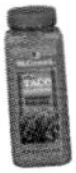

	C	F	Cb
Auromatic Bitters *(Angostua)*, 1 tsp	15	0	4
Bacon Bits, average, 1 Tbsp	35	2	2
Bacon Chips *(Durkee)*, 1 Tbsp	30	1	2
Bac-Os *(Betty Crocker)*, 1Tbsp	30	1.5	2
Blends *(Mrs Dash)*, 1 tsp	0	0	0
Butter Buds, 1 tsp	5	0	2
Flavor Enhancer *(Accent)*, 1 tsp	0	0	0
Flavor Sprinkles *(Molly McButter)*, Natural/Cheese, 1 tsp	5	0	1
Garlic Bread Sprinkle, 1 tsp	8	0.5	1
Garlic Salt, 1 tsp	2	0	0
Italian Seasoning, 1 tsp	4	0	1
Lemon Pepper Seasoning, 1 tsp	7	0	1
Meat Tenderizer, av., 1 tsp	7	0	1
Salad Crunchies *(McCormick)*, 1 tsp	10	0.5	2
Salt, Reg., Sea Salt, Lite Salt	0	0	0
Seasoning *(Old Bay)*, ¼ tsp	0	0	0
Seasoning Mix *(Vegit)*, ¼ tsp	0	0	0
Seasoning Mixes, av., ¼ pkg	70	1	9
Taco Seasoning, av., ¼ pkg	30	0.5	4
Bragg's, Liquid Aminos	0	0	0
Old El Paso: Chili Season. Mix, 1 Tbsp	8	0.5	1.5
Cheesy Taco Seasoning Mix, 1 Tbsp	10	0.5	2
Taco/Burrito Seasoning Mix, 2 tsp	15	0	4
Fajita Seasoning Mix, 1 tsp	5	0	1.5

Spices & Herbs

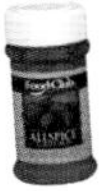
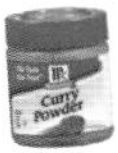
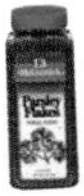
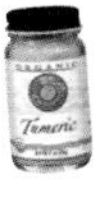

	C	F	Cb
Average all types, 1 tsp	5	0	1
All Purpose, 1 tsp	0	0	0
Allspice, ground	5	0	1
Chili Powder	8	0	1
Cinnamon, ground	6	0	2
Curry Powder	6	0	1
Garlic Powder	9	0	2
Nutmeg, ground	12	0	1
Onion Powder	7	0	2
Parsley, dried	4	0	1
Pepper, average	6	0	1
Saffron	2	0	0
Salt-Free Blends, 1 tsp	0	0	0
Tumeric, ground	8	0	1
Seeds: Fenugreek	12	1	2
Mustard, Poppyseed	15	1	1
Other varieties, average	7	0	1

Home-Popped Popcorn

	C	F	Cb
Popping Corn Kernels,			
2 Tbsp, 1 oz	110	1	26
(makes approximately 5 Cups)			
Air-popped, without oil: Plain,.1 oz	110	1	22
1 Cup, 0.2 oz	20	0	5
Oil-popped: Plain, 1 oz	145	8	16
1 Cup, 0.4 oz	55	3	6
Popcorn Oil, 1 Tbsp	120	14	0

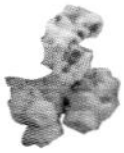

Microwave Popcorn

	C	F	Cb
Average all Brands: *Per 1 Cup Popped, Unless Indicated*			
Butter: Regular, 1 Cup	35	2	4
Light, 1 Cup	25	1	4
Act II Popcorn:			
Butter,			
Microwave, 2.75 oz bag	130	6	19
Butter Lovers: 1 Cup	30	1.5	4.5
4.5 Cups	140	7	20
Movie Theatre Butter/ Buttery Kettle Corn:			
1 Cup	35	2	4.5
4.5 Cups	150	8	19
Xreme Butter: 1 Cup	30	2	4
5 Cups	160	9	20
BodyKey *(Amway)*, Slim Popcorn,			
Sea Salt, 1 bag, 0.7 oz	110	7	10
Jolly Time:			
Blast O Butter, 1 Cup	45	3	4
Crispy 'n White Light, 1 Cup	25	1	4
Xtra Butter: 1 Cup	40	2.5	4
4 Cups	160	10	16
Newman's Own: *Per 3½ Cups*			
Microwave: Butter Flav.	150	8	16
Tender White	150	9	16
Sea Salt	150	9	16
Organic Butter	150	4.5	23
Orville Redenbacher's:			
Butter: 4½ Cups	170	12	17
Light, 6 Cups	160	6	27
Movie Theater Butter, 5 Cups	160	10	18
Ultimate Butter, 4½ Cups	160	9	19
Naturals, Simply Salted, 4½ Cups	170	11	18
Sweet & Savory:			
Cheddar Cheese, 4½ Cups	190	13	18
Melt On Caramel, 3 Cups	180	8	26
Pop Secret: *Per Cup*			
94% Fat-Free, Butter	20	0	3
Double Butter	40	2	3
Skinnygirl *(Orville Redenbacker's)*,			
Butter/ Lime & Sea Salt, 6 cups	160	6	28

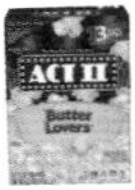

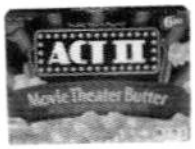

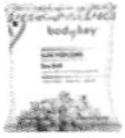
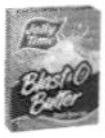
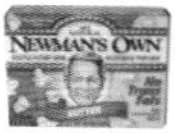

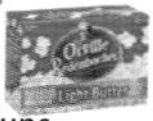
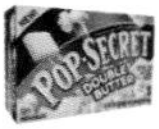

Bagged Popcorn

	C	F	Cb
Average All Brands (Ready-to-Eat)			
Regular/Plain: ½ oz package	80	5	8
1 oz package	160	10	16
4 oz package	640	40	64
2 oz Box (store/airport)	320	16	32
3 oz Bag (9" high x 5" wide)	480	24	48
Caramel Popcorn,			
with nuts, 1 Cup, 1.5 oz	230	12	39

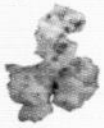

Bagged Popcorn ~ Brands

	C	F	Cb
Boston's, Lite, 3½ Cups, 1 oz	140	4.5	20
Cracker Jack: Original, 1 Cup, 2 oz	240	4	46
Chocolate & Caramel, 1 Cup, 2 oz	220	1	50
Crunch 'N Munch:			
Buttery Toffee: ⅔ cup, 1.1 oz	150	5	24
1 Cup, 1.65 oz	225	7.5	36
Caramel: ⅔ cup, 1.1 oz	160	7	22
1 Cup, 1.65 oz	240	10	33
fiddle faddle:			
Butter: ⅔ Cup	130	2	26
1 Cup	195	3	39
Caramel: ⅔ Cup	120	2	24
1 Cup, 2 oz	180	3	36
Popcorn Indiana:			
Kettlecorn: Maple, 1 oz	160	11	14
Sweet & Salty, 1 oz	130	7	16
Popcorn:			
Aged White Cheddar, 1 oz	130	10	12
Movie Theater, 1 oz	140	11	11
Sea Salt, 1 oz	150	9	15
Poppycock:			
Bags: Cashew Lovers, ½ Cup, 1 oz	150	6	20
Pecan Delight, ½ Cup, 1 oz	150	6	22
Cannisters, Orig./Pecan Delight, av:			
½ Cup, 1.1 oz	155	7	21
1 Cup, 2.2 oz	310	14	42
Skinny Pop:			
Original/Cheddar, avg., ¼ bag, 1 oz	150	10	15

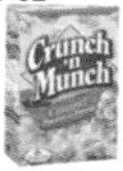

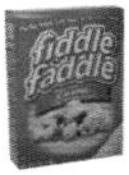

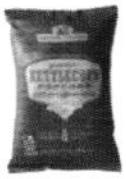
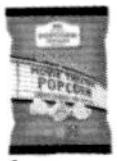

Movie Theater Popcorn

	C	F	Cb
Small, (7 Cups): Plain	385	21	44
with Butter (3 pumps, 0.8 oz)	570	42	44
Medium, (15 Cups): Plain	825	45	94
with Butter (4 pumps, 1 oz)	1075	73	94
Large, (20 Cups): Plain	1100	60	124
with Butter (6 pumps, 1.5 oz)	1485	102	124
Butter: 1 Pump, 0.3 oz	65	7	0
4 Pumps (2 Tbsp), 1 oz	250	28	0

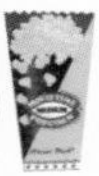

Corn & Tortilla Chips

	C	F	Cb
Average All Brands			
Corn Chips:			
Average all types: 1 oz	**150**	8	18
8 oz bag	**1200**	64	144
Fritos, Original, 32 chips, 1 oz	**160**	10	16
Tortilla Chips: Average, 1 oz	**140**	7	18
(1 oz = approx. 12 chips or 13 strips)			
Doritos: Original, 1 oz	**140**	7	18
Nacho Chse; Salsa Verde, av., 1 oz	**145**	8	18
Popchips: Barbecue, 1 oz	**130**	4.5	20
Buffalo Ranch, 1 oz	**120**	4	20
Snyder's:			
El Restaurante, all flavors, 1 oz	**150**	8	17
Yellow Corn/White, av., 1 oz	**135**	5	21
Tostitos:			
Average all flav., 1 oz	**145**	7	19
Baked! Scoops, 1 oz	**120**	3	22
Utz, Bar-B-Q Flavor Corn Chips	**150**	9	16

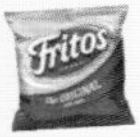
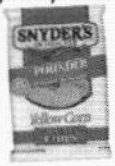
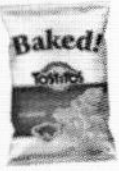

Potato Chips/Crisps

	C	F	Cb
Average All Brands			
Regular:			
Plain or flavored, (4 chips)	**30**	2	3
1 oz package (20 chips)	**150**	10	15
4 oz quantity	**600**	40	60
14 oz package	**2100**	140	210

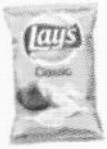
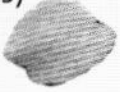

Chips/Crisps ~ Brands

	C	F	Cb
Hippeas, Chick Pea Puffs,			
average all flavors, 0.78 oz	**90**	4	11
Lay's *(Fritolay):*			
Classics; Wavy Originals, 1 oz	**160**	10	15
Kettle Cooked, Original, 1 oz	**150**	9	17
Pringles:			
All Flavors: 1 oz	**150**	9	16
Large can, 6 oz	**900**	54	96
Reduced Fat, Original, 1 oz	**140**	7	18
Ruffles: Regular, av. all flavors, 1 oz	**150**	9	15
Double Crunch, all flavors, 1 oz	**150**	8	17
Simply7, Hummus/Lentil Chips,			
average all flavors, 1 oz	**135**	5	19
Sun Chips: Original, 16 crisps, 1 oz	**140**	6	19
Whole Grain, Garden Salsa, 1 oz	**140**	6	19

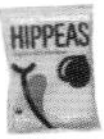
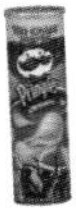

Pretzels

	C	F	Cb
Average All Brands			
Hard-Baked Pretzels: *Each*			
1 oz quantity	**110**	1	23
Sticks, thin, 2¼" (9/oz)	**12**	0	3
Twists, thin, ¼" thick, (5/oz)	**25**	0	5
Dutch (2¾"x 2⅝"), 0.5 oz	**55**	1	11
Snyders, Sourdough, 1 oz	**110**	0	23
Soft Pretzel Twists, average: *Each*			
Plain: Small, 2 oz	**210**	2	43
Medium, 4 oz	**390**	3.5	80
Large, 5 oz	**485**	4.5	100
Big Cheese, 1.8 oz	**130**	3	22
New York Street Vendors, 7 oz	**660**	6	135
Trader Joe's, Peanut Butter filled, 1 oz	**140**	8	14
Snyder's: Milk Chocolate Dips, 1 oz	**150**	7	20
White Creme Dips, 1 oz	**140**	6	21

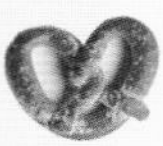

Pretzels ~ Brands

	C	F	Cb
Flipz: Milk Choc, 8 pieces, 1 oz	**140**	5	21
White Fudge, 7 pcs, 1 oz	**140**	5	21
Rold Gold *(Frito-Lay):*			
Braided Twists,			
Honey Wheat (8), 1 oz	**110**	1	23
Pretzel Thins, Orig. (9), 1 oz	**110**	1	23
Rods, Original (3), 1 oz	**110**	1	22
Tiny Twists, Original, (18), 1 oz	**110**	0	23
Sticks, Original, 1 oz	**100**	0	23
Snackwell's Pretzels, Minis:			
Fudge Dipped, 1 pack	**100**	4	16
Yogurt Dipped, 1 pack	**100**	5	16
Snyder's of Hanover:			
Butter Snaps, (24), 1 oz	**120**	1	25
Gluten Free, Sticks (32), 1 oz	**120**	3	24
Mini Pretzels,(20), 1 oz	**110**	0	25
Sticks, (26), 1 oz	**110**	1	23
Special K, Salted Choc. Coated, 1 oz	**100**	3	18
SuperPretzel:			
6 Count Soft, Original (1), 2.3 oz	**160**	0	34
Bites, (3), 2 oz	**160**	4.5	21
Softstix, (2), 1.76 oz	**130**	3.5	21
Utz:			
Sourdough Pretzels: Extra Dark, 1 oz	**110**	1	21
Hard (1)	**90**	0	18

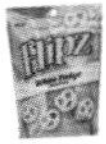
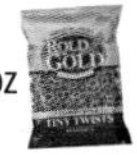
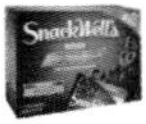
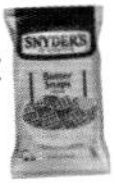
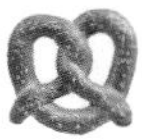

Snacks

Note: Actual weight of packaged snacks is usually 5-10% more than label Net Wt. For accuracy, weigh snack and allow extra calories, fat and carbs for any extra weight.

Snacks	C	F	Cb
Apple Chips *(Seneca)*, av., 1 oz	**140**	7	20
Bagel Crisps *(N.Y. Style)*, 6 crisps, 1 oz	**130**	6	17
Baguette Chips, 1 oz	**130**	5	19
Banana Chips *(T.Joe's)*, 13 chips, 1 oz	**160**	11	13
Beef Jerky *(Jack Link's)*, av., 1 oz	**80**	1	6
Beef Sticks:			
Slim Jim, Giant, Smoked, 1 oz	**130**	10	5
Jack Link's, Original (1), 1.5 oz	**190**	16	3
Beet Chips *(Rhythm)*, Sea Salt, 1oz	**130**	4	20
Trader Joes, 1.3 oz	**140**	0.5	29
BodyKey *(Amway)*:			
Zesty Protein Snack, 1 oz	**120**	3.5	15
Bugles, Orig.; Nacho Cheese, 1 oz	**150**	6.5	18
Cheese Balls *(Utz)*, 1 oz serving	**150**	9	16
Cheese Bites *(Tr. Joes)*, 1 oz	**170**	12	0.5
Cheese Nips *(Nabisco)*, (29), 1 oz	**150**	6	19
Cheese Puffs, average, 1 oz	**160**	10	15
Cheetos:			
Crunchy: Av. all flavors, 1 oz	**165**	10	15
4 oz package	**640**	40	60
Baked!; Fantastix, av., 1 oz	**130**	5	19
Simply Puffs, Wh. Cheddar, 1 oz	**160**	9	16
Cheez-It *(Sunshine)*:			
Snack Mix: Classic, ½ cup, 1 oz	**140**	5	20
Double Cheese, ½ cup, 0.9 ozz	**120**	5	17
Sweet & Salty, ½ cup, 1oz	**140**	5	21
Chester's: Fries, Flamin' Hot, 1 oz	**150**	8	17
Puffcorn, Cheese, 1 oz	**160**	11	13
Chex Mix *(General Mills)*:			
Muddy Buddies, Mint Choc, 0.9 oz	**120**	3.5	21
Traditional, 1 oz	**130**	3.5	23
Chicharrones ~ *See Pork Skins*			
Crackers *(Tr. Joes)*, Mini Edaname (28)	**120**	2	21
Churro Bites *(Great Value)*, Cinn., 1 oz	**100**	5	12
Combos, Crackers, av., ⅓ cup, 1 oz	**140**	6	18
Cool Cuts, Carrot & Ranch, 2.3 oz	**60**	5	6
Corn Chips ~ *See Page 149*			
Corn Nuts: Av all flav., 1 oz	**130**	4.5	20
1.7 oz bag	**210**	8	34
Corn Puffs, Buttery C'rml, 1 oz	**130**	4.5	22
Edamame,			
Seapoint Farms, Dry Roasted, 1 oz	**130**	5	9
Fritos,			
Corn Chips, Orig.; Flamin' Hot, 1 oz	**160**	10	16

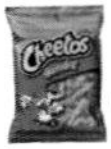

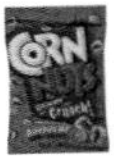

Snacks (Cont)	C	F	Cb
Fruit Snacks ~ *See Page 102 & 151*			
Funyuns, Onion Flavored, 1 oz	**140**	6	19
Goldfish, Crackers, av., 1 oz	**140**	5	20
Gold-n-Chees *(Lance)*:			
Snack Crackers, 1 oz	**140**	6	18
Gripz *(Sunshine)*, Mighty Tiny (1)	**120**	6	15
Flamin Hot Peanuts *(Munchies)*, 1 oz	**170**	15	5
Kale Chips *(Rhythm)*:			
Kool Rancch, 1 oz	**130**	9	6
Zesty Nacho, 1 oz	**130**	9	8
Lance ~ *See Sandwich Crackers Page 151*			
Munchies *(Frito-Lay)*,			
Snack Mix, all flavors, 1 oz	**140**	7	18
Munchos *(Fritolay)*, all flavors, 1 oz	**160**	10	16
Newtons:			
Single Serve: 2 oz pkg	**200**	4	42
Fat-Free, 2 oz package	**180**	0	46
Nutella, w/ Breadsticks/Pretzels (1)	**270**	14	35
Nutter Butter, Sandwich Cookies:			
2 Cookies	**120**	5	17
Bites, 1 pack	**130**	5	20
Wafers (5), 1.2 oz	**160**	9	19
Oreo Cookies, all Creme Fillings:			
Double Stuf (2), 1 oz	**145**	7	21
Mini: 1 Pack, 1 oz	**135**	5.5	20
Snak-Sak (9), 1 oz	**140**	6	21
Oriental Mix Rice Snacks, 1 oz	**125**	3.5	21
Peanut Butter Nuggets, (10), 1 oz	**140**	6	15
Pepitas, dried or roasted,			
¼ cup, 1 oz	**155**	14	3
Pirate's Booty: 1 oz	**140**	6	18
Aged White Cheddar, 4 oz	**560**	24	72
Veggie, 4 oz bag	**560**	28	72
Pita Chips *(Stacy's)*, (10), 1 oz	**130**	5	9
Plaintain Chips *(Goya)*, 1 oz	**150**	8	19
PopChips Ridges, av., 1 oz	**130**	5	19
PopCorners, Kettle, 1 oz	**125**	3.5	20
Popcorn ~ *See Page 148*			
Pork Cracklins, 1 oz	**160**	12	0
Pork Skins/Rinds: 1 oz	**160**	10	0
Baken-ets, Traditional, 0.5 oz	**80**	5	0
Mission, Chiccarones, 4 oz package	**640**	40	0
Potato Chips ~ *See Page 149*			
Potato Skins Chips *(TGI Friday)*,			
all flavors, 16 chips, 1 oz	**140**	8	16
Puffed Wheat,			
Sabritones, Chili & Lime, 1 oz	**140**	8	16
Pretzels ~ *See Page 149*			

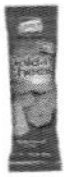

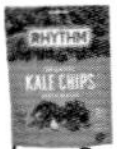

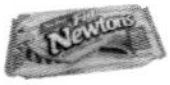

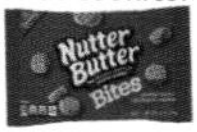

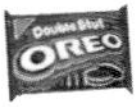

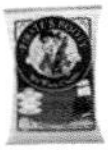

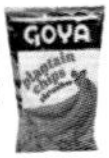

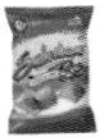

Snacks (Cont)

	C	F	Cb
Rice Cakes:			
Lundberg: Honey Nut (1)	80	0.5	19
Thin Stackers, Brown Rice (4), 1 oz	110	1	4
Quaker:			
100% Whole Grain, lightly salted (1)	35	0	7
Chocolate (1)	60	1	12
Rice Chips,			
Lundberg, average, 1 oz	135	6	18
Sandwich Crackers:			
Austin, Cheese Sandwich Crackers:			
w/ Cheddar, 1.4 oz	190	9	24
w/ Peanut Butter, 1.3 oz	190	9	24
Cheese Crackers, with PB, 0.8 oz	130	6	15
Lance: Nekot Lemon Creme, 1pkg	240	11	35
Toasty, PB, 1 pkg	180	9	21
Toast Chee, PB, 1.5 oz	220	10	25
Ritz Bits: Cheese (13), 1 oz Pkg	160	9	19
P'nut Butter:,1.5 oz pkg	220	13	24
Sesame Sticks, Salted,			
SunRidge Farm, 1 oz	170	11	14
Smart Puffs,			
Pirates Booty, 1 oz	140	7	17
Soybeans in Pods,			
AFC, ½ Cup, 3.2 oz	90	5	3
Soy Crisps, average, 1 oz	120	3	17
Soy Nuts: Dry Roasted, 1/4 cup, 1 oz	130	6	9
Choc-Coated, 1 oz	140	7	13
Sun Chips,			
Fritolay, average, 1 oz	140	6	19
Takis: Crunchy Fajitas, 1 oz	140	8	17
4 oz package	560	32	68
Tings *(Robert's)*, 2 oz bag	300	16	36
Toasted Chips *(Ritz)*, av. all, 1 oz	130	5.5	20
Tortilla Chips, White,			
Garden of Eatin, Touch of Lime, 1 oz	130	7	17
Trail Mix (Nuts/Seeds/Dried Fruit):			
Regular, 3 Tbsp, 1 oz	140	9	13
Tropical, 3 Tbsp, 1 oz	130	7	16
Turkey Jerky: Teriyaki, 1 oz	80	1	8
Trader Joe's, Original, 1 oz	60	0.5	6
Veggie Crisps,			
Snyder's, 1 oz	150	8	19
Wheat Thins *(Nabisco)*, av. all, 1 oz	135	5	21
Woats, Oatsnack, av., 1/4 cup, 1 oz	120	5	17
Yogurt Pretzels *(Larissa)*, 5 pces, 1 oz	150	8	20
Yogurt Raisins, Vanilla,			
Sun-Maid, 1 oz	120	4.5	20

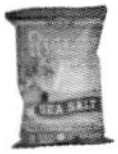
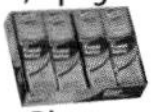
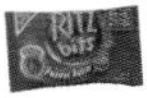
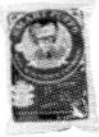
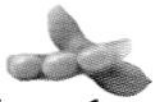
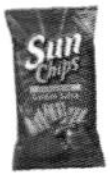
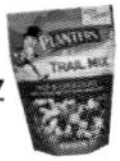

Fruit Snacks

	C	F	Cb
Betty Crocker: Fruit Gushers, 0.9 oz	80	1	18
Fruit by the Foot, 1 roll, 0.8 oz	80	1	17
Fruit Roll Ups, 1 roll, 0.5 oz	50	1	11
Sunkist:			
Fruit Lover's Trail Mix:			
Pineapple Coconut Blend, 1 oz	120	5	18
Straweberry Banana, 1 oz	110	4	19

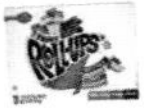

Fruit Snack Cups ~ See Page 102

Vending Machines

	C	F	Cb
Bugles, Nacho Cheese, 1 oz	150	9	18
Cheese Balls *(Utz)*, 1 oz	150	9	16
Cheetos, Crunchy, av., 1 oz	165	10	15
Cheeze-It, Classic Snack Mix, 1 oz	140	5	20
Chester's, Flamin' Hot Fries, 1 oz	150	8	17
Choc Chip Cookies:			
Chips Ahoy, 2 oz pkg	280	14	38
Famous Amos, 1.2 oz pouch	170	8	23
Grandma's, (1), 1.4 oz	200	10	25
Chocolate Bars:			
Hershey's, Milk Choc.,1.5 oz	220	13	26
Kit Kat, 1.5 oz	210	11	28
Snickers, 1.7 oz bar	250	12	32
Donut, plain cake, 1.4 oz	160	9	18
Doritos, av. all flavors, 1 oz	145	8	18
Fritos, Corn Chips, Orig., 2.75 oz	440	28	44
Fruit Pie,			
Hostess, Apple, 4.5 oz	430	17	67
Granola/Cereal Bars, av., 1 oz	140	3	26
M & M's:			
Milk Chocolate, 2 oz	280	10	40
Peanuts, 2 oz	280	14	34
Oreo Cookies, (3), 1.2 oz	160	7	25
Peanut Butter Cups,			
Reese's, 1.5 oz	210	12	24
Popcorn, plain, 1 oz	160	10	16
PopChips Ridges, 1 oz	130	5	19
Pork Skins, 1.5 oz	240	15	0
Potato Chips: 1 oz	150	10	15
Baked! *(Ruffles)*, Orig.,1 oz	120	3	22
Potato Skins Chips *(TGI Friday's)*,			
all flavors, 1 oz	140	8	16
Pretzels *(Snyder's)*, Olde Tyme, 1 oz	120	1	24
Raisins, 0.5 oz package	45	0	11
Rice Krispies Treat, Original, 0.78 oz	90	2	17
Skittles, Original,1 oz	110	1	26
Starburst, Fruit Chews, Orig., 1 oz	120	2.5	24
Tortilla Chips, 1 oz	140	7	18

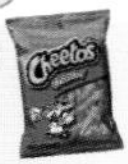
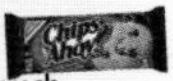
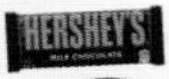
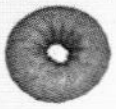
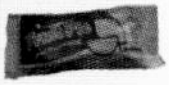
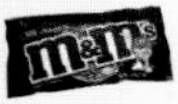
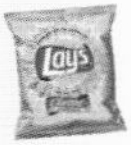
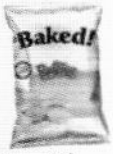

S Soups

Homemade & Restaurant

Restaurant & Take-Out:

Average All Recipes: *Per 1 Cup, 8 fl oz*
For 12 fl.oz Serving: Add 50% of figures
For 16 fl oz Serving: Double the figures

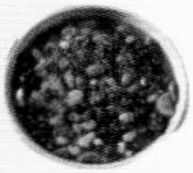
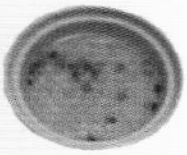
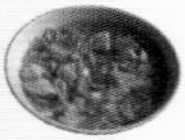
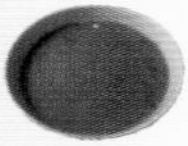
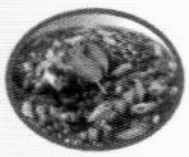
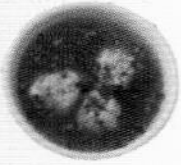
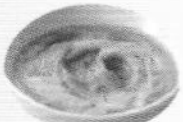
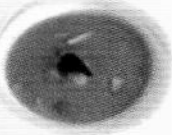

	C	F	Cb
Bean Medley	200	3	34
Beef Consomme	30	0	2
Borscht, w/ Sour Cream	130	8	14
Bouillabaisse	400	15	10
Chicken & Corn	290	14	20
Chicken & Wild Rice	80	4	9
Chicken Consomme	50	0	2
Chicken Curry	180	8	18
Chicken Jambalaya	160	7	8
Chicken Noodle	80	2	12
With Chicken	160	4	12
Chicken Soup	80	2	6
Chili with Beans	250	12	25
Clam Chowder	240	15	17
Corn & Crab	120	3	18
Corn Chowder	150	8	16
Cream of Broccoli	200	12	20
Cream of Potato	150	6.5	17
Cream of Mushroom	200	13	15
Fish Chowder	220	15	6
French Onion	420	15	25
Gazpacho	50	0	5
Lentil Soup	250	9	28
Lobster Bisque	320	15	10
Matzo Ball Soup	180	7	24
Minestrone	125	2.5	20
Mulligatawny	300	15	8
Pea & Ham	240	10	25
Potato & Bacon	170	7	19
Pumpkin, Creamy	210	10	26
Shark Fin Soup	100	4	8
Spicy Shrimp Soup, 1 bowl	160	7	10
Split Pea Soup	180	2.5	30
Vegetable (Fat Free)	75	0	18
Vegetable Beef	80	2	10
Vichyssoise	200	9	15
Watercress	90	4	13

Other Soups ~ *See International & Fast-Foods Sections (Arby's, Au Bon Pain, Boston Market, Dunkin' Donuts, Denny's, Schlotzsky's, Sizzler, Souplantation, Sweet Tomatoes, Zoup!)*

Homemade Soups: *Calculate calories, fat and carbohydrates from recipe ingredients.*

Bouillon Cubes & Powders

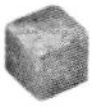
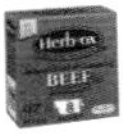

Bouillon Cubes: *Average all types*	C	F	Cb
Regular, 1 cube	5	0	1
Extra Large, 1 cube	20	1	1
Powders, average, 1 tsp	10	0	1
Herb-Ox:			
Instant Broth & Seasoning,			
Beef, 1 envelope, 0.14 oz	5	0	1
Chicken, 1 envelope, 0.14 oz	5	0	1

Soup ~ Brands

Amy's:

Heat & Serve (Organic): *Per 1 Cup,*

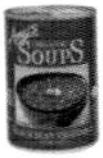
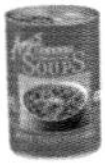
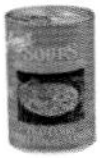

	C	F	Cb
Alphabet	110	2	21
Black Bean Vegetable	140	1.5	26
Chunky Vegetable	70	1.5	11
Carrot Ginger	200	13	18
Cream of M'shrm, 3/4 cup	150	9	13
Lentil Vegetable	160	4	24
Rustic Italian Vegetable	250	9	35
Southwestern Vegetable	140	5	20
Split Pea	110	1	19
Thai Coconut	210	14	15
Thai Curry Sweet Pot. Lentil	280	20	20
Tuscan Bean & Rice	170	4.5	28

Campbell's:

Chunky: *Per Cup, Unless Indicated*

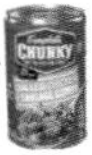

	C	F	Cb
Baked Potato w/ Ched. & Bacon Bits	190	9	22
Baked Potato with Steak & Cheese	190	9	21
Beef with Country Vegetables	110	1.5	16
Buffalo-Style Chicken Soup	150	7	15
Chicken Corn Chowder	190	9	20
Chipotle Chkn & Corn Chowder	180	8	20
Classic Chicken Noodle	120	3	14
Creamy Chkn & Dumplings	170	9	14
Grilled Chicken & Sausage Gumbo	140	3.5	21
Hearty: Bean & Ham, Smoked	150	1.5	27
Jambalaya Chkn, Ssg & Ham	140	4	20
Manhattan Clam Chowder	100	2.5	15
Old Fashioned Vegetable	110	2	16

Campbell's (Cont):

Condensed Soup: *Per ½ Cup*

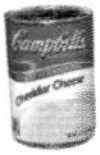
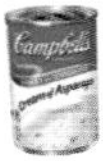
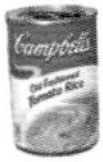
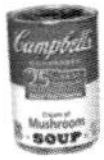

	C	F	Cb
Beef Broth	15	0	1
Beef Consume	20	0	1
Beef with Veggie & Barley	100	1	18
Broccoli Cheese	100	5	11
Cheddar Cheese	90	4	14
Chicken Gumbo	70	2	12
Cream of: Asparagus	100	7	8
Celery	100	7	8
Mushroom with Roasted Garlic	90	5	9
Onion	120	7	12
French Onion	70	1.5	13
Golden Mushroom	80	3.5	10
Mega Noodle	60	2	8
Old Fashioned Tom. Rice	120	1.5	25
Tomato	90	0	20
25% Less Sodium,			
Cream of Mushroom	100	7	8
98% Fat Free:			
Broccoli Cheese	80	2.5	11
Cream of: Celery	60	2.5	9
Chicken	60	2	8
Mushroom	60	2	9

Healthy Request: *Per ½ cup, Unless Indicated*

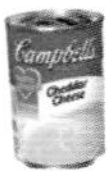

	C	F	Cb
Beef with Country Vegetables	110	1.5	17
Cheddar Cheese	60	1	12
Chicken Corn Chowder	140	3	22
Chicken Noodle	110	3	13
Golden Mushroom	70	2.5	10
Old Fashioned Vegetable Beef	110	2	17

Homestyle: *Per Cup*

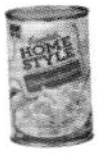

	C	F	Cb
Chicken Noodle	60	2	8
Chkn w/ Whole Grain Pasta	70	1.5	10
Harvest Tomato with Basil	110	1	23
Mexican-Style Chkn Tortilla	130	2	20
New England Clam Chowder	170	10	15
Savory Chicken with Brown Rice	110	2.5	16

Soup on the Go: *Per Container*

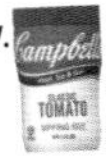

	C	F	Cb
Cheesy Chicken Tortilla	100	4	13
Cheesy Potato w/Bacon Flav.	130	6	16
Classic Tomato	140	0.5	32
Creamy Tomato	230	10	30
Creamy Tomato Parmesan Bisque	230	8	35

Campbell's (Cont):

Slow Kettle Style: *Per Container*

	C	F	Cb
Baked Potato with Smoked Bacon	440	32	32
Creamy Broccoli Cheddar Bisque	370	28	23
Mediterranean Vegetable	180	2	34
Rstd Red Pepper & Gouda Bisque	320	20	30
Tomato & Sweet Basil Bisque	550	33	56
Vegetarian Black Bean	340	3	61

Health Valley Organics: *Per Cup*

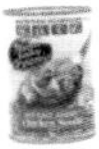
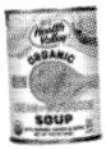
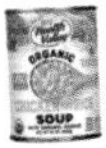
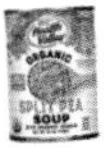

	C	F	Cb
40% Less Sodium:			
Chicken Noodle	80	2	11
Vegetable	90	0	18
Creamed:			
Cream of Chicken	120	3	17
Cream of Mushroom	90	1.5	16
No Salt Added:			
Chicken & Rice	100	1.5	19
Chicken Noodle	80	2	11
Lentil	150	1.5	27
Minestrone	100	2	18
Split Pea	160	2.5	26
Tomato	110	2	22
Vegetable	90	2	15

Healthy Choice:

Canned: *Per Cup*

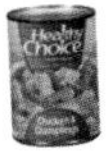
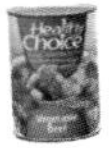

	C	F	Cb
Chicken & Dumplings	150	3	22
Chicken Noodle	90	2	12
Chicken with Rice	110	3	15
Country Vegetable	100	0.5	21
Vegetable Beef	120	1	21

Imagine:

Broths, Organic: *Per Cup*

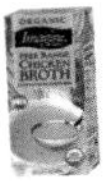

	C	F	Cb
Beef	20	1	2
Free Range Chicken	20	1	2
Vegetable, unsalted	20	0	4
Vegetarian, No-Chicken	15	0	2

Chunky Style, Organic: *Per Cup*

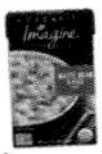

	C	F	Cb
Italian Style Wedding	150	5	20
Italian Vegetables & Beans	130	2	25
Loaded Baked Potato	120	5	18
Moroccan Chickpea & Carrot	100	1	1
Tomato Bisque	80	3	15
White Bean & Kale	110	1	21

Continued Nex Page...

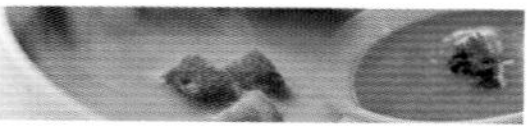

Imagine (Cont):	C	F	Cb
Creamy: *Per 8 fl.oz Cup*			
Butternut Squash	100	2	20
Broccoli	70	1	14
Garden Tomato, Light Sodium	80	1	16
Potato Leek	90	3	14
Portobello Mushroom	80	3	12
Tomato; Tomato Basil, av.	85	1	16
Kettle Cuisine: *Per 8 fl.oz Cup*			
Albondigas Meatball Soup	150	7	17
Beef, Barley & Vegetable	110	3	13
Broccoli Cheddar	320	24	16
Buffalo Chicken	240	15	14
Carrot Ginger	110	4	18
Chicken Tortilla	120	3	15
Chipotle Sweet Potato	150	6	22
Classic Gazpacho	60	1	10
Cream of Crab	290	22	16
Hot Honey & Butternut Squash	140	4	26
Lobster Bisque	250	18	18
Manhattan Clam Chowder	120	3	16
Minestrone	80	2	14
North Atlantic Haddock Chowder	260	17	14
Organic, Split Pea	80	1	13
Portuguese Kale with Linguica	170	7	23
Knorr:			
Cubes: *Per ½ Cube, 1 Cup, Prepared*			
Beef; Chicken; Vegetable, average	12	1	0.5
Homestyle Stock: *Per 1 Tsp*			
Beef	10	0.5	1
Chicken	10	1	0.5
Lipton:			
Cup-a-Soup: *Per Envelope, 6 fl.oz Prepared*			
Chicken Noodle, White Meat	50	1	8
Cream of Chicken Flavor	70	1.5	12
Recipe Secrets:			
Onion, 1 Tbsp	20	0	4
Onion Mushroom, 1⅔ T.	35	0	7
Savory Herb w/ Garlic, 1 T.	30	0	6
Manischewitz:			
Dry Soup Mix:			
Matzo Ball, 0.5 oz	40	0	8
Tetra Pack: *Per 1 cup*			
Chicken Broth	15	0.5	1
Maruchan:			
Instant Lunch, average all flavors, 1 pkg	290	12	38
Ramen, all flavors, 1 pkg, 3 oz	380	14	52

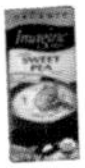
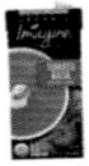
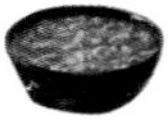
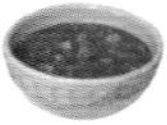
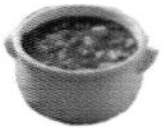
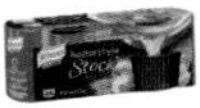
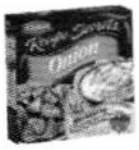
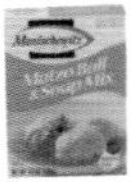
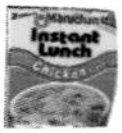

Nissin:	C	F	Cb
Soup'd Up Cup Noodles: *Per Package*			
Roasted Chicken Flavor, 2.57 oz	330	12	45
Savory Shrimp Flavor, 2.57 oz	330	13	45
Souper Meal, Beef, 1.45 oz pkg	550	22	753
Pacific Foods:			
Condensed: *Per Container*			
Cream of Chicken	190	6	23
Cream of Mushroom	190	8	27
Creamy: *Per 1 Cup*			
Golden Cauliflower	120	6	13
Moroccan Sweet Potato	130	5	19
Tomato Basil	90	2	13
Hearty Organic: *Per 1 Cup*			
Butternut Squash Bisque	120	3	22
Cashew Carrot Ginger Bisque	140	5	22
Coconut Curry	200	9	28
Rosemary Potato Chowder	170	8	22
Progresso: *Per Cup*			
Broths: Beef	15	0	1
Classic Chicken	5	0	0
Vegetable	5	0	1
Rich & Hearty:			
Beef Pot Roast w/ Country Vegetables	110	1.5	16
Chicken & Homestyle Noodles	110	2.5	14
Chkn Pot Pie w Dumplings	130	4	17
Lasagna Style w Ital Ssc	170	7	20
Minestrone w/ Italian Ssg	150	5	17
New England Clam Chowder	170	7	23
Steak & Vegetables	100	1.5	16
Traditional: *Per 1 Cup*			
Cheese Tortellini Garden Vegetable	100	1	20
Chickarina	110	4	12
Chicken & Rotini	90	1.5	13
Italian-Style Wedding	120	4	15
Manhattan Clam Chowder	100	2	17
Potato, Broccoli & Cheese	210	13	19
Vegetable Classic: *Per 1 Cup*			
Creamy Mushroom	130	9	12
Green Split Pea w/ Bacon	150	1.5	29
Minestrone	110	2	20
Tuscan-Style White Bean	130	1.5	23
Light: *Per 1 cup*			
Beef Pot Roast	70	1	9
Broccoli Cheese	120	6	11
Chicken Noodle	60	0.5	9
Vegetable	70	0	15

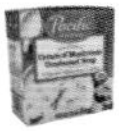
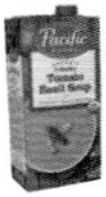
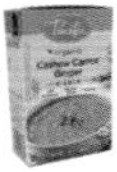
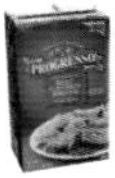
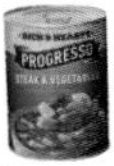
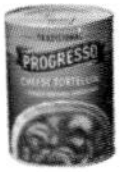
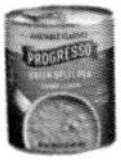
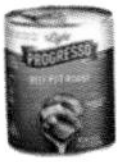

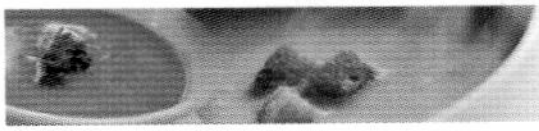

Swanson:	C	F	Cb
Broth: *Per 8 fl.oz Cup*			
Beef, unsalted	15	0	1
Chicken/Chicken unsalted	10	0	1
Organic Chicken	15	0	0.5
Vegetable	10	0	2
Stock: Beef	15	0	1
Chicken	20	0	1
Vegetable	15	0.5	2
Tabatchnick:			
Frozen:			
Dairy: *Per 7.5 oz Pouch*			
Corn Chowder	130	4.5	21
Cream of Mushroom	100	5	11
New England Potato	140	4.5	21
Gluten Free: *Per 7.5 oz Pouch*			
Balsamic Tomato & Rice	100	1.5	20
New England Potato	140	4.5	21
Old Fashioned Potato	100	1.5	21
Southwest Bean	220	5	36
Split Pea	180	0.5	33
Tuskany Lentil	160	0	29
Wilderness Wild Rice	90	0.5	19
Low Sodium: *Per 7 .5oz Pouch*			
Barley & Mushroom	80	0.5	17
Split Pea	110	1.5	20
Vegetable	110	1.5	20
Meat: *Per 7.5 oz Pouch*			
Chkn Broth with Noodles & Dumplings	120	4	16
Chkn Broth NY Style w/ Noodles & Veg.	70	1.5	12
Frenchman's Onion	60	1.5	11
Pareve: *Per 7.5 oz Pouch*			
Barley & Mushroom	80	0.5	17
Black Bean	220	2.5	38
Cabbage	90	0.5	21
Minestrone	110	1.5	19
Vegetarian Chili	200	3.5	32
Yankee Bean	180	1.5	32
Thai Kitchen:			
Rice Noodle Soup Bowls: *Per Bowl*			
Hot and Sour Rice Noodle	250	4	51
Lemongrass & Chili	250	3.5	52
Roasted Garlic	250	3	52
Spring Onion	260	4.5	50
Thai Ginger	260	3	52

Trader Joe's:	C	F	Cb
28 fl.oz Cans: *Per Cup*			
Chunky, Low Fat:			
Lentil with Vegetables	140	3	21
Minestrone	110	2.5	19
14.5 oz Cans: *Per Cup*			
Organic: Black Bean	140	1.5	26
Lentil Vegetable	160	4	24
Split Pea	100	0	19
10.75 oz Can,			
Low Sodium, Minestrone	200	4	37
15 oz Can,			
Low Fat, Chicken Noodle, 1 cup	90	1	14
32 fl oz. Cartons: *Per Cup*			
Butternut Squash	90	2	16
Carrot & Ginger	80	1	17
Creamy Corn & Rstd Pepper	110	2	23
Latin Style Black Bean	70	1	12
Sweet Potato Bisque	130	1	28
Organic: Butternut Squash	70	0	17
Tomato & Rstd Red Pepper	100	3.5	15
Low Sodium, Creamy Tomato	90	3.5	15
17.6 fl.oz Cartons: *Per Cup*			
Beef, Barley with Veggies	100	0.5	16
Chicken Noodle with Veggies	100	1	16
Ramen Soups: *Per 43g Container*			
Chicken	180	4	29
Miso	180	3	31
Whole Foods: *Per Cup*			
365 Organic:			
Caribbean Black Bean	170	0	35
Chicken Noodle	70	0	10
Lentil	100	0	18
Minestrone	140	1.5	23
Sthwestern Black Bean	120	1	23
Vegetable Medley	70	0	16
Condensed,			
Cream of Mushroom, ½ cup	60	1.5	10
Wolfgang Puck: *Per Cup*			
Organic:			
Chicken with White & Wild Rice	130	4	18
Classic Minestrone	120	2.5	20
Creamy Butternut Squash	140	11	10
Old Fashioned Potato	170	10	20
Thick Hearty Lentil Vegetable	160	1	29
Tomato with Basil	150	6	21
Tortilla	160	3.5	27
Vegetable	130	5	19

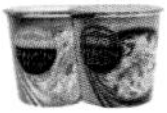

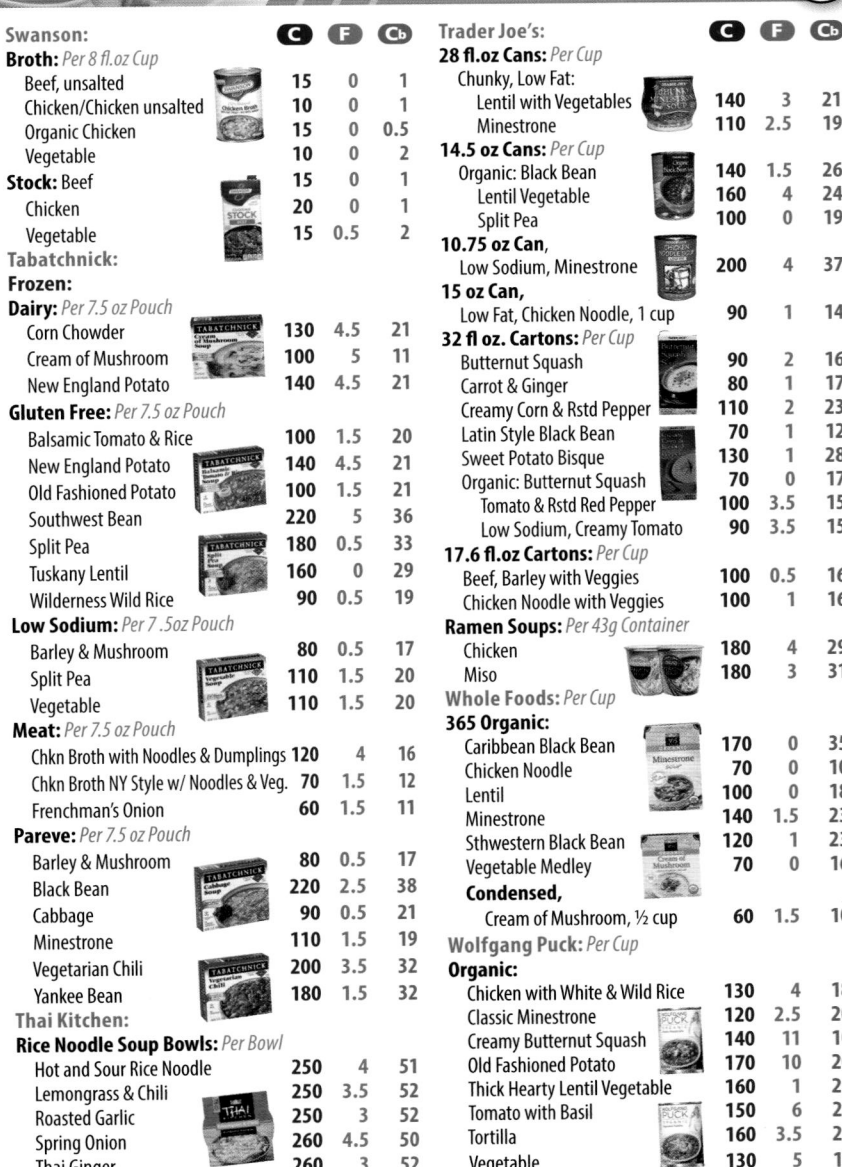

Soybean Products

	C	F	Cb
Cheeses (Soy) ~ *See Page 78*			
Miso Soy Bean Paste:			
Cold Mountain: Light Yellow, 1 tsp	10	0	1
Mellow Red, 1 tsp	15	0	3
Red, 1 tsp	10	0	1
Miso Soup (dry mix):			
1 Tbsp., dry mix	35	1	5
1 cup, prepared	35	1	5
Natto, ½ cup, 3 oz	160	7	14
Okara (Tofu fiber residue), ½ c., 2 oz	47	1	8
Tempeh: 1 piece, 3 oz	180	8	12
Fried, 3 oz	250	14	14
Seitan *(Westsoy)*, Strips, 3 oz	120	2	4
Soybean Protein *(TVP)*, 1 oz	95	0	8
Soy Bean Paste, 1 tsp	10	0	2
Soy Beans ~ *See Page 160*			
Soy Drinks ~ *See Page 49*			

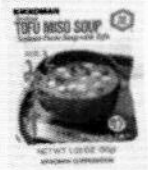

Tofu ~ Brands

	C	F	Cb
Azumaya Tofu:			
Extra Firm; Firm, av., 3 oz	70	4	2
Firm (Silken), 3.2 oz	50	2.5	2
House Foods: *Per 3 oz*			
Premium: Firm	70	4	2
Extra Firm	80	4.5	2
Grilled, Super Firm	80	4.5	3
Medium Firm	60	3	2
Soft (Silken)	60	3	2
Super Firm, cubed	80	4.5	2
Organic Tofu: Firm	70	4	2
Extra Firm	70	3.5	2
Grilled, Super Firm	70	3.5	3
Mori-Nu Tofu: *Per 3 oz*			
Extra Firm	45	1.5	1
Firm Silken	50	2	1
Lite	30	1	0
Organic, Silken	45	2	1
Soft	45	2	1
Nasoya: *Per 3 oz*			
Organic: Extra Firm	80	4	3
Firm	70	3.5	2
Silken	45	2	1
Organic Tofubaked: *Per 3.5 oz*			
Sesame Ginger	150	8	5
Teriyaki	140	7	6
Organic Toss'ables, Garlic & Herb, 3 oz	150	8	5

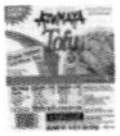

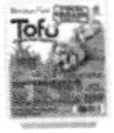

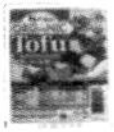

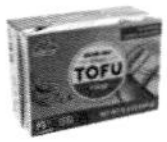

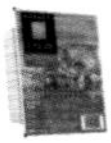
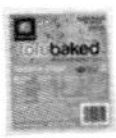

Supplements

	C	F	Cb
Aloe Vera Juice, undiluted, 2 fl.oz	5	0	1
Flakes, 1 heaping Tbsp, 0.3 oz	30	0.5	4
Powder, 1 heaping Tbsp, 0.5 oz	50	0.5	6
Tablets, 2 tabs	4	0	0.5
Calcium Chews: *CVS*, 1 chew	20	0	3
Trader Joe's, Chocolate, 1 chew	20	1	3
Cod Liver Oil, 1 Tbsp	125	13	0
Fiber Choice, 2 tabs	15	0	4
Fiber,			
Fibersure, 1 heaping tsp	25	0	6
Fish Oil Capsules, (1), av.	10	1	0
Flax Oil:			
Capsules (2)	10	1	0
Barlean's, softgels (3)	110	11	0
Garlic Tablets/Capsules, each	3	0	0
Glowelle:			
Beauty Drink, 8 fl.oz	100	0	24
Powder Stick (1)	50	0	12
Lecithin Granules, 1 Tbsp	55	4	0.5
Metamucil, Powder:			
Orange (Smooth Texture), 1 rounded Tbsp	45	0	12
Sugar-Free, 1 rounded tsp	20	0	5
Pink Lemonade, Sugar-Free, 1 rounded tsp	20	0	5
Capsules: Heart & Digestive (6)	10	0	3
Strong Bones (5)	10	0	3
Meta, Fiber Wafers (2)	100	4.5	16
Protein, Powders, av., 1 oz	100	0.5	0
Seaweed: Dried, 1 oz	85	0.5	22
Soaked, drained, 1 oz	15	0.5	3
Spirulina, 1 tablet	2	0	0.5
Vitamins/Minerals: Tabs/Caps (1)	2	0	0
Vitamin E Capsules, each	5	0.5	0
Viactiv Chews, Choc. (1)	20	0.5	4

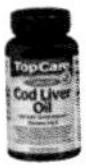

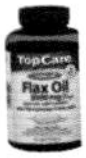

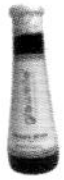
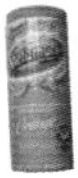
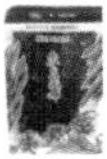
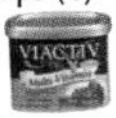

Cough & Pharmaceutical

	C	F	Cb
Antacids: Av., 1 tablet	4	0	1
Liquid, 1 Tbsp	6	0	1
Antacid Sodium Counts ~ *See Page 280*			
Cough/Cold Syrups:			
Regular: With sugar, 1 Tbsp	35	0	9
With alcohol, 1 Tbsp	46	0	9
Diabetic Tussin, Sugar Free, 1 T.	0	0	0
Cough Drops/Lozenges ~ *See Page 75*			
Sudafed, Syrup 1 tsp	14	0	3
Tylenol, Liquid: Child, 1 tsp	17	0	4
Extra Strength, 1 tsp	11	0	3

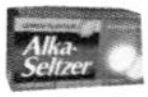

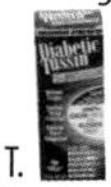

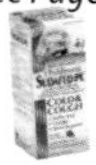

Sugar

	C	F	Cb
White Sugar, granulated:			
1 level teaspoon, 4g	15	0	4
1 heaping teaspoon, 6g	25	0	6
1 Tablespoon, 12g	50	0	12
1 ounce, 1 oz	110	0	28
1 cup, 7 oz	775	0	200
1 lb (16 oz)	1760	0	454
Single Portion Packages:			
1 stick	15	0	4
1 packet	15	0	4
1 cube	10	0	2.5
Brown Sugar: 1 Tbsp	50	0	13
1 ounce, 1 oz	110	0	28
1 cup, not packed, 5 oz	550	0	140
1 cup, packed, 7.8 oz	835	0	216
Powdered Sugar:			
Sifted, 1 cup, 3.5 oz	390	0	100
Unsifted, 1 cup, 4¼ oz	470	0	120
Coconut Palm Sugar, 1 tsp, 4g	15	0	4
Dextrose, 1 tsp	12	0	3
Fructose, powder, 1 tsp	12	0	3
Glucose Powder, 1 oz	110	0	27
Glucose Tablets, (1)	20	0	5
Palm Sugar, 3 Tbsp	45	0	11
Piloncillo, (Brown Sugar), 3oz	325	0	81
Turbinado Sugar, 2 Tbsp, 1 oz	110	0	27

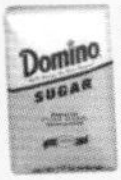
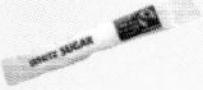
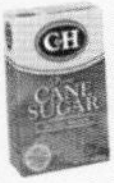
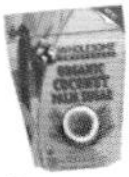

Sugar Substitutes

	C	F	Cb
Agave, 1 Tbsp, 0.7 oz	60	0	16
DiabetiSweet, 1 teaspoon	9	0	4.5
Note: Carb figure includes 4.5 g sugar alcohol			
Domino, Light, ½ tsp	5	0	2
Equal: Tablet (2)	0	0	0
Granular, 1 tsp	0	0	0
Packet (1)	0	0	0
Next, 1 packet	0	0	0
Nectresse, 1 packet	0	0	0
NutraSweet, 1 tsp	0	0	0
Splenda, Granulated No Calorie Sweetener:			
1 tsp	0	0	0
1 cup	95	0	24
Packets, all flavors	0	0	0
Sugar Blend,Orig/Brown, ½ cup	385	0	96
Stevia, single serving	0	0	0
Sugar Twin, 1 packet	0	0	0
Sweet 'N Low, 1 packet	0	0	0
Truvia, 1 packet	0	0	0
Walgreens, Wal-Sweet, 1 packet	0	0	0
Whey Low, 1 tsp	4	0	1

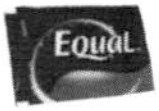

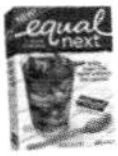
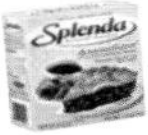

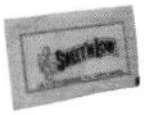

Syrups, Molasses, Agave

Syrups- Plain: *Average All Brands (Corn/Rice/Maple/Pancake/Sundae/Waffle) Includes Aunt Jemima, Cary's, Karo, Hershey's, Hungry Jack, IHOP, Log Cabin, Mrs Butterworth's*

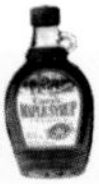

	C	F	Cb
Regular/Dark/Light Color:			
1 Tbsp, 0.5 fl.oz	55	0	14
¼ cup (4 Tbsp)	220	0	55
Single Portion, 1.5 oz pkg	170	0	42
Lite, 1Tbsp, 1 oz	25	0	6
Sugar-Free: 2 Tbsp, 1 oz	18	0	5
Maple Grove, Cozy Cottage, 2 Tbsp	10	0	3
IHOP, 4 Tbsp, 2 oz	20	0	7
Fruit Syrups, *(IHOP)*, ¼ cup, 2 oz	200	0	52
Honey Cream Syrup, ¼ cup, 2 oz	220	0	55
Molasses: Dark/Light: 1 T, 0.7 oz	60	0	15
1 cup, 12 oz	975	0.5	252
Blackstrap, 1 Tbsp, 0.8 oz	47	0	13
Agave Nectar, av. all flavors, 1 Tablespoon, 0.8 oz	60	0	15

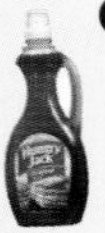
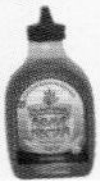

Flavored Syrups/Ice Cream Toppings

	C	F	Cb
Hershey's: *Per 2 Tbsp*			
Double Chocolate,	200	0	50
Choc.; Strawb; Caramel, av.	95	0	25
Sugar Free	10	0	6
Smuckers: *Per 2 Tbsp*			
Magic Shell, average all flavors	215	16	16
Spoonables: Hot Caramel/Fudge, av	140	3.5	27
Sugar Free: Caramel; Hot Fudge	90	0.5	24
Strawberry	30	0	10
Note: Carb figures include 9g-17g sugar alcohol			
Sundae Syrups: Regular, av. all flavors	105	0	25
Sugar Free, average all flavors	95	0.5	24
Note: Carb figures includes 15g-16g sugar alcohol			

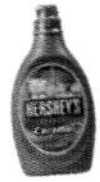

Honey, Jam, Preserves

Average all Brands

	C	F	Cb
Honey: 1 tsp, 0.23 oz	20	0	5.5
1 Tbsp, 0.7 oz	60	0	17
1 oz	85	0	24
½ cup, 6 oz	515	0	145
Single Portion, 0.5 oz package	45	0	12
Jams/Jellies/Marmalade/Preserves:			
Regular: 1 tsp, 0.3 oz	20	0	5
1 Tbsp, 0.8 oz	55	0	14
1 ounce, 1 oz	80	0	20
Single Portion, 0.5 oz pkg	40	0	11
Apple/Fruit Butters, 1 T., 0.6 oz	20	0	6
Fruit Spreads: Regular, 1 tsp	15	0	4
Low Sugar, 1 tsp	8	0	2
Jelly: Regular, average, 1 tsp	18	0	4.5
Imitation, Low Calorie, 1 tsp	4	0	1

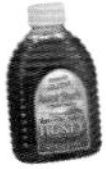
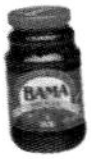

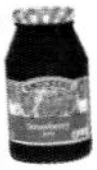

V Vegetables & Legumes ~ Fresh

Vegetables	C	F	Cb
Alfalfa Sprouts, ½ cup, 0.5 oz	5	0	0.5
Artichokes, Globe/French: 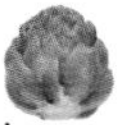			
1 medium, 4.5 oz	60	0	13
1 large, 5.7 oz	75	0	17
Artichoke Heart, plain, 2 pieces	15	0	3
Asparagus, raw/frozen: 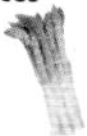			
Cuts & Tips, ½ cup, 4.3 oz	20	0	3
Spears, 3 medium	10	0	2
Bamboo Shoots, cooked, ½ cup, 2 oz	7	0	1
Beans, Green/Snap/String: 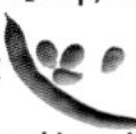			
10 beans (4" long), 2 oz	20	0	4
Pieces, ½ cup, 3 oz	30	0	7
Dried Beans (Kidney, Brown, Lima, Navy, Pinto, White):			
Raw: 2 Tbsp, 1 oz	95	0.5	18
1 cup, 7 oz 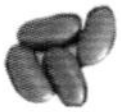	665	3	126
Cooked: 1 oz	35	0	7
½ cup, 3 oz	105	0	21
Bean Sprouts, average, ½ cup, 2 oz	15	0	3.5
Beets (Beetroot): 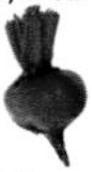			
Raw, 1 beet (2" diam.), 4 oz	35	0	8
Cooked, 1 cup, slices, 3 oz	35	0	8
Canned ~ *See Page 161*			
Beet Greens, cooked, ½ cup, 2.5 oz	20	0	4
Bell Pepper ~ *See Peppers*			
Bitter Melon/Gourd, 1 cup, 1.5 oz	15	0	1.5
Blackeye Peas, cooked, ½ cup, 3 oz	100	0.5	18
Bok Choy (Chinese Chard), 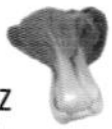			
cooked, 3 oz	10	0	1.5
Breadfruit, ¼ small fruit, 3 oz	100	0	26
Broadbeans (Fava Beans):			
Green, raw, (in pod): 4 pods			
(3.5 oz with shells, 1.2 oz beans)	30	0	6
1 cup beans, without shell, 4.5 oz	110	1	22
Mature Seeds: Raw, 1 cup, 5.3 oz	510	2.5	87
Cooked, ½ cup, 3 oz	95	0	17
Broccoflower, ⅕ head, 3.5 oz	35	0	7
Broccoli: Raw, chopped, 1 cup, 3 oz	30	0	6
3 Florets, 2.5 oz	25	0	5
1 Spear (5" long), 1.oz	10	0	2
1 Whole: Medium, 14 oz 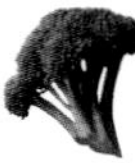	135	1.5	26
Large, 21 oz	205	2	40
1 Head (no stalk), 11 oz	105	1	21
1 Stalk, small (5" long), 5.3 oz	50	0.5	10
Brocco Sprouts, ½ cup, 1 oz	15	0	2
Brussels Sprouts: 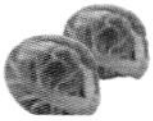			
Cooked, ½ cup, 2.8 oz	30	0.5	6
2 Sprouts, 1.5 oz	15	0	3
Butterbeans, cooked, ½ cup, 3 oz	90	0	16
Cabbage, average other flavors: 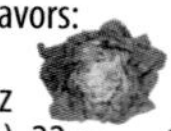			
Raw: 1 leaf, large, 1 oz	5	0	2
Shredded, 1 cup, 2.5 oz	15	0	4
½ large head (7" diam), 22 oz	150	1	35
Cooked, shredded, ½ cup, 2.5 oz	15	0.5	3.5

Vegetables (Cont)	C	F	Cb
Cactus Leaf (Nopales): 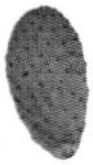			
1 leaf, 4.5 oz	20	0	4
1 cup (slices), 3 oz	15	0	3
Carrots, regular thick variety: 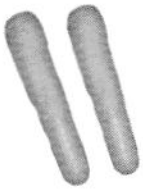			
1 small, 4 oz	45	0	11
1 medium, 6 oz	70	0	16
1 large, 8 oz	95	0	22
Chopped, 1 cup, 4.5 oz	50	0	12
Grated, 1 cup, 4 oz	45	0	11
Slices, 1 cup, 4.5 oz	50	0	12
Sticks (4"), 4-5, 1.5 oz	20	0	4
Long thin variety, 1 medium, 2.2 oz	25	0	6
Baby: Snack size, 3 medium, 1 oz	10	0	2.5
Snack Pack, 3 oz	30	0	7
Cassava, raw, 1 cup, 2.5 oz	330	0.5	78
Cauliflower, raw: 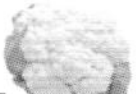			
Pieces, 1 cup, 3.5 oz	25	0	5
½ medium head, 10 oz	70	0	15
Cooked, 3 florets, 2 oz	10	0	2
Celeriac, ½ cup, raw, 2.8 oz 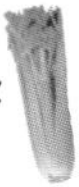	35	0	7
Celery: 1 large stalk, 11", 2.2 oz	10	0	2
4 Strips, thin sticks, 0.5 oz	5	0	1
Chopped, 1 cup, 3.5 oz	15	0	3
Chard (Swiss), ½ cup, cooked, 3 oz	20	0	3.5
Chayote Squash: 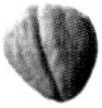			
1 medium, 7 oz	40	0	9
Pieces, 1 cup, 4.5 oz	25	0	6
Chickpeas, (Garbanzo Beans): 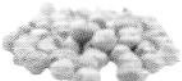			
Dry, 1 cup, 7 oz	730	12	121
Cooked, 1 cup, 5.8 oz	270	4	45
Chicory Greens, 1 cup, 1 oz	7	0	1.5
Chili Peppers ~ *See Peppers*			
Chinese Long Bean, slices, 1 cup, 3.2 oz	45	0	8
Chives, chopped, 1 Tbsp 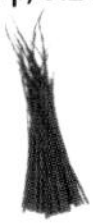	1	0	0
Choy Sum, 3 oz	15	0	3
Cilantro, (Coriander), 1 cup	5	0	0.5
Collards, cooked, ½ cup, 3 oz	25	0	5
Corn, Yellow/White:			
Raw: Kernels, ½ cup, 3 oz	80	0.5	19
Ear (5"x 1¾"), 5.5 oz	155	1	37
Cooked: Kernels, ½ cup, 3 oz 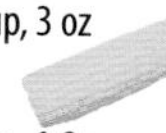	77	0.5	18
Cob, small, 2.3 oz	60	0.5	14
Ear, large, 5.5 oz	120	1	28
Cress, garden, raw, 1 cup, 1.8 oz	15	0	3
Cucumber, average other flavors: 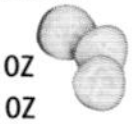			
Slices, ½ cup, 2 oz	10	0	2
Green, 1 medium (9"), 11 oz	45	0	11
Persian, 1 medium (8"), 6 oz	25	0	5
Daikon Radish, ½ cup, slices, 2 oz	9	0	2
Dandelion Greens, raw, ½ cup, 1 oz	10	0	2.5
Edamame, (Immature green soybeans): 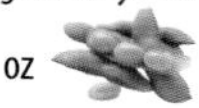			
Shelled, ½ cup, 2.6 oz	110	5	8
With shells, 10 pods, 1.3 oz	30	1	3

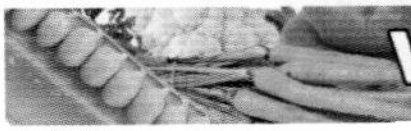

Vegetables (Cont)	C	F	Cb
Eggplant, raw: 4 oz	30	0	7
½ cup, 1" pieces, 1.5 oz	10	0	2
1 slice, fried, 1 oz	75	4	10
Endive, Belgian/French: Raw,			
1 medium head (6"), 2.5 oz	12	0	3
Fennel, 1 cup, sliced, 3 oz	25	0	7
Gai Choy Cabbage, cooked, 1 cup, 6 oz	20	0	3
Gai Lan, (Chinese Kale), cooked, 1 cup	35	0.5	7
Garbanzo Beans ~ *See Chick Peas*			
Garlic, 1 clove	4	0	1
Ginger: ¼ cup slices, 1 oz	20	0	5
Crystallized (sugared), 7 pieces, 1.5 oz	130	0	35
Horseradish, raw, 1 pod, 0.5 oz	5	0	1
Jerusalem Artichoke, raw, ½ cup	55	0	13
Jicama, raw, sliced, ½ cup, 2.3 oz	25	0	6
Kale, 1 cup, chopped, 2.5 oz	35	0.5	7
Kalettes, 1 cup, 2 oz	30	0	4
Kohlrabi, cooked, ½ cup, 1.8 oz	17	0	5
Leek, cooked, 1 whole, 4.5 oz	40	0	9
Lentils, green/brown: Dry, 1 oz	100	0.5	17
1 cup, 6.8 oz	675	3	115
Cooked, ½ cup, 3.5 oz	115	0.5	20
Lettuce: 1 cup, chopped/shredded, 2 oz	7	0	1
Butterhead, 2 leaves, 0.5 oz	2	0	0.5
Cos/Romaine, shredded, 1 cup	10	0	2
Iceberg: 1 outer leaf, 0.5 oz	2	0	0.5
1 medium head, 16 oz	75	1	16
Lima Beans, baby, cooked, ½ cup, 3 oz	105	0	20
Lotus Root, cooked, 10 slices, 3 oz	60	0	14
Mung Bean Sprouts, ½ cup, 2 oz	15	0	3
Mushrooms, average all varieties:			
Raw, diced/siced, 1 cup, 3 oz	20	0	3
Pieces, 1 cup, 1.3 oz	8	0	1
Fried/Sauteed, 6 oz	220	16	10
Grilled, pieces, ½ cup, 2.5 oz	20	0.5	4
Shitake, dried, 1 oz package	90	0	22
Mustard Greens, raw, ½ cup, 1 oz	7	0	2
Okra: Raw, 8 pods, 4 oz	30	0	7
Cooked, ½ cup, 2.8 oz	20	0	4
Onions, Raw: 1 small, 2.5 oz	30	0	7
1 medium, 4 oz	50	0	11
1 large, 5.5 oz	65	0	15
1 jumbo, 16 oz	190	0.5	46
Chopped: ½ cup, 3 oz	35	0	8
1 Tbsp, 0.4 oz	5	0	1
Slices: 1 cup, 4 oz	50	0	12
1 medium slice (⅛"), 0.5 oz	5	0	1
1 large slice (¼"), 1.3 oz	15	0	4
Flakes, dried ¼ cup, 0.5 oz	50	0	12
Rings, breaded & fried, 2 rings	80	5	9
Scallions, ½ cup, 2 oz	15	0	3
Spring, chopped, ½ cup, 2 oz	15	0	3

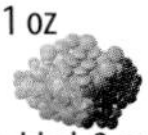
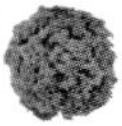

Vegetables (Cont)	C	F	Cb
Parsley, chopped, ½ cup, 1 oz	10	0	2
Parsnip: 1 medium, 4 oz	85	0	20
Cooked, slices, ½ cup, 2.8 oz	55	0	13
Peas: Green, raw, ¼ cup, 1.5 oz	30	0	5
With pods, 0.5 lb	70	0	13
Snow Peas, 10 pods, 1.2 oz	15	0	3
Split: Dry, hulled, 1 oz	100	0.5	17
Cooked, 1 cup, 7 oz	230	1	42
Peppers:			
Sweet, 1 medium, 4.2 oz	30	0	7
Bell: 1 medium, 4.2 oz	30	0	7
raw, chopped, ½ cup, 2.5 oz	20	0	5
2 rings (5" diam. x ¼" thick)	3	0	1
Chili: Green/Red, 1.5 oz	20	0	5
Habanero, 1 only, 0.3 oz	10	0	2
Pigeon Peas, cooked, ½ cup, 3 oz	95	1	17
Pimientos, 3 medium, 3.5 oz	25	0	5
Poi, ½ cup, 4.2 oz	135	0	33
Potatoes:			
Raw (with skin):			
1 baby, 2 oz	45	0	10
1 small, 6 oz	135	0	30
1 medium, 8 oz	180	0	40
1 large, 12 oz	270	0	60
1 extra large, 16 oz	360	0	80
Baked, (no added fat), 1 medium:			
Plain: With skin, 7 oz (cooked wt)	185	0	42
Without skin, 5.5 oz (cooked wt)	145	0	34
With Skin/Toppings:			
With 2 tsp fat	255	8	42
With Grated Cheese, 1 oz	300	9	42
With Plain Yogurt, 2 Tbsp	220	2	45
With Sour Crm & Chives, 2 Tbsp	240	5	43
Mashed:			
With milk plus fat, ½ cup, 4 oz	120	4.5	18
KFC Style without gravy, 4 oz	90	3	15
Loaded (fat/cream/cheese/bacon):			
Side serving, 6 oz	180	9	22
Large serving, 12 oz	360	18	44
Roasted, with oil:			
Whole, 1 small, 3 oz	140	5	20
Diced, 1 cup, 5 oz	180	8	30
Potato Skins, baked w/ cheese topping,			
½ whole, 4 oz	240	13	22
French Fries: Small serving, 2.6 oz	250	13	30
Medium serving, 4 oz	380	20	47
Frozen, uncooked, 18 fries, 4 oz	165	5.5	28
Oven-heated, 18 fries, 4 oz	165	5.5	28
Take-Out, 1 cup, 5 oz	440	25	60
Au Gratin, ½ cup, 4.3 oz	160	9	14
Scalloped, 8.5 oz	220	9	26

 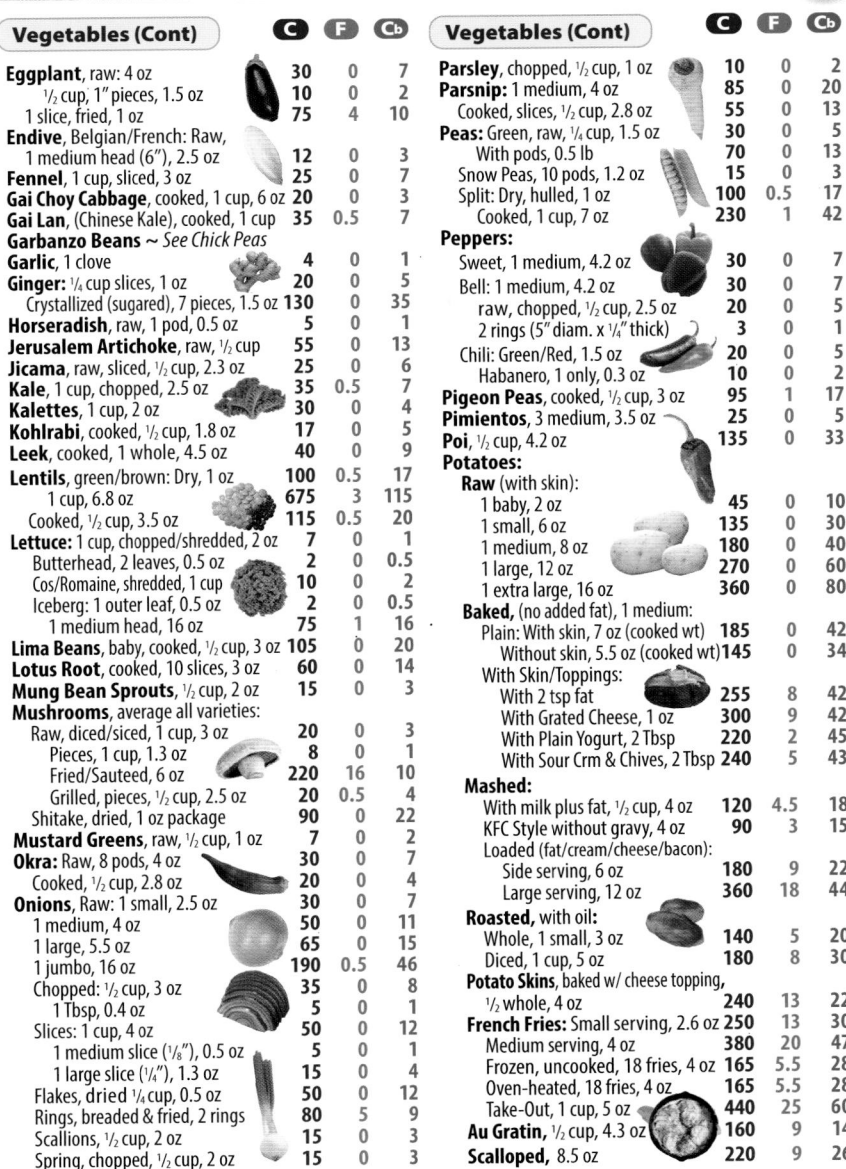

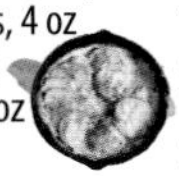

Vegetables (Cont)

Food	C	F	Cb
Pumpkin:			
Raw, 1" cubes, 1 cup, 4 oz	30	0	7
Cooked:			
Baked, without fat, 4 oz	90	7	9
Mashed: 1 scoop, 2 oz	10	0	2
½ cup, 4.3 oz	25	0	6
Pumpkin Flowers, 1 cup, 1.2 oz	5	0	1
Purslane: Cooked, ½ cup, 2 oz	10	0	2
Raw, 1" cubes, 1 cup, 1.5 oz	5	0	1.5
Radicchio: 2 leaves, 0.5 oz	5	0	1
Shredded, 1 cup, 1.5 oz	20	0	4
Radishes: 1 small	0	0	0
10 medium/5 large, 1.6 oz	5	0	1
Slices, ½ cup, 2 oz	10	0	2
Rhubarb, raw, ½ cup, 2 oz	15	0	3
Rutabaga, cubes, cooked, ½ cup, 3 oz	30	0	7
Salsify, cooked, slices, ½ cup, 2.5 oz	50	0	11
Sauerkraut, ½ cup, 2.5 oz	15	0	3
Seaweed: Dried, 1 oz	5	0	2
Soaked, drained, 1 oz	15	0	4
Nori/Laver, dried, 6 sheets, 0.5 oz	35	0	5
Shallots, chopped, 1 Tbsp, 0.5 oz	5	0	1
Sorrel, raw, ½ cup, 4 oz	20	0	4
Soybeans: Dry, ½ cup, 3.3 oz	390	18	28
Mature, dry, 1 oz	120	5.5	9
Cooked, ½ cup, 3 oz	150	7.5	8
Soy Products/Tofu/Tempeh ~ *See Page 156*			
Spinach: Cooked, ½ cup, 3 oz	20	0	4
Creamed, av., ½ cup, 4.5 oz	190	15	8
Raw: 3 leaves, 1 cup, 1 oz	7	0	1
1 Bunch, 12 oz	80	1.5	12
Baby Spinach, 1 cup, 1 oz	5	0	1
Squash:			
Summer: Raw, ½ cup, 2.5 oz	10	0	2
Cooked, slices, ½ cup, 3 oz	15	0	3
Winter, cooked:			
Acorn: Cubes, ½ cup, 3.5 oz	35	0	9
½ medium (10 oz raw weight)	115	0	30
Butternut: Cubes, ½ cup, 3.5 oz	40	0	10
¼ medium (9 oz raw weight)	115	0	30
Spaghetti, ½ cup, 1.8 oz	15	0	3
Succotash, cooked, ½ cup, 3.3 oz	110	1	23
Sweetcorn ~ *See Corn*			
Sweet Potatoes:			
Cooked with skin (w/o fat), 1 medium, 4 oz	105	0	24
Without skin, mashed, ½ cup, 5.5 oz	125	0	29
Fries (Alexia, Julienne syle), approximately 12 pieces, 3 oz	140	5	24

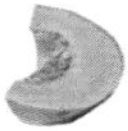
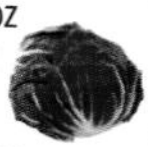
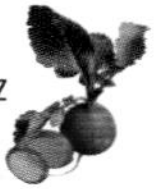
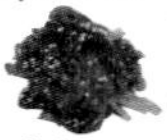
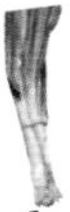
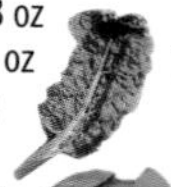
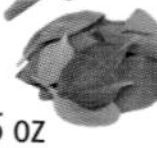

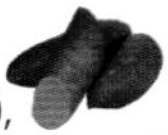

Vegetables (Cont)

Food	C	F	Cb
Swiss Chard, cooked, chopped, 1 c., 6 oz	35	0	7
Taro, cooked, ½ cup, 2.3 oz	95	0	23
Tomatoes: 1 small (2¼" diam.), 3 oz	15	0	3
1 medium (2¾" diameter), 5 oz	25	0	5
1 large (3½" diameter), 8 oz	40	0.5	9
1 extra lge (4" diam.), 12 oz	60	0.5	14
Chopped, 1 cup, 6.5 oz	35	0.5	7
Tomatillo: 1 medium, 1.2 oz	10	0	2
1lb quantity for recipe	135	4.5	27
Turnip: Cooked, ½ cup, 2.8 oz	15	0	4
Greens, cooked, ½ cup, 2.5 oz	15	0	3
Water Chestnuts: 5-6 nuts, 1 oz	56	0.5	13
Raw, slices, ½ cup, 2.3 oz	60	0	15
Canned, 1 oz	15	0	3
Watercress, 10 sprigs, 1 oz	3	0	0.5
Yams: Cooked, steamed, ½ cup, 2.5 oz	80	0	19
Baked:			
1 medium (6") 8 oz	265	0.5	63
1 large (9") 12 oz	400	0.5	94
Yardlong Bean, 1 pod, 0.5 oz	5	0	1
Yucca Root, raw, ½ cup, 3.5 oz	165	0	39
Zucchini: Raw, 1 medium, 7 oz	30	0.5	7
1 large, 12 oz	60	1	12
Cooked, slices, ½ cup, 3 oz	15	0	4

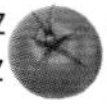
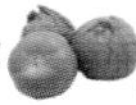
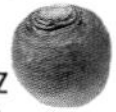
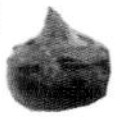
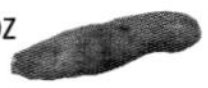
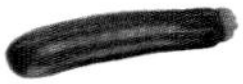

Frozen Vegetables

Food	C	F	Cb
Birds Eye:			
Flavor Full:			
Buffalo Cauliflower, 3.3 oz	50	2	7
Ranch: Broccoli, 3 oz	50	1.5	5
Cauliflower, 3.3 oz	50	2	6
Salt & Vinegar Potatoes, 3.9 oz	150	4	25
Steakhouse Green Beans, 3 oz	60	2.5	6
Teriyaki Broccoli, 3 oz	50	1.5	7
Steamfresh:			
Asparagus Spears (6)	20	0	3
Chopped Kale, 3.1 oz	25	0	4
Cut Green Beans, 3 oz	30	0	5
Mixtures: Brocc. Cauliflower, 3 oz	25	0	4
Brocc, Cauliflower, Carrots,	30	0	5
Italian Blend, 2.7 oz	30	0	5
Roasted Red Potato Blend, 2.7 oz	50	0	11
Power Blends: Barley Kale, 10 oz	240	3.5	40
Black Rice & Edamame, 10 oz	290	4.5	48
Chickpea & Spinach, 10 oz	320	7	51
Quinoa & Spinach, 10 oz	310	5	57

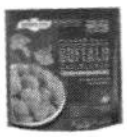
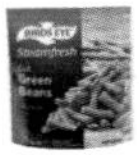

Frozen Vegetables (Cont)

Frozen Vegetables (Cont)	C	F	Cb
Green Giant:			
Grilled, Zucchini, 3.17 oz	40	0.5	7
Mashed Cauliflower: Original, 4.2 oz	80	5	7
Cheddar & Bacon, 4.2 oz	90	6	6
Garlic & Herb., 4.2 oz	80	4.5	8
Marinated Veggies: *Per ⅓ Package*			
Eggplant, Peppers & Zucchini, 4.33 oz	70	3	7
Mushrooms, 3.3 oz	80	7	4
Riced Veggies: *Per ¼ Cup, 1.76 oz*			
Chickpea, Cauliflower	180	2.5	32
Red Lentils, Green Pea, Chickpea	180	1.5	32
Roasted Veggies:			
Brussels Sprouts, 3 oz	30	0	6
Corn, 3 oz	120	1.5	25
Simply Steam: *Prepared*			
Baby Bruss. Sprouts & Butter Sce, ½ c.	50	1.5	8
Baby Lima Beans, 1/2 cup	80	0	14
Chopped Spinach, ⅓ cup	20	0	3
Garden Vegetable Medley, ½ cup	70	0.5	14
Riced Cauliflower & Cheese Sce, ½ c.	70	3	10
Sugar Snap Peas, ½ cup	40	0	9
Sweet Peas, ½ cup	60	0	12
Ore-Ida: *Per 3 oz Unless Indicated*			
Fries:			
Classic: Golden Crinkles	90	4.5	12
Golden Fries	90	4	13
Steak Fries	80	3	13
Extra Crispy:			
Fast Food Fries	130	7	16
Golden Crinkles	130	7	16
Seasoned Crinkles	150	6	22
Flavored:			
Country Style French Fries	90	4	13
Garlic & Bl. Pepper Steakhouse Fries	150	8	16
Zesty Curly Fries	150	9	17
Zesty Straight Fries	140	8	16
Hash Browns:			
Golden Patties (1)	120	8	10
Potatoes O'Brien	50	0	12
Shredded Hash Brown Potatoes	60	0	13
Mashed Potatoes: Bites (8)	170	10	17
Homestyle Steam 'n' Mash, 3.35 oz	60	0	15
Onion:			
Gourmet Rings, 2.7 oz	185	9	24
Onion Ringers, 2.85 oz	180	10	21
Sweet Potato Straight Fries	150	7	19
Tater Tots, Reg., Crispy Crowns, av.	135	9	12

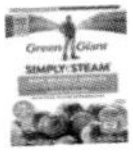
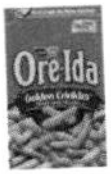
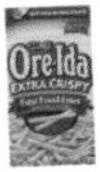
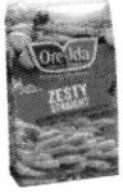
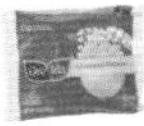

Canned/Bottled

Canned/Bottled	C	F	Cb
Solids & Liquid			
Artichoke Hearts:			
Fancifoods: Plain, 1 oz (1)	8	0	1
Marinated, ¼ bottle, 1 oz	25	1.5	2
Asparagus: Drained, 3 spears	10	0	1.5
Pieces, ½ cup, 4.3 oz	25	0.5	3
Bamboo Shoots, 1 cup, 4.5 oz	25	0	4
Bean Salad, ½ cup, 4.4 oz	90	0	20
Beans: Baked, ½ cup, 4.5 oz	120	0.5	27
Butter, ½ cup, 4.5 oz	90	0	16
Green, ½ cup, 2.5 oz	15	0	3
Italian, ½ cup, 4.5 oz	30	0	6
Kidney, ½ cup 3.5 oz	105	0.5	19
Lima, ½ cup, 4.5 oz	80	0	15
Pinto, ½ cup, 4.5 oz	105	1	18
Beets: Sliced, ½ cup, 3 oz	25	0	6
Crinkle/Pickled, ½ cup	80	0	20
Carrots: Sliced, ½ cup, 2.5 oz	20	0	4
Del Monte, Honey Glazed, ½ cup	75	0	18
Corn: Kernels, ½ cup, 4.5 oz	80	0.5	18
Creamed style, ½ cup, 4.5 oz	90	0.5	23
Garbanzo/Chick Peas, ½ c, 4.2 oz	145	1.5	27
Hearts of Palm, (1), 1.2 oz	7	0	1
Mushrooms: ½ cup, 2.5 oz	20	0	4
In Butter Sauce, 2 oz	20	1	2
Onions: Cocktail (1)	0	0	0
Pickled, 1 medium, 0.5 oz	10	0	2
Peas, ½ cup, 3 oz	60	0.5	10
Peppers: Hot Chili, Jalapeno (1), 1 oz	5	0	1
Red/Green, 1 oz	5	0	1
Sweet, undrained, 2.5 oz	13	0	3
Jalapeno, with liquid, ½ cup chopped	20	0.5	3
Fried, drained, 2 Tbsp, 1 oz	60	5	3
Salsa, average all varieties, 2 Tbsp	10	0	2
Sauerkraut, drained, 1 cup, 5 oz	25	0	6
Spinach, ½ cup, 3.5 oz	25	0.5	3.5
Succotash: Cream Style, ½ cup	100	0.5	23
w/ whole kernels, undrained, ½ cup	80	0.5	18
Sweetcorn ~ *See Corn*			
Sweet Potato, ½ cup, 3.5 oz	90	0	24
Tomatoes, Sundried: Nat., 5-6 pieces	20	0	5
In Oil, drained, 6 pieces, 0.5 oz	40	2.5	4
Tomato Products ~ *See Page 144*			
Vegetables, mixed, ½ cup, 4 oz	45	0	8
Yams: In Light Syrup, ½ cup, 4 oz	105	0	25
Candied, ½ cup, 5 oz	170	0	46
Zucchini, in Tomato Sauce, ½ cup, 4 oz	30	0	8

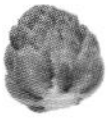
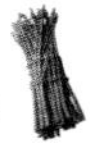
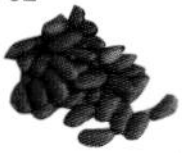
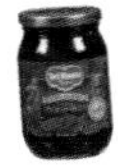
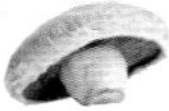
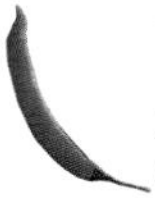

Quick Guide

	C	F	Cb
Yogurt: *Average All Brands: Per 8 oz Container*			
Plain Yogurt: Whole	140	8	10
Low-Fat	145	3.5	16
Fat-Free	125	0.5	17
Fruit Flavored: Whole	225	8	32
Low-Fat	230	3	43
Fat-Free, regular	215	0.5	43
Fat-Free, no sugar added	80	0	15
Yogurt Parfait/Deli Cups:			
With Fruit Pieces: (2/3 Yogurt + 1/3 Fruit)			
Small, 8 oz cup	140	3	20
Large, 12 oz cup	210	4.5	30
With Fruit + Granola:			
Small, 8 oz cup (+ 0. 75 oz Granola)	235	7	30
Large, 12 oz cup (+ 1.3 oz Granola)	400	13	58

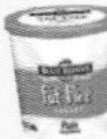
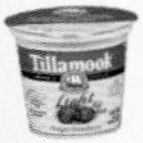

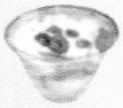

Yogurt ~ Brands

	C	F	Cb
Activia:			
Dairy Free, all flavors	120	4	18
Probiotic Yogurts: *Per 4 oz Container*			
60 Calorie, all flavors	60	0	10
Greek: Vanilla	140	0	23
Other Flavors	120	0	17
Less Sugar, all flavors	130	4.5	11
Lacatose Free, Strawberry	90	2	15
With Fiber, Strawberry	90	0	22
With Fruit, average all flavors	85	1.5	15
With Fruit On The Bottom, all	90	2	15
Axelrod:			
32 oz Ctn: Regular Plain, 8 oz	160	8	15
Fat Free, Plain, 8 oz	130	0	19
6 oz Containers:			
Low Fat, Fruit flavors, av.	180	1.5	36
NonFat Vanilla	90	0	17
Brown Cow:			
Cream Top: *Per 5.3 oz Ctn*			
Whole Milk: Plain	130	7	11
Cherry Vanilla; Choc	160	5	26
Coffee; Vanilla	150	6	19
Average Other Flavors	155	6	23

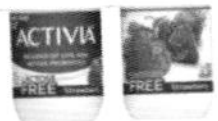

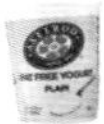
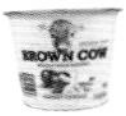

	C	F	Cb
Cabot: *Per 8 oz Serving*			
Greek Style:			
Whole Milk, Plain	230	16	9
Lowfat (2%): Plain	130	3.5	8
Strawberry; Vanilla Bean	180	2.5	26
Triple Cream, Vanilla Bean	260	13	26
Nonfat, Plain	80	0	13
Chobani Greek Yogurt: *Per 5.3 oz Unless Indicated*			
Blended: Coconut	140	4.5	15
Mixed Berry	140	2.5	17
Coconut Based: Plain, slightly swt	130	8	16
Average Other flavors	140	7	20
Creamy Blended, average	150	4.5	17
Flip: Almond Coco Loco	230	10	23
Coffee Brownie Bliss	180	4	25
Fruit On The Bottom:			
Apricot; Mango; Strawb Banana, av,	130	2.5	16
Strawberry/Blueberry	110	0	16
Gimmies, average all flavors, 4 oz	145	4	20
Less Sugar, all flavors, 5.3 oz	120	2.5	11
Nut Butter, average all flavors, 5.3 oz	165	7	15
Plain, 32 oz Ctn:: Lowfat, 8 oz	130	3.5	7
Nonfat, 8 oz	90	0	6
Whole Milk, 8 oz	170	9	7
Dannon:			
Activia ~ *See Activia*			
Creamy, Strawberry, 4 oz	70	0	14
Fruit On The Bottom, all flavors, 5.3 oz	130	1.5	25
Lowfat: Plain, 6 oz	100	2.5	12
Coffee; Vanilla, 6 oz	140	2	24
Plain, 32 oz Ctn: Lowat, 8 oz	110	2.5	12
Nonfat, 8 oz	80	0	13
Whole Milk, 8 oz	110	6	7
Fage Greek Yogurt:			
Best Self: Plain, 5.3 oz	110	3	5
Blueberry, 5.3 oz	120	2.5	14
Strawberry, 5.3 oz	110	2.5	12
Vanilla, 5.3 oz	100	2.5	11
Total: Plain 5% Milk Fat, 7 oz	190	10	6
Plain, 2% Milk Fat, 7 oz	140	4	6
Plain, 0% Milk Fat, 6oz	90	0	5
Total Split Cups: *Per 5.3 oz*			
5% Milk Fat: Fruit Flav., av.	150	6	13
Honey	210	6	28
2% Milk Fat: Fruit Flavors	120	2.5	13
Honey	180	2.5	28
Tru Blend: *Per 5.3 oz*			
Fruit Flavors	110	2.5	10
Vanilla; Coconut	110	2.5	9

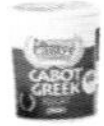

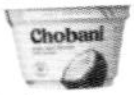

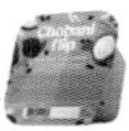
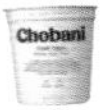

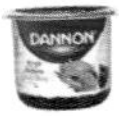

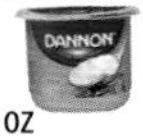

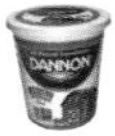

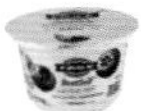
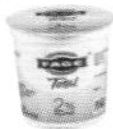
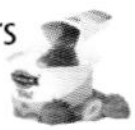
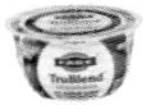

Yogurt Brands (Cont)

	C	F	Cb
Great Value *(Walmart):*			
Greek, Fat Free,			
32 oz Ctn, Plain, 6 oz	90	0	7
Greek Non Fat Light: *Per 5.3 oz Ctn*			
Banana Cream; Peach; Vanilla	80	0	9
Strawberry	80	0	9
Original Lowfat:			
5.3 oz, Blueberry	120	1	23
6 oz, Strawberry; Peach	130	1.5	26
32 oz, Vanilla, 6 oz	130	1.5	26
Kemps:			
5 lb Containers:			
Lowfat: Plain, Sweeetened, 6 oz	120	2	15
Nonfat: Raspberry, 6 oz	130	0	27
Strawberry; Blueberry, 6 oz	120	0	26
Vanilla, 6 oz	130	0	28
Kroger, CarbMaster, all flavors, 6 oz	70	1.5	5
La Yogurt: *Per 6 oz Container*			
Low Fat: Orig., Fruit Flavors, av.	155	1.5	30
Rich & Creamy, Fruit Flav., av.	180	1.5	33
LALA:			
Blended Yogurt: Plain, 6 oz	110	1.5	14
Fruit Flavors, average, 6 oz	155	1	29
Lavva *(Dairy Free):*			
Pili Nut Yogurt: *5.3oz Ctn*			
Blueberry	160	11	10
Original	185	14	11
Raspberry	140	11	9
Lucerne:			
Greek Nonfat, Plain, 8 oz	130	0	14
Low-Fat, Blueberry Flav., 6 oz	140	2	26
Light Nonfat, Blueberry, 6 oz	100	0	18
Nonfat, Vanilla Flavored, 8 oz	190	0	32
Mountain High: *Per 8 oz*			
32 oz Containers:			
Whole Milk Original: Plain	170	7	15
Strawberry; Vanilla, av.	200	7	27
Lowfat: Plain	130	2.5	16
Vanilla	170	2.5	28
Fat Free: Plain	110	0	16
Vanilla	160	0	28
Nancy's:			
Natural:			
Whole Milk, Honey, 8 oz	170	8	17
Lowfat: Fruit flavors, av., 5.3 oz ctn	120	2	18
Plain, 8 oz	140	3	16
Vanilla, 5.3 oz ctn	100	2.5	13
Nonfat: Plain, 8 oz	120	0	17
Vanilla, 6 oz	90	0	15

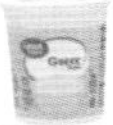
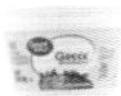
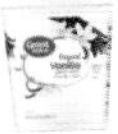
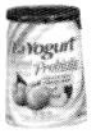
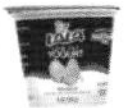
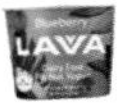

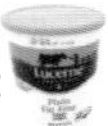
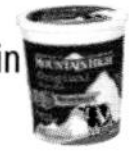
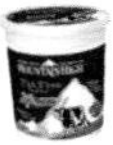
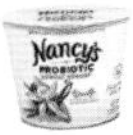

Oikos *(Dannon): Per 5.3 oz Single Sve*	C	F	Cb
Protein Crunch:			
Vanilla with Blueberries	160	1	21
Other Flavors	150	2	17
Nonfat, Plain	80	0	6
Triple Zero Greek: Av all flavors	110	0	12
Go Pack: Strawberries & Crm, 4.5 oz	80	0	13
Fruit Flavors, 4.5 oz	80	0	11
Whole Milk, av. all flav.	160	4	20
O Organics *(Vons):*			
Greek, Nonfat Strained, Vanilla, 6 oz	130	0	15
Whole Milk: Plain, 6 oz	130	6	11
Vanilla, 6 oz	160	6	22
Siggi's:			
Skyr: *Per 5.3 oz Unless Indicated*			
0%: Plain	90	0	6
Fruit Flavors	110	0	13
2%: Coconut	160	5	14
Fruit Flavors, average	140	3	14
4%: Fruit flavors, 4.4 oz	130	4.5	11
Fruit, no added sugar, av., 4.4 oz	95	2	8
Plant Based, Fruit Flavors, average	180	10	12
With Almond Butter, average, 5 oz	255	14	14
Silk: *Per 5.3 oz Containers*			
Almond Yogurt: Plain	170	13	10
Fruit flavors, average	180	11	18
Vanilla	190	11	19
Oat Yeah, Vanilla	80	0	17
Soy Yogurt: Fruit flavors, av	125	3.5	19
Vanilla	140	3.5	21
So Delicious:			
Coconut Milk: *Per 5.3 oz*			
Blueberry	140	4	24
Chocolate	140	4.5	24
Plain: Regular	130	5	19
Unsweetened	89	5	8
Vanilla, Regular	130	4	22
Stonyfield Organic:			
Dairy Free (Soy):			
Fruit Flav., 5.3 oz	150	2.5	26
Vanilla	130	2.5	20
0% Fat Fruit On The Bottom:			
Blueberry On The Bottom, 5.3 oz	100	0	18
Chocolate Underground, 5.3 oz	110	0	22
Low Fat: Plain, 6 oz	90	1.5	11
Strawberry, 5.3 oz	100	1.5	16
Vanilla, 6 oz	110	0	20
Whole Milk: Strawb.; Van., av., 5.3 oz	140	5	18
32 oz Ctn: Plain, 6 oz	120	7	9
Vanilla, 6 oz	150	6	20
Greek: Plain, 6 oz	150	6	7
Vanilla Bean, 6 oz	170	5	18

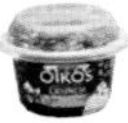

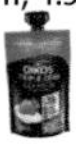
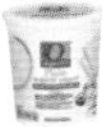
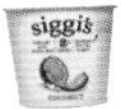

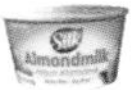
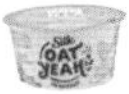
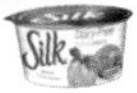

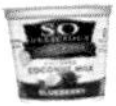
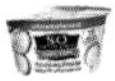
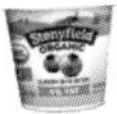
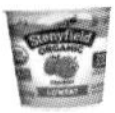
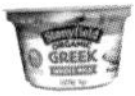

Yogurt Brands (Cont)

	C	F	Cb
Trader Joe's:			
Organic: Greek, Nonfat, Plain	80	0	6
Whole Milk, Strawb., 5.3 oz 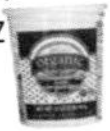	150	5	17
Lowfat, av. all flavors, 6 oz	150	2.5	26
Nonfat, plain, 6 oz	80	0	6
Greek, Lowfat (2%):			
Almond Butter coconut, 5.3 oz	170	6	16
Plain, 1 cup, 8 oz	120	0	7
Greek, Whole Milk: 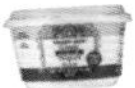			
5.3 oz Cups, av. all flavors	180	6	18
16 oz Ctn: Plain, 1 cup, 8 oz	280	22	12
Icelandic Style: 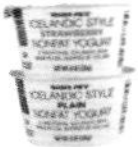			
Non Fat: Plain, 8 oz	130	0	10
Strawberry, 8 oz	190	0	26
Low Fat:			
Vanilla with Almonds, 4.6 oz 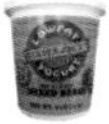	160	7	20
Prestirred, Strawberry, 8 oz	220	3	40
European Style:			
Organic, Plain: Whole Milk, 1 cup, 8 oz	170	7	14
Nonfat, 1 up, 8 oz 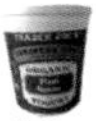	120	0	17
Voskos:			
Greek:			
2x Protein (0%), Exotic Fig, 5.3 oz	160	0	28
Real Fruit: Fruit Flavors, av., 6 oz	140	0	19
Coconut Cream, 6 oz 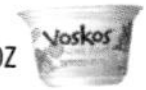	160	0	22
16 oz Tubs: Orig. Plain, 8 oz	280	20	15
Nonfat Vanilla, 8 oz	200	0	30
Wallaby Organic: 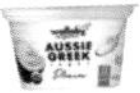			
Lowfat Greek, Plain, 5.3 oz	100	2	7
Nonfat, Plain, 5.3 oz	90	0	7
Whole Milk: Fruit Flavors, av., 5.3 oz			
Aussie Smooth,			
Fruit Flav., av., 5.3 oz 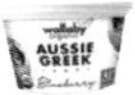	145	4	21
Wegmans:			
Fruit On The Bottom, Lowfat:			
Blueberry; Cherry Vanilla, 6 oz	160	2	29
Average other Fruit Flavors, 6 oz	175	2	34
Greek Non-Fat: Plain, 5.3 oz	80	0	5
Fruit flavors, av., 5.3 oz 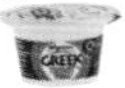	125	0	18
Vanilla, 5.3 oz	100	0	11
Whole Foods (365 Orgainic):			
Whole Milk: Plain, 8 oz	170	9	13
Unsweetened, 6 oz 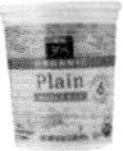	120	6	9
Blueberry, 5.3 oz	150	4.5	15
Vanilla, 5.3 oz	140	5	18
Low-Fat, European Style, 6 oz	110	2	13
Greek Nonfat, 6 oz	100	0	7
YoCrunch: *Per 4 oz Container*			
Lowfat Vanilla Yogurt: 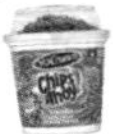			
Chips Ahoy; Twix, av.	185	4	32
M&M's; Oreo, av.	125	3	22

Yogurt Brands (Cont)

	C	F	Cb
Yoplait: 			
Single Serve Cups: *Per 6 oz*			
Original, all Flavors, average	150	2	29
Lactose Free, av. all flavors, 6 oz	150	2	26
Light, 6 oz cup, average all flavors	90	0	17
FruitSide, all flavors, 5.3 oz	160	4	25
Greek 100 Protein, av. all flav., 5.3 oz	100	0	11
Go-Gurt: Tube, 2 oz	50	0.5	10
Dunkers, all flavors, 2.2 oz tray	120	2	22
Simply, all flavors, 2 oz 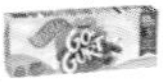	45	0.5	8
Just 3, av. all flavors, 5 oz	175	9	19
Lactose Free, av. all flavors, 6 oz	150	2	27
Light, av. all flavors, 6 oz 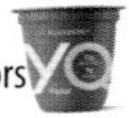	90	0	18
Starburst, average all flavors	160	1.5	29
Whips!:			
Regular: Coconut Crème,4 oz	160	4	24
Chocolate, 4 oz 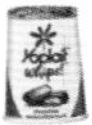	160	4	25
Sea Salt Caramel, 4 oz	170	4	27
Average other flav., 4 oz	140	2.5	25

Yogurt Drinks & Probiotics

	C	F	Cb
Dannon: 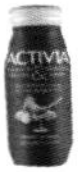			
Activia Probiotics:			
Dailies, all flavors, 3.15 fl.oz	70	1.5	11
Drinks, av. all flavors, 7 fl oz	160	35	25
Smoothies, av. all flavors, 7 fl.oz	135	4	18
DanActive Dailies, all flav., 3.1 fl.oz	75	1	13
Danimals Smoothies: All flavors, 3.1 fl.oz	50	0	11
Pouches, all flavors,3.5 oz	80	1	13
Organic, all flavors, 3.1 fl.oz 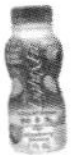	45	0	8
Wild, all flavors, 7 fl.oz	90	1	17
Glen Oaks, all flavors, 6 fl.oz	150	2.5	27
Lifeway:			
Kefir: *Per 8 fl.oz*			
Organic Whole Milk: Plain	160	8	12
Other Flavors	190	8	20
Organic Lowfat: Plain 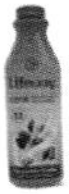	110	2	12
Other flavors	140	2	20
Plantiful: Plain	90	1	9
Other Flavors	110	1	14
Probugs, 3.5 fl.oz	80	3	11
Stonyfield:			
Smoothies: Low Fat, av., 6 oz 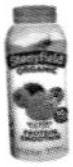	110	1.5	17
10 oz bottle, average	180	3	29
Daily Probiotics, all flav., 3.1 fl.oz	60	1	11
Yakult: Regular, 2.7 fl.oz bottle	50	0	12
Light, 2.7 fl.oz	25	0	6

Cafeteria-Style Foods

	C	F	Cb
Average All Preparations:			
Beef Stroganoff, 5 oz	195	13	7
Beef Stroganoff, with 4 oz noodles	350	14	36
Chicken Lasagna, 1 piece	300	11	32
Chicken Chop Suey, with 4 oz rice	245	4	37
Deep Dish Burrito, 7 oz	265	13	20
Ground Beef Casserole, 2 scps, 6 oz	245	13	17
Italian Meat Sce, for Spaghetti, 5 oz	150	9	9
with 5 oz Spaghetti	350	10	49
Lasagna, 1 piece	275	11	25
Meatloaf, 3 oz	205	13	4
Ranch Beans, 2 scoops, 6 oz	350	11	45
Red Beans & Rice, 7 oz	280	9	37
Scalloped Potato/Ham, 2 scoops, 6 oz	160	6	20
Stuffed Shells in Sauce, (1)	105	3	17
Swedish Meatballs, (3)	205	12	9
Sweet & Sour Pork/Rice, 9 oz	240	3	40
Swiss Steak, w/ Mushroom Gravy, 6 oz	280	11	4
Tator Tot Casserole, 2 scoops, 6 oz	260	15	20
Tenderloin Tips/Mshrm Gravy: 5 oz	210	13	3
With 5 oz noodles	395	15	38
Tuna Noodle Casserole, 2 scoops, 6 oz	180	6	17
Turkey Tetrazzini, 2 scoops, 6 oz	195	7	17
Vegetable Lasagna, 1 piece	250	13	21

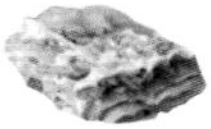

Croissants

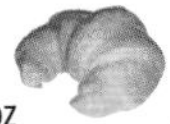

	C	F	Cb
Unfilled, medium 1.5 oz	180	10	21
Filled: With Ham (2 oz), garnish	280	14	24
With Ham (2 oz), Cheese (2 oz)	470	30	20
With Chick (2 oz) Cheese (2 oz)	470	30	20
With Turkey/Ham/Cheese (2 oz ea.)	580	36	20
Au Bon Pain: Ham & Cheese	390	21	35
Spinach & Cheese	290	17	28

7-Eleven ~ *See Page 236*

Bagels

	C	F	Cb
Plain: Large, 4 oz (without filling)	320	2	65
With 2 oz Cream Cheese	500	27	54
With 2 oz Lox (Smoked Salmon)	400	4	65

Also see Bagels Section ~ *Page 56*
Fast-Foods Restaurants ~ *Page 175*
Au Bon Pain ~ *Page 178*
Bruegger's ~ *Page 185*
Einstein Bros Bagels ~ *Page 199*

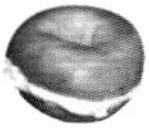

Sandwiches

	C	F	Cb
No Spreads Unless Indicated:			
Includes 2 Slices Bread ~ 3 oz			
BLT, (5 strips Bacon, 2 Tbsp Mayo)	600	40	46
Breaded Chicken & Garnish	540	28	46
Chicken Salad, with Mayo., 5 oz	580	30	49
Chopped Liver, Egg Mayonnaise	630	25	44
Corned Beef with Mustard, 5 oz	560	28	44
Egg Salad, with Mayonnaise	570	29	49
Egg Salad Club, with Bacon & Mayo,	780	53	49
Grilled Cheese, (3 oz)	540	30	44
Ham, (4 oz), Cheese (4 oz), & Mayo.	910	56	44
Lobster Salad, (4 oz), w/ Mayo.	530	25	45
Overstuffed Tuna Salad, (7 oz)	870	39	75
Philly Cheese Steak Sandwich	550	23	42
Reuben, (6 oz Beef/Pastrami, 2 oz Cheese, 2 Tbsp Dressing)	920	60	28
Roast Beef, (4 oz), with Mustard	460	12	45
Roast Pork, (4 oz), with Apple Sauce	500	16	55
Shrimp Salad Club, w/ Bacon & Mayo	800	57	48
Sloppy Joe with Sauce, (7 oz)	600	30	45
Steak Sandwich, (5 oz cooked)	680	32	41
Triple Cheese Melt, (4 oz)	720	45	46
Tuna Salad, (5 oz), with Mayonnaise	610	30	49
Turkey Breast, (5 oz), w/ Mayo.	460	18	44
Turkey Breast, (5 oz,) with Mustard	360	7	44
Turkey Club, with Bacon & Mayo.	830	38	31
Vegetarian, with Avocado & Cheese	820	49	72

7-Eleven ~ *Page 236*
Schlotzsky's ~ *Page 237*
Subway ~ *Page 245*

Wraps & Roll-Ups

	C	F	Cb
Average All Types			
Meat/Chicken/Fish/Veggie:			
Small, approximately 9 oz	500	25	48
Regular, approximately 15 oz	830	40	80
Large, approximately 22 oz	1400	70	134

Fast-Foods Restaurants ~ *Page 175*
Au Bon Pain ~ *Page 178*
Sonic Drive-In ~ *Page 241*
Subway ~ *Page 245*
WAWA ~ *Page 254*

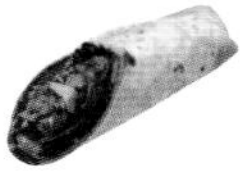

Fair & Carnival Foods

	C	F	Cb
Barbeque Chicken/Meats:			
Chicken, ½ chicken, 15 oz	740	24	34
Grilled Chicken Pita, with dressing	680	19	82
Teriyaki Chicken, on stick, w/ dress.	250	6	4
Pork Ribs, 18 oz	1360	68	21
Turkey Leg: Regular, 19 oz	1135	54	0
Caveman (2lb Turkey Leg, with 1lb Bacon)	2360	177	3
Bacon: Fried, on-a-stick, with syrup	230	16	5
Choc-covered Bacon, 4.5 oz dish	640	43	30
Beef Stew over Rice, 2 cups	440	14	61
Butter Balls, deep fried, 4 Balls	460	38	24
Cheese Curds, Breaded & fried, *Culver's*, 6.7 oz	670	38	54
Corn Dogs: Regular, 4 oz	250	14	23
Jumbo, 6 oz	375	21	36
Pretzel-Wrapped Dog	300	16	30
Papa Pup, on-a-stick	400	24	32
Pronto Pup, on-a-stick	170	9	16
Corn On The Cob, 8" (1), 16 oz	200	1	42
Finger Foods:			
Artichoke, fried, 9 pieces	250	14	24
Chicken Nuggets, (6)	340	17	26
Chicken Strips, (4), 4.5 oz	445	21	33
Onion Rings, 3 rings	310	13	40
Onion Flower	1320	72	140
Shrimp, Fried, 10-12 pieces, 5 oz	555	30	36
Spam, deep-fried in batter, 2 pieces	330	24	18
Gator:			
Big Gator, Nuggets/Hushpuppies	550	31	54
Stick Gator, 1 sausage	250	20	4
Greek:			
Baklava, 2" square	245	13	32
Falafel, 11.6 oz	660	27	85
Greek Salad, 14 oz	520	48	17
Gyro, 7.5", 12 oz	680	40	55
Spanakopita, 8 oz	200	7.5	23
Hamburgers:			
⅓ Pound Burger, 7.5 oz	670	41	26
Cheeseburger, 6 oz	550	36	25
Hot Dogs: *With Bun*			
Regular: No extras	215	14	28
With Chili, 6 oz	450	32	32
With Chili & Cheese, 7.3 oz	500	36	31
⅓ Pound Hot Dog	550	41	31
Foot Long Hot Dog	470	26	41
Jumbo, Bratwurst/Kielbasa, average	800	60	28

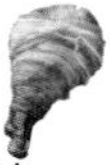
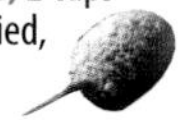
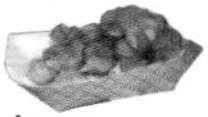

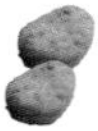
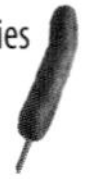
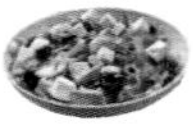
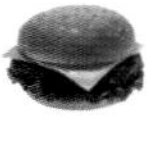

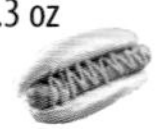

Fair & Carnival Foods (Cont)

	C	F	Cb
Mexican:			
Burrito, with Bean/Beef, 17 oz	1100	41	104
Carne Asada, 14.5 oz	820	44	58
Cheese Quesadilla, 1.8 oz	480	27	40
Chicken Taco, 3.3 oz	210	12	16
Fish Taco, 5 oz	270	13	31
Jalapeno Pepper, choc-covered (3)	270	15	31
Nachos with Cheese, 9" plate	860	59	70
Tamale, 3.5 oz	180	8	21
Taquito, 5 oz	370	17	43
Pizza:			
Pizza Bread, Pepperoni, ½ loaf, 12 oz	1115	32	151
Pizza on-a-stick, 1 piece	535	28	55
Personal Pizza: *Per 7"*			
Cheese	670	24	80
Pepperoni	795	35	80
Ham & Pineapple	800	31	87
Potatoes & Fries:			
Australian Battered Potatoes	1290	66	155
Baked Potato, 14 oz	435	0.5	100
Fries: French, 7 oz	560	24	79
Cheese Fries, 10 oz	645	38	62
Chili Fries, 10 oz	700	36	83
Curly Fries, 7 oz	620	30	78
Jamaican Jerk Fries, 7 oz	640	34	77
Sweet Potato, baked, 14 oz	405	0.5	97
Tornado, on-a-stick	210	15	18
Salads/Sides:			
Chili, 1 cup	280	11	24
Cole Slaw, 5 oz	350	21	37
Pickle, whole (6")	30	0	8
Potato Salad, 5 oz	290	15	35
Sandwiches: *7½" Roll*			
Ham, 11 oz	645	39	47
Hot Pastrami, 9 oz	760	17	62
Roast Beef, 11 oz	620	36	46
Philadelphia Cheese Steak, 13 oz	680	36	49
Turkey, 11 oz	665	24	65
Drinks:			
Icee, 16 fl.oz	235	0	59
Shakes, average, 16 fl.oz	690	33	85
Slushies: Horchata, 16 fl.oz	280	8	50
Lemonade, 18 fl.oz	210	0	52
Orange Julius, 20 fl.oz	490	10	96
Strawberry Julius, 20 fl.oz	430	0	98
Soft Frozen Lemonade, 12 fl.oz	300	0	78
Smoothies, Berry Flavors, 16 fl.oz	350	1	80

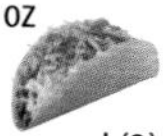
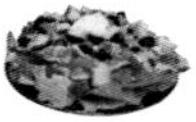
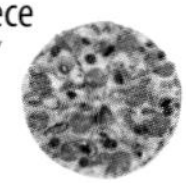
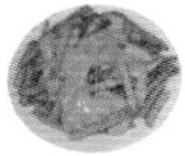
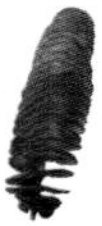
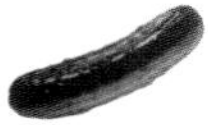
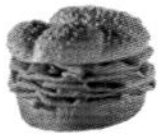
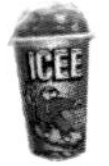

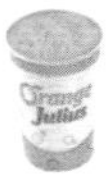

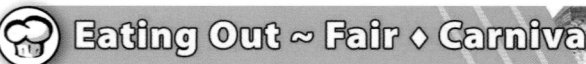

Fair & Carnival Foods (Cont)

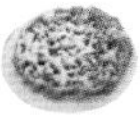
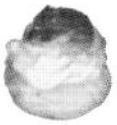
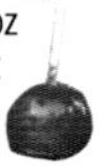
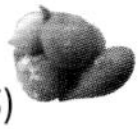
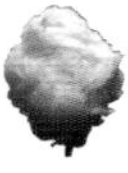
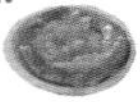
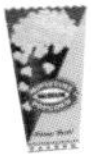
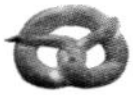

Cakes, Pastries:	C	F	Cb
Funnel Cake, Plain (1)	760	44	80
Toppings:			
Apple Cinnamon, 2 oz	85	3	16
Cinnamon & Sugar, 2 tsp	40	0	10
Strawberry & Cream, 2 oz	70	0	16
Cheesecake on-a-stick, 6 oz	655	47	56
Churro, (1), 9", 1.6 oz	170	8	22
Cream Puff, 4.3 oz	500	43	22
Fried Twinkie, (1)	420	34	45
Puff-on-a-Stick, (4), 8.6 oz	995	86	44
Strawberry Crepe, 4.3 oz	280	14	36
Twinkie Dog, (Sundae)	500	14	89
Candied Apple, 7 oz	330	0	80
Cookies:			
Sweet Martha, (1), 0.8 oz	90	4	14
Deep Fried: Oreos, tray (5)	890	48	108
Cookie Dough on stick, 3 pieces	670	32	89
Cotton Candy:			
Small, 1 oz	110	0	27
Large, 2.3 oz	250	0	62
Family Size, 5.5 oz	610	0	151
Dirt Dessert, 1 cup, 9.3 oz	405	12	69
Donuts, Jumbo Twist, (1), 7.5 oz	905	49	109
Fried Dough/FryBread:			
Plain: 7", 3.7 oz	390	19	47
9", 4 3/4 oz	510	25	61
Toppings: Cinnamon Sugar, 2 tsp	40	0	10
Butterscotch; Caramel, 2 Tbsp	115	0	29
Hot Fudge, average, 2 Tbsp	110	4	22
Cheese Powder, 2 tsp	70	3	2
Honey, 1 Tbsp, 0.8 oz	65	0	17
Fudge, 1.5 oz	200	11	25
Ice Cream & Frozen Treats:			
Deep-fried Klondike Bar, w/ syrup	430	16	18
Dippin' Dots Ice Cream, 6 oz cup	380	20	46
Frozen Banana, choc. coated, 5 oz	240	4	53
Frozen Yogurt, in sugar cone, 14 oz	475	2	94
Ice Cream: Small, sugar cone, 10 oz	775	42	83
Large, sugar cone, 14 oz	935	54	96
Sherbet, 8 oz	270	4	59
Snow Cone, with 3 oz syrup	270	0	68
Strawberry, Choc. Dipped, 1 piece	125	7	15
Popcorn:			
Plain: Small, 3 oz	450	24	48
Large, 6 oz	900	48	96
Kettle Corn: Small, 5 oz	600	15	110
Large, 10 oz	1200	30	220
Pretzels, Soft, 4.5 oz	340	2	70
S'more, on stick	275	16	27

Stadium Foods

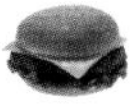
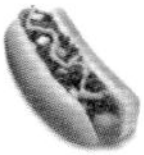
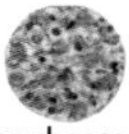
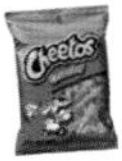

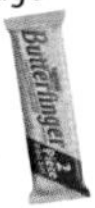

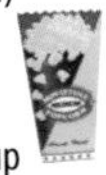
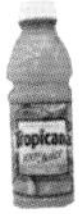
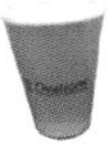
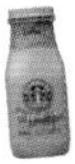

Burgers:	C	F	Cb
Bacon Burger, 8.3 oz	470	25	34
Cheeseburger, 8.3 oz	450	23	33
Hamburger, 7.8 oz	400	19	33
French Fries, 6.4 oz	470	34	39
Fruit Cup, 6 oz	80	0	20
Hot Dogs:			
Chili Dog, 7.7 oz	520	29	45
Hot Dog, 6.4 oz	465	21	50
Jumbo Dog, 6 oz	440	25	38
Kraut Dog with Sauerkraut, 7.8 oz	490	27	41
Individual Pan Pizza (6"): *Per Pizza*			
BBQ Chicken	630	24	71
Cheese	630	27	71
Pepperoni	660	30	70
Nachos, 40 chips, with 4 oz cheese	1100	59	132
Sandwiches:			
Chicken: With Bacon, 8.3 oz	530	31	41
With Cheese, 8.3 oz	510	29	40
Without Cheese, 7.7 oz	460	25	40
Polish Sausage Sandwich, 7 oz	565	33	46
Snacks:			
Brownie, 2.5" x 4.5"	360	18	44
Cheese Sauce, 1.3 oz	100	8	4
Cheetos, 2.8 oz package	440	28	42
Chocolate Chip Cookie, 2.3 oz	280	12	40
Churro, (1), 10", 2 oz	210	10	26
Doritos, Nacho, 2.8 oz package	390	20	48
King Size Candy:			
Butterfinger, 3.8 oz	480	18	75
Nestle Crunch, 2.8 oz	390	21	85
Lay's, Chips, 2.8 oz package	440	28	42
Peanuts, in shell, 8 oz	930	80	24
Popcorn: Small (9 cup size)	575	35	56
Large (15 cup size)	950	58	93
Pretzel, Soft, Reg., 5.5 oz	490	3.5	101
Red Vines, 5 oz box	500	0	117
Snow Cone: With 3 oz syrup	270	0	68
With 6 oz syrup	540	0	136
Beverages:			
Orange Juice, 12 fl.oz	180	0	2
Beer:			
Heineken, 16 fl.oz	200	0	16
Miller: Draft, 16 fl.oz	195	0	17
Lite, 16 fl.oz	125	16	4
Jack Daniels, Punch, 12 fl.oz	235	0	34
Wine, White, 9 fl.oz	190	0	6
Soda, (with 1/2 ice), average:			
20 fl.oz	160	0	40
32 fl.oz	260	0	65
Starbuck's, Coffee, Frappuccino, 9.5 fl.oz	200	3	37

Restaurant & International Foods

Asian & Chinese Dishes

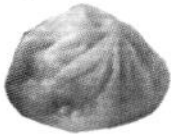
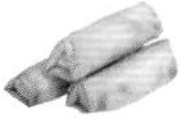
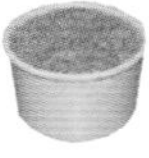
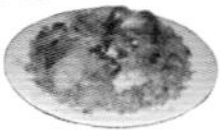
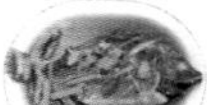

Asian & Chinese Dishes	C	F	Cb
Appetizers:			
Crab Cake, 2.3 oz	125	10	1
Dumplings: *Per Dumpling*			
Pork: Steamed	80	4.5	5
Fried	90	6	5
Vegetable, steamed	35	1	5
Egg Rolls, Mini, 3 rolls	100	3	11
Spring Roll:			
Small, 1.5 oz	85	4	9
Medium, 3 oz	170	8	17
Large, 5 oz	290	15	29
Wonton, 1 only	75	4	5
Soup: Egg Flower, bowl 12 oz	90	2	16
Hot & Sour Soup, bowl 12 oz	110	3.5	14
Rice: Plain,1 cup, 6.5 oz	320	2	66
2 Cups, 13 oz	640	4	132
Fried: 1 cup, 5 oz	365	11	55
Large dish, 16 oz	950	28	67
Noodles, Chinese Egg, cooked, 1 cup	200	4	37
Entrees & Mains: *Per Serving*			
Almond Chicken, 6 oz	270	10	21
BBQ Pork, 5.5oz	440	23	15
Beef in Black Bean Sauce, 8.5 oz	390	17	17
Broccoli Beef, 6 oz	370	21	13
Chicken & Broccoli, 5.5 oz	160	8	10
Chicken Skewers, 3 oz	210	9	18
Chop Suey:			
Chicken, 5 oz	140	9	2
Pork, 5 oz	170	12	3
Chow Mein, Beef/Chicken, 8 oz	390	12	59
Crab Puff/Rangoon, 1 dumpling	190	11	13
Crispy Fried Chicken, 8 oz	485	33	12
Egg Drop Soup: With Noodles, 1 cup	110	3	16
Without Noodles, 1 cup	60	3	4
Egg Foo Yung with Sauce, 1 cup	270	15	16
Kung Pao Chicken, 5.5 oz	240	15	12
Lemon Chicken, 5 oz	525	21	57
Lo Mein, stir-fried, 8 oz	705	42	49
Omelet, Chicken/Shrimp, 16 oz	990	82	10
Orange Chicken, 5.5 oz	500	27	42
Steamed Whole Fish, ½ Sockeye Salmon	646	36	23
Sweet & Sour:			
Fish, 20 oz	1160	58	106
Pork, 5.5 oz	400	23	35
Vegetable Combo, with oil, 6 oz	367	5	66
Vegetables, Steamed, without oil, 6 oz	135	1	29
Sauces: Mandarin Sauce 1.5 oz	70	0	17
Potsticker Sauce, 1.5 oz	35	0	8
Bubble Tea, average, 12 fl oz	280	0.5	68
Fortune Cookie, each	32	0.5	7

Cajun & Creole

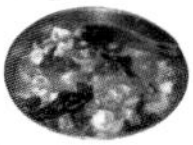

Cajun & Creole	C	F	Cb
Alligator, cooked, 4 oz	160	2	0
Baked Herb Chicken, 1 serving	850	53	2
Bouillabaisse	400	15	10
Cajun Fried Turkey, 1 serving	630	25	0
Cocktail Sauce, 2 Tbsp	30	0	6
Couche-Couche, ½ cup	80	0	17
Crawfish Bisque, 1 serving	500	10	10
Crawfish, cooked, 2 oz	45	0.5	0
Creole Jambalaya, 1 serving	550	30	15
Frog Legs, steamed (2)	45	0	0
Guinea Fowl, flesh, 4 oz, cooked	160	4	0
Hogshead Cheese, ¼ cup	80	5.5	0
Jambalaya, Shrimp & Crabmeat	520	14	12
Red Beans & Rice, 1 serving	400	17	52
Roasted Quail, with Bacon, on Toast	550	25	15
Remoulade Sauce, 2 Tbsp, 1 oz	110	11	2
Shrimp Creole, 1 serving	450	20	10
Stuffed Smothered Steak, with 1 cup Rice	890	50	50
Turtle, cooked, 3 oz	120	3	0

Canadian Foods

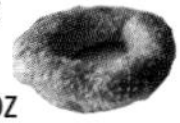
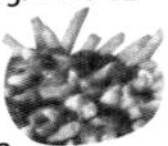
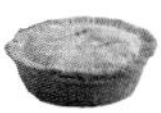

Canadian Foods	C	F	Cb
Bagels, Montreal-Style:			
Plain, 100g/3.5 oz	300	2	60
Poppyseed, 100g/3.5 oz	310	4	58
Sesame, 100g/3.5 oz	320	6	56
Bannock: Plain 33g/1.2 oz	120	3	20
With currants/raisins, 85g/3 oz	215	9	32
Meals:			
Baked Beans in Maple Syrup, 1 cup, 250g/8.8 oz	320	1	62
Donnairs (*Pizza Delight*):			
Famous, regular, 250g/8.8 oz	510	21	60
Super, regular, 310g/11 oz	685	34	62
Poutine:			
A&W, 330g/12 oz	610	33	58
Boston Pizza, regular, 400g/14 oz	610	30	67
Burger King, Classic, 330g/11.6 oz	680	36	72
Harvey's, 240g/8.5 oz	730	41	63
McDonald's, 1 serving	510	29	44
Swiss Chalet, Chalet -Style, 340g/12 oz	150	12	195
Shish Taouk:			
Chicken: 1 skewer, 200g/7 oz	270	25	9
Wrap, 455g/16 oz	1150	12	195
Tassot:			
Beef, 283g/10 oz	430	28	12
Goat, 100g/3.5 oz	360	36	9
Toutiere, 170g/6oz	600	42	35

Canadian (Cont)

	C	F	Cb
Pastries:			
Beaver Tails:			
Cheese & Garlic, 80g/2.8 oz	390	30	28
Cinnamon & Sugar, 80g/2.8 oz	315	13	30
Butter Tart, mini, 1 tart	120	3	16
May West,			
Original, 54g/1.9 oz	240	11	34
Nanaimo Bar, 56g/2 oz	270	16	30
Snacks: Maple Syrup Taffy, 40g/1.4 oz	130	0	33
Potato Chips: Dill Pickle Flav., 40g	160	10	15
Ketchup Flavor, 50g/1.8 oz	260	16	26

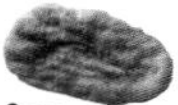
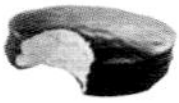

French Foods

	C	F	Cb
Blanquette d' Agneau, (Lamb Stew)	800	30	17
Brioche, 1 cake	280	14	34
Bouillabaisse	400	15	10
Coq au Vin, leg/thigh	700	28	31
Coquilles St. Jacques	320	13	36
Crème Brulée, 1 serving	460	40	21
Baguette, 3 slices, 2.2 oz	150	1	35
Creme Caramel, (Caramel Custard)	260	10	38
Crepe Suzette, 1x6" crepe with sauce	220	10	13
Duck a l'Orange, ¼ duck, 22 oz	970	44	19
Escargot, (Snails), in garlic butter (6)	200	10	4
Frog Legs, fried, 4 medium pairs	400	20	10
Lamb Noisettes, fried, 2 chops	500	40	1
Potage Creme Crecy, (Carrot Soup)	360	18	14
Salade Nicoise, (Tuna/Olives/Vegs)	450	13	14
Veal Cordon Bleu, (Veal/Ham)	650	25	18
Vichyssoise, (Potato /Leek Soup), 1 c.	200	9	15

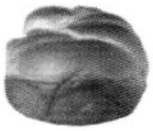
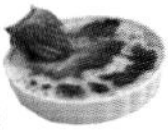

Baguette & French Stick ~ *Page 54*

German Foods

	C	F	Cb
Beef: Goulash with Veggies	520	20	46
Weiner Schnitzel, 1 medium	750	35	38
Chicken: Fried, Viennese-style	530	20	28
Livers with Apple/Onion, 6 oz	460	28	10
Herring, pickled: Rollmops, 4 oz	260	16	3
With Sour Cream, 4 oz	310	20	3
Pork, Sauerbraten (Pot Roast)	650	35	15
Sausage: Bratwurst, grilled, 6 oz	450	37	2
Hot Sausage Curry	300	7	6
Cakes:			
Black Forest, 1 slice	380	16	30
Bavarian Bread Dumpling, 3 small	330	10	28
Kugelhupf Cake, 1 large slice, 4 oz	400	23	40
Torte: Linzer (Almond/Raspb. Jam)	430	18	58
Sacher (Chocolate/Apricot Jam)	260	12	23

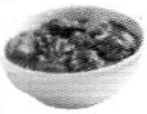
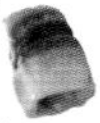
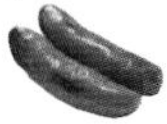

Greek Foods

	C	F	Cb
Baklava Pastry: Small	240	13	32
Large, 3.8 oz	400	21	45
Calamari, deep fried, 1 cup	300	13	17
Chicken Kebob Plate	345	13	8
Dolmades, 2 rolls, 6 oz	200	5	13
Galactobureko, 1 only			
(Filo, Custard, Pastry in Syrup)	360	15	48
Greek Chicken Salad	400	18	9
Gyros: 6" Pita, 8 oz	475	32	35
7½" Pita, 12 oz	680	40	55
Hummus & Pita, 4 oz	260	12	30
Kataifi, (Filo, Nut, Pastry in Syrup)	350	11	56
Moussaka: Small serving, 8 oz	350	22	22
Large serving, 16 oz	700	44	44
Soup, Avgolemono (Egg & Lemon			
with Chicken & Rice), 1 cup	85	6	5
Souvlaki, (Lamb), each, 2 oz	120	6	1
Stuffed Tomatoes, (2)	250	12	17
Taramosalata, 1 T., 0.5 oz	40	3	2
Tyropita, (Filo/Egg/Cheese Pastry)	350	26	31

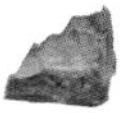

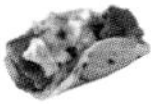
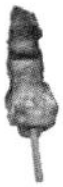
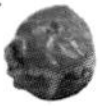

Hawaiian

	C	F	Cb
Ahi Tuna, grilled w/o fat, 6 oz fillet	220	2	0
Chicken Long Rice, 1 cup, 7 oz	240	14	12
Gyoza, 1 only	55	2	6
Haupia, (Coconut Pudd.), 1 pce, (4"x 2½")	120	6	17
Hawaiian Sweet Bread, ½" slice, 2 oz	180	4.5	29
Kalua: Chicken, 4 oz	280	16	0
Pork, 4 oz	350	24	0
Kim Chee, (pickled cabbage), ½ cup, 4 oz	20	0	5
Kulolo, (Taro Pudding), 1 slice	125	5	19
Lau Lau:			
Chicken (1), 7 oz	280	21	3
Pork (1), 7 oz	320	26	5
Loco Moco, (rice/burger/egg/gravy)	650	27	63
Lomi Salmon, ¼ cup, 4 oz	20	1	2
Malasadas, (Donut), 2 oz	240	13	26
Manapua, (Char Siu Pork Bun), 2.3 oz	180	8	25
Poi ,(mashed cooked taro), 1 cup., 8.5 oz	270	0.5	65
Poke, average all types, 3 oz	90	1	0
Portuguese Sausage, 2 oz	180	15	2
Potato Salad, ½ cup, 5 oz	170	10	17
Shave Ice, *(Matsumoto),* all flavors:			
With Ice Cream, 1 large	300	4	64
With Beans, 1 large	290	0	72
Spam Musubi:			
With Regular Spam	265	11	34
(4 oz rice+1.3 oz Spam/7-Eleven Hawaii)			
Homemade, w/ Lite Spam (50% less fat)	220	5	34
Taro Pancake Mix, ⅓ cup (makes 2)	140	2	26

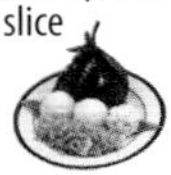
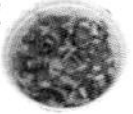
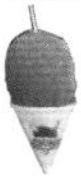

Hawaiian (Cont)

	C	F	Cb
Plate Lunches:			
Chicken Katsu, (9 oz:) With Rice	1110	48	108
+ Macaroni Salad, 3/4 cup	1360	68	123
or Tossed Salad + 2 T. French Dress.	1240	61	111
Hamburger, (5 oz): With Rice	710	24	81
Gravy + Macaroni Salad	1135	49	112
Mahi Mahi, (7 oz): With Rice	650	12	90
+ Macaroni Salad + Tartar Sce	1150	58	109
or Macaroni Salad, w/o Tartar ce	935	34	108
or Tossed Salad + 3 Tbsp Fr. Dress.	815	27	96
or Tossed Salad, without dressing	670	12	93
Teri Beef, (5 oz): With 2 scoops Rice	790	23	94
+ Macaroni Salad, 3/4 cup	1095	47	113
or Tossed Salad, without dressing	800	23	95

Indian & Pakistani

Per Serving, Meat dishes allow 4 oz meat/serving

	C	F	Cb
Aloo Samosa, each	155	12	12
Alu Gosht Kari, (Meat/Potato Curry)	600	40	23
Chicken Korma	500	35	6
Chicken Pilaf	700	53	50
Chicken Tikka	260	16	2
Chicken Vindaloo	400	20	8
Chapati/Roti, 7" diameter, 1 piece	60	0.5	11
Dahl, (Lentil Puree):			
1 cup, without oil	230	1	37
1 Tbsp Tadka (oil topping)	120	13	0
Dhakla, (Lentil Dish), 1" square, 1 oz	105	5	13
Dhansak, ½ cup	105	3.5	11
Gosht Kari	460	25	17
Lamb Pilaf	520	35	40
Lassi, (Sweet or Mango), 1 cup, 8 oz	160	4	24
Masala Gosht, (Beef/Tomato/Gravy)	400	25	18
Mulligatawney Soup	300	15	8
Murgh Tikka, 1 cup	300	4	7
Naan Flatbread, 2 oz	160	3.5	29
Pappadum, 1 large/2 small	50	3	5
Pesrattu, (Lentil Crepe), 9", 2.6 oz	130	5	15
Pork Vindaloo Curry, without Rice	620	47	3
Rajmah, 1 cup	225	5	35
Rogan Josh,			
without Rice/Potatoes	500	30	3
Shahi Korma, (Braised Lamb)	430	28	3
Tandoori Chicken:			
Breast	260	13	5
Leg/Thigh portion	300	17	6

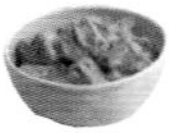
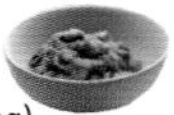
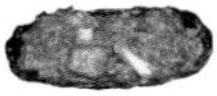
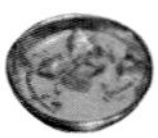
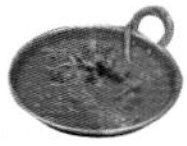
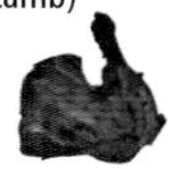

Italian Dishes

	C	F	Cb
Entrees:			
Baked Ziti: Small	370	27	32
Regular	575	42	49
Breadstick, 2 oz piece	120	2.5	25
Broccoli Fettucine Alfredo, regular	815	23	125
Bruschetta, 2 slices	380	17	53
Calzones, av. all varieties	840	34	101
Cannelloni, 1 tube, 6 oz	280	15	18
Cheese Breadstick, 2.4 oz piece	180	8	20
Cheese Ravioli, with sauce	495	17	65
Chicken Alfredo	775	29	82
Chicken Parmigiana, 11 oz	520	22	16
Chicken Scallopine, dinner	1110	71	68
Eggplant Parmigiana	900	39	78
Fettucine Alfredo: Lunch, 9 oz	885	65	63
Dinner, 15 oz	1475	108	104
Linquine & Seafood, dinner	1130	71	79
Manicotti Formaggio	800	38	57
Meat Lasagne:			
Small, 10 oz	440	23	39
Large, 16 oz	700	36	60
Meat Ravioli	725	22	102
Minestrone Soup, 1 bowl	110	2	18
Penne Rustica: Lunch	1300	71	76
Dinner	1540	80	101
Ravioli, over-stuffed, average	990	67	57
Panini Sandwich:			
Chicken, 16 oz	900	38	81
Meats, average, 18 oz	940	39	81
Vegetarian, 15 oz	750	31	83
Pizza, Ready-To-Eat ~ *See Page 135*			
Spaghetti & Meatballs:			
With Tomato Sauce: Kids	500	20	58
Medium/Lunch	1080	63	89
Large/Dinner	1430	81	119
With Meat Sauce: Kids	550	25	56
Medium/Lunch	1300	79	84
Large/Dinner	1700	103	110
Veal Marsala, dinner	1320	66	132
Veal Parmigiana, dinner	1270	65	116
Vegetable Primavera	610	8	116
Salad,			
Caprese, 11 oz	445	34	10
Desserts:			
Gelato: Vanilla (Milk Base), 1/2 cup	200	15	18
Choc. Hazelnut (Milk), 1/2 cup	370	29	26
Water Base, 1/2 cup	100	0	25
Lemon Ice,	180	0	45
Tiramisu, 1 piece, 5 oz	400	29	30

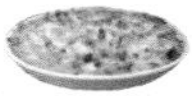
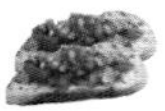
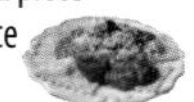
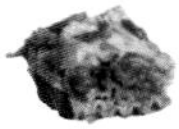
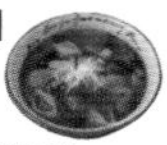
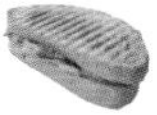
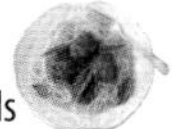
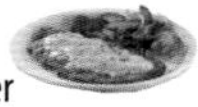
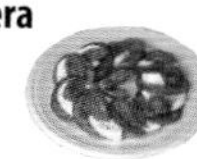
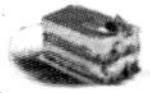

Further listings ~ *See Fast-Foods Section*

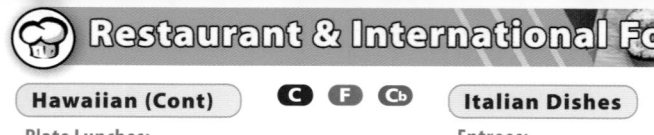

Japanese

	C	F	Cb
Sashimi: (Sliced Raw Seafood/Beef)			
Ika (Squid), 4 oz	**105**	2	0
Hamachi (Yellowtail), 4 oz	**165**	6	0
Maguro (Yellowfin Tuna), 4 oz	**120**	1	0
Niku (Beef), 5 oz	**200**	10	0
Saba (Mackerel), 4 oz	**160**	7	0
Suzuki (Sea Bass), 4 oz	**110**	0.5	0
Tako (Octopus), 4 oz	**95**	1	0
Sushi Rice: Cooked, 1 Tbsp	**25**	0	5
1 cup, 5.3 oz	**380**	3	82
Sushi (Maki) Rolls: *Per Piece*			
Average all types (California Rolls; Cream Cheese with Crab; Eel; Salmon; Shrimp; Tuna; Yellowtail; Vegetable)			
Small (1.2″ diam. x 1.2″ high), 0.8 oz	**25**	0.5	3.5
Medium (1¾″ diam. x 1¾″ high), 1.6 oz	**50**	1	7
Large (2¼″ diam. x ⅞″ high), 2 oz	**60**	1.5	9
Sushi Packs: *Per Pack*			
Average all types: 6 large pieces	**370**	5	55
9 medium pieces	**360**	6	60
12 small pieces	**265**	3	45
Futomaki (thick roll), 6 pieces	**380**	5	72
Hand Roll (Cone), 4 oz	**120**	2	18
Inari (rice filled soybean pocket), 4 pces	**420**	9	73
Sushi-Nigiri, (fish on rice), average all varieties, 1 piece	**70**	0.5	12
Sushi Plate, Assorted: 6 pieces	**420**	3	36
Combination (Sushi & Sushi Rolls) 2 Sushi + 6 small & 3 medium rolls	**400**	7	72
Dipping Sauces: Average, 2 Tbsp	**30**	0	7
Ginger Vinegar Dressing, 2 Tbsp	**20**	0	5
Edamame: (young green soybeans):			
Boiled beans (no pods), 4 oz	**160**	7	12
Steamed (in pods), 4 oz	**60**	3	5
Katsu-don, Pork with Rice	**1100**	39	141
Miso Soup, with Tofu pieces, 1 cup	**85**	3	11
Sake Wine, (16% alcohol), 3 fl.oz	**115**	0	7
Seaweed Salad, 1.5 oz	**20**	2	0
Sukiyaki, (Beef/Tofu/Veggies), 8 oz	**400**	24	32
Tempura:			
3 large shrimp & veggies	**320**	18	25
1 shrimp only	**60**	4	3
Teppan Yaki, (Steak, Seafood & Veggies), 10 oz serving	**470**	30	15
Teriyaki: Beef, 4 oz	**350**	25	4
Chicken, 4 oz	**260**	9	7
Salmon, medium, 6 oz	**270**	8	3
Yakatori, 1 skewer, 2.5 oz	**140**	5	1

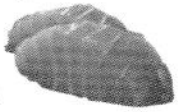
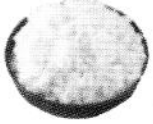
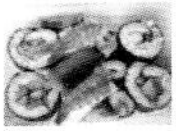
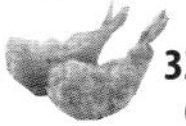
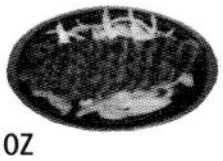

Kosher/Deli Foods

	C	F	Cb
Bagel/Bialy, 1 small, 2 oz	**160**	2	32
Beiglach, (Cheese Knish)	**350**	17	35
Blintzes: Average, 1 only	**120**	1	25
With Sour Cream & Preserves	**370**	10	30
Borscht, (Without Sour Cream): 1 cup	**85**	3	14
Diet/Reduced Calorie, 1 cup	**30**	1	7
Cabbage Rolls, (meat/rice), 5 oz	**170**	6	21
Chicken Broth: 1 cup	**80**	8	0
With vegetables	**100**	8	5
With noodles	**150**	9	16
Lowfat, plain, 1 cup	**25**	1	0
Cholent, 1 medium serving, 1 cup	**350**	16	48
Chopped Liver: 1 serving, 3 oz	**110**	6	5
With Egg Salad, ¼ cup	**100**	7	3
Farfel, dry, ½ cup	**90**	0.5	21
Gefilte Fish Balls:			
Regular, 2 oz	**55**	2	4
With Jelled Broth	**80**	2	6
Cocktail size, 1 oz	**30**	1	2
Sweet: Medium, 2 oz	**65**	2	4
With Jelled Broth	**95**	2	9
Hallah, (Yeast Bread), 1 slice, 1 oz	**85**	2	14
Herring: Smoked, 2 oz	**120**	8	0
In Sour Cream, 2 oz	**150**	10	0
Kasha, cooked, ½ cup	**100**	0.5	20
Kipfel, (Vanilla/Almdond Cookie), 1 pce	**60**	2	7
Knaidlach ~ *See Matzo Balls*			
Knish: Kasha/Potato, 1 only	**130**	4	22
Cheese, 1 only	**350**	17	35
Kreplach, beef, 1 piece	**40**	1	6
Kugel, potato/noodle, 1 serving	**300**	20	25
Latkes, (Potato Pancake): 2 oz	**200**	11	22
3 Latkes w/ Sour Cran Apple Sauce	**750**	25	95
Lochshen: Plain, 1 cup	**130**	2	26
Pudding, 1 cup	**380**	13	48
Lox, (Smoked Salmon), 2 oz	**65**	2	0
Mandelbrot, (Almond Bread), 1 slice, ¼″ thick	**45**	2	5
Matzo, 1 oz board	**110**	0.5	21
Matzo Balls: 2 small, or 1 large, 2″	**90**	3	12
Extra large ball, 3″	**180**	6	24
Matzo Ball Soup:			
Cup w/ 2 small or 1 large ball	**150**	5	27
Bowl w/ Chkn & Noodles	**325**	13	34
Jerry's Deli, large bowl	**560**	17	56
NY Cheesecake, 4 oz	**350**	24	26
Pierogi, potato/cheese, 1 piece	**90**	4	11
Reuben S'wich, w/ ½ lb Corned Beef	**920**	60	28
Schmaltz, (Rend'd Chicken Fat), 1 T.	**90**	10	0

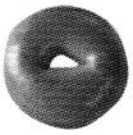
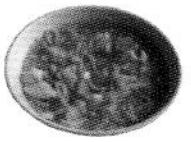
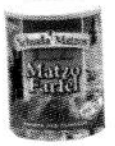

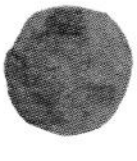
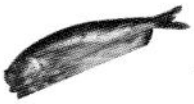
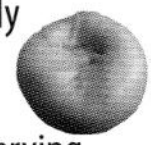
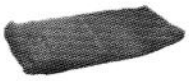
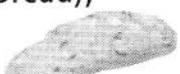
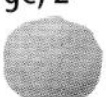
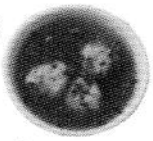

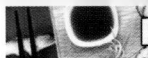

Korean Food	C	F	Cb
Bibimbab, (Veg. & Beef on Rice), 1 cup	565	15	89
Bulgogi, (Barbeque Beef), 3.5 oz	325	12	15
Galbi (Short Ribs), 16 oz	975	61	16
Gujeolpan, (Pancake with Meat & Vegetables), 1 cup with 1 pancake	340	11	39
Japchae, (Noodle w/ Veggies & Meat), 1¼ cups	365	19	34
Sides:			
Kimchee, (Cabbage Relish), ½ cup	30	0	6
Namool, (Assorted Vegetables), 1 cup	125	6.5	9
Soups: *Per Serving*			
Muguk, (Radish & Chive Soup), 6 oz	105	7	6
Samgyetang, (Ginseng Chkn Soup):			
Without Chicken Skin, 1 cup	520	11	60
With Chicken Skin, 1 cup	725	35	60
Yuk Gae Jang, (Spicy Beef Soup), 1¼ cups	180	13	5
Lebanese/Middle East			
Baba Ghannouj, 2 Tbsp, 1 oz	70	6	2
Baklava, (Pastry, Nuts, Syrup), 1 pastry, 1¾ oz	245	18	18
Cabbage Rolls, (Cabb. Leaf, Meat, Rice), 1 roll, 3 oz,	100	3	12
Cous Cous, (Semolina, Milk, Fruit, Nuts), 1 cup	400	21	43
Falafel, (Chick Pea Fritter), Fried, 1 medium, 1 oz	60	4	4
Hummus, ¼ cup, 2.2 oz	105	3	5
Fried Kibbi, (Wheat, Meat Pinenuts), 1 piece, 3 oz	180	8	15
Kafta, (Ground Lamb, Ssge on Skewer), 1 skewer, 1.5 ozoz	85	5	2
Kibbeh Naye, (raw Lamb, Bulgur & Spice) 1 cup, 9 oz	450	18	28
Lebanese Omelet, 1 serving, 4 oz (Egg, Spinach, Pinenuts, Onion)	200	12	13
Pilaf, (Rice, Onion, Raisins, Apr., Spice) 1 cup	400	11	60
Shawourma, (Spit-Roast Beef), 4 oz serving	280	15	2
Shish Kabob, 1 stick, 2.5 oz	130	7	2
Spinach Pie, 1 piece, 3.5 oz	290	21	20
Sweet Almond Sanbusak, (Pastry, Almonds, Spices), 1 piece	200	15	11
Tabouli, 1 serving, 4 oz	125	7	13
Tahini Sauce, average, 1 Tbsp	90	8	2

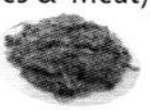
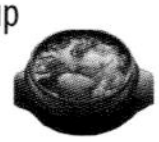
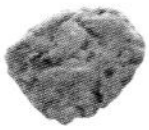
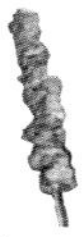

Mexican Food	C	F	Cb
Burritos *(Taco Bell):* Bean	370	10	56
Supreme Beef	420	16	53
Chili, plain, ¼ cup	90	6	8
Chili con Carne: With Beans, 1 cup	310	17	15
Without Beans, 1 cup	370	28	10
Chimichangas, Beef, 5 oz	400	19	43
Chorizo Sausage, 2 oz	265	23	0
Churro, (1), 1.5 oz	150	8	18
Corn Chips, ½ cup, 1 oz	160	10	17
Enchilada, average	330	10	49
Fajitas, Chicken	200	7	20
Guacamole, average, 2 Tbsp, 1 oz	45	4	2
Horchata: *(Don Jose)*, 1 cup, 8 fl.oz	140	4	25
Cacique, 1 pint bottle, 16 fl.oz	320	7	62
Margarita, with 1.5 oz Tequila	160	0	6
Masa, (Pre-mixed for Tamales), 1 oz	80	5	9
Menudo:			
With Hominy, 1 cup	240	9	19
Without Hominy, 1 cup	170	9	2
Nachos: With cheese, peppers, 1 portion, 6-8 nachos, 7 oz	600	33	60
With cheese, beans, beef, peppers, 1 portion, 6-8 nachos, 9 oz	570	31	56
Del Taco: Regular, 4 oz	300	19	30
Macho Nachos, 17 oz	1000	56	94
Taco Bell, BellGrande®, 10.8 oz	780	40	84
Nopal Cactus Salad, 1 cup	130	9	11
Papas Fritas, (1), 6 oz	325	18	40
Piloncillo, (Brown Sugar):			
1 Tbsp, 0.5 oz	50	0	13
Cone, small, 3", 3 oz	325	0	81
Quesadilla, Cheese	490	28	39
Queso Fresco, ¼ cup	80	4.5	8
Refried Beans, ¾ cup, 6 oz	160	3	26
Rice Pudding, (Arroz Con Leche), 4 oz	140	3	24
Soup, Black Bean, 1 bowl	200	3	34
Tacos *(Taco Bell):*			
Crunchy: Regular	170	10	12
Supreme	200	12	15
Soft: Crispy Potato	270	13	31
Grilled Steak	250	14	19
Taco Salad with Salsa	840	52	85
Taco Sauce, average, ¼ cup	15	0	3
Taco Shell, regular	50	2	8
Tamales, Beef/Chicken, av. 4.5 oz	250	11	27
Taquitos, Beef & Cheese, 4.5 oz	330	15	36
Tostada *(Taco Bell)*	250	10	29
Tortilla, Corn, 6" diameter	70	1	14
Tortilla Chips, 1 oz	150	8	18
Soup, Black Bean, 1 bowl	200	3	34

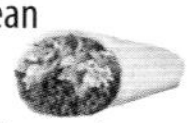
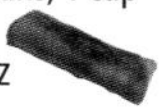
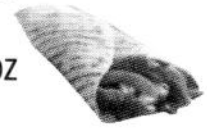
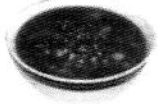
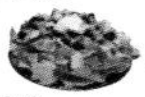
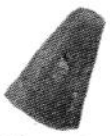
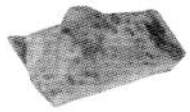
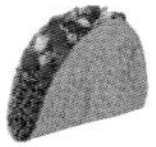
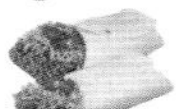
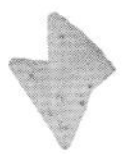

Extra Food Listings ~ See Fast Food Section
(Examples: Del Taco, Taco Bell, Taco Cabana, Taco Time)

Mexican (Cont)

	C	F	Cb
Breads:			
Bolillos, 1 roll, 3.5 oz	240	4	42
Mexican Cornbread, 4" square	210	11	19
Pan de Leche, 1 roll, 1.3 oz	110	2.5	20
Telera, 2 oz	150	1.5	19
Cakes· Cookies· Pastries Pan Dulce:			
Banderilla, 1 piece	140	10	8
Bigotes, 7"	570	22	44
Capirotada, (Bread Pudding), 10 oz	810	38	107
Cinnamon Cookies, 2	125	8	13
Concha, av. all varieties:			
Small (3" diameter), 2.5 oz	250	8	38
Medium (4" diameter), 3.5 oz	350	11	53
Large (5" diameter), 5.5 oz	550	18	84
Cream Puff, with Custard, 4.3 oz	255	14	25
Cuernos, (Horns), 3 oz	340	17	41
Donut, large, 4", 3.5 oz	440	21	58
Elotes, 3.5 oz	450	24	51
Empanadas, average all varieties:			
Medium, 3 oz	300	14	42
Large, 4 oz	400	19	56
Fiesta Cookie, (1), 2.3 oz	280	8	47
Galletas Mixtas:			
Small, 1 oz	100	2.5	16
Medium, 2 oz	200	5	32
Large, 3 oz	300	7.5	48
Guayaba, 3.3 oz	360	14	53
Jelly Roll, (1), 3.3 oz	240	4	46
Mantecadites, 4.5 oz	670	42	64
Mini Cupcake, (1),1.8 oz	180	8	25
Muffins/Nino Enbuelto, large, 6 oz	465	11	48
Nuez, 3.3 oz	380	17	52
Ojo de Buey, 4 oz	360	15	55
Orejas, 1 medium, 3 oz	310	15	38
Pan Dulce, 1 bun	330	10	45
Panquecitos, 2.5 oz	260	11	36
Piedras, 4 oz	470	15	76
Polvorones: Small, 1.5 oz	180	9	24
1 large, 3 oz	370	18	48
Pound Cakes, mini, 3.5 oz	380	16	52
Puerquitos, 3.5 oz	350	12	55
Rebanadas, 3.5 oz	390	18	51
Roles De Canela, (Cinn. Roll), 4.5 oz	490	15	81
Roscas, 1 piece, 2.8 oz	360	18	44
Semitas *(Bimbo)*, 1 piece, 2.2 oz	210	6	33
Sopapillas, (flaky pastry puffs): 1 piece	100	7	10
With Honey & Cream	200	14	18
Strawberry Crema Roll, 2.5 oz slice	240	5	45

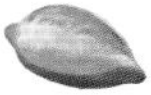
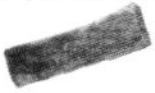
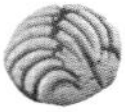
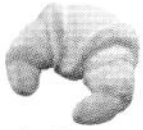
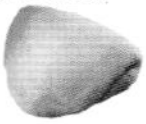
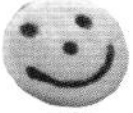
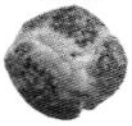
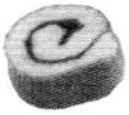
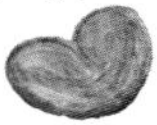

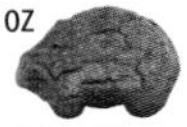

Extra Food Listings ~ *See CalorieKing.com*

Polish

	C	F	Cb
Cabbage Rolls, w/ Sour Cream, 2 small	220	10	30
Chicken Casserole, w/ Mshrms, 1 cup	520	27	5
Kielbasa, (Sausages, Onions, fried), 2 large	350	28	2
Meatballs,			
in sour cream, 3 x 1½" balls	300	16	11
Pierogi, Fruit/Vegetables, 3" ball	80	2	15
Pork Goulash, (Pork/Vegetable Stew)	550	21	38
Pot Roast, with Vegetables	630	21	28

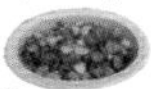

Soul Foods

	C	F	Cb
Breakfast Sausage, fried, 2 patties	250	17	0
Brunswick Stew, 1 cup, 8.5 oz	320	14	19
Cornbread, homemade, 3 oz	200	7.5	28
Fatback, 0.5 oz	110	11	0
Ham Hock, pickled, 3 oz	200	12	0
Hog Maw, 1 oz	70	4.5	0
Hominy, cooked, ¾ cup	110	0.5	25
Hush Puppies, 5 pieces	260	12	35
Kale, cooked, ½ cup	20	0.5	4
Opossum, roasted, without bone, 3 oz	190	9	0
Oxtail, cooked, without bone, 2 oz	85	4.5	0
Pig's Ear, ¼ ear	50	3	0
Pig's Foot, ½ foot	70	4.5	0
Pig's Tail, ⅓ tail	115	10	0
Poke Salad, cooked, ½ cup	16	0.5	3
Pork Brains, braised, 3 oz	115	8	0
Pork Chitterlings, simmered, 3 oz	260	25	0
Pork Cracklings, 0.5 oz	80	6	0
Pork Neck Bones, cooked, no bone, 2 oz	100	4.5	0
Pork Skin, 1 cup	70	4.5	0
Pork Tongue, ⅓ tongue	75	5.5	0
Sousemeat, 1 oz	60	4.5	0
Succotash, ½ cup	80	1	17
Sweet Potato Pie, ⅛ of 9" pie	250	12	34
Tripe, 2 oz	55	2	0
Vienna Sausage:			
2 small, 1 oz	90	8	1
1 small, 0.5 oz	45	4	0.5

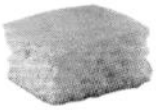
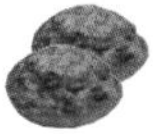
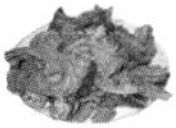
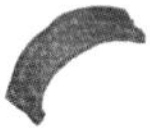
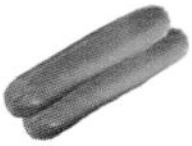

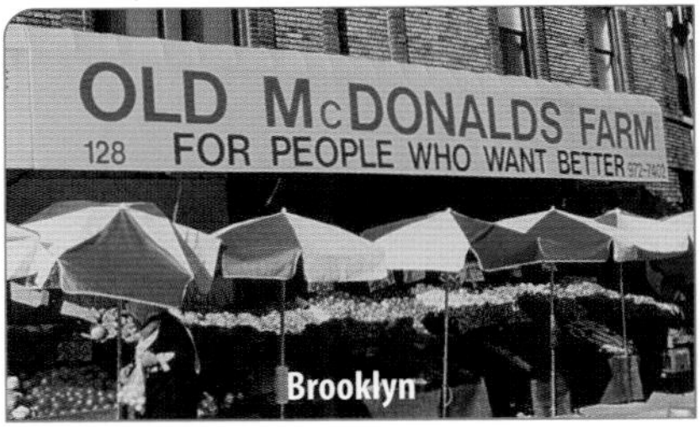

Brooklyn

Spanish

	C	F	Cb
Arroz Abanda, (Fish with Rice)	340	8	31
Arroz Con Pollo, (Rice/Chkn Salad)	500	23	50
Clams Marinara, 8 clams	330	16	22
Cochifrito, (Lamb with Lemon/Garlic)	650	25	5
Cochinillo Asado, (Rst Suckling Pig), 2 slices	300	15	3
Cocido Madrileno, (Madrid-Style Boiled Dinner)	450	27	18
Flan de Leche, (Caramel Custard)	325	9	52
Fritadera de Ternera, (Sauteed Veal)	450	27	2
Gazpacho, 1 bowl	60	0	15
Mole Poblano, ½ cup	205	14	16
Paella a la Valenciana, (Chicken & Shellfish Rice)	900	42	70
Pollo a la Espanola, (Chicken)	475	30	4
Ternera al Jerez, (Veal with Sherry)	660	29	6
Zarzuela, (Fish & Shellfish Medley)	530	27	40

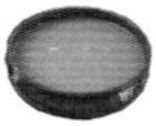

Thai Foods

	C	F	Cb
Appetizers: Satay Pork, 1 oz	100	4	2
Spring Roll, 1.3 oz	110	6	13
Soups, Tom Yam (Hot & Sour):			
Spicy Shrimp/Seafood:			
1 cup	100	4	6
1 bowl	160	7	10
Vegetarian, 1 cup	50	0	11
Curries: Chicken with Ginger, 1 cup	390	34	4
Thick Red Curry with Beef, 1 cup	600	50	7
Thai Chicken Curry, 1 cup	340	23	4
Massaman Curry, 1 cup	680	57	8
Green Curry with Pork, 1 cup	480	44	5
Pad Thai, large serving, 18 oz	990	38	125
Fish: Steamed with Spicy Thai Sce	450	8	46
Crispy Fried, 5 oz	290	15	9
Spicy Chicken, stir-fry	450	22	14
Spicy Garlic Tofu, stir-fry	340	18	18
Sticky Thai Rice: Plain 1 cup, 6 oz	170	0.5	36
With Coconut & Sesame Seeds, 1 cup	880	28	120
Stir-fried Rice Noodles, 1 cup 5.5 oz	270	9	40
Stir-fried Vegetables, 1 cup	100	3	18
Salads: Green Papaya Salad	160	0	40
Spicy Prawn, 9 shrimp	170	3	15
Thai Beef Salad, 1 serving	260	9	15
Thai Chicken, 1 serving	330	9	17
Thai Noodle, 1 serving	410	13	45
Satay Chicken & Peanut Sauce, 1 satay stick	390	24	20
Sauce, Peanut Satay, ½ cup, 4 oz	160	10	13

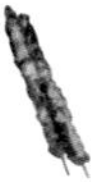
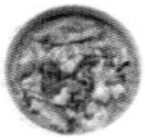
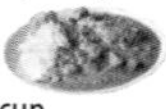
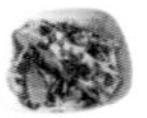
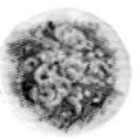
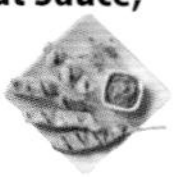

Vietnamese

	C	F	Cb
Banh Cuon, (Steam Rice w/ Pork), 1 roll	105	7	8
Bo Nuong, (Beef Satay), 2 sticks	265	9	4
Bo Xao Dau Phong, (Ginger Beef with Onion, Fish Sce)	750	30	10
Ca Chien Gung, (Whole Snapper/Ginger)	600	16	6
Canh Chay, (Vegetable/Tofu Soup)	80	3	13
Cari Chicken, 1 cup	475	29	16
Cari Chicken, with Rice Noodle, 1 cup curry & 1 cup noodles	660	29	60
Cari Chicken, with Steamed Rice, 1 cup curry & 1 cup rice	650	29	55
Cuu Xao Lan, (Curried Lamb and Veggies in Coconut)	900	40	80
Ga Chien, (Crisp Chick + Plum Sauce)	900	40	105
Ga Nuong, (Chicken Satay + Sauce)	240	10	4
Ga Xao Rau, (Marinated Chicken Braised with Vegetables)	800	26	100
Gio Lua, (Lean Pork Pie), ⅙ of pie	245	12	0
Goi Cuon, (Cold Spring Rolls), 1 roll	60	1	7
Rau Cai Xao Chay, (Stir Fried Veggies)	400	15	65
Thit Bo Vien, (Beef Balls), 6 balls	225	14	2
Thit Heo Goi Baup Cai, (Spicy Cabb. Rolls with Pork), 1 roll	200	7	11
Soup: *Per Bowl, ½ Cup*			
Bun Bo Hue, (Hot & Spicy Soup):			
Without Pork Feet	340	9	35
With Pork Feet	830	45	35
Chicken & Rice Noodle Soup	400	3	55
Pho Bo, (Beef Noodle Soup)	410	7	59
Pho Ga, (Chicken Noodle Soup)	460	6	58
Pho Tai, (Rare Beef & Noodle Soup)	440	7	73
Salad, Goi Du Du, (Green Papaya), ½ cup	155	3	29
Sauce, Nuoc Cham (Hot Sauce)	5	0	1

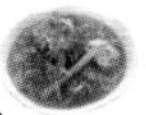
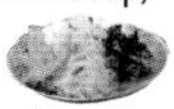

Gourmet & Miscellaneous

	C	F	Cb
Ants Eggs/Larvae, 1 Tbsp	20	0	0
Ants, chocolate coated, 3 Tbsp	140	7	2
Bee Maggots, canned, 3 Tbsp	65	2	0
Caviar, black/red, 1 Tbsp	40	3	0
Caterpillars, canned, 2 oz	60	2	0
Frog Legs, fried, 1 pair (large)	125	7	0
Haggis, boiled, 4 oz	350	24	22
Locusts, roasted, 1 oz	35	1	0
Silkworms, raw, 1 oz	60	2	0
Snails in garlic butter, 6 large	200	10	4
Snake, roasted, 4 oz	160	6	0

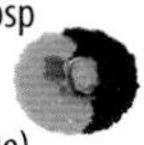
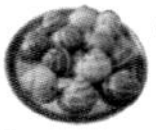

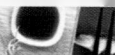

Nutritional data is based on U.S. outlets

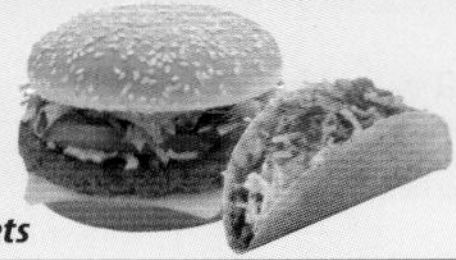

For More Restaurants & Full Nutritional Data ~ See CalorieKing.com

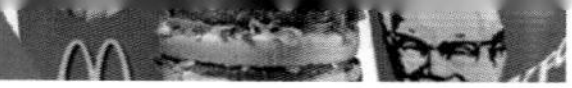

A&W® (Jun '21)

Burgers:	C	F	Cb
Original Bacon Cheeseburger:			
Single	460	23	40
Double	650	36	41
Cheeseburger	400	16	42
Double Cheeseburger	590	29	42
Hamburger	350	11	41
Papa Burger: Single	450	22	42
Double	640	35	42
Sandwiches: Crispy Chicken	480	20	51
Chicken Sliders (2)	460	16	42
Cod Sliders (1)	260	11	41
Grilled: Chicken	410	12	38
Chicken Club	470	17	39
Chicken Tenders, breaded, 3 pcs	260	9	5
Corn Dog Nuggets, 10 pieces	540	26	40
Hot Dogs: Plain	310	18	28
Coney	320	19	26
Coney Cheese Dog	360	22	29
Footlong Hotdog	610	34	52
Fries: Chili Cheese Fries, 7 oz	410	18	51
French Fries:			
Small/Kids, 2.5 oz	210	8	29
Regular, 4 oz	310	13	45
Large, 5.5 oz	430	17	61
Onion Rings, 5.1 oz	280	4	53
Dipping Sauces: *Per 1 oz Cup*			
BBQ	40	0	10
Buttermilk Ranch	130	14	1
Honey Mustard	45	0	10
Spicy Papas	130	12	6
A&W Root Beer Float:			
Regular: 16 oz Cup	310	5	61
20 oz Cup	340	5	68
32 oz Cup	610	11	119
Diet Root Beer, 16 oz	160	5	24
Cones: Chocolate, regular, 5.5 oz	290	7	51
Root Beer, regular, 5.5 oz	260	8	41
Freeze:			
A&W Root Beer: 16 oz	380	9	68
20 oz	520	12	92
Diet Root Beer, 16 oz	270	9	41
Polar Swirls: M&M, 12 oz	810	29	123
Oreo, 12 oz	660	17	100
Reese's Peanut Butter Cup, 12 oz	690	29	95
Shakes: Chocolate/Vanilla, av., 16 oz	540	17	87
Strawberry, 16 oz	520	17	81
Sundaes: Chocolate, regular	360	11	61
Hot Fudge/Hot Caramel, reg., av.	385	13	63

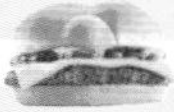
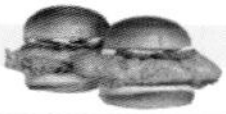
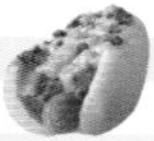
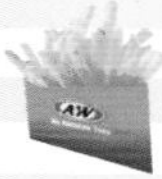

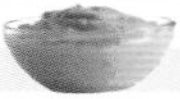
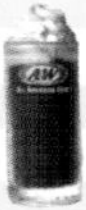

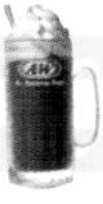

Applebees® (Jun '21)

Appetizers: As Served	C	F	Cb
Boneless Wings, plain	640	32	48
Dressings: Bleu Cheese	190	21	0.5
Ranch	150	15	3
Sauces: Honey BBQ	190	0	46
Sweet Asian Chili	250	2.5	56
Brew Pub Pretzels & Beer Chse Dip	1170	47	151
Chipotle Lime Chicken Quesadillas	1120	69	78
Chicken Wonton Tacos	590	27	50
Crunchy Onion Rings	1220	55	165
Mozzarella Sticks	830	40	81
Neighborhood Nachos, Chicken	1830	118	119
Spinach & Artichoke Dip	990	61	89
Burgers: *With Fries*			
Classic	1150	67	95
Classic Bacon Cheeseburger	1340	82	97
Classic Cheeseburger	1250	75	96
Quesadilla	1650	108	102
Whisky Bacon	1650	102	122
Chicken: *With Menu Set Sides*			
Bourbon Street Chicken & Shrimp	810	46	51
Chicken Tenders Plate	1120	62	102
Chicken Tenders Platter	1430	80	129
Fiesta Lime Chicken	1170	61	97
Grilled Chicken Breast	600	28	46
Fajitas: Loaded Chicken	1510	76	129
Loaded Shrimp	1390	74	130
Loaded Sirloin Steak	1620	88	130
Sandwiches & More: *With Fries*			
Bacon Cheddar Grilled Cheese S'wch	1250	65	99
Chicken Fajita Rollup	1410	77	120
Clubhouse Grille	1450	79	133
Oriental Chicken Salad Wrap	1910	114	180
The Prime Rib Dipper	1370	71	128
Pasta: *As Served, with Breadstick*			
Broccoli Blackened Shrimp Alfredo	1310	76	104
Broccoli Grilled Chicken Alfredo	1420	78	102
Three Cheese Chicken Penne	1320	71	96

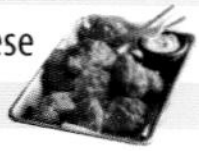
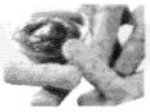
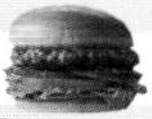
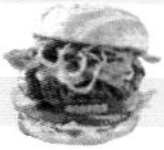
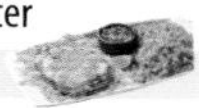
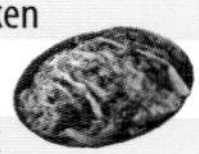
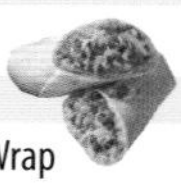

Applebees® cont... (Jun '21)

Seafood: With Menu Set Sides	C	F	Cb
Blackened Cajun Grilled Salmon	660	35	50
Double Crunch Shrimp	1160	51	143
Hand Battered Fish & Chips	1490	103	100
Steaks & Ribs: *With Menu Set Sides*			
6 oz Top Sirloin	620	32	46
8 oz USDA Sirloin	690	36	46
12 oz USDA Ribeye	1010	65	46
Bourbon Street Steak	860	53	49
Double Glazed Baby Back Ribs:			
Full Rack	1450	91	71
Half Rack	880	52	57
Riblets: Plate	900	50	61
Platter	1310	76	76
Shrimp & Parmesan Sirloin, 8 oz	980	60	50
Salads: *Per Regular, with Set Dressing, without Bread*			
Caesar: with Blackened Shrimp	880	60	56
with Grilled Chicken	990	62	54
Crispy Chicken Tender	1220	78	87
Oriental Grilled Chicken	1440	91	105
Strawberry Balsamic Chicken	870	51	56
Soup: Chicken Tortilla	280	15	25
French Onion	380	23	27
Tomato Basil	230	14	23
Fries & Sides:			
Baked Potato: with Sour Cream	530	31	59
Loaded	590	35	59
Breadstick	190	7	25
Classic Fries	430	20	57
Crunchy Onion Rings	510	28	60
Four-Cheese Mac & Cheese w/ Bacon	410	21	34
Garlic Mashed Potatoes	320	17	40
Garlic Mashed Potatoes, loaded	490	33	43
Garlicky Green Beans	160	13	10
Steamed Broccoli	100	8	6
Desserts: *As Served*			
Blue Ribbon Brownie	1410	68	188
Brownie Bite	320	15	45
Sizzlin' Crml Apple Blondie	1230	49	186
Triple Choc. Meltdown	830	37	118

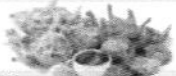
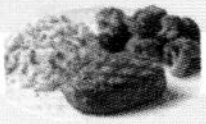
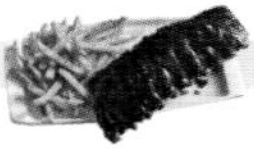
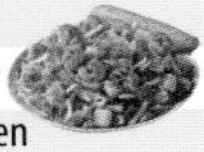
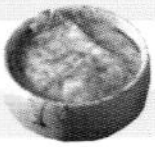
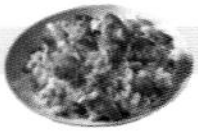
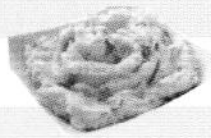
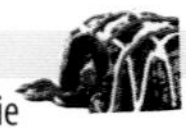

Arby's® (Oct '21)

Sandwiches:	C	F	Cb
Beef 'n Cheddar: Classic	450	20	45
Double	630	32	48
½ Pound	740	39	48
Roast Beef: Classic	360	14	37
Double	510	24	38
½ Pound	610	30	38
Smokehouse Brisket	600	35	42
Chicken: Buffalo Chicken	500	23	48
Chicken Bacon & Swiss	610	30	51
Classic Crispy Chicken	510	25	48
Roast Buffalo Chicken	360	14	36
Roast Chicken Bacon Swiss	480	21	39
Signature: Greek Gyro	710	44	55
Reuben	680	31	62
Roast Beef Gyro	550	29	48
Roast Turkey Gyro	470	20	48
Turkey:			
Roast Turkey & Swiss	720	28	79
Roast Turkey Gyro	470	20	48
Roast Turkey, Ranch & Bacon	810	35	79
Wraps: Creamy Medit. Roast Chicken	540	29	40
Japapeno Bacon Ranch Rst. Chicken	600	33	42
Roast Chicken Club	650	35	47
Sliders: Buffalo Chicken	300	14	31
Chicken 'n Cheese	270	11	30
Jalapeno Roast Beef 'n Cheese	220	9	21
Roast Beef 'n Cheese	210	9	21
Roast Turkey 'n Cheese	180	5	21
Chicken Tenders: 3 pieces	370	18	28
5 pieces	610	30	47
Dipping Sauces: Buffalo, 1 oz	10	1	2
Honey Mustard, 1 oz	130	13	5
Ranch, 1 oz	100	10	1
Tangy BBQ , 1 oz	45	0	10
Crinkle Cut Fries: Small	390	19	49
Medium	530	26	68
Large	620	30	79
Curly Fries: Small	410	22	49
Medium	550	29	65
Large	650	35	77
Sides: *Without Sauce*			
Jalapeno Bites:			
5 pieces	290	17	31
8 pieces	470	27	50
Mozzarella Sticks: 4 pieces	440	23	37
6 pieces	650	35	56

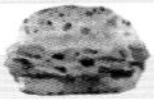
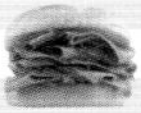
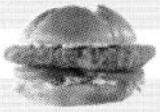
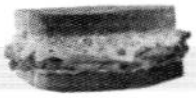
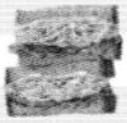
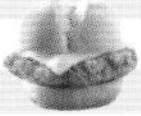
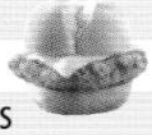
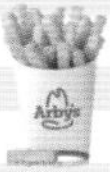

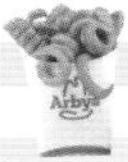

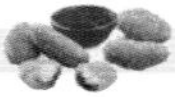
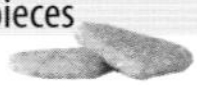

continued next page...

Arby's® cont... (Oct '21)

	C	F	Cb
Salads: Without Dressing			
Crispy Chicken	430	25	27
Roast Chicken	250	14	8
Side Salad	70	5	4
Dressings: Per 1.5 oz Packet			
Balsamic Vinaigrette	130	12	4
Buttermilk Ranch	210	22	2
Dijon Honey Mustard	180	16	7
Light Italian	15	1	2
Kids Menu: Buffalo Chicken Slider	300	14	31
Chicken 'N Cheese Slider	270	11	30
Curly Fries	250	13	29
Premium Chicken Nuggets: 4 pcs	210	10	12
6 pieces	310	15	18
Roast Beef 'n Cheese Slider	210	9	21
Breakfast: Per Serving			
Biscuits: Bacon	340	17	36
Bacon, Egg & Cheese	470	28	38
Chicken	390	18	44
Ham	340	16	37
Ham, Egg & Cheese	460	24	38
Sausage	500	33	36
Sausage, Egg & Cheese	630	44	39
Croissants: Bacon, Egg & Cheese	430	26	29
Ham, Egg & Cheese	410	23	30
Ssge, Egg & Cheese	580	43	30
Potato Cakes: 2 Cakes	250	14	23
3 Cakes	370	21	35
4 Cakes	490	28	46
Sourdoughs:			
Bacon, Egg & Cheese	470	22	46
Ham, Egg & Cheese	460	18	47
Sausage, Egg & Cheese	630	38	47
Wraps: Bacon, Egg & Cheese	490	26	42
Ham, Egg & Cheese	470	23	43
Sausage, Egg & Chse	620	40	42
Sauces: Arby's, 0.5 oz	15	0	3
Bronco Berry, 1 oz	60	0	15
Cheddar Cheese, 1.5 oz	50	3.5	4
Horsey, 0.5 oz	60	5	3
Ketchup, 0.3 oz	10	0	3
Marinara, 1 oz	20	0	4
Spicy Three Pepper, 0.5 oz	25	1	3
Tangy BBQ, 1 oz	45	0	10
Desserts:			
Apple Turnover	430	18	65
Cherry Turnover	390	13	65
Salted Caramel & Chocolate Cookie	430	18	63
Triple Chocolate Cookie	450	21	60
Shakes: Per Medium			
Chocolate; Jamocha	830	24	135
Vanilla	690	23	103

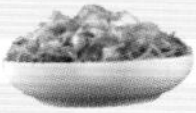
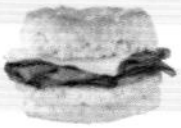
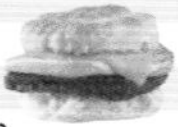
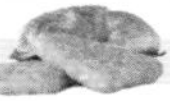
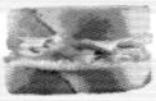
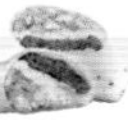
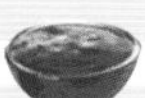
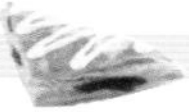

Atlanta Bread Co® (Jun '21)

	C	F	Cb
Breakfast Bagel Sandwiches:			
Egg & Cheese	525	17	69
Egg, Cheese & Ham	505	13	69
Egg, Cheese & Turkey Sausage	500	14	68
Side, Breakfast Potatoes	170	9	20
Paninis: Chicken Pesto	735	30	76
Cuban	845	41	75
Steakhouse	725	33	68
Sandwiches: Chicken Salad	745	42	57
Grilled Caprese	700	36	64
Roast Beef	475	16	52
Roasted Turkey	510	16	58
Tuna Salad	720	38	60
Salads: Per Full Size, with Dressing, without Bread			
Balsamic Blue	605	44	40
Caesar	790	5	60
Chopstix Chicken	855	46	80
Cobb	355	17	32
Greek	700	51	40
Sides, Black Beans & Corn	190	9	24

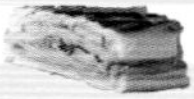
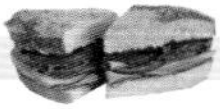
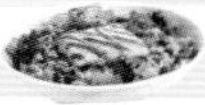

Au Bon Pain® (Jun '21)

	C	F	Cb
Bagels: Per Bagel			
Asiago Cheese, 4 oz	310	5	54
Cinnamon Raisin, 3.7 oz	270	1	57
Everything, 3.6 oz	270	1.5	54
Plain, 3.5 oz	260	0.5	53
Sesame Seed, 3.6 oz	280	2	54
Whole Wheat Skinny , 1.6 oz	90	1	21
Breakfast Sandwiches:			
2 Eggs on a Bagel	400	11	54
with Bacon	450	15	55
with Bacon & Cheese	510	20	55
Egg Whites On Skinny Wheat Bagel:			
Cheddar	210	7	22
Cheddar & Avocado	360	23	25
Smoked Salmon & Avocado	470	16	62
Classic Oatmeal, 12 oz	260	5	47
Fruit Cup, large, 12 oz	140	0.5	36
Yogurt Parfait:			
Blueb. Yog. & Wild Blueb. 10.2 oz	370	9	65
Greek Van. Yog. & Wild Blueb., 10.2 oz	320	8	44
Sandwiches: Per Whole Sandwich			
Cafe: Extra Bacon BLT	510	24	54
Tuna Salad on Croissant	480	23	34
Turkey Club	580	25	49
Signature: Chipotle Turkey & Avoc.	770	43	59
Toasted Chicken & Avocado	620	24	67

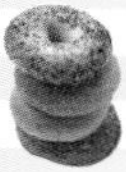
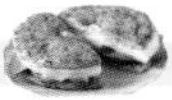
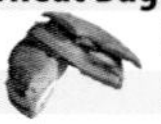
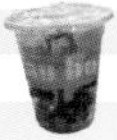
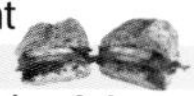

Au Bon Pain® cont... (Jun '21)

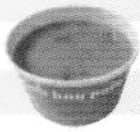
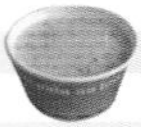
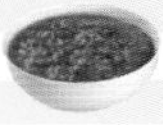
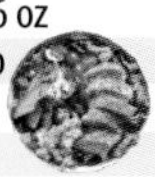

Harvest Hot Bowls:	C	F	Cb
Mayan Chicken	560	11	85
Mediterranean Chicken	670	26	76
Roasted Vegetarian	640	32	75
Teriyaki Steak	700	12	107
***Soups:** Per 12 fl.oz*			
Baked Stuffed Potato	390	24	34
Broccoli Cheddar	340	24	20
Chicken Noodle	120	2.5	15
Clam Chowder	350	20	32
Corn & Green Chili Bisque	270	16	26
Harvest Pumpkin	230	13	24
Lemon Orzo Chicken	230	12	20
Roasted Eggplant	190	6	25
Wild Mushroom Bisque	190	9	23
***Salads:** Without Dressing*			
Chicken Caesar Asiago, 9.6 oz	270	8	21
Chicken Cobb, w/ Avocado	440	24	17
Chef	280	13	10
Mediterranean	350	24	24
Dressings: Bals. Vinaig., 1.5 fl.oz	100	9	5
Caesar, 1.5 fl.oz	220	24	1
Chili Lime Vinaigrette, 1.5 fl.oz	120	10	8
Ranch, 1.5 fl.oz	200	20	4
Cake, Cookies, Croissants, Danish, Dessert:			
Cake, Iced Lemon Pound, 4.5 oz	470	21	66
Cinnamon Swirl Roll, 5.2 oz	530	25	73
Cookies:			
Chocolate Chip, 2.8 oz	370	18	54
Oatmeal Raisin, 2.2 oz	290	11	46
Croissants: Almond, 4 oz	490	25	59
Apple & Cinnamon, 3.4 oz	220	8	33
Chocolate, 4 oz	470	25	55
Plain, 2.4 oz	280	16	28
Danish, Sweet Cheese, 4.4 oz	410	20	50
Muffins:			
Banana Walnut, 4.2 oz	520	29	56
Blueberry, 4.3 oz	420	21	53
Chocolate Chip, 4.2 oz	490	25	61
Scone, Cinnamon Chip, 3.7 oz	460	25	50
Beverages:			
Hot: Caffe Latte, 16 fl.oz	140	7	12
Caramel Macchiato, 16 fl.oz	270	8	41
Chocolate, 16 fl.oz	350	12	51
Iced: Caramel Macchiato, 16 fl.oz	270	8	41
Mocha Latte, 16 fl.oz	300	9	45
Vanilla Latte, 16 fl.oz	230	7	35
Strawb. Banana Smoothie, 16 fl.oz	290	0	68

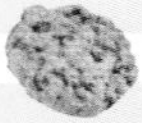
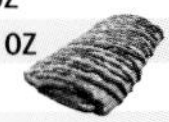
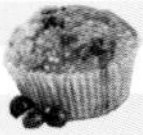
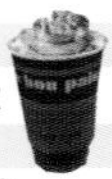

For Complete Items ~ See CalorieKing.com

Auntie Anne's® (Jun '21)

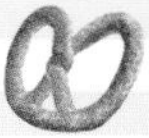
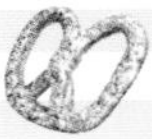
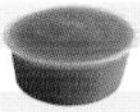
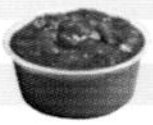
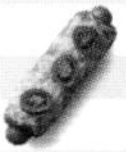

***Pretzels:** With Butter*	C	F	Cb
Cinnamon Sugar	470	12	84
Jalapeno	330	5	63
Original	340	5	65
Pepperoni	480	16	65
Roasted Garlic & Parm.	380	8	68
Sour Cream & Onion	380	8	68
Sweet Almond	390	6	74
Dipping Sauces:			
Caramel, 1.7 oz	170	2	37
Cheese, 1.4 oz	90	8	2
Hot Salsa Cheese, 1.4 oz	90	8	2
Light Cream Cheese, 1.25 oz	80	6	1
Marinara, 2 oz	45	1	7
Melted Cheese, 2 oz	150	12	6
Sweet Glaze, 1.7 oz	150	0	39
Sweet Mustard, 1.5 oz	90	3	14
***Pretzel Dogs:** With Butter*			
Original	360	20	33
Cheese	370	20	33
Jalapeno Cheese	370	20	34
Mini Pretzel Dogs (10)	630	35	56
Pretzel Nuggets, Orig., w/ Butter, 16 oz	390	5	75
Beverages, Frozen Lemonade Mixer, Blue Raspberry; Strawb., 16 fl.oz	230	0	58

Back Yard Burgers® (Jun '21)

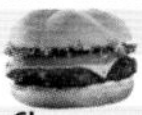
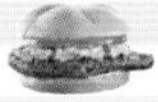

***Black Angus Burgers:** On Brioche Bun*	C	F	Cb
Back Yard Burgers: *Without Cheese Unless Indicated*			
Classic	760	47	49
Double Classic	1210	84	49
Black Jack w/ Pepper Jack Cheese	840	57	44
Black & Bleu w/ Blue Cheese Crumbles	940	65	46
Chipotle with Cheddar Cheese	1000	67	56
Mushroom Swiss with Swiss Cheese	850	56	44
***Chicken Sandwiches:** On Brioche Bun*			
Blackened Chicken w/out cheese	620	27	51
Black Jack Chicken Club w/ P. Jack	710	37	47
Grilled Chicken w/out cheese	460	11	46
Hawaiian Chicken, w/out cheese	530	11	64
Specialties:			
Breaded Chicken Tender Basket, w/o Toppings, Chse, Sce or Bread	540	36	27
Veggie Burger, Brioche Bun, w/o Chse	430	10	68
***Turkey Burgers:** On Brioche Bun*			
Classic, without cheese	540	28	42
Club with Swiss Cheese	660	38	43
Wild with Pepper Jack Cheese	610	33	44

continued next page ...

Back Yard Burgers® cont... (Jun '21)

Fries:	C	F	Cb
Chili Cheese Fries, seasoned, reg.	**790**	59	52
Seasoned Fries: Regular, 4.5 oz	**480**	36	38
Large, 6 oz	**640**	47	50
Sweet Potato Fries, regular, 6 oz	**450**	29	40
Waffle Fries: Reg., 6 oz	**820**	56	66
Large, 8 oz	**1100**	75	88
Sides: Back Yard Chili	**310**	18	15
Creamy Cole Slaw	**200**	16	15
Loaded Baked Potato	**420**	21	45
Panko Onion Rings, regular, 4 oz	**340**	13	47
Salads: Without Dressing			
Back Yard: with Blackened Chicken	**450**	21	22
with Grilled Chicken	**350**	10	21
Cranberry Pecan w/ Blackened Chkn	**770**	41	52
Side Salad with Cheddar Cheese	**140**	6	14
Dressings:			
Bleu Cheese	**220**	24	1
Caesar	**260**	26	4
Gorgonzola Vinaigrette	**170**	15	6
Honey Mustard	**200**	20	7
Ranch, Homestyle	**150**	16	1
Dessert/Cobblers: Apple/Cherry	**390**	16	58
Apple/Cherry Cobbler A La Mode	**540**	24	78
Ice Cream, A La Carte	**150**	8	20
Milk Shakes: With Whole Milk & Whipped Topping			
Chocolate: Vanilla, av.	**745**	35	98
Chocolate Oreo	**850**	40	115
Peanut Butter	**830**	51	79

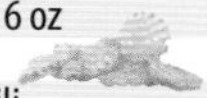
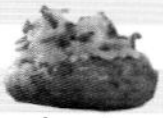
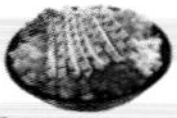
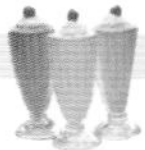

Baja Fresh® (Oct '21)

Baja Bowls: With Black Beans	C	F	Cb
Carnitas	**680**	18	92
Chicken	**700**	22	82
Shrimp	**660**	20	83
Steak	**690**	22	82
Veggie	**540**	14	90
Burritos: With Standard Components			
Baja: with Carnitas	**800**	41	63
with Chicken	**820**	46	53
with Steak	**810**	45	53
Mexicano: *With Black Beans*			
Chicken	**800**	27	94
Roasted Veggie	**640**	19	102
Steak	**790**	26	94
Ultimo: Carnitas	**950**	45	88
Chicken	**970**	50	78
Steak	**960**	50	78
Nachos: Large Size, with Black Beans			
Chicken	**1960**	105	162
Shrimp	**1920**	104	164
Steak	**1950**	105	162

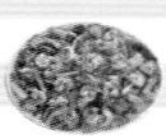
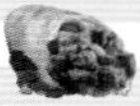
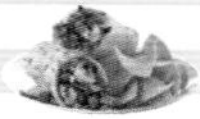
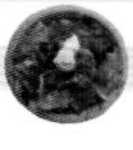

Baja Fresh® cont... (Oct '21)

Fajitas: With Pinto Beans	C	F	Cb
Chicken: with Corn Tortilla	**1060**	39	121
with Flour Tortilla	**1250**	44	146
Shrimp: with Corn Tortilla	**990**	35	123
with Flour Tortilla	**1180**	41	148
Steak: with Corn Tortilla	**1050**	38	121
with Flour Tortilla	**1240**	44	146
Wahoo: with Corn Tortilla	**990**	35	121
with Flour Tortilla	**1180**	40	146
Tacos: With Standard Toppings			
Americano, Soft Taco: Carnitas	**220**	9	21
Chicken	**230**	11	19
Baja, meat/fish varieties, average	**160**	6	17
Wahoo Crispy Taco	**250**	15	24
Salads: Without Dressing			
Baja Ensalada:			
with Chicken	**260**	11	18
with Shrimp	**280**	12	19
with Steak	**250**	11	17
Tostada: *With Pinto Beans*			
Chicken	**1030**	53	89
Shrimp	**1000**	51	90
Steak	**1030**	53	88
Sides: Guacamole, 8 oz	**310**	27	19
Queso, 8 oz	**470**	37	13
Rice & Black Beans, 17.4 oz	**580**	13	91
Rice & Pinto Beans, 17.4 oz	**600**	13	96
Tortilla Chips, 5 oz	**710**	28	99

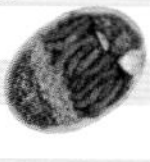
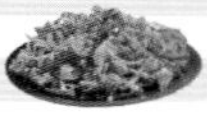
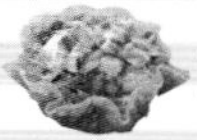

For Complete Nutritional Data ~ see CalorieKing.com

Baskin Robbins® (Oct '21)

Cones:	C	F	Cb
Cake	**25**	0	5
Fancy Waffle Cone, with Sprinkles	**310**	13	46
Fresh-Baked Waffle	**155**	4	29
Sugar	**50**	0.5	10
Ice Creams: Per 4 oz Scoop			
Classic Flavors: Baseball Nut	**260**	14	29
Caramel Macchiato	**280**	15	34
Cherries Jubilee	**240**	11	31
Chocolate	**240**	14	26
Chocolate Almond	**280**	18	25
Chocolate Chip	**250**	16	23
Cotton Candy	**230**	12	28
Jamoca Almond Fudge	**260**	15	27
Made with Snickers Bars	**270**	14	32
Mint Chocolate Chip	**250**	16	23
Mom's Makin' Cookies	**310**	15	41
Nutty Coconut	**290**	19	24

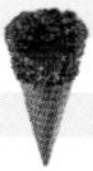
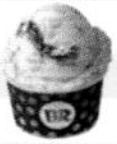
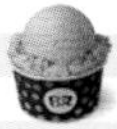
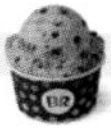

Baskin Robbins® cont... (Oct'21)

Ice Creams (Cont): Per 4 oz Scoop	C	F	Cb
Classic Flavors Cont:			
Old Fashioned Butter Pecan	280	18	25
Oreo Cookies 'n Cream	260	15	28
Peanut Butter 'n Chocolate	300	20	25
Oreo 'n Cold Brew	320	18	35
Pistachio Almond	270	19	21
Pralines 'n Cream	270	14	31
Quarterback Crunch	300	17	33
Reese's P'nut Butter Cup	280	17	27
Rocky Road	290	15	35
Strawberry Cheesecake	250	13	29
Vanilla	240	16	21
Very Berry Strawberry	200	11	24
World Class Chocolate	260	16	25
No Sugar Added:			
Caramel Turtle Truffle	200	8	38
Pineapple Coconut	160	6	29
Note: Carbohydrate figures include 14-25 g sugar alcohol			
Non Dairy:			
Choc. Chip Cookie Dough	270	14	36
Salted Fudge Bar	250	11	41
Strawberry Streusel	230	7	42
Wild 'n Reckless Sherbet	130	2	26
Ice Cream Quarts: *Per ⅔ Cup, 3.46 oz*			
Chocolate/ Mint Chocolate Chip, av.	210	13	21
Gold Medal Ribbon	210	11	25
Peanut Butter 'n Choc.	260	18	22
Pralines 'n Cream	250	13	29
Vanilla	210	14	18
Very Berry Strawberry	180	9	21
Sundaes: Banana Royale	690	28	103
Choc. Chip Cookie Dough	1130	48	164
Made with Snickers	1110	43	165
Oreo Layered	920	44	122
Reese's Peanut Butter Cup	1250	85	106
Bakery, Brownie, 2.2 oz	240	9	36
Beverages: *Per Medium, 24 fl.oz*			
Blasts: Caramel Cappuccino	790	25	130
Mocha Cappuccino	590	22	97
Oreo Cookies 'n Cream	730	31	105
Turtle	820	23	148
Milkshakes: Chocolate Chip	1030	54	118
World Class Chocolate	1060	55	123
Smoothie: Mango Banana	600	1	145
Strawberry Banana	520	1	126
Tropical Banana	540	1	127

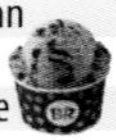
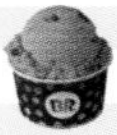
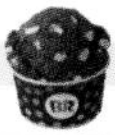
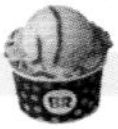
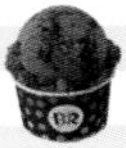
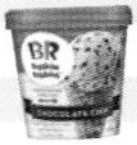
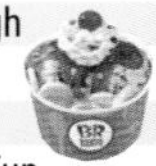
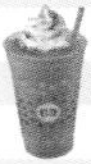
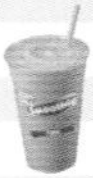

Big Apple Bagels® (Oct'21)

Bagels:	C	F	Cb
Asiago Melt; Swiss Melt	370	6	65
Cinnamon Sugar	370	2	78
Everything	340	3	66
Plain or Salt	320	2	64
Cream Cheese: *Per 1.5 oz*			
Cheddar & Bacon	140	13	4
Plain/Salsa/Scallion, average	135	12	2
Plain, Lite	100	9	2
Strawberry	130	11	5
Tomato-Basil/Lox/Dill Garlic, av.	140	13	3
Muffins: *With Whole Egg*			
Mini: Blueberry; Lemon Poppyseed	90	4.5	12
Cinnamon Swirl Cheesecake	90	5	9
Large:			
Blueberry	590	28	78
Choc. Cheesecake, 6 oz	650	38	70
Breakfast Sandwiches:			
French Toast with Egg:			
on BAB Bagel	1020	55	107
On MFM Bagel	1060	55	117
Salads:			
Caesar, with Caesar Dressing	450	34	19
Chicken Club, with Ranch Dressing	760	59	18
Mediterranean Bread Salad, with Balsamic Vinaigrette	740	41	63
Beverages: *Per Medium, 16 fl.oz*			
Hot Chocolate	440	12	71
Mocha; White Chocolate Latte, av.	380	8	67
Vanilla Creme Latte	310	7	50

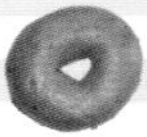
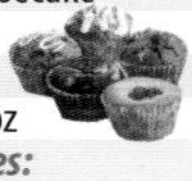
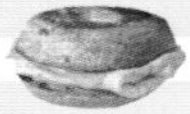

Biggby Coffee® (Jun '21)

Hot Drinks: *Per Tall, 16 fl.oz, without Whipped Cream*	C	F	Cb
Cafe au Lait: with 2% Milk	100	4	9
with Nonfat Milk	65	0	9
with Soy	90	3	11
Caffe Latte: with 2% Milk	175	7	16
with Nonfat Milk	115	0	16
with Soy	160	5	19
Cappuccino: with 2% Milk	105	5	10
with Nonfat Milk	70	0	10
with Soy	95	3	11
Chai Latte: with 2% Milk	315	7.5	51
with Nonfat Milk	255	0	51
Dark Hot Chocolate: w/ 2% Milk	320	9	50
with Non-Fat Milk	260	2	50
Creme Freeze Smoothies: *Per 16fl.oz w/out Wh. Crm*			
Banana Berry	405	6	89
Mango	540	5	118
Peachberry	410	5.5	76
Raspberry Zinger	385	5	85

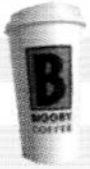
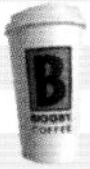
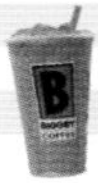

BJ's Restaurant® (Dec'20)

Shareable Appetizers: Full Order	C	F	Cb
Ahi Poke	320	10	24
Chicken Lettuce Wraps	490	19	46
Crisp Potato Skin Platter	1300	60	137
Mozzarella Sticks	810	39	76
Root Beer Glazed Ribs	560	17	85
Sliders	800	30	81
Spinach Stuffed Mushrooms	290	20	17
Burgers: With French Fries			
Brewhouse: Bacon Cheeseburger	1260	74	94
Black & Bleuhouse	1240	73	94
Brewhouse	1090	60	93
Loaded Burgers: Crispy Jalapeno	1430	87	105
Mushroom Swiss Burger	1600	105	102
Brunch: Avocado Toast	410	20	47
Buttermilk Pancakes, short stack	910	31	143
Calif. Scramble, w/ sourdough	1210	69	90
Enlightened Veggie Omelette w/ Fruit	250	8	23
Enlightened Entrees: Includes Menu Set Sides			
Cherry Chipotle Glazed Salmon	580	26	40
Lemon Thyme Chicken	630	19	52
Mediterranean: Chicken Pita Tacos	720	24	80
Spiced Chicken	750	50	21
Seared Ahi Salad	570	31	42
Turkey Burger	850	45	72
Pasta: Includes Garlic Knot			
Deep Dish Ziti	1400	91	99
Grilled Chicken Alfredo	1460	71	129
Italiano Veggie Penne	700	28	91
Jumbo Spaghetti & Meatballs	1600	82	161
Shrimp Scampi	1660	100	130
Deep Dish Pizza: Per Slice, 1/8 Med. Pizza			
BBQ/Buffalo Chicken, average	310	10	35
Classic Combo; Pepperoni Extreme, av.	335	17	32
Gourmet Five Meat	360	18	33
Sweet Pig; Vegetarian, average	265	10	34
Tavern Crust Pizza: Per Slice (1/12 Pizza)			
Brewhouse; Italian Market, average	115	6	9
Garlic Chicken Pesto	100	5	9
Spicy Pig; Old Country Tomato, average	80	4	9
Sandwiches: With French Fries			
Brewhouse Philly	1490	90	108
California Chicken Club	1310	69	91
Slow Roasted Turkey Club	1560	99	104
Ribs & Steaks: Without Sides			
Baby Back Pork Ribs, half rack, with Peppered BBQ Sauce	710	34	74
Classic Rib-Eye	1080	67	5
Dble Bone In Pork Chop	610	38	13
Prime Rib Dinner	1310	106	6
Soups: Chicken Tortilla, Bowl	280	12	30
Clam Chowder: Bowl with Crackers	510	31	37
Sourdough Loaf with Crackers	1470	42	219

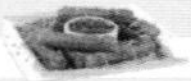
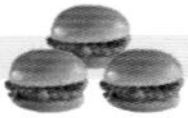
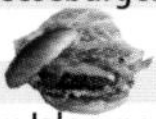
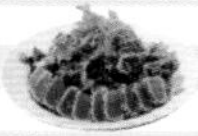
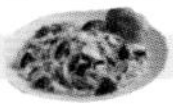
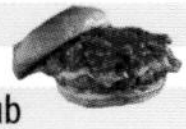
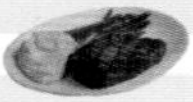

BJ's Restaurant® cont...(Dec'20)

Salads: With Dressing & Toppings	C	F	Cb
BBQ Chicken Chopped Salad	930	47	64
Caesar Salad	810	64	44
Derby-Style Chicken Cobb Salad	940	69	20
Honey-Crisp Chicken Salad	1360	103	75
Tri-Tip Wedge Salad	1300	91	68
Sides: Broccoli	40	0	6
Classic Baked Potato	590	28	70
French Fries	350	19	40
Honey Sriracha Brussels Sprouts	160	4	23
Rice Pilaf	230	6	39
White Cheddar Mashed Potatoes	330	18	33
Desserts: Baked Beignet	640	25	93
Monkey Bread Pizookie	1380	67	182
Salted Caramel Pizookie	1380	56	204
Soda Floats, Black Cherry/Or. Crm	535	19	83

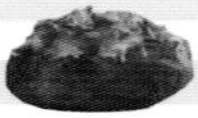

Blimpie® (Oct'21)

Cold Deli Subs:	C	F	Cb
Per Regular, 6" White Sub, with Standard Menu Board Toppings			
Blimpie Best; Turkey & Prov., av.	465	16	54
Club; Ham & Swiss	430	14	54
Roast Beef & Provolone	460	14	53
Tuna	480	22	48
Wraps, average	580	30	52
Hot Deli Subs: Per Regular White Sub with Standard Menu Board Toppings Unless Indicated			
BLT	510	27	48
Meatball Parmigiana	740	38	59
Philly Cheesesteak	570	28	49
Salads: Regular, without Dressing			
Buffalo Chicken; Grilled Chicken, av.	170	7	7
Garden	40	0	8
Macaroni	290	21	22
Potato	190	10	24
Ultimate Club	310	16	11
Dressings: Per 1.5 oz			
Blue Cheese; B'mlk Ranch, average	245	26	3
Creamy Ital.; Pepp. Ranch, average	240	25	2
Thousand Island; Creamy Caesar, av.	205	21	4
Soup: Chicken Noodle	210	4	29
Cream of Broccoli with Cheese	190	11	15
Crm of Potato w/ Bacon	190	9	24
New Eng. Clam Chowder	170	3	28
Vegetable Beef with Barley	100	3	14
Breakfast:			
Biscuits: Bacon, Egg & Cheese	410	22	37
Sausage, Egg & Cheese	560	36	37
Bluffin, Egg & Cheese	240	8	29
Burritos: Ham, Egg & Cheese	570	27	51
Sausage, Egg & Cheese	710	43	50
Sandwich, Grilled Bacon	520	23	49

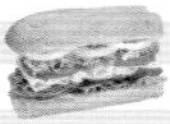
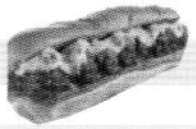
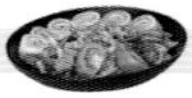
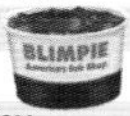

Bob Evans® (Jun '21)

Burgers:	C	F	Cb
Big Farm Burgers:			
Bacon Cheeseburger	810	48	47
Rise & Shine	1300	77	102
Steakhouse	1040	60	56
Sandwiches:			
Farmhouse Chicken	530	32	41
Slow Roasted:			
Pot Roast	810	49	47
Turkey Bacon Melt	670	33	45
Dinners:			
Best Farmhouse Dinners: *With Menu Set Sides*			
Down-Home Country Fried Steak	730	45	58
Fork-Tender Pot Roast	950	62	62
Heartland Chicken Pot Pie	1430	87	106
Herb Rubbed Turkey & Dressing	820	40	81
Craveable Classics: Without Sides			
Great Alaska Cod with Tartar Sauce	640	39	39
Grilled Chicken Breast (2)	270	4	2
Lemon Sole, 2 fillets	380	18	25
Homestyle: *Without Sides*			
Boneless Fried Chicken Breast (2)	580	27	19
Fried Chicken Tenders (3)	640	36	46
Sirloin & Shrimp with Cocktail Sce	710	36	39
USDA Choice Sirloin with Toppings	660	45	10
Sides: Baked Potato	330	12	51
Bread & Celery Dressing	340	15	42
Broccoli, with Butter	110	10	5
Carrots	90	4.5	13
Coleslaw	200	14	19
Corn	170	10	20
French Fries	330	14	47
Green Beans with Ham	30	1.5	4
Hashbrowns	220	12	28
Homefries	250	17	24
Mac & Cheese	250	12	25
Mashed Potatoes: w/ Chicken Gravy	210	14	19
with Country Gravy	170	10	17
Salads: Regular Size, with dressing			
Cranberry Pecan Chicken	920	59	55
Wildfire: without Chicken	390	22	44
with Grilled Chicken	660	26	46
with Homestyle Chicken	970	49	63

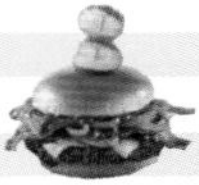
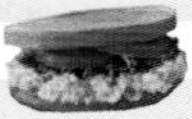
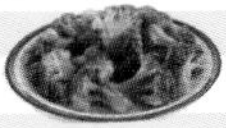
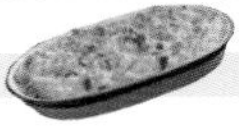
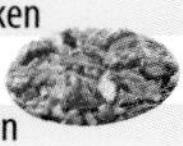

Bob Evans® cont... (Jun '21)

Soups: Per Bowl, with 4 Saltine Crackers	C	F	Cb
Cheddar Baked Potato	390	21	32
Chicken N Noodles	290	15	26
Hearty Beef Vegetable	230	5	36
Kid's: With Menu Set Sides			
Chicken & Noodles with Broccoli	150	7	14
Cheeseburger with Fries	760	36	84
Gr. Cheese S'wch & Tomato Basil Soup	430	22	43
Gr. Chicken w/ Broccoli, Roll, Apple Jce	360	6	52
Grilled Cheese Triangles w/ Fresh Fruit	330	15	40
Mac & Cheese with Broccoli	280	12	31
Turkey Lurkey w/ Mshd Pot., Carrots & Chicken Gravy	410	23	34
Breakfast: As Served with Menu Set Sides			
Country Fried Steak, Eggs & Gravy	540	33	38
Everything Breakfast	1130	73	63
Three Meat Omelet without Bread	1210	94	21
Western Omelet without Bread	650	50	11
Hotcakes: *With Menu Set Toppings*			
Buttermilk (4)	1150	28	209
Cinnamon Supreme (4)	1070	26	190
Brioche Fr. Toast, w/ butter & syrup	830	25	134
Doule Blueberry Hotcakes (4)	1090	23	203
Double Chocolate (4)	1120	27	199
Multigrain (4)	1200	31	214
Pot Roast Hash, w/out Eggs or Bread	580	39	28
Sunshine Skillet without Bread	760	59	27
Breakfast Sides:			
Eggs: Egg White	60	0	0.5
Freshly Cracked	200	16	0.5
Scrambled	160	11	1
Home Fries	250	17	24
Grits with butter	240	21	13
Hardwood Smoked Bacon	190	14	0.5
Hashbrowns	220	12	28
Hickory-Smoked Ham	100	2.5	2
Sausage Links (3)	190	16	0
Sausage Patties (2)	320	26	2
Turkey Sausage Links (2)	140	7	2
Dessert: Cherry Pie, plain, slice	610	31	75
Chocolate Peanut Butter Pie, 1 slice	680	41	74
Double-Crust Apple Pie, 1 slice	530	24	77

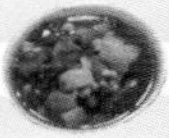
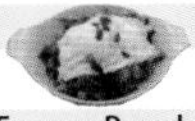
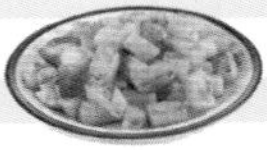
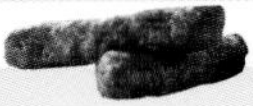

Bojangles® (Oct '21)

Biscuit:	C	F	Cb
Bacon, Egg & Cheese	510	27	40
Cajun Filet	570	27	57
Country Ham	460	25	38
Gravy Biscuit	430	21	49
Sausage	470	28	38
Sausage & Egg	550	34	38
Southern Filet	550	27	54
Steak	620	40	48
Biscuit Add Ons: American Cheese	40	3.5	1
Egg	80	6	0
Chicken: Breast (1)	540	29	24
Leg (1)	190	13	8
Thigh (1)	240	10	14
Wing (1)	150	8	8
Homestyle Tenders, 4 pieces	490	24	39
Supremes, 4 pieces	500	25	33
Sandwiches: Bo's Chicken	670	36	95
Grilled Chicken	570	33	36
Grilled Chicken Club	690	39	39
Fixins': Per Individual Size, Unless Indicated			
Bo-Tato Rounds, medium	390	24	40
Cole Slaw	170	11	20
Green Beans	20	0	5
Macaroni & Cheese	280	18	21
Mashed Potatoes 'N Cajun Gravy	120	3	18
Seasoned Fries: Small	360	21	39
Medium	450	26	49
Picnic	670	38	73
Salads: Without Dressing or Croutons			
Chicken Supreme	490	28	28
Garden	120	9	3
Grilled Chicken	270	14	4
Dressings: Blue Cheese, 1.5 fl.oz	230	24	2
Buttermilk Ranch, 1.5 fl. oz	200	20	2
Honey Dijon, 1.5 fl.oz	120	7	14
Sweets: Bo-Berry Biscuit (1)	370	17	49
Cinnamon Twist (1)	380	24	38
Sweet Potato Pie	350	20	41

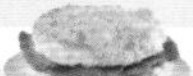
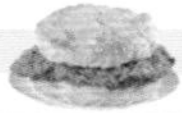
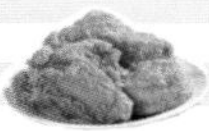
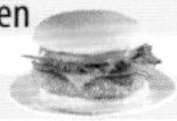
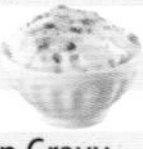
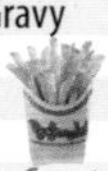
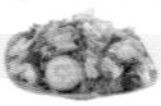
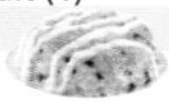

Boston Market® (Oct '21)

Sandwiches: Per Whole Sandwich, with Standard Ingredients	C	F	Cb
Chkn Avocado Club on Ciabatta Roll	1110	66	75
Chkn Salad Carver on Multigr. Roll	870	51	63
Rstd Turkey Carver on Ciabatta Roll	970	55	73
Sthwest Chkn Carver on Ciabatta Roll	1110	65	76
Individual Meals: Without Sides or Corn Bread			
Meatloaf, regular	470	33	17
Parmesan Rotisserie Half Chicken	590	28	12
Roasted Garlic & Herb Half Chkn	650	35	13
Rotisserie Prime Rib	630	47	0
Sesame Half Chicken	630	30	18
Turkey Pot Pie	710	38	64

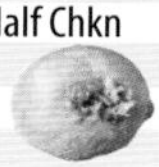

Boston Market® cont...(Oct '21)

Salad Bowls: With Dressing	C	F	Cb
Chicken Caesar	770	51	33
Southwest Cobb	760	53	30
Sides: Cornbread	160	3	31
Creamed Spinach	240	17	12
Fresh Steamed Veggies	60	3.5	7
Fresh Vegetable Stuffing	220	10	28
Garlic Dill New Potatoes100	100	2	20
Macaroni & Cheese	310	10	41
Mashed Potatoes	270	11	37
Steamed Brocoli	35	0	6
Sweet Corn,	160	7	20
Sweet Potato Casserole	460	12	87
Soup, Chicken Noodle	240	9	20
Kid's: Without Sides or Corn Bread			
Chicken: Dark, 1 thigh, 1 drumstick	230	13	0.5
White, 1 breast, 1 wing	270	11	0
Meatloaf	240	16	9
Turkey	80	2.5	0
Sauce: Cranberry Walnut Relish	140	2	31
Gravy, Beef/Au Jus/Chicken	10	0	2
Horseradish	60	3	6
Zesty BBQ	40	0	10
Desserts: Apple Pie, 1 slice	560	32	66
Chocolate Brownie (1)	340	14	53
Chocolate Cake, 1 slice	570	33	66
Chocolate Chunk Cookie (1)	370	18	53

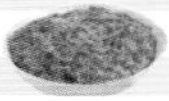
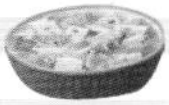
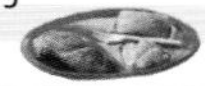
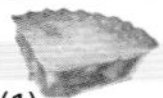

For Complete Nutritional Data ~ see CalorieKing.com

Boston Pizza® (Oct '21)

Starters:	C	F	Cb
Bourbon Poutine	880	28	128
Nonna's Meatballs	1280	67	116
Spinach & Artichoke Dip	1260	58	137
Burgers: Black Bean Veggie	510	19	74
Boston Brute	800	24	108
The Big Dipper	1200	60	116
Vegan	460	16	73
Mains:			
Bowls: Honey Dill Chicken, grilled	1080	34	143
Salmon Power	930	26	135
Vegan	1050	33	167
Chicken Parmesan	780	33	76
NY Striploin Steak	800	56	48
Pizzas: Per 8" Individual Pizza			
Original Crust: Boston Royal	820	28	97
Deluxe	720	24	92
Hawaiian	660	16	100
Pepperoni	710	25	89
Vegetarian	620	15	94
Thin Crust Pizzas: *Per Slice of 13" Medium Pizza*			
Fiesta Chicken, 2.86 oz	200	11	18
Pesto Caprese	230	13	18
Pizza Bella, 2.3 oz	150	6	17

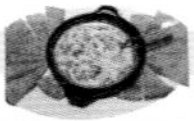
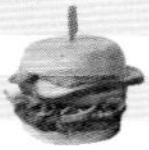
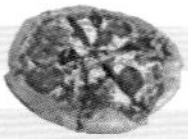
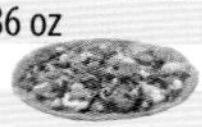

Boston Pizza® (Oct'21)

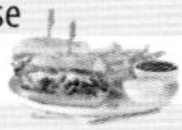

Sandwiches: Without Sides	C	F	Cb
Grilled Chicken Clubhouse	1040	44	98
Kick'n Memphis Chicken	1210	75	86
Montreal Smoked Meat	910	59	40
Wrap, Thai Chicken, grilled	820	33	87
Salads: Chicken Caesar	680	49	13
Pineapple, Beet & Goat Cheese	390	24	36
Thai Chicken	720	24	86
Desssert:			
NY Cheesecake	580	37	54
The Panookie, with Ice Cream	940	45	125

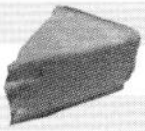

For Complete Nutritional Data ~ see CalorieKing.com

Braum's® ~ *see CalorieKing.com*

Bruegger's® (Oct'21)

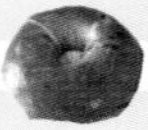

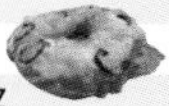

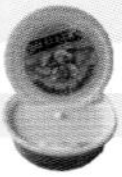

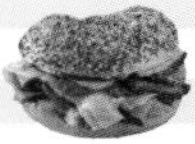

Bagels:	C	F	Cb
Blueberry, 4.1 oz	310	2	63
Cinnamon Sugar, 4.1 oz	320	2	63
Everything, 4.1 oz	310	2.5	62
Five Cheese, 4.1 oz	350	9	53
Jalapeno Cheddar, 5.5 oz	440	9	75
Plain, 4.1 oz	300	2	60
Rosemary Olive Oil, 4.1 oz	330	6	59
Sesame, 4.1 oz	310	3	60
***Cream Cheese:** Per 1.5 oz*			
Bacon Scallion; Jalapeno, average	140	12	5
Honey Walnut	150	12	8
Light Herb Garlic/Plain	100	6	4
Plain; Garden Veggie	130	11	6
Smoked Salmon; Strawberry	145	13	3
***Breakfast Bagel S'wiches:** With Standard Toppings*			
Egg, Cheese & Bacon	500	24	64
Egg, Cheese & Ham	510	16	65
Egg, Cheese & Turkey Sausage	510	23	63
Egg, Cheese & Sausage	590	34	63
***Deli Sandwiches:** Plain Bagel With Standard Toppings*			
BLT	530	23	64
Garden Veggie	360	2	72
Ham	410	7	64
Tuna Salad	550	21	65
***Signature & Bagel Sandwiches:** W/ Standard Toppings*			
Herby Turkey on Sesame Bagel	570	15	75
Hot Pastrami on Everything Bagel	590	19	66
Hot Tuna on Ciabatta	500	24	51
Leon. da Veggie on Asiago Parm. Bagel	490	14	70
Sm. Salmon Egg Salad on Pumpnkl Bgl	570	21	64
Turkey Chipotle Club on Evrythng Bagel	810	45	66

Bruegger's® cont... (Oct'21)

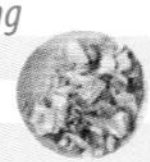

***Salads:** Without Dressing*	C	F	Cb
Chicken Caesar	200	8	14
Garden with Chicken	270	14	22
Mixed Green Base	20	0	4
Dressings: Balsamic Vinaigrette, 1 oz	60	6	3
Caesar, 1 oz	80	7	2
Sides, Twice Baked Hashbrowns	170	11	12
Soup: Chicken & Wild Rice, 8 oz	230	16	14
Chicken Spaetzle, 8 oz	140	3.5	14
Dessert: Blueberry Muffin, Main St.	490	28	54
Marshmallow Chew, 2.7 oz	290	7	54

For Complete Menu & Data ~ see CalorieKing.com

Burgerville® (Oct'21)

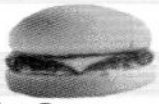

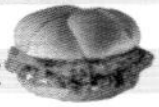

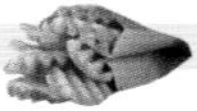

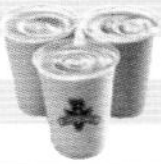

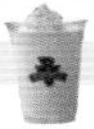

***Burgers:** With Standard Ingredients*	C	F	Cb
Colossal on Non Seeded Bun	540	28	40
½ lb Colossal On Non Seeded Bun	790	46	40
Double Cheeseburger on Plain Bun	490	28	31
Original: Hamburger on Plain Bun	340	17	31
Cheeseburger on Plain Bun	380	21	31
Northwest Cheeseburger			
on Non Seeded Bun	590	33	38
Number 6 Burger on Brioche Bun	620	37	30
Pepper Bacon on Non Seeded Bun	660	39	37
Walla Walla Wonder on Non Seeded Bun	450	18	40
Chicken & Chips, without sauce	770	43	71
Halibut Fish & Chips, w/out sauce	690	33	73
***Sandwiches:** Without Cheese*			
Best Coast Chkn on Non Seeded Bun	430	16	36
Crispy Chkn, on Non Seeded Bun	610	32	61
Halibut Fish on Plain Bun	460	27	40
French Fries: Small, 2.8 oz	220	11	28
Regular, 5 oz	400	19	50
Large, 6.5 oz	510	25	65
Waffly Fries, regular	280	14	34
Farm Salad:			
with Blue Cheese Crumblies	120	8	3
with Grilled Chicken Breast	100	2	4
with Smoked Salmon	90	2.5	3
Dressing: Balsamic Vinaigrette	180	18	5
Blue Cheese	180	18	2
Ranch	190	20	2
***Bliss Shakes (Non Dairy):** Per 16 oz w/out Wh. Cream*			
Chocolate	840	31	143
Mint Patty	940	38	148
Oregon Strawberry	860	38	129
Sweet Cream	610	28	89
***Ice Cream Milkshakes:** Per 16 oz with Whipped Cream*			
Chocolate Hazelnut	1080	72	98
Portland Cold Brew	910	55	89
Sweet Cream	930	57	92

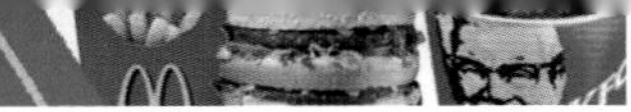

Burger King® (Oct '21)

Flame Gr. Burgers & Sandwiches:

	C	F	Cb
Burgers:			
Bacon Cheeseburger	315	16	27
Double	405	22	27
Cheeseburger	285	13	27
Double	390	21	28
Hamburger	240	10	26
Rodeo	330	14	38
Sandwiches:			
Bacon King: Combo/Single Size	1430	74	53
Regular	2105	93	52
Double Quater Pound King	1065	67	53
Garlic Bacon King, Combo size	1135	75	59
Whopper: Regular	660	40	49
Double Whopper	900	58	49
with Cheese	980	64	50
Impossible Whopper	630	34	58
Texas Double Whopper	1875	136	58
Triple Whopper with Cheese	1300	89	52
Whopper Jr	315	18	27
Burrito, Egg-Normous	805	44	69
Chicken Sandwiches:			
Original	660	40	48
Ch'King: Regular	800	39	69
Deluxe	890	54	70
Spicy	950	60	72
Spicy Deluxe	1050	69	74
Jr: Regular	450	30	34
BLT	490	32	37
Spicy	385	21	37
Chicken Nuggets: Without Sauce			
4 pieces	225	11	23
10 pieces	480	27	39
Dipping Sauces: BBQ	40	0	11
Buffalo	80	8	2
Ranch; Zesty Onion Ring, av.	145	15	2
Fish Sandwich,			
Big Fish	515	28	51
Platters: Pancake	440	16	71
with Sausage	605	31	72
Sides:			
Cheesy Tots, 8 pieces	315	16	35
Chicken Fries, 9 pieces	430	32	21
Onion Rings: Small	470	31	44
Medium	565	36	56
Large	655	40	67

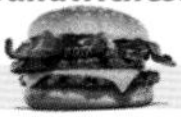
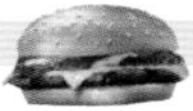
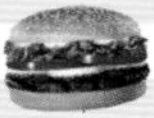
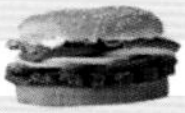
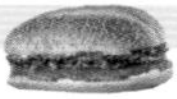
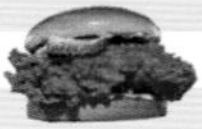
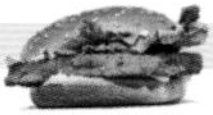
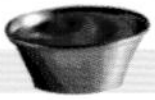
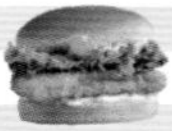
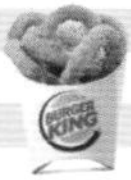

Burger King® cont... (Oct '21)

Fries:	C	F	Cb
Classic Fries: Small, 4.3 oz	320	13	49
Medium, 5.8 oz	385	17	53
Large, 7 oz	435	19	60
Breakfast:			
Biscuits:			
Bacon, Egg & Cheese	385	25	29
Egg & Cheese	475	30	33
Fully Loaded Buttermilk	615	42	31
Ham, Egg & Cheese	370	23	29
Sausage	430	30	30
Sausage, Egg & Cheese	520	37	29
Double	910	69	35
Croissan'wich:			
Bacon, Egg & Cheese	335	18	30
Bacon, Sausage, Egg & Cheese	580	40	31
Fully Loaded	570	37	32
Ham, Egg & Cheese	335	16	31
Sausage, Egg & Cheese	515	35	30
Double	795	59	32
French Toast Stick:			
3 pieces	230	11	29
5 pieces	380	18	49
Hash Browns: Small, 3 oz	250	16	24
Medium, 6 oz	505	33	48
Large, 8 oz	670	44	65
Desserts:			
Chocolate Chip Cookie	160	8	24
Pie, Hershey's Sundae	305	19	32
Sundae, Chocolate Fudge	270	7	47
Vanilla Soft Serve: Cone	140	4	24
Cup	170	4.5	28
Shakes:			
Chocolate	760	21	131
Chocolate Oreo	685	18	118
Oreo	715	20	118
Strawberry	645	15	113
Vanilla	585	15	98
Beverages:			
Iced Coffee: Mocha, 16 fl.oz	240	10	35
Vanilla, 16 fl.oz	200	10	27
Fat Free Milk, glass	90	0	13
Low Fat Chocolate Milk, glass	160	2.5	26
Orange Juice, 10 fl.oz	140	0	33
Sweet Tea, medium	300	0	75

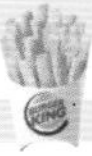
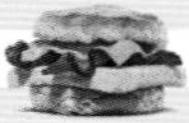
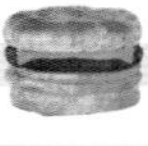
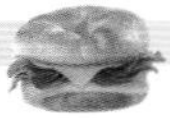
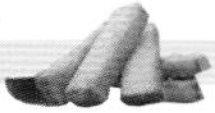
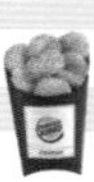
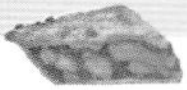
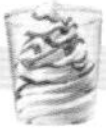
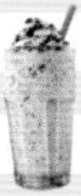
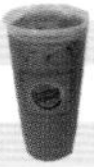

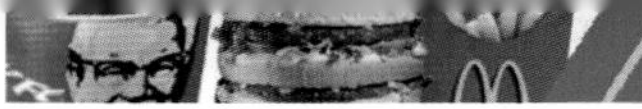

Captain D's Seafood® (Oct '21)

From The Grill: Without Sides, Rice, Hushpuppies or Breadstick	C	F	Cb
Blackened Tilapia	210	7	1
Grilled Wild Salmon	230	10	2
Grilled White Fish & Shrimp Skewer	280	11	3
Lemon Pepper White Fish Fillet	180	8	1
Shrimp Skewers (2)	200	6	2
***Variety Meals:** W/out Sides Or Hush Puppies*			
Butterfly Shrimp (15)	900	64	58
Deluxe Seafood Platter	1100	75	67
Fish & Shrimp	810	56	45
Supreme Sampler	1180	79	68
White Fish, Shrimp & Crab	940	64	52
***Salads:** Without Dressing or Breadstick*			
Grilled Tilapia	310	13	9
Southern Style Breaded Chicken	290	17	20
***Add-Ons:** Per Item/Serving*			
Baked Potato, plain, (1)	210	0	48
Loaded	400	15	49
Coleslaw	180	13	15
French Fries	330	22	28
Hush Puppy	80	4	9
Jalapeno Poppers	510	36	40
Mac & Cheese	170	8	18
Okra	320	20	31
Dessert, Chocolate Cake, 1 order	300	11	49

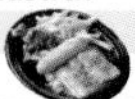
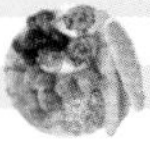
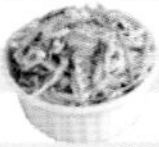

Caribou Coffee® (Oct '21)

With Standard Recipe Ingredients.

Hot Beverages:	C	F	Cb
Cappuccino: Small, 12 fl.oz	90	3.5	9
Medium, 16 fl.oz	110	4.5	10
Large, 20 fl.oz	130	5	11
Chai Tea Latte, 16 fl.oz	310	7	48
Chocolate, 16 fl.oz	450	22	49
Crafted Press Coffee:			
Small, 12 fl.oz	90	6	7
Medium, 16 fl.oz	160	9	12
Large, 20 fl.oz	190	11	17
***Cold Beverages:** Per Medium 20 fl.oz, without Whipped Cream*			
Smoothies:			
Mango Orange Key Lime	420	0	106
Strawberry Banana	360	0	87
Coolers:			
Berry White Mocha	770	24	126
Caramel High Rise	720	27	113
Mint Condition	790	27	121

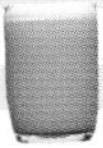
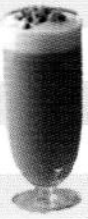
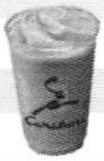
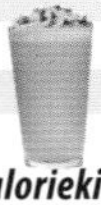

For Complete Menu ~ See Calorieking.com

Carl's Jr.® (Oct '21)

California menu only. Please check instore for further nutritional information.	C	F	Cb
Charbroiled Burgers:			
Beyond Famous Star w/ Cheese	770	44	61
Famous Star w/ Cheese	670	37	57
Spicy Beyond BBQ Cheeseburger	790	37	81
Super Star w/ Cheese	920	56	59
The Big Carl	920	58	56
Western Bacon Cheeseburger	760	35	74
Double	1020	54	75
Thickburgers: ⅓ lb Original	820	51	56
⅓ lb Jalapeno	830	54	53
⅔ lb Monster Angus	1290	89	53
Chicken Sandwiches:			
Bacon Swiss Crispy Chicken Fillet	810	45	58
Big Chicken Fillet	680	36	56
Fiery Chicken	550	33	45
Charbroiled: BBQ Chicken	370	5	49
Chicken Club	600	27	46
Santa Fe Chicken	550	25	45
Chicken Stars: 6 pieces	270	15	19
9 pieces	410	23	29
Chicken Tenders, Hand Breaded:			
3 pieces, without sauce	260	13	13
5 pieces, without sauce	440	21	21
Breakfast:			
Biscuit: Bacon, Egg & Cheese	590	37	44
Monster Biscuit	850	61	46
Sausage, Egg & Cheese	710	50	44
Breakfast Burger, Single	830	44	67
Burritos: Bacon, Egg & Cheese	580	35	32
Beyond Sausage	680	36	41
Loaded Breakfast	760	48	46
Steak & Egg Burrito	600	33	37
Sandwiches: Grilled Bacon & Cheese	740	33	77
Grilled Ham & Cheese	690	28	77
Grilled Sausage & Cheese	840	45	77
Hash Rounds: Small, 2.75 oz	250	17	23
Medium, 4 oz	360	24	34
Large, 5.5 oz	510	34	47
Fries: CrissCut Fries, 4.5 oz	410	26	39
Natural Cut: Small, 3.5 oz	300	15	39
Medium, 6 oz	420	21	55
Large, 6.5oz	460	22	59
Fried Zucchini, 5 oz	330	20	34
Onion Rings, 4.5 oz	520	28	61
***Salads:** Without Dressing*			
Charbroiled Chicken	280	9	19
Garden, side	140	7	15
Dessert: Choc. Chip Cookie, 1.4 oz	200	10	26
Chocolate Cake, 3 oz	290	11	46
Strawb. Swirl Cheesecake, 3.5 oz	320	17	35
***Shakes:** With Ice Cream*			
Oreo Cookie	710	39	79
Vanilla; Choc.; Strawberry, av.	690	35	85

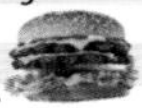
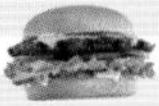
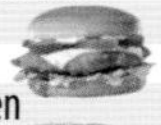
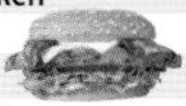
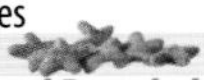
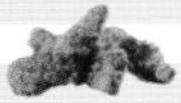
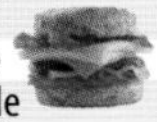
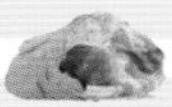
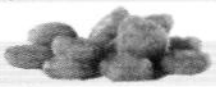
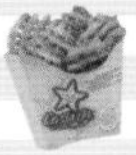
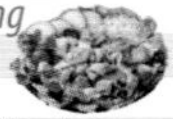
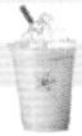

Carvel® (Oct'21)

	C	F	Cb
Carvelanche:			
M&M'S: Small, 12 oz	650	32	73
Regular, 16 oz	850	43	97
Large, 24 oz	1320	66	152
Classic Sundaes: *Per Small, 12 oz*			
Hot Caramel	620	27	79
Hot Fudge	620	32	72
Strawberry	530	26	61
Sundae Dashers: *Per Regular, 16 oz*			
Banana's Foster	1050	33	171
Fudge Brownie	1250	62	166
Mint Chocolate Chip	1080	56	144
Peanut Butter Cup	1850	110	174
Strawberry Shortcake	880	37	125
Ice Cream Scoops: *Per Medium*			
Butter Pecan	750	51	57
Chocolate	520	27	59
Mint Chcolate Chip	670	35	78
Peanut Butter Treasure	680	41	73
Thick Shakes: *Per 16 oz*			
Chocolate; Vanilla, av.	650	27	90
Coffee	720	27	58
Strawberry	590	27	73

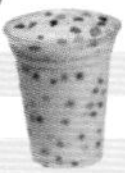
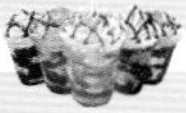
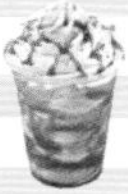
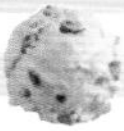
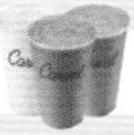

Charley's Philly Steaks® (Oct'21)

	C	F	Cb
Philly Cheessesteaks: *Per Regular witht Toppings*			
Bacon 3 Cheesesteak	850	43	58
Chicken Buffalo/Teriyaki, average	735	30	62
Chicken California	800	40	56
Pepperoni Steak	890	49	58
Philly Cheesesteak	780	38	58
Chicken Wings: *Per Piece Without Sauce or Rubs*			
Boneless: Plain/Buffalo/Habanero	110	7	6
Garlic Parmesan	160	12	8
Nashville Hot	180	14	9
Thai Chili	150	7	16
Classic: Plain	120	9	0
Angry Ghost	140	10	3
Buffalo/Cajun Rub/Smokin Habanero	130	9	1
Nashville Hot	190	16	2
Thai Chili	160	9	10
Fries:			
Original, regular	400	22	46
Gourmet: Cheese & Bacon	680	41	63
Cheese	550	30	62
Ultimate	790	54	61
Sides:			
Celery Sticks with Ranch Dip	210	21	3
Texas Toast, 1 piece	170	6	26
Breakfast: Bacon, Egg & Chse S'wich	490	26	36
Sausage, Egg & Cheese Burrito	650	40	49
Veggie Omelet Platter	790	46	62

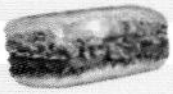
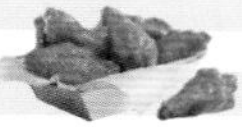
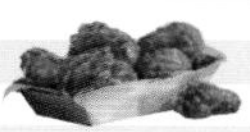
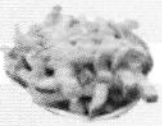

For Complete Menu & Data ~ see CalorieKing.com

Cheesecake Factory® (Oct'21)

	C	F	Cb
Cheesecake: *Per Slice*			
Original	830	59	63
Godiva Chocolate	1400	105	110
Reese's P.B. Chocolate Cake	1530	94	157
White Chocolate Raspberry Truffle	1220	89	92
Appetizers: Avocado Eggrolls	930	48	111
Buffalo Blasts	1670	93	129
Chicken Pot Stickers	420	14	42
Fried Macaroni & Cheese	1310	96	70
Thai Lettuce Wraps w/ Satay. Chkn	850	27	105
Spicy Ahi Tempura Roll	770	51	44
Small Plates: Beets & Avoc. Salad	290	12	40
Chicken Samosas	480	28	29
Crispy Fried Cheese	1080	75	50
Korean Fried Cauliflower	1150	71	113
Stuffed Mushrooms	510	42	19
Flatbread Pizza: Cheese	1000	50	86
Margherita	760	30	85
Pepperoni	1110	61	87
Glamburgers: *Without Sides*			
American Cheeseburger	1400	93	79
Bacon-Bacon Cheeseburger	1680	116	77
Classic Burger	1340	87	69
Impossible Burger	930	53	80
Macaroni & Cheeseburger	1340	85	81
Mushroom Burger	1470	102	72
Veggie Burger	1310	84	114
Glamburger Sides: French Fries	530	23	76
Green Salad	130	12	5
Sweet Potato Fries	510	20	78
Fish & Seafood:			
Fish & Chips	1860	121	133
Shrimp Scampi	1350	77	123
Seared Ahi Tuna	1090	54	107
Sandwiches: Club	1210	60	111
Cuban	1190	71	64
Sthwst Chicken	1040	57	80
Specialties: Baja Chicken Tacos	1250	53	123
Cajun Chicken "Littles"	2070	107	167
Chicken Bellagio	1790	100	135
Chicken Madeira	1210	69	71
Crispy Chicken Costoletta	1800	120	104
Factory Burrito Grande	2150	129	161
Grilled Fish Tacos	1030	42	121
Grilled Steak Tacos	1060	49	124
Pasta Carbonara	2070	143	141
Sides: Broccoli	280	21	13
French Fries	1060	46	152
Green Beans	150	12	9
Mac & Cheese	1550	109	92
Mashed Potatoes	450	25	49
Sauteed Spinach	250	20	12
Sweet Potato Fries	1010	52	125

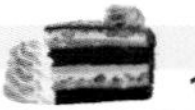
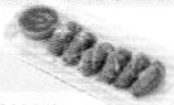
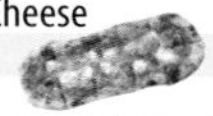
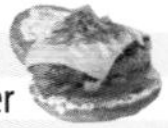
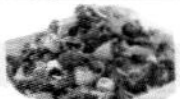
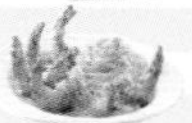
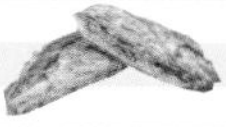
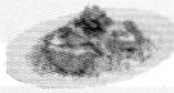
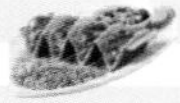

Chick-fil-A® (Oct '21)

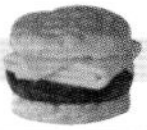
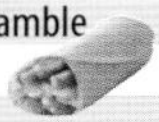

Breakfast:	C	F	Cb
Biscuits: Plain, buttered	290	15	37
Bacon, Egg & Cheese	420	23	38
Chicken	460	23	45
Egg White Chicken Grill	290	8	30
Sausage, Egg & Cheese	610	42	38
Bowl, Hash Brown Scramble	470	30	19
Burrito, Hash Brown Scramble	700	40	51
Chick-n-Minis, 4 pieces	360	13	41
Hash Browns, 2.7 oz	270	18	23
Parfait, Greek Yogurt, fruit topping	270	9	36

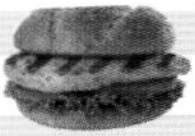
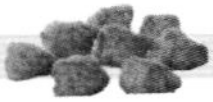

Sandwiches: Without Sauce	C	F	Cb
Chick-fil-A: Chicken	440	17	41
Deluxe	500	22	44
Grilled Chicken	320	6	41
Grilled Chicken Club	520	22	44
Spicy Deluxe	550	25	47
Breaded Chick-n-Strips, 3 count	310	14	16
Nuggets: 5 count	160	7	7
8 Count	250	11	11

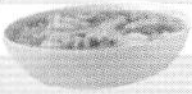
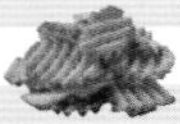

Salads:	C	F	Cb
Cobb: *With Avocado Lime Dressing*			
with Chick-n Strips	910	63	40
with Grilled Filet (warm)	700	51	25
Market: *With Zesty Apple Cider Vinaigrette*			
with Nuggets	690	41	51
without Chicken	440	29	40
Spicy Southwest: *With Creamy Salsa Dressing*			
with Grilled Nuggets	720	50	29
with Spicy Grilled Filet (cold)	690	49	29
Sauces: BBQ	45	0	11
Chick-fil-A	140	13	7
Honey Mustard Sauce	50	0	12
Sweet & Spicy Sriracha Sauce	45	0	11
Sides: Fruit Cup, medium	60	0	15
Chicken Noodle Soup, cup	145	3.5	21
Side Salad, with toppings & dressing	470	42	16
Mac & Cheese: Small	270	17	17
Medium	450	29	28
Waffle Potato Chips	220	13	25
Dessert: Chocolate Chunk Cookie	370	17	49
Frosted Coffee	250	6	43
Milkshakes: Chocolate, 14 oz	590	22	90
Cookies & Cream, 14.5 oz	630	25	90
Vanilla, 14.4 oz	580	23	82

Chili's® (Oct '21)

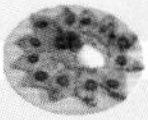
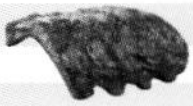

Appetizers: As Served	C	F	Cb
Classic Nachos: Beef	1390	87	55
Chicken	1170	70	57
Southwestern Eggrolls	800	41	82
Texas Cheese Fries, full order	1650	110	99
Triple Dipper: *Serving for One*			
Awesome Blossom Petals	760	50	70
Big Mouth Bites	780	54	41
Original Chicken Crispers	510	34	23
Baby Back Ribs: *Full Rack, without Sides*			
Dry Rub	1480	107	30
Original BBQ	1430	106	21
Honey Chipotle BBQ	1520	106	47
House BBQ	1440	107	21
Burgers: *Without Side Fries*			
Just Bacon Beef	1030	71	43
Oldtimer, with Cheese	860	55	42
Southern Smokehouse	1260	83	68
Crispers & More: *As Served, with Set Sides*			
Cajun Pasta with Grilled Chicken	1180	53	110
Orig. Tempura, with Honey Mustard	1320	67	120

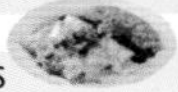
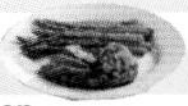
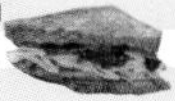
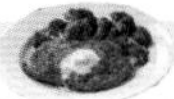
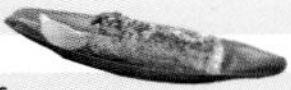
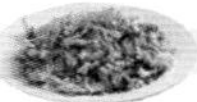
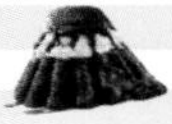

Fresh Mex: *As Served*	C	F	Cb
Bacon Ranch Chicken Quesadilla	1570	117	71
Brisket Quesadilla	1600	122	77
Chipotle Chicken Bowl	1000	49	80
Ranchero Chicken Tacos	1020	44	100
Guiltless Grill: *As Served*			
Ancho Salmon	620	30	42
Grilled Chicken Salad	430	23	22
Mango Chile Chicken	510	20	50
Margarita Grilled Chicken	650	17	68
Sirloin (6 oz), with Grilled Avocado	340	16	13
Sandwiches: *Without Fries*			
Bacon Avocado Chicken	1160	61	75
Buffalo Chicken Ranch	960	51	81
CA Turkey Club	1030	59	78
Steaks: *Without Sides*			
Classic Ribeye	630	40	0
Classic Sirloin, 6 oz	260	13	1
Country-Fried Steak, with gravy	600	36	29
Sides: Asparagus	35	1	5
Black Beans	120	1	20
Coleslaw	250	19	14
Homestyle Fries	420	17	60
Loaded Mashed Potatoes	350	20	33
Mexican Rice	160	4.5	27
Roasted Street Corn	390	27	31
Steamed Broccoli	40	0	8
Sweet Corn on the Cob	180	6	29
Salads: *As Served*			
Boneless Buffalo Chicken	1020	64	60
Caribbean with Seared Shrimp	600	26	81
Quesadilla Explosion	1410	94	82
Sweet Stuff: *Per Slice*			
Cheesecake	720	43	74
Molten Chocolate Cake	1170	59	155

Chipotle® (Oct '21)

Tortillas:	C	F	Cb
Burrito Size Flour Tortillas (1)	320	9	50
Tacos: Crispy Corn Tortilla (3)	200	9	29
Soft Flour Tortillas (3)	250	8	40
Meal Components:			
Barbacoa, 4 oz	170	7	2
Black/Pinto Beans, average, 4 oz	130	1.5	22
Cilantro Lime: Brown Rice, 4 oz	210	6	36
White Rice, 4 oz	210	4	40
Carnitas, 4 oz	210	12	0
Chicken, 4 oz	180	7	0
Fajita Vegetables, 2.5 oz	20	0	5
Guacamole, 3.5 oz	230	22	8
Monterey Jack, 1 oz	110	8	1
Romaine Lettuce	5	0	1
Sofritas, 4 oz	150	10	9
Steak, 4 oz	150	6	1
Condiments:			
Queso Blanco, 2 oz	120	9	4
Salsa: Chili Corn, 3.5 oz	80	1.5	16
Green Tomatillo, 2 oz	15	0	4
Red Tomatillo, 2 oz	15	0	4
Sour Cream, 2 oz	110	8	1
Extras, Chips, 4 oz	540	25	73

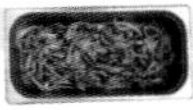
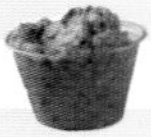
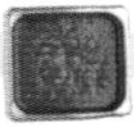

Chuck E. Cheese® (Oct '21)

Appetizers:	C	F	Cb
Cheesy Bread	140	6	15
French Fries, 8 oz	420	13	67
Sub Sandwiches: Per Half Sub Without Fries			
Chicken Bacon Ranch	290	13	24
Ham & Cheese	280	13	25
Italian	290	14	24
Specialty Pizzas: Per Slice, 1/10 Medium Pizza			
5 Meat	210	10	18
Supreme	190	9	19
Veggie	160	6	19
Traditional Wings: Per 12 oz Wings with 2 oz Sauce			
Small, with BBQ or Sweet Chili Sauce	680	34	44
Desserts: Giant Warm Cookie, 1/8th	200	9	28
Unicorn Churros (5)	485	25	62

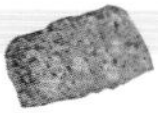
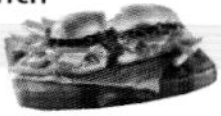
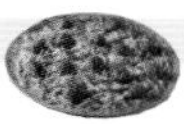

Church's Chicken® (Oct '21)

Chicken: Per Piece	C	F	Cb
Original: Breast, 1 piece	250	14	9
Leg, 1 piece	150	8	6
Thigh, 1 piece	360	27	12
Wing, 1 piece	290	18	8
Spicy: Breast, 1 piece	280	17	12
Leg, 1 piece	160	9	9
Thigh, 1 piece	380	25	21
Wing, 1 piece	350	20	19
Texas Tener, average, 1 piece	120	6	7
Sides: Per Regular Serving			
Baked Macaroni & Cheese, 4.7 oz	210	12	19
Cole Slaw, 4.2 oz	170	11	16
French Fries, 2.6 oz	210	9	29
Honey Butter Biscuit, 2.2 oz	230	15	25
Jalapeno Cheese Bombers (4)	220	11	24
Mashed Potatoes & Gravy, 4.5 oz	110	1	24
Okra, 3.4 oz	260	15	30
Sauces: Honey BBQ, pkt	45	0	11
Creamy Jalapeno, pkt	120	13	2
Honey Mustard/Ranch, av., pkt	140	14	3
Dessert, Apple Pie	270	13	37

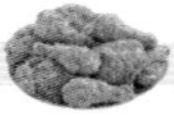
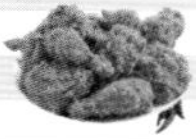
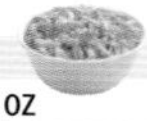
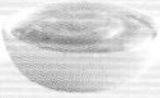

Cici's Pizza® (Oct '21)

Pizza:	C	F	Cb
Regular Crust: *Per Slice, 1/10 of Large 14" Pizza*			
Alfredo; Zesty Ham & Cheddar, av.	170	6	22
Pepperoni	200	8	23
Flatbread: Chicken Bacon Club	150	7	14
Honey BBQ Chicken	140	4.5	19
Spinach Alfredo	140	7	14
Stuffed Crust, Cheese; Pepperoni	190	8	21
Saucy Wings: BBQ (5)	260	12	16
Buffalo (5), average	215	14	3
Garlic Parmesan (5)	270	18	5
Sides: Chicken & Pasta Soup, 8 oz	90	2.5	13
Garlic Cheesy Bread, 2 slices	70	3	9
Pasta with Marinara Sce	300	4	56
Dessert: Brownie, 1 square	140	6	21
Apple/Barvarian Pizza, 1 slice	130	3	23

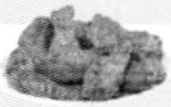

Cinnabon® (Oct '21)

	C	F	Cb
Cinnabon Classic Roll (1)	880	37	129
MiniBon Roll (1), 3.4 oz	350	15	52
Cheese Roll Paninis:			
Grilled Cheese	480	24	46
Black Forest Ham	540	25	48
Smoked Turkey Club	530	24	49
Chillata: Per 16 fl.oz			
Chocolate Mocha	380	13	61
Oreo Cookies & Cream	710	27	109
Strawberries & Cream	530	18	86

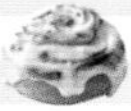
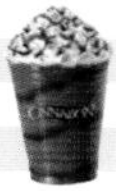

Claim Jumper® (Oct '21)

Appetizers: As Served	C	F	Cb
Beef Sliders with Cheese	740	35	67
Chips & Salsa	540	10	90
Spinach & Artichoke Dip, share	1735	64	233
Burgers: *Without Sides*			
Bacon & Mac	950	48	89
Classic Hamburger	750	40	60
Impossible Burger	1230	75	91
Widow Maker Burger	1565	89	126
Meals: *As Per Menu Description*			
Classics: After The Goldrush	890	47	47
Country Fried Steak	1175	50	116
Fish & Chips	1115	37	148
Meatloaf & Mashed Potatoes	1180	73	83
Combo Plates: Steak & SHrimp	770	52	17
Tri-tip Prospector	765	42	9
Pasta: Black Tie Pasta	1895	97	161
Shrimp Fresca	2005	143	110
Seafood: Blackened Salmon	405	26	3
Coconut Shrimp	1305	36	202
Grilled Shrimp	550	22	53
Wood Fired Pizza, Classic Crust: *Per Whole Pizza*			
BBQ Chicken, 8 slices	1960	80	230
Sausage & Pepperoni, 8 slices	2010	100	190
Sides: Baked Potato with Butter	635	27	82
Brussels Sprouts	190	14	11
Charbroiled Asparagus	235	19	7
Chili French Fries	580	35	44
Loaded French Fries	550	35	39
Mac & Cheese	460	25	40
Mashed Potatoes	270	16	28
Roasted Veggies	55	3	6
Sweets: Chocolate Motherlode Cake	3415	158	459
Raspberry Cream Cheese Pie	1570	97	147

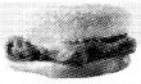
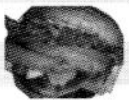
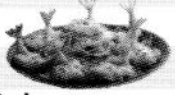
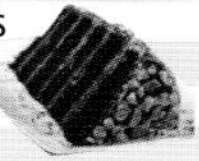

Cold Stone Creamery® (Oct '21)

Ice Cream:	C	F	Cb
Amaretto: Like it	340	21	36
Love it	550	33	57
Gotta have it	820	49	85
Chocolate: Like it	330	20	34
Love it	520	31	54
Gotta have it	780	47	81
Sorbet:			
Strawberry Mango Banana:			
Like it, 5 oz	210	0	54
Love it, 8 oz	340	0	87
Gotta have it, 12 oz	510	0	130
Shakes: *Per 20 oz With Whipped Topping*			
Cake Batter 'n Shake	1440	76	176
Oh Fudge; Very Vanilla, average	1320	76	149
Savory Strawberry	1200	71	133
Sundaes: Banana Split Decision	650	37	77
Who You Callin' Shortcake	560	31	68

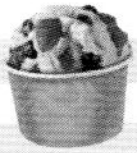
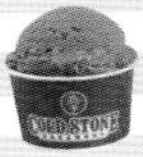

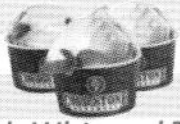

Costco Food Court® (Sept '19)

(Approximate Figures Only)	C	F	Cb
Baked Potato, with Chicken Chili	840	24	120
French Fries, 11 oz	870	45	106
Hot Dogs: Hebrew National	550	34	42
KS	570	33	46
Sinai	540	30	48
Pizza: *Per Slice*			
Cheese Pizza, 9.8 oz	700	28	70
Combo Pizza, 10.7 oz	680	29	72
Pepperoni Pizza, 8.9 oz	620	24	68
Chicken Bake, 12.75 oz	770	25	78
Wrap, Turkey, 14.4 oz	810	38	65
Salad, Chicken Caesar, w/ Dressing	650	40	34
Sandwiches: Hebrew Sausage	540	32	44
Italian Sausage	700	42	46
KS Polish/Sinai Sausage, av.	570	33	47
Desserts: California Churro	410	18	51
Ice Cream Bar	870	65	60
J&J Churro	470	22	61
Yogurt, 12 oz	390	0	82
Smoothies: Fruit, 16 fl. oz	290	0	72
Strawberry Banana, 16 fl.oz	300	0	74
Sundae, Berry, 12.3 oz	410	0	87
Beverages: Hot Latte, 9.6 fl.oz	190	5	24
Hot Mocha, 11.3 fl.oz	310	9	45

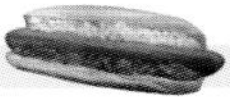
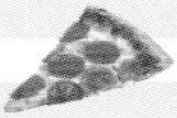
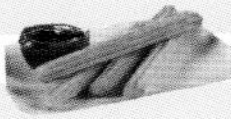

Cousins Subs® (Oct '21)

Subs: *Per 7.5", Standard Toppings*	C	F	Cb
Grilled To Order:			
Chkn Bacon Cheddar	610	23	53
Chicken Cheese Steak	560	18	52
Double Steak Cheese Steak	800	31	56
Classics:			
Club, with Mayo	670	32	53
Italian Special, with Oil	830	48	52
Tuna with Mayo	650	36	51
Deli Fresh:			
Ham & Provolone, with Mayo	630	32	51
Roast Beef & Cheddar, with Mayo	740	37	52
Turkey Breast with Mayo	550	25	53
Cheese Curds: Regular, 5 oz	680	56	13
Large, 10 oz	1380	113	26
French Fries:			
Regular, 4.5 oz	240	12	29
Large, 9 oz	470	24	57
Soup: *Per Cup*			
Broccoli Cheese	150	9	12
Chicken Noodle	100	2	15
Potato with Bacon	170	8	20

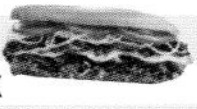
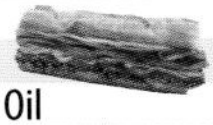
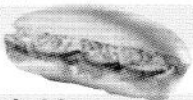
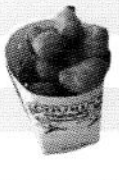
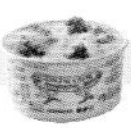

For Complete Nutritional Data ~ see CalorieKing.com

Culver's® (Oct '21)

ButterBurgers:	C	F	Cb
Original: Single	390	17	38
Double	560	30	38
Triple	730	43	38
Bacon Deluxe: Single	610	38	40
Double	850	56	41
Triple	1090	76	42
Cheddar:			
Single	460	23	39
Double	700	42	40
Culver's Deluxe:			
Single	570	34	41
Double	810	53	42
Mushroom & Swiss, Single	500	26	40
Sourdough Melt, Single	490	25	42
Wisconsin Swiss Melt: Single	470	24	39
Double	720	43	40
Harvest Veggie Burger	590	25	72
Homestyle Favorites:			
Beef Pot Roast	500	18	46
Chopped Steak Dinner	610	38	32
Sandwiches:			
Beef Pot Roast	410	13	40
Crispy Chicken	460	14	56
Grilled Chicken	390	8	40
Sides:			
Coleslaw, regular	200	16	15
Mshd Pot. & Gravy, reg.	130	1	25
Steamed Broccoli	40	0	7
Fries, Regular	360	14	53
Dinner: With Dinner Role, Butter & Menu Set Sauce			
Butterfly Jumbo Shrimp, 6 pieces	380	18	42
North Atlantic Cod, Fried, 2 pieces	920	68	42
Soup: Broccoli Cheese	220	12	17
Chicken Noodle	100	2	15
Potato with Bacon	240	10	28
Salads: Without Dressing			
Chicken Cashew with Gilled Chicken	450	24	13
Cranberry Bacon Bleu, with Grilled Chicken	360	14	14
Garden Fresco with Grilled Chicken	360	14	15
Side Salad	50	2	5
Dressings: Chunky Bleu Cheese	310	33	2
French	190	13	19
Honey Mustard	130	6	20
Ranch	180	19	2
Raspberry Vinaigrette	45	0	11
Kid's Meals:			
Corn Dog	240	14	23
Grilled Cheese Sourdough Sandwich	360	17	39
Original Chicken Tenders, 2 pieces	270	12	21

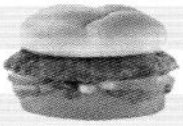
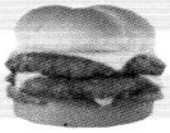
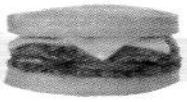
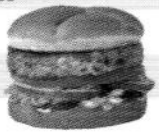
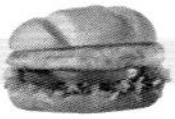
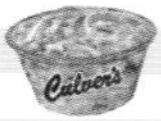

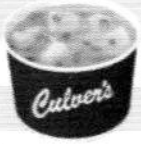

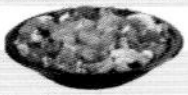
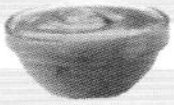
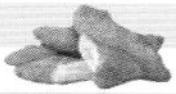

Culver's® cont... (Oct '21)

Concrete Mixers: No Toppings	C	F	Cb
Chocolate & PB Cups, reg.	980	51	116
Vanilla, with Oreo, regular	950	53	105
Sundaes: Per 2 Scoops			
Banana Split	1090	61	122
Caramel Cashew	1000	52	121
Turtle	1040	61	111
Shakes: Chocolate, regular	820	38	108
Mint, regular	840	38	114
Peanut Butter, regular	1040	74	78
Strawberry, regular	720	38	84

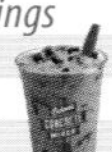
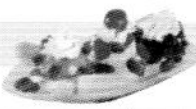
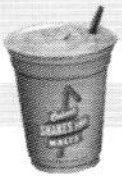

D'Angelo® (Oct '21)

Deli Sandwiches: Per Medium			
Italian Sub Bread	310	3.5	57
Add Chicken Salad	700	62	3
Add Ham & Cheese	310	24	6
Add Tuna Salad	570	58	0
Wraps: Per Medium			
Tortilla Wrap Only	250	6	42
Add Buffalo Chicken	520	38	13
Add Chicken Caesar	600	41	20
Add Greek	390	31	17
Fresh Entree Salads: With Dressing, without Pokket			
Entree: Caesar	490	39	24
Greek	520	45	19
Grilled Topped:			
Chicken Cobb	810	59	25
Steak Cobb	880	65	25
Steak Greek	780	62	20
Soup: Per Bowl			
Beef Stew	330	12	34
Broccoli & Cheddar	370	28	18
Main Lobster Bisque	540	43	24
New England Clam Chowder	480	27	46

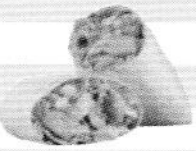
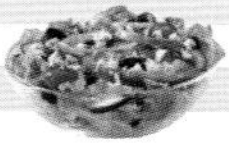
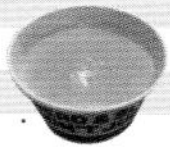

For Complete Menu & Data ~ see CalorieKing.com

Dairy Queen® (Oct '21)

Burgers:			
Cheeseburger	400	18	36
GrillBurgers: ¼ lb Bacon Cheese	630	36	44
½ lb with Cheese	800	49	44
½ lb Flame Thrower	980	70	40
Stackburgers: Orig. Cheeseburger	370	17	34
Double	580	33	36
Bacon Two Cheese Deluxe Double	730	45	36
FlameThrower Double	710	46	35
Loaded A.1. Steakhouse Double	830	50	49
Sandwiches:			
Chicken: Bacon Ranch	500	28	49
Crispy Chicken	550	28	49
Grilled Chicken	390	15	34
Turkey, BLT	580	28	45

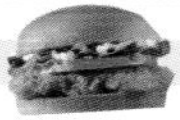

Dairy Queen® cont... (Oct '21)

Hot Dogs:	C	F	Cb
Cheese Dog	390	24	27
Chili Dog	360	22	27
Chili Cheese Dog	420	26	28
Classic Hot Dog	330	19	25

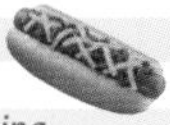

Salads: Without Dressing	C	F	Cb
Chicken BLT:			
Chicken Strip	360	18	28
Crispy Chicken	400	21	28
Grilled Chicken	280	11	12
Side Salad	25	0	5
Dressing: Balsamic Vinaigrette	130	12	4
Blue Cheese	200	21	2
Creamy Caesar	180	18	2
Light: Italian	15	1	2
Ranch	60	2.5	9

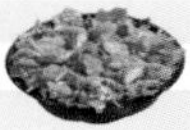

French Fries:	C	F	Cb
French Fries: Regular	290	13	39
Large	470	21	63
Sides:			
Cheese Curds: Regular	500	34	26
Large	1000	67	52
Onion Ring: Regular	360	16	48
Large	540	24	71
Pretzel Sticks with Zesty Queso	330	9	52

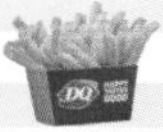

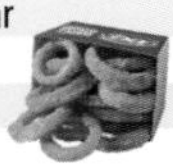

Desserts: Per Medium	C	F	Cb
Blizzard Treats:			
Choco Brownie Xtreme	810	36	111
Choc. Chip Cookie Dough	1030	41	151
M&M's	800	27	124
Oreo Cookie	790	31	117
Reese's: P'nut Butter Cup	750	31	102
Turtles with Pecan	900	48	105
Curl On Top Treats:			
Banana Split	520	14	94
Brownie & Oreo Cupfection	720	23	122
Peanut Buster Parfait	710	31	95
Triple Chocolate Brownie	540	25	74
Dipped Cone, Chocolate	460	22	58
DQ Sundaes: Caramel	430	11	73
Hot Fudge	430	15	66
Strawberry	340	10	56
MooLatte: Caramel	620	18	103
Mocha	620	23	94
Vanilla	560	17	93
Shakes: Caramel	750	25	115
Chocolate	710	23	110
Strawberry	630	23	92
Vanilla	660	23	97
Treatzza Pizza: Choco Brownie, sl.	190	10	26
Reese's Peanut Butter Cup, slice	200	10	24

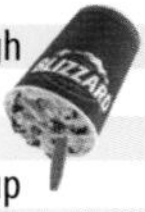

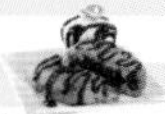

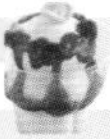

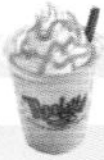

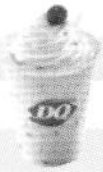

Daphne's Greek Cafe® (Dec '20)

California Menu Only. Check Instore for Latest Information

Starters:	C	F	Cb
Fire Feta & Warm Pita	340	17	39
Hummus & Warm Pita	320	12	47
Classic Pita Sandwiches: *Without Tzatziki Sauce*			
with Chicken	410	16	41
with Crispy Shrimp	410	17	48
with Falafel	640	17	96
with Gyro	680	45	49
Plates: *Without Pita or Tzatziki Sauce*			
Cali-Greek Bowls:			
with Crispy Shrimp	930	38	117
with Falafel	1160	39	165
with Gr. Chicken	930	37	109
with Grilled Shrimp	1060	46	91
Mediterranean Veggie	1300	56	161
Surf & Turf	690	25	85
Classic Greek Salads: *W/ Dressing, w/o Pita & Sauce*			
Crispy Shrimp	440	31	25
Falafel	670	31	74
Grilled Chicken	440	30	18
Add, Pita & Tzatziki	130	3	21
Sides: Cucumber-Tomato Salad	120	11	5
Fire Roasted Vegetables	70	3	12
French Fries	440	22	55
Greek Salad, small	140	12	7
Lemon Chicken Soup	280	12	37
Moroccan Carrot Salad	180	13	15
Pita Chips	220	6	36
Pita Bread	190	3	36
Seasoned Rice	360	8	68
Tabouli	220	15	20
Dessert, Traditional Baklava	250	9	36

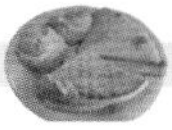

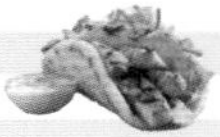

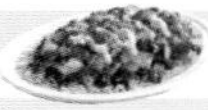

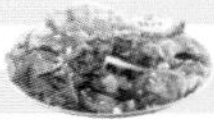

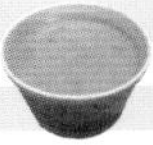

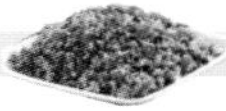

Davanni's® (Oct '21)

Hot Hoagies: *Per Half, with 6" White Bun & Standard Toppings*	C	F	Cb
Assorted	490	30	39
Cheese	500	31	39
Chicken & Bacon, w/ Honey Mustard	505	22	46
Chicken Parmigiana	445	16	40
Club	495	27	40
Pastrami	470	27	40
Roast Beef	470	25	39
Southwestern Chicken	535	26	43
Tuna Melt	645	44	42
Turkey Bacon Chipotle	565	33	39
Pasta: *As Served, with Garlic Toast*			
Chicken Florentine, half portion	610	28	56
Lasagna, half portion	625	43	37

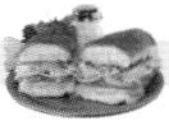

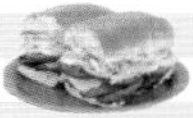

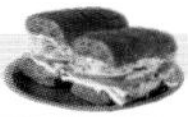

continued next page...

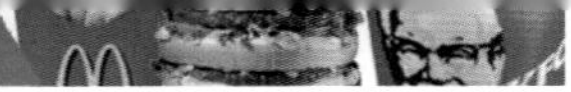

Davanni's® cont... (Oct '21)

Pizzas: Per 1/8 Medium Pizza, with Red Sauce	C	F	Cb
Five Meat: Thin Crust	255	13	19
Traditional Crust	305	13	30
Gluten Free Crust	215	12	16
Veggie: Thin Crust	220	10	19
Traditional Crust	275	10	30
Works: Thin Crust	265	14	19
Traditional Crust	315	15	30

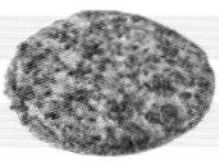

Del Taco® (Oct '21)

Breakfast:	C	F	Cb
Burritos: Bacon	520	26	37
Carne Asada	460	20	39
gg & Cheese	390	17	36
Epic Scrambler: Bacon	1040	62	71
Carne Asada	960	54	73
Hash Brown Sticks, 5 pieces	230	17	18
Roller: Bacon	290	14	24
Egg & Cheese	250	12	24
Egg & Cheese			
Burgers: Without Fries			
Bacon Double Del Cheeseburger	760	51	35
Del Cheeseburger	470	28	34
Double Del Chseburger	690	47	35
Burritos:			
Bean & Cheese, red	470	10	69
Beyond 8 Layer	550	21	60
Classic Grilled Chicken	530	33	40
Del Beef	500	24	40
Del Combo	470	17	54
Epic Cali Bacon: Beyond Meat	1120	67	75
Carne Asada	1060	23	73
Epic Fresh Guacamole:			
Beyond Meat	820	32	91
Carne Asada	730	26	88
Epic Loaded Queso:			
Beyond Meat	980	51	78
Chicken	880	45	74
Crunchtadas: Chicken Guacamole	480	26	43
Queso Beef	440	22	40
Tostada	330	14	38
Fries: Carne Asada	810	59	46
Chilli Cheddar	570	35	42
Crinkle Cut, medium	320	19	34
Queso Loaded Nachos: Per Regular			
Beef; Carne Asada, average	570	30	52
Chicken	550	28	52
Quesadillas: 3 Layer Queso	270	11	36
Cheddar	460	26	31
Chicken/Cheddar or Spicy Jack, av.	550	31	34

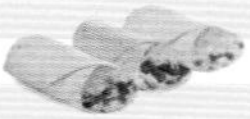
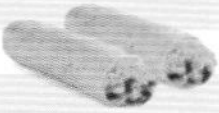
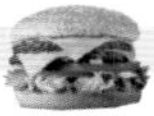
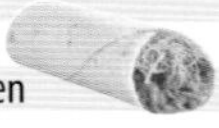
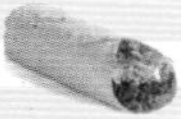
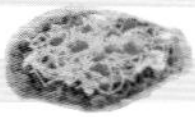

Del Taco® cont... (Oct '21)

Tacos:	C	F	Cb
Beer Battered Crispy Fish	230	12	26
Beyond: Guacamole	240	2	24
Original	300	19	15
Chicken Al Carbon	150	4.5	19
Grilled Chicken	210	12	16
Habero Crispy Chicken	240	15	18
Ranch Crispy Chicken	230	14	19
Salads:			
Chicken, Bacon Guac.: w/ Ranch	530	38	26
with Caesar	580	44	24
Signature Taco w/ Fresh Guacamole	510	26	36
Sides, Bean & Cheese Cup, 7.8 oz	220	3	34
Desserts:			
Caramel Cheesecake Bites (2)	460	28	43
Mini Cinnamon Churros (2)	200	10	25
Premium Shakes: Per Regular			
Chocolate	510	8	102
Strawberry; Vanilla, av.	465	6.5	92

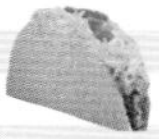
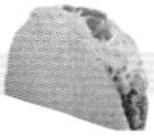
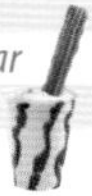

Denny's® (Oct '21)

Breakfast:	C	F	Cb
Classic Favorites: *With Scrambled Eggs & Hash Browns*			
Country Fried Steak w/ Engl. Muffin	1150	68	89
Moons Over My Hammy	950	60	57
Santa Fe Sizzlin' Skillet, no H. Browns	940	70	36
T'Bone Steak with English Muffin	1250	73	62
The Grand Slamwich	1490	93	110
3 Egg Omelettes: *With Hash Browns & Wheat Toast*			
Loaded Veggie	900	61	53
Mile High Denver	1060	71	55
Ultimate	1110	83	49
Pancakes: *With Bacon, Scrambled Eggs & Hash Browns*			
Choconana	1010	44	144
Cinnamon Roll	1500	64	205
Double Berry Banana	1030	47	120
Hearty 9 Grain	900	48	85
Red White & Blue	1070	49	122
Salted Caramel & Banana Cream	1630	64	224
Slams: *With 4 Bacon Strips*			
All American with Hash Browns & 2 P'cakes	870	67	19
French Toast, w/ Scrambled Eggs	1020	63	66
Lumberjack, w/ 2 B'milk Pancakes & Scrambled Eggs	880	44	80
Original Slam, with Over Easy Eggs, & 9 Grain Pancakes	810	43	70

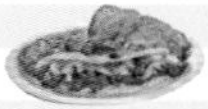
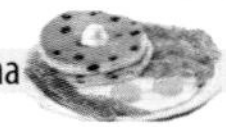

Denny's® cont... (Oct '21)

Breakfast Sides:	C	F	Cb
Bacon Strips (4)	**210**	16	2
1 Egg: Over Easy/Medium/Hard	**125**	11	0
Scrambled	**110**	9	1
Scrambled with Cheese	**160**	14	1
English Muffin without Margarine	**130**	1	25
Fries, Wavy Cut	**400**	22	46
Hash Brown:			
Regular (1)	**170**	12	15
Cheddar Cheese (1)	**250**	18	15
Pancakes, Buttermilk (2)	**450**	11	77
Sausages, 4 links	**310**	30	2
Toast: Wheat, with Margarine , 2 sl.	**230**	11	29
White, with Margarine, 2 slices	**240**	10	31
Appetizers: *Without Dipping Sauce*			
Beer Battered Onion Rings	**400**	27	35
BBQ Boneless Chicken Wings	**770**	36	80
Loaded Bacon Cheddar Tots	**730**	50	45
Prem. Chicken Tenders	**680**	40	38
Zesty Nachos	**1660**	106	170
Condiments: Pico de Gallo, 2 oz	**15**	0	3
Sour Cream, 1 oz	**45**	4	1
Tomato Sauce, 1.5 oz	**25**	1	3
Whipped Margarine, 0.5 oz	**40**	4.5	0
Dipping Sauces: *Per 1.5 oz*			
All American	**200**	21	1
Blue Cheese	**160**	16	2
BBQ	**110**	16	2
Bourbon	**110**	0	26
Buffalo	**110**	12	1
Honey Mustard	**180**	15	12
Nashville Hot Sauce	**70**	4.5	9
Ranch	**200**	21	1
Burgers: *Without Sides*			
America's Diner Single	**2010**	127	101
Bourbon Bacon	**910**	51	64
Double Cheeseburger:			
with Cheddar Cheese	**1140**	68	50
with Swiss Cheese	**1200**	70	52
Slamburger	**870**	51	55
Chicken Dinners: *Without Sides or Sauce*			
Bourbon Chicken Sizzlin Skillet	**840**	35	69
Premium Chkn Tenders & Dinner Bread	**860**	47	63
New Additions: *Without Sides*			
Chicken Addiction Bowl with Bread	**870**	39	84
Mama D's Pot Roast Bowl with Bread	**760**	32	65
Nashville Hot chicken Melt	**1260**	81	84
The Big Dipper Melt	**1140**	69	63
Sandwiches: *Without Sides*			
All American Patty Melt	**1100**	70	69
Chick 'n Honey	**770**	40	70
The Super Bird	**680**	35	44

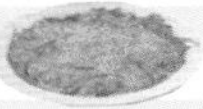
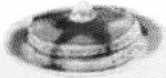
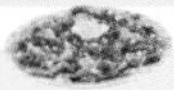
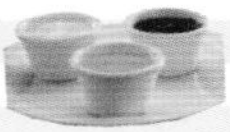
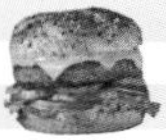
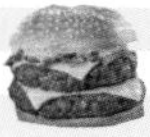
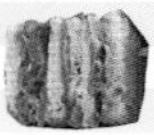

Denny's® cont... (Oct '21)

Seafood & Steak: *W/ Dinner Bread, without Sides or Toppings*	C	F	Cb
Fried Fish Platter	**1010**	68	65
Sirloin Steak	**530**	25	27
T-Bone Steak	**680**	38	26
Wild Alaskan Salmon	**530**	31	26
Lunch/Dinner Sides:			
Beer Battered Onion Rings	**400**	27	35
Broccoli, 3 oz	**35**	0	5
Garden Salad, without dressing	**170**	9	16
Red Skinned Potatoes	**200**	8	26
Mashed	**120**	5	17
Seasoned Fries	**490**	26	57
Seasonal Fruit	**110**	0	27
Sweet Petite Corn	**210**	13	20
Wavy-Cut Fries	**400**	22	46
Whole Grain Rice	**240**	2.5	48
Fit Fare: *With Set Menu Components*			
Fit Slam	**590**	11.5	81
Loaded Veggie Omelette	**510**	14	58
55 & Over: *Without Extras*			
B'fast, Scrambled Eggs & Cheddar	**1010**	58	80
Gr. Cheese Sandwich & Veg Beef Soup	**640**	28	66
Wild Alaska Salmon w/ Dinner Bread	**530**	31	26
Salads: *Without Dressing*			
House Salad:			
without Meat	**190**	9	19
with Chicken Tenders (3)	**600**	33	42
with Grilled chicken	**390**	18	19
with Wild Alaska Salmon	**500**	28	21
Dressings: Balsamic Vinaigrette	**130**	4	24
Blue Cheese	**160**	16	2
Honey Mustard	**180**	15	12
Light Italian	**30**	0	8
Thousand Island	**155**	16	7
Desserts: *As Served*			
New York Style Cheesecake, plain	**520**	35	43
Signature Skookie	**820**	40	108
Beverages:			
Chocolate Milk	**290**	5	60
Hot Chocolate	**190**	3	37
Lemonade	**100**	0	23
Orange Juice	**210**	0	27
Raspberry Tea	**110**	0	28
Milk Shakes: *Per 16 fl.oz*			
Cake Batter	**1090**	52	147
Chocolate	**870**	43	111
Oreo	**1050**	56	125
Strawberry	**760**	34	110

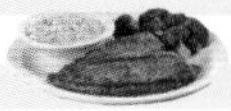
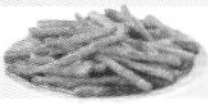
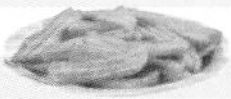
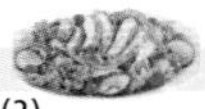
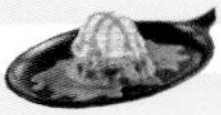
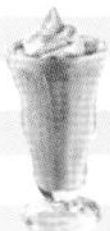

Dippin' Dots® (Oct '21)

Ice Cream: Per ⅔ Cup, 3.4 oz	C	F	Cb
Chocolate	190	9	25
Chocolate Chip Cookie Dough, 3.5 oz	230	10	31
Cookies 'N Cream	210	10	18
Cotton Candy	170	9	15
Ultimate Brownie Batter	220	10	30
Ice, Rainbow, ⅔ cup, 3.35 oz	110	0	28

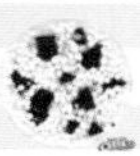

Donatos Pizza® (Oct '21)

Pizzas: Per Slice	C	F	Cb
Cauliflower Crust, 10":			
Spinach Mozzarella	80	4	5
Other varieties, average	65	3	5
Hand Tossed Signature Pizzas: *Per Slice of 14" Pizza*			
Chicken Spinach Mozzarella	330	15	31
Founder's Favorite	330	14	33
Mariachi Beef	300	12	34
Mariachi Chicken	300	11	34
The Works	320	14	34
Thick Crust Signature Pizzas: *Per Slice of 14" Pizza*			
Chicken Spinach Mozzarella	150	7	15
Double Bacon Pepperoni	200	10	16
Founders Favorite	170	8	16
Margherita	160	8	14
Serious Meat, Ground Beef	190	9	16
The Works	170	8	17
Oven Baked Subs:			
Big Don with Marinara Sauce	600	25	63
Chicken Bacon Ranch	740	35	62
Fresh Vegy	490	19	63
Ham & Smoked Prov.	560	21	62
Meatball	850	38	80
Salad: *Entree Size, with Menu Set Dressing*			
Chicken Caprese	400	25	17
Italian Chef	500	42	12
Side: Caprese	220	18	11
Italian	330	31	7
Wings: *Per 6 pieces, without Dipping Sauce*			
Boneless Chkn:			
Mild/Hot Scauce, average	415	23	26
BBQ Sauce	400	17	39
Dessert: Cinnamon Bread, ¼ bread	280	10	44
Fudge Brownie (1)	360	21	39
Triple Chocolate Chunk Cookie (1)	320	23	22

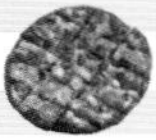

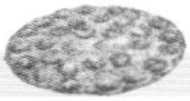

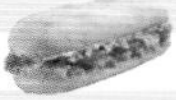

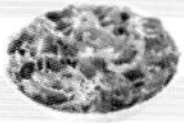

For Complete Nutritional Data ~ see CalorieKing.com

Domino's® (Oct '21)

With Regular Cheese Base	C	F	Cb
12" Hand Tossed: *Per Slice, ⅛ Pizza, with Honey BBQ Sauce Unless Indicated*			
Bacon, Beef, & Italian Sausage	290	15	26
Beef, Green Peppers, Onions, & Mshrm	210	8	27
Black Olives, Green Peppers, Onions, Mshrm &Tomatoes, Marinara Sauce	190	7	25
Ham & Pineapple, no sauce	190	7	23
Italian Sausage	240	11	26
Italian Sausage, Beef & Pepperoni	280	14	26
Pepperoni & Ital. Sausage, no Sauce	230	12	22
14" Brooklyn: *Per Slice, ⅙ Pizza, with Honey BBQ Sauce Unless Indicated*			
Beef, Green Pepp., Onions & Mshrm	300	13	33
Black Olives, Green Peppers, Onions, Mushrooms, Tomatoes	290	11	34
Ham & Pineapple, no sauce	260	11	26
Italian Sausage	330	19	24
Pepperoni, no sauce	290	15	24
Pepperoni & Italian Sausage, no sauce	340	20	24
14" Thin Crust: *Per Slice, ⅛ Pizza, with Honey BBQ Sauce Unless Indicated*			
Bacon, Beef & Italian Sausage	320	20	21
Beef, Green Pepp., Onions & Mshrm	220	11	21
Black Olives, Green Peppers, Onions, Mushrooms & Tomatoes	210	10	22
Ham & Pineapple, no sauce	190	9	17
Italian Sausage	260	15	21
Pepperoni, no sauce	210	12	15
Pepperoni & Ital. Sausage, no sauce	250	16	15
12" Specialty Handmade Pan: *Per Slice, ⅛ Pizza*			
Cali Chicken Bacon Ranch	380	23	29
Deluxe	320	17	29
Memphis BBQ Chicken	340	17	34
Spinach & Feta	310	17	29
12" Specialty Hand-Tossed: *Per Slice, ⅛ Pizza*			
Deluxe	220	10	24
ExtravaganZZa	280	14	25
MeatZZa	270	13	24
Philly Cheeese Steak	230	14	16
Ultimate Pepperoni	260	14	24
14" Specialty Thin Crust: *Per Slice, ⅛ Pizza*			
Cali Chicken Bacon Ranch	330	23	17
Deluxe	230	14	18
Honolulu Hawaiian	260	14	19
Memphis BBQ Chicken	280	15	22
Wisconsin 6 Cheese	260	15	18

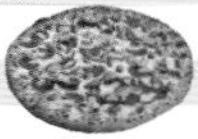

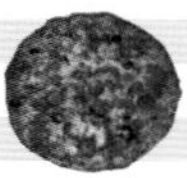

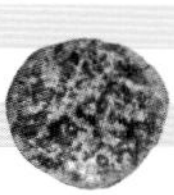

Domino's® cont... (Oct '21)

	C	F	Cb
***Chicken Wings:** Without Sauce*			
Honey BBQ, 4 wings	**310**	20	22
Hot Buffalo, 4 wings	**260**	20	9
Chicken Dipping Cups:			
Blue Cheese, 1.25 oz	**200**	21	2
Honey BBQ, 1.25 oz	**70**	0	17
Hot Buffalo, 1.25 oz	**15**	1	1
Ranch, 1.5 oz	**160**	17	1
Sweet Mango Habanero, 1.25 oz	**70**	0	17
***BreadBowl Pasta:** Per 1/2 Bowl*			
Chicken Alfredo, 10.5 oz	**690**	25	92
Chicken Carbonara, 11.6 oz	**730**	28	93
Italian Sausage Marinara, 11.85 oz	**740**	28	96
Pasta Primavera, 11 oz	**660**	23	92
***Oven Baked Sandwiches:** Per Sandwich*			
Buffalo Chicken	**840**	42	74
Chicken Bacon Ranch	**880**	44	70
Chicken Parmesan	**760**	30	72
Italian	**820**	40	70
Mediterranean Veggie	**700**	30	76
Philly Cheese Steak	**720**	30	74
Sweet & Spicy Chicken Habanero	**800**	32	84
Pasta In Dish: Chkn Alfredo, 11.5 oz	**600**	29	60
Chicken Carbonara, 13 oz	**690**	34	63
Italian Sausage Marinara, 13.5 oz	**700**	36	68
Pasta Primavera, 11.9 oz	**530**	26	62
***Salads:** Without Dressing*			
Chicken Caesar	**220**	8	14
Classic Garden	**80**	4	8
***Salad Dressings:** Per 1.5 oz Package*			
Caesar Dressing	**230**	25	1
Italian	**160**	17	4
Light Balsamic Dressing	**100**	8	5
Ranch Dressing	**190**	20	2
Bread Side Items:			
Garlic Bread Twists, 2 pcs	**220**	11	27
Jalap. Bacon Stuffed Cheesy Bread (1)	**170**	8	16
Parmesan Bread Bites, 4 pieces	**220**	10	27
Spin. & Fetta Stuffed Cheesy Bread, 1 piece	**160**	7	16
Stuffed Cheesy Bread, 1 piece	**150**	7	16
***Bread Dipping Sauces:** Per Container*			
Garlic, 1 oz cup	**250**	28	0
Marinara, 2 oz cup	**30**	0	6
Dessert: Choc. Lava Crunch Cake, 3 oz	**360**	19	46
Marbled Cookie Brownie, 1.5 oz	**200**	10	26
Sweet Icing, Dipping Cup, 2.25 oz	**220**	4	52

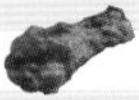
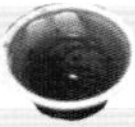
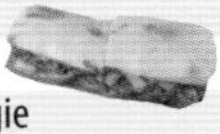
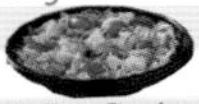
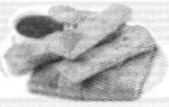

Dunkin'® (Oct '21)

	C	F	Cb
***Bagels:** Per Bagel*			
Plain	**300**	1	64
Cinnamon Raisin	**320**	1	67
Everything	**340**	3	67
Multigrain	**380**	8	63
Sesame Seed	**350**	5	64
White Cheddar Twist	**390**	8	64
Donuts: Apple 'n Spice	**230**	10	31
Apple Crumb	**290**	11	44
Bavarian Kreme	**240**	11	31
Bismark	**480**	22	63
Boston Kreme	**270**	11	39
Butternut	**430**	21	57
Chocolate Butternut	**440**	23	55
Chocolate Dipped French Cruller	**280**	15	33
Chocolate Frosted Cake	**360**	20	41
Chocolate Headlight	**310**	14	41
Chocolate Long John	**320**	15	41
Cinnamon	**330**	20	34
Coconut; Coffee Roll, average	**400**	20	49
Coffee Roll	**390**	19	48
Double Chocolate	**370**	22	40
French Cruller	**230**	14	21
Glazed	**240**	11	33
Glazed Chocolate	**360**	22	39
Glazed Jelly	**280**	10	44
Jelly	**250**	10	36
Lemon	**230**	10	31
Maple Creme	**290**	14	38
Maple Frosted	**260**	11	35
Maple Vanilla Creme	**330**	15	45
Old Fashioned	**310**	19	30
Peanut	**470**	27	50
Plain Stick	**410**	30	31
Powdered	**330**	20	34
Strawberry Frosted	**260**	11	35
Sugared	**210**	11	24
Toasted Coconut	**430**	22	52
Vanilla Creme	**300**	15	37
Muffins: Blueberry	**460**	15	77
Chocolate Chip	**550**	21	85
Coffee Cake	**590**	24	88
Corn	**460**	16	73
Munchkins: Cinnamon	**60**	3.5	6
Glazed	**60**	3	7
Glazed Chocolate	**60**	3.5	8
Jelly	**60**	3	8
Old Fashioned	**60**	3.5	6
Powdered	**60**	3.5	6
Other Bakery Items:			
English Muffin	**190**	2	35
Plain Croissant	**340**	19	37

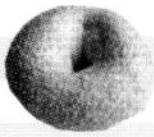
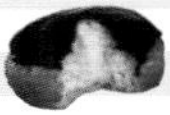
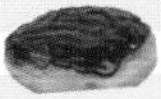
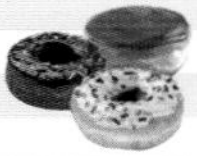
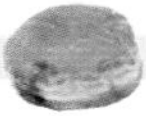
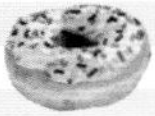
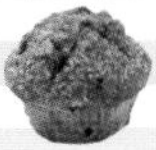
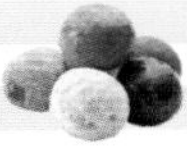
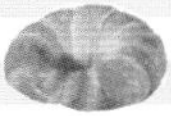

...continued next page

Dunkin'® cont... (Oct '21)

Sandwiches:	C	F	Cb
Plain Bagel Sandwiches:			
Bacon, Egg & Cheese	520	18	67
Egg & Cheese	460	13	66
Ham, Egg & Cheese	500	15	68
Sausage, Egg & Cheese	680	34	68
Tuna Salad on Plain Bagel	510	17	64
Veggie Bacon, Egg & Cheese	510	17	68
Beyond Sausage Sandwich	510	26	39
Biscuit, Chicken Sandwich	460	22	46
Croissants: Bacon, Egg & Cheese	560	36	41
Egg & Cheese	500	31	40
Ham, Egg & Cheese	540	33	41
Sausage, Egg & Cheese	720	52	42
English Muffin Sandwiches:			
Bacon, Egg & Cheese	400	19	39
Ham, Egg & Cheese	370	15	39
Sausage, Egg & Cheese	560	35	40
Wake-Up Wraps:			
Bacon, Egg & Cheese	220	13	15
Beyond Sausage	280	18	15
Egg & Cheese	180	10	14
Turkey Sausage & Egg	240	15	15
Veggie Egg White & Bacon	190	10	15
Hash Browns, 6 pieces	130	6	12
Hot Beverages: Per Medium			
Chocolate: Original	330	10	59
Mint	300	10	52
Dunkaccino	350	15	52
Iced Drinks: Per Medium, without Sugar			
Iced Cappuccino:			
with Skim Milk	70	0	10
with Whole Milk	120	6	10
Iced Latte:			
with Almond Milk	100	3	17
with Whole Milk	170	9	14
Iced Macchiato:			
with Coconutmilk	40	3	3
with Oatmilk	90	2.5	17
Frozen Drinks: Per Medium			
Butter Pecan Swirl Frozen Coffee:			
with Skim Milk	680	5	150
with Whole Milk	720	9	150
Frozen Chocolate, Butter Pecan Swirl, whole milk	720	9	150
Frozen Matcha Latte:			
with Skim milk	360	0	83
with Whole milk	390	5	83

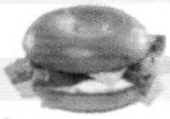
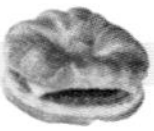
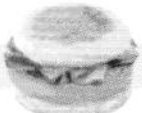
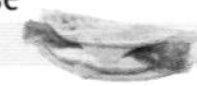
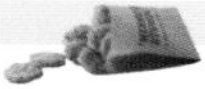
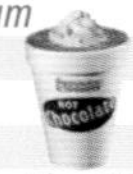
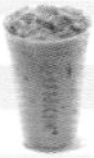
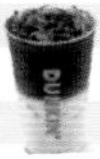
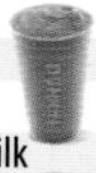
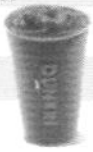

Eat 'N Park® (Oct '21)

Breakfast: Without Extras	C	F	Cb
Bananas Foster French Toast	440	6	88
Country Fried Steak & Eggs	580	23	51
Home Made French Toast, with Maple Syrup & Sugar, 2 slices	300	10	38
Omelettes: Ham & Cheese	660	47	6
Mushroom & Swiss	490	25	5
Pancakes: Blueberry (2)	330	3	64
Buttermilk (2)	320	2.5	65
Scramblers:			
All-American with Sausage	740	42	58
Philly Steak & Egg	620	24	59
Appetizers:			
Fried Cheese Sticks	590	35	41
Fresh Potato Chip Basket	620	40	63
Southwest Chicken Quesadilla	1010	47	84
Burgers: Without Sides			
Bacon Cheeseburger	810	51	37
Eat 'N Park Beyond	850	60	45
Mushroom & Onion	790	48	41
Superburgers: Black Angus	1100	71	39
Original	670	42	37
Sandwiches: Without Sides			
Bacon Grilled Cheese	800	43	70
Chargrilled Chicken	470	18	41
Classic Grilled Cheese	720	37	70
Grilled Chicken Club	810	49	39
Philly Cheesesteak	800	42	50
Shredded Pot Roast	540	31	28
Turkey Club	850	46	48
Whale of a Cod Fish	930	35	96
Dinners: Without Sides or Sauces			
Baked Chicken Parmigiana, with Marinara Sauce	920	41	84
Baked Cod, 1 fillet	220	12	3
Breaded Shrimp	430	18	39
Chicken Bruschetta, 1 breast	500	27	27
Fried Chicken, 4 pieces	1650	97	79
Nantucket Cod & Stuffing, 1 piece	400	28	10
Rosemary Chicken, 1 piece	240	9	5
Whale & Mac	1080	52	83
Whale of a Cod	620	30	39

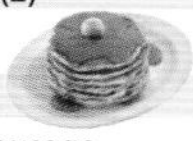
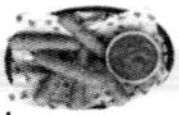
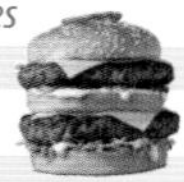
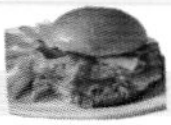
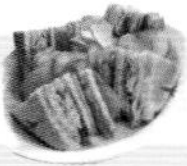
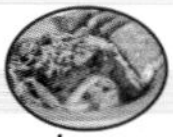
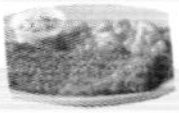

Eat 'N Park® cont... (Oct '21)

Salads: *Without Dressing*	C	F	Cb
Chef's Cobb	**690**	45	11
Chkn & Strawb. w/ Sesame Dressng	**510**	25	35
Chicken Fiesta w/ Chip. Lime Dressng	**660**	31	53
Sides: Broccoli	**40**	0	8
Carrots	**40**	1	9
Coleslaw	**120**	8	12
French Fries Alone	**350**	17	47
Dinner Portion	**175**	8	24
Mac'n Cheese	**450**	22	44
Mashed Potatoes	**110**	6	13
Tater Tots	**250**	14	30
Soup Bowls: *Per Bowl*			
Chicken Noodle	**270**	8	34
Clam Chowder	**420**	18	48
Cream of Broccoli	**300**	12	39
Cream of Potato	**310**	14	39
Desserts: *Per Slice, without Whipped Cream*			
Pies: Apple Pie	**390**	14	65
Bananas Foster Creme Pie	**560**	29	74
Chocolate Cream Pie	**510**	28	58
Dutch Apple Pie	**410**	16	65
Peachberry	**390**	17	55

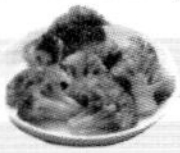
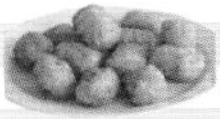
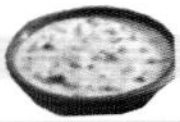
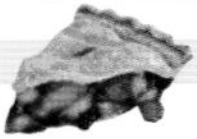

Edo Japan® (Oct '21)

Chop Chop Bowls: *Without Teriyaki Top Sauce*	C	F	Cb
Beef	**680**	21	80
Chicken	**565**	9	80
Chicken & Beef	**620**	15	80
Tempura Shrimp	**600**	17	92
Veggie	**390**	3	77
Noodle Meals: *W/ Asian Veggies, w/out Teriyaki Top Sauce*			
Beef Noodleful	**795**	37	72
Chicken Noodleful	**680**	25	72
Shrimp	**625**	22	71
Veggie	**550**	20	79
Yakisoba: Beef	**615**	23	61
Chicken	**505**	11	62
Chicken & Beef	**560**	17	62
Rice Meals: *With Asian Veggies, w/out Teriyaki Top Sauce*			
Beef & Shrimp	**825**	34	80
Chicken & Beef	**570**	12	76
Chicken & Shrimp	**715**	22	80
Fresh Grilled Vegetables	**445**	1	96
Hawaiian Chicken	**505**	6	75
Sizzling Shrimp	**470**	4	78
Teriyaki Salmon	**540**	8	79
Sushi: *Per 4 Rolls without Sauce*			
Beef	**165**	5	23
California Rolls	**170**	4	27
Dynamite Rolls	**180**	6	26
Salmon	**145**	2	22

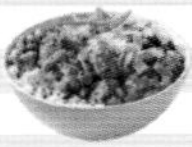
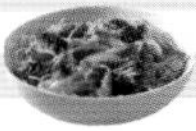
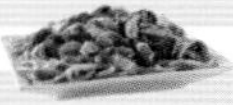
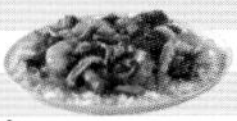
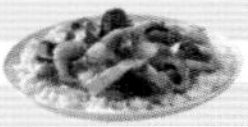
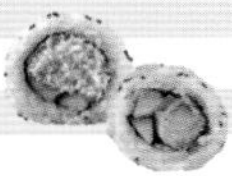

Einstein Bros® (Jun '21)

Bagels: *For Nutritional Information on Menu Items at Licensed Locations ~ see In Store*

	C	F	Cb
Bagels: Ancient Grain	**290**	5	50
Asiago Cheese	**300**	4	54
Blueberry	**280**	1	60
Chocolate Chip	**280**	3	56
Cinnamon Sugar	**300**	2	61
Cranberry	**310**	4	59
Everything	**280**	1	57
French Toast	**380**	7	70
Honey Whole Wheat	**280**	3	51
Onion	**280**	0.5	58
Plain. 3.5 oz	**270**	0.5	56
Poppy Seed	**280**	2	56
Sesame Seed	**290**	2	56
Thintastic: Ancient Grain	**190**	2.5	35
Everything	**200**	1	41
Honey Whole Wheat	**200**	3	37
Plain	**200**	0	41
Lunch Hot & Toasty Sandwiches:			
Pizza Bagel Cheese	**440**	14	58
Pizza Bagel Pepperoni	**530**	23	59
Lunch Signature Sandwiches:			
Avocado Veg Out	**420**	12	68
Ham & Swiss/Plain Bagel	**550**	20	63
Nova Lox /Plain Bagel	**480**	17	60
Tasty Turkey/Asiago Bagel	**520**	15	66
Cream Cheese: *Per 1.2 oz Schmear*			
Garlic & Herb	**110**	9	5
Plain	**120**	12	2
Onion and Chive	**110**	10	4
Reduced Fat:			
Garden Veggie	**100**	9	5
Honey Almond; Strawberry, av.	**120**	9	10
Smoked Salmon	**110**	10	3
Breakfast:			
Chef's Creation 2 Egg Sandwiches:			
All-Nighter on Hash Brown Bagel	**880**	55	65
Chorizo Sunrise	**870**	52	63
Farmhouse	**640**	27	64
Classic 1 Egg Sandwiches: *On Plain Bagel*			
Applewood Bacon & Cheddar	**450**	15	57
Turkey Sausage & Cheddar	**480**	15	58
Signature Egg Sandwich:			
Bacon, Avocado & Tomato	**420**	19	47
Texas Brisket Egg Sandwich	**830**	51	55
Sides, Twice Baked Hash Brown	**170**	11	12

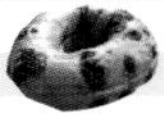
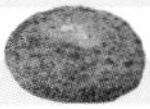
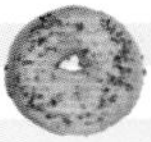
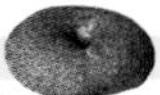
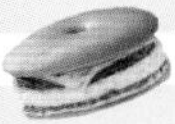
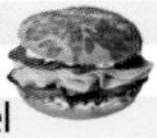

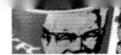

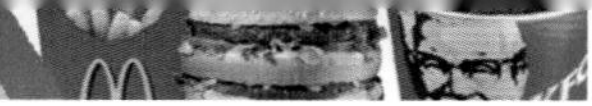

El Pollo Loco® (Oct '21)

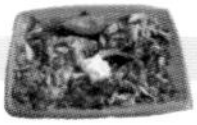
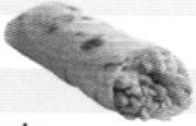
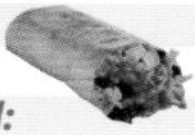
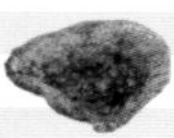
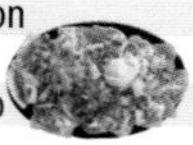
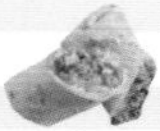
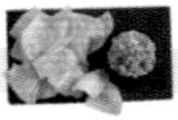
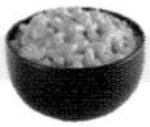
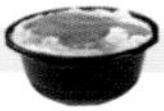
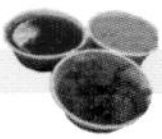

	C	F	Cb
Bowl:			
Original Chicken	530	7	81
Double Chicken	850	27	86
Double Protein Avocado Chicken	390	16	15
Grand Avocado Chicken	760	26	89
Burritos:			
Chicken Avocado	850	45	71
Chickenless Pollo	740	33	86
Chipotle Chicken Avocado	870	39	86
Original BRC	400	11	62
Vegan Chickenless	550	16	82
Chicken, Fire-Grilled:			
Breast with skin, 4.3 o	220	9	0
Leg with skin,1.6 oz	80	4	0
Thigh with skin, 3.1 oz	210	15	0
Wing with skin,m1.3 oz	90	5	0
Fire-Grilled Combos:			
Chicken Tacos Al Carbon	430	13	51
Chicken Nachos	830	48	68
Classic Chicken Burrito	580	17	68
Original Pollo Bowl	530	7	81
Extras:			
Chicken Taco Al Carbon	140	4	17
Classic Chicken Burrito	480	13	65
Fried Tortilla Chips, 5 oz	760	44	83
Chips & Guacamole:			
5.9 oz	490	32	49
11.8 oz	990	63	98
Tortilla Soup: Small	250	9	19
Large	450	17	34
Sides:			
Black Beans: Small, 6 oz	140	1	25
Large, 16 oz	370	2.5	65
Coleslaw, small, 4 oz	130	10	9
Loco Side Salad, small	170	15	8
Macaroni & Cheese: Small, 6 oz	310	19	24
Large, 15 oz	770	48	60
Mashed Potatoes & Gravy:			
Small, 6 oz	105	1	20
Large, 17 oz	340	4.5	69
Pinto Beans, small	150	2.5	24
Spanish Rice: Small, 4.5 oz	160	1.5	33
Large, 10.75 oz	380	3.5	78
Condiments:			
Salsa: Avocado, 1.3 oz	30	2.5	2
House; Pico de Gallo, Roja,1.3 oz	10	0	2
Sour Cream, 1.3 oz	80	7	1
Dessert, Two Cinnamon Churros	280	17	29

Fatburger® (Oct '21)

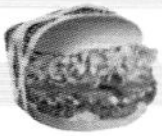
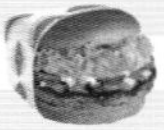
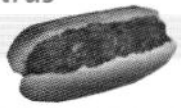
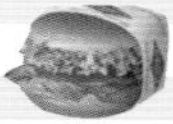
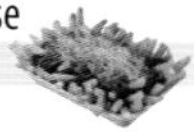
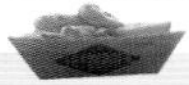
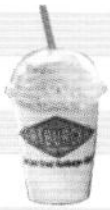

	C	F	Cb
Burgers: *Without Extras*			
Fatburger: Baby Fat	400	21	37
Original	590	31	46
Kingburger	850	41	69
Impossible Burger	525	13	54
Thousand Island	770	47	46
Turkeyburger	480	21	50
Veggieburger	510	20	60
Hot Dogs: *Without Extras*			
Chili Cheese	480	27	35
Regular Hot Dog	320	15	32
Sandwiches: *Without Extras*			
Bacon & Egg	350	16	37
Chicken: Crispy	660	16	91
Grilled	430	14	42
Sausage & Egg	780	53	47
Spicy Chicken	520	21	58
Fries: Fat Fries	380	18	47
with Chili & Cheese	590	33	53
Skinny Fries	390	15	58
with Chili Cheese	600	30	64
Sweet Potato	480	24	66
Wings & Tenders: Bone In Wing (1)	60	4	2
Boneless Wing (1)	50	3	2
Chicken Tender (1)	110	5	2
Sides: Chili Cup	200	11	10
with Cheese & Onions	320	20	12
Onion Rings	540	29	64
Shakes: Chocolate	910	45	115
Maui Banana	940	44	126
Strawberry	880	44	111
Vegan Strawberry/Vanilla, av	540	24	81

For Complete Nutritional Data ~ see CalorieKing.com

Fazoli's® (Oct '21)

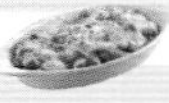

	C	F	Cb
Oven-Baked Pasta: *Per Serving*			
Baked Lasagna	630	25	69
Chicken Broccoli Penne	860	38	74
Chicken Parmigiano	840	25	114
Penne with Creamy Basil Chicken	900	45	70
Spicy Baked Ziti with Sausage	1040	61	79
Classic Pastas:			
Chicken Fettuccine Alfredo	870	28	106
Fettuccine Alfredo	690	22	104
Spagh. with Marinara	510	4	108
Spaghetti with Meatballs	740	21	113
Breadstick, Garlic, (1)	130	8	16

Fazoli's® cont... (Oct '21)

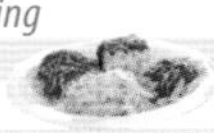
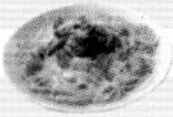
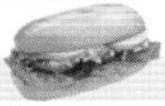

Samplers: Per Serving	C	F	Cb
Classic	820	25	120
Oven Baked	930	35	116
Ultimate	1050	30	163
Signature Pasta:			
Chicken Carbonara	940	33	110
Three Cheese Tortellini Alfredo	890	35	78
Submarinos:			
Meatball da Vinci	920	56	65
Primo Italiano	840	45	60
Salads: *With MenuSet Dressing*			
Chicken Bacon Caesar	740	51	26
Crispy Chicken Bacon Caesar	970	75	37

For Complete Nutritional Data ~ see CalorieKing.com

Firehouse Subs® (Oct '21)

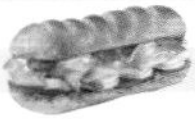
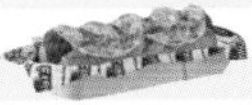
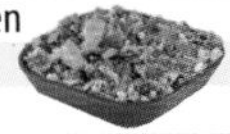

Hot Subs: *Per Medium White Sub, with Standard Toppings*	C	F	Cb
Cajun Chicken	710	35	54
Chicken Gyro Hero	810	44	58
Club on a Sub	770	40	63
Engineer	690	35	60
Hook & Ladder	720	36	63
Italian	940	58	65
Meatball	830	51	59
Steak & Cheese	830	51	53
Sides, Chili, Bowl without Chips	300	15	22
Under 500 Calorie Salads:			
Firehouse Chopped: *Without Dressing*			
with Grilled Chicken	380	10	14
with Ham	310	10	27
with Turkey	220	7	15
Italian, with Grilled Chicken	410	22	14

Five Guys® (Oct '21)

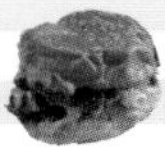
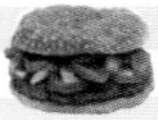
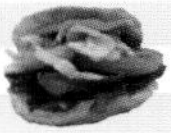

Burgers: *Without Toppings or Sauce*	C	F	Cb
Bacon Burger	920	50	39
Bacon Cheeseburger	1060	62	40
Cheeseburger	980	55	40
Hamburger	840	43	39
Little Burgers: Bacon Burger	620	33	39
Bacon Cheeseburger	690	39	40
Hamburger	540	26	39
Hot Dogs: Bacon	600	42	40
Bacon Cheese	670	48	41
Cheese	590	41	41
Sandwiches: BLT	600	34	42
Cheese Veggie	420	21	61
Grilled Cheese	470	26	41
Veggie	280	15	60

Five Guys® cont... (Oct '21)

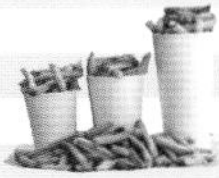

Burger Sauces:	C	F	Cb
A.1 Original	15	0	3
Bar-B-Que	50	0	15
Ketchup	30	0	5
Mayo	110	11	0
Fries: Little, 8 oz	530	23	72
Regular, 14.5 oz	955	41	131
Large, 20 oz	1315	57	181

Flame Broiler® (Oct '21)

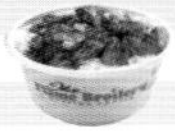
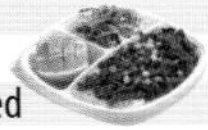

Bowls: *Regular Single Protein with White Rice, without Toppings or Cooking Sauce*	C	F	Cb
Beef, marinated	660	10	103
Chicken	650	12	84
Tofu	550	9	88
White Meat Chicken	590	6	82
Plates: *Regular Single Portion with White Rice, without Toppings or Added Sauce*			
Beef, marinated	850	5	126
Chicken, without sce	840	18	100
Rib (beef), marinated	1000	35	107

Freshens® (Oct '21)

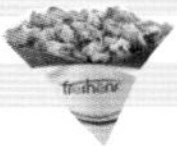
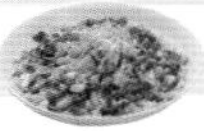
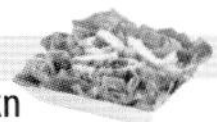
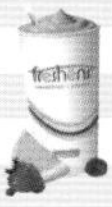

	C	F	Cb
Crepes: Buffalo Chicken	410	22	25
Cheesecake Supreme	450	21	55
Chicken Caesar	600	44	25
Chipotle Ranch Turkey Melt	520	31	25
Denver, with Bacon	520	29	27
Honey Mustard Chkn	460	22	36
Pesto Chicken	490	29	27
Southwest Chicken	580	33	36
Rice Bowls: Baja Queso	680	33	74
Buffalo Chicken	600	23	70
Florence	610	14	80
KC BBQ	610	11	97
Mexican	710	29	83
Power Protein	810	30	94
Spicy Korean	520	8	90
Salads: Buffalo Chkn	480	27	29
Gr. Chicken Caesar	520	37	26
Roadhouse BBQ Chkn	420	17	42
Strawberry & Kale	490	15	56
Smoothies: *100% Juice*			
Blended Fruit Classics: *Per 20 fl.oz*			
Bangin' Berry	330	0	80
Caribbean Craze	300	0	73
Jamaican Jammer	330	0	70
Peach On The Beach	330	2.5	75
Peanut Butter Protein	480	12	69
Tropical Therapy	530	4	81
Vegan PowerUp	320	0	71

Godfather's Pizza® (Oct '21)

Golden Crust Pizza: Per Slice	C	F	Cb
Cheese: Medium, ⅛ pizza	210	8	26
Large, 1/10 pizza	240	10	28
Combo: Medium, ⅛ pizza	280	13	28
Large, 1/10 pizza	310	15	30
Super Combo:			
Medium, ⅛ pizza	310	16	28
Large, 1/10 pizza	360	18	31
Mozza-Loaded:			
All Meat Combo: Medium, ⅛ pizza	340	18	29
Large, 1/10 pizza	380	20	31
Original Crust Pizza:			
BLT: Small, ⅙ pizza	300	14	30
Medium, ⅛ pizza	320	15	33
Jumbo, 1/12 pizza	440	21	43
Buffalo Chicken: Small, ⅙ pizza	250	9	30
Medium, ⅛ pizza	270	9	33
Jumbo, 1/12 pizza	380	14	43
Taco Pie: Small, ⅙ pizza	300	12	33
Medium, ⅛ pizza	340	14	36
Jumbo, 1/12 pizza	460	20	47
Thin Crust Pizza:			
BBQ Chicken: Medium, ⅛ pizza	200	8	20
Large, 1/10 pizza	240	10	24
Pepperoni: Medium, ⅛ pizza	200	11	15
Large, 1/10 pizza	230	13	18
The Don: Medium, ⅛ pizza	250	14	16
Large, 1/10 pizza	290	17	19
Sides: Baked Beans, 4 oz	120	1	25
Biscuit, 1 oz	90	4	13
Cheesy Potatoes, 4 oz	300	19	30
Coleslaw, 4 oz	210	17	12
Gravy, 2 oz	30	1	4
Mashed Potatoes, 4 oz	100	3	17
Mixed Vegetables, 4 oz	90	0	18
Potato Wedges, 4 oz	180	7	26

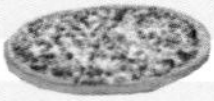
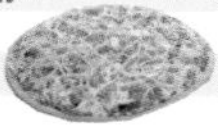
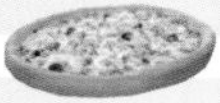

Gold Star Chili® (Oct '21)

Burgers: Per Single	C	F	Cb
Bacon Cheeseburger	870	58	46
Chili Burger	680	39	50
Classic Burger	560	33	44
Coneys, Original Chili: Plain	210	11	21
Cheese	300	18	21
Chili Cheese Sandwich (no dog)	140	4	20
Ways, Original Chili:			
Regular: 3-Way	760	41	56
5-Way	850	41	74
Regular Veggie: 3-Way	730	40	58
5-Way	830	40	74
Gorditos: Orig.	590	30	62
Vegetarian Chili	590	29	62

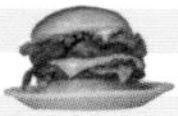
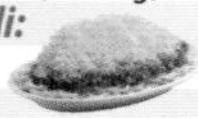
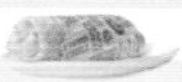

Gold Star Chili® cont...(Oct '21)

Double Deckers: With White Bread	C	F	Cb
Ham & Bacon	1080	80	46
Ham & Turkey	760	46	46
Turkey & Bacon	1070	78	46
Salads: Full Salad, without Dressing			
BBQ Chicken	490	24	36
Harvest Pecan Chkn	340	16	25
Fries: French, regular	460	19	67
Chili	490	22	63
Chili Cheese	840	51	64
Garlic Parmesan	870	62	71
Vegetarian Chili	540	24	71

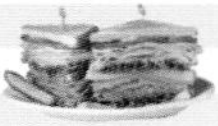
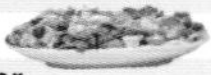
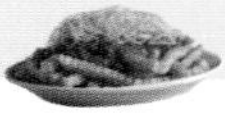

Golden Corral® (Oct '21)

Breakfast:	C	F	Cb
Corned Beef Hash, ½ cup	230	15	14
Egg& Sausage Casserole, ½ cup	240	6	11
Hasbbrown Casserole, ½ cup	110	4	14
Sausage & Egg Burrito	320	19	22
Hot Lunch Favorites: Without Sides			
Beef: Pot Roast, ½ cup	150	7	8
Roast, flat, 3 oz	180	10	1
Smoked Beef Short Ribs, 3 oz	340	27	0
Steak, Smothered Chopped, 5.9 oz	290	18	4
Chicken: Buffalo Chicken S'wich	200	9	21
Fried Chicken, 3 oz	240	15	6
Orange Chicken, 6 oz	390	15	40
Smoked White Meat Chicken, 3 oz	150	6	0
Fish: Baked, 3 oz	150	8	1
Fried Catfish, 3 oz	180	10	12
Pork: Baby Back Ribs, 3 oz	190	13	3
Sweet & Sour, 6 oz	220	11	18
Sides: BBQ Baked Beans, ½ cup	160	1	35
Creamed Spinach, ½ cup	170	12	10
Fries, Seasoned Wedges (10)	190	12	21
Fried Okra (10)	110	7	10
Mac & Cheese, ½ c.	180	10	19
Mshd Potatoes,½ c.	160	8	20
Rice Pilaf, ½ cup	130	5	18
Salad Buffet: Per ½ Cup Unless Indicated			
Caesar, without dressing, 1 cup	110	8	8
Chicken	250	22	3
Coleslaw	110	9	6
Macaroni	280	11	41
Marinated Vegetable	35	2	3
Potato	150	5	26
Romaine Lettuce, 1 cup	10	0	2
Seafood	140	10	9
Spinach, 1 cup	15	0	2
Strawberry Spinach, 1 cup	40	3	5
Tuna	190	12	4

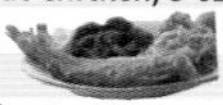
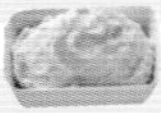
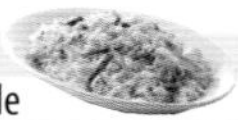

Great American Bagel Co® (Oct '21)

Bagels:	C	F	Cb
Asiago Cheese	520	16	72
Cheddar Herb	390	8	66
Cinnamon Raisin	380	4	76
Jalapeno Cheddar	370	7	63
Plain	360	4	71
Spinach Tomazzo	640	20	86
Tomazzo	520	13	77
Cream Cheese Filling: *Per 1 oz*			
Plain	100	10	1
Strawberry; Vegetable, average	95	8	4
Paninis: *With Set Menu Ingredients On Regular Baguette*			
Chicken Pesto	770	35	70
Ham & Swiss	600	26	58
Philly Beef	920	40	92
Turkey Club	680	29	67
Sandwiches: Asiago Omelet	720	29	80
BLT	550	17	72
Chicken Parmigiana	740	22	81
Ham	460	9	71
Roast Beef	465	9	71
Turkey	435	5	72
Pastries:			
Cookies: Chocolate Chunk, 4 oz	110	4	19
Oatmeal Raisin, 4 oz	120	5	18
Muffins: Banana Nut, 4.25 oz	430	18	61
Blueberry, 4.25 oz	430	16	64

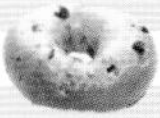
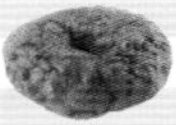
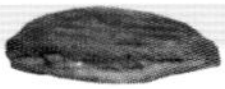
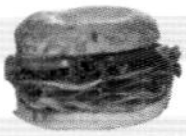

Green Burrito® (Oct '21)

Burritos:	C	F	Cb
Bean & Cheese	660	25	76
Bean, Rice & Cheese	730	26	93
Green: Chicken	930	38	96
Steak	940	38	96
Grilled, Beef; Chicken; Steak, av.	835	31	88
Quesadillas: 4 Cheese	640	64	53
Chicken	780	40	56
Steak	790	39	56
Super Nachos: Regular	670	41	51
Beef/Chicken/Steak, average	735	44	53
Tacos: Crunchy Beef/Chkn/Steak, av.	210	11	15
Soft Beef/Chicken/Steak, av.	255	13	18
Taco Salad, Beef/Chicken/ Steak, av.	880	53	61
Sides: Chips, 2 oz	300	17	35
Guacamole, 2.7 oz	100	8	5

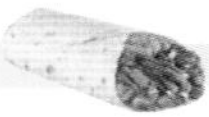
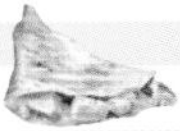
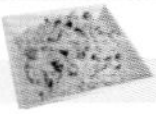

(The) Great Steak® (Oct '21)

Cheesesteaks:	C	F	Cb
Regular 7": Chicagoland	610	24	59
Great Steak	790	45	55
Original Philly	510	17	55
Super Steak	800	45	57
Large 12": Chicagoland	1050	41	97
Great Steak	1360	79	92
Original Philly	840	26	91
Super Steak	1380	80	95
Chicken Philly Sandwiches: *Per Regular 7"*			
Original	490	15	56
Buffalo Chicken	720	37	58
Teriyaki Chicken	800	42	66
Ultimate Chicken	780	43	58
Grilled Sandwiches: *Per Regular 7"*			
Chicken Bacon Ranch	800	43	58
Veggie Delight	490	19	61
Baked Potatoes:			
Bacon & Cheese	440	23	36
Broccoli & Cheese	250	6	45
Sour Cream & Chives	250	10	38
The Great Potato:			
Chicken	440	18	47
Ham	450	19	52
Steak	470	20	46
Turkey	430	17	48
The King	540	32	38
Fries:			
Bacon Ranch: Regular	880	44	55
X Large	1600	95	148
Cheese: Regular	440	22	54
Large	660	33	82
Chili Cheese: Regular	530	24	65
Large	780	36	97
Great Fry: Regular	370	18	48
Large	590	28	77
King Fry, regular	510	29	55
Philly, large	1090	48	131
Salads: *Without Dressing*			
Great Salad:			
Grilled Chicken	350	21	14
Grilled Ham	360	22	19
Turkey	350	20	19
Salad Dressings: Mayo, reg., 1 oz	200	22	0
Ranch, 1 oz	150	16	2
Thousand Island, 1 oz	130	12	4
Sauce: BBQ, 1 oz	50	0	12
Buffalo, 1 oz	10	0	1
Honey Mustard, 1 oz	40	1	7
Teriyaki, 1 oz	25	0	3

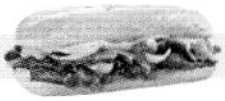
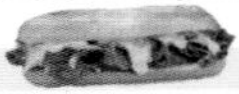
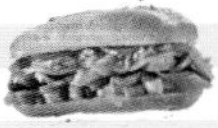
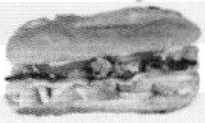
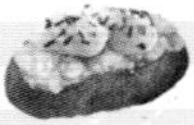
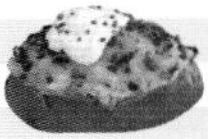
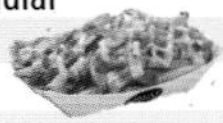
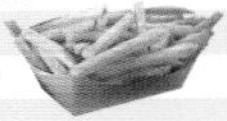
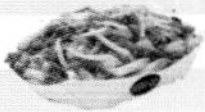
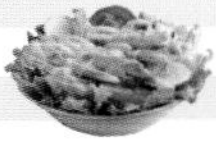

Haagen-Dazs® (Dec '20)

Classic Flavors: Per ⅔ Cup	C	F	Cb
Bourbon Praline Pecan	380	21	42
Bourbon Van. Bean Truffle	340	20	36
Butter Pecan	370	28	26
Caramel Cone	400	25	38
Cherry Vanilla	290	18	29
Chocolate	260	17	22
Chocolate Chocolate Chip	380	24	34
Chocolate Peanut Butter	450	29	36
Coffee; Cookies & Cream, av.	310	21	27
Cold Brew Espresso Chip Heaven	220	9	27
Double Belgian Chocolate Chip	330	21	30
Dulce de Leche	350	20	36
Green Tea	310	21	25
Honey Salted Caramel Almond	350	22	33
Irish Cream Brownie	360	21	37
Mango	330	17	40
Mint Chip	360	23	33
PB Chocolate Fudge	380	19	47
Pineapple Coconut; Rose & Crm. av.	300	17	33
Pistachio	280	19	22
Rocky Road; Rum Tres Leches, av.	365	21	38
Rum Raisin; Vanilla, av.	310	20	27
Sea Salt Caramel Truffle	300	17	32
Strawberry	240	15	22
Vanilla Choc. Chip/Swiss Alm., av.	370	24	32
Whisky Hazelnut Latte	380	25	32
Light: Chocolate Sea Salt Heaven	230	8	30
PB Chip Heaven	230	10	26
Strawberry Waffle Cone Heaven	210	6	33
Non Dairy: Per ⅔ cup			
Amaretto Black Cherry Almond Toffee	320	12	49
Chocolate Salted Fudge Truffle	270	11	40
Peanut Butter Chocolate Fudge	380	19	47
Trio Crispy Layers: Per ⅔ cup			
Coconut Caramel Chocolate	370	24	34
Coffee Vanilla Chocolate	360	25	29
Lemon Raspberry White Chocolate	360	22	36
Salted Caramel Chocolate	300	20	26
Triple Chocolate Trio	290	19	26
Van. Blackberry Chocolate	280	19	24

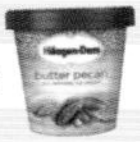
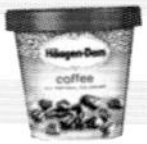
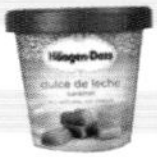
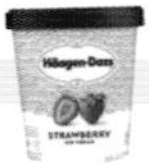
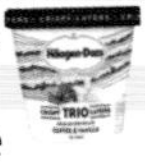

Ice Cream Bars/Cones ~ See Page 109

Hardee's® (Oct '21)

Charbroiled Burgers:	C	F	Cb
Famous Star with Cheese	660	37	55
Super Star w/ Cheese	920	56	59
The Big Hardee	920	58	55
Western Bacon Cheeseburger	810	38	80
Cheeseburgers: Big	540	23	56
Double	530	26	56
Thickburgers: Original, ⅓ lb	820	51	56
Bacon Cheese, ⅓ lb	790	49	54
Frisco, ⅓ lb	760	50	43
Monster Double, ⅔ lb	1400	97	53
Mushroom 'N' Swiss, ⅓ lb	620	33	52
Original Beyond Meat	780	46	61
Double	1110	70	66
All Star Meals: Per Set Menu, without Dipping Sauce			
Double Cheeseburger:			
w/ Spicy Chicken	1280	71	131
w/ Jumbo Hot Dog	1160	64	111
Sandwiches:			
Beef: Big Roast Beef	500	22	49
Monster Roast Beef	870	33	52
Big Hot Ham 'N' Cheese	530	20	51
Chicken: Big Chicken Fillet	590	29	61
Charbroiled Chicken Club	650	29	53
Chicken Tenders: Without Sauce			
Hand Breaded:			
3 pieces, 4.5 oz	260	13	13
5 pieces, 7.5 oz	440	21	21
Boxes: 10 Pieces	880	42	42
15 Pieces	1320	63	63
20 Pieces	1760	84	84
Chili Dog, Jumbo	390	26	23
Natural Cut Fries:			
Kid's, 3 oz	240	12	31
Small, 3.7 oz	300	15	39
Medium, 5.9 oz	420	21	55
Large, 6.5 oz	460	22	59
Sides:			
Beer Battered Onion Rings	670	35	77
Crispy Curls:			
Small, 4.1 oz	310	15	39
Medium, 5.36 oz	420	21	53
Large, 6.5 oz	460	23	58
Side Salad	120	7	7

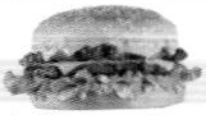
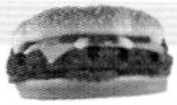

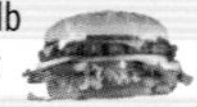
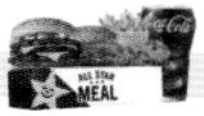
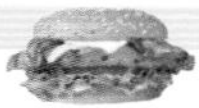
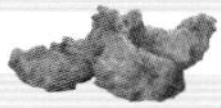
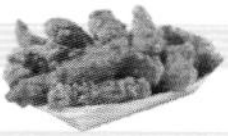
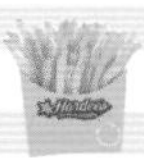
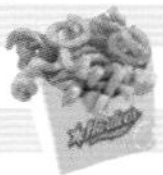

Hardee's® cont... (Oct '21)

Breakfast:	C	F	Cb
Bowls:			
Loaded Hash Round	510	36	30
Low Carb	760	68	0
Burritos: Beyond Sausage	730	41	51
Loaded	580	30	46
Southwest Omelet	690	41	44
Made From Scratch Biscuits:			
Bacon, Egg & Cheese	620	40	44
Beyond Sausage	480	26	44
with Egg	600	35	47
Biscuit 'N' Gravy	600	38	54
Chicken Fillet	660	43	50
Country Ham	510	32	42
Country Fried Steak	650	44	49
Loaded Omelet	630	41	46
Monster	890	63	45
Pork Chop 'N' Gravy	550	34	48
Sausage	630	45	42
with Egg	700	50	44
Smoked Sausage, Egg & Cheese	700	48	45
Platters: With Bacon	1050	68	76
With Chicken Fillet	980	58	63
With Country Ham	990	61	75
With Country Steak	970	60	62
With Pork Chop	990	56	66
With Sausage	1150	79	76
Sandwich, Frisco Breakfast	430	19	42
Sunrise Croissant: Bacon	420	26	29
Ham	390	23	29
Sausage	550	40	30
Breakfast Sides:			
Hash Rounds: Small, 2.9 oz	240	14	21
Medium, 4.2 oz	370	22	33
Large, 5.8 oz	490	29	43
Desserts:			
Apple Turnover, w/out Cinnamon Sugar	270	13	35
Chocolate Chip Cookie, 1.5 oz	200	10	26
Ice Cream Shakes: *Per 14 oz*			
Hand Scooped: Chocolate	690	36	84
Strawberry	690	35	83
Vanilla	700	35	86

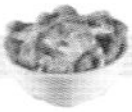
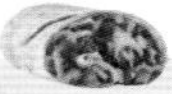
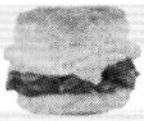
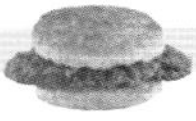
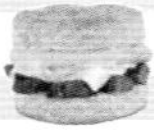
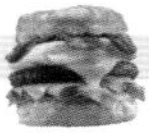
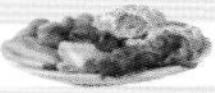
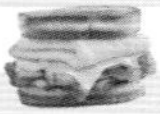
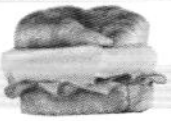
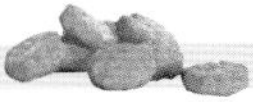
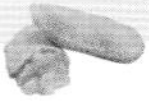
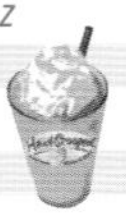

Hissho Sushi® (Oct '21)

Natural Food Store Menu Items	C	F	Cb
Maki Sushi Rolls: *Per Package*			
California, 11.5 oz	330	7	60
Dazzling Dragon, 13 oz	510	22	52
Krispy Krab, 9.8 oz	410	19	53
Living Color, 10.6 oz	340	11	40
Philadelphia, 11.4 oz	470	20	62
Rising Sun, 13.4 oz	680	40	50
Salmon Lover, 12.4 oz	600	34	41
Spicy California, 13 oz	440	16	66
Spicy Pepper, 8.9 oz	250	9	40
Spicy Salmon, 12 oz	420	15	53
Spicy Tuna, 12 oz	390	9	53
Tempura Shrimp, 12.87 oz	520	23	70
TNT, 10.3 oz	440	19	42
Veggie, 12 oz	320	7	60
Veggie TNT, 10.3 oz	220	5	43
Wasabi Crunch, 9.45 oz	290	9	43

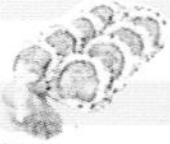
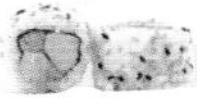
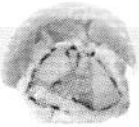
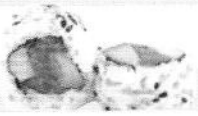
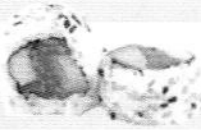

Hot Dog on a Stick® (Oct '21)

Menu Items:	C	F	Cb
On A Stick: American Cheese	260	16	20
Beef Hot Dog	330	21	25
Pepper Jack Cheese	260	15	22
Turkey Hot Dog	240	5	27
Veggie Dog	200	6	26
Fish & Zucchini Platter	470	15	53
Fish Platter with Tartar Sauce	320	14	27
Zucchini Platter with Ranch Sauce	420	23	45
Condiments: Ketchup, 0.5 oz	10	0	3
Mayo, 0.5 oz	80	9	0
Sweet Relish, 0.3 oz	10	0	3
Yellow Mustard, 0.2 oz	5	0	1
French Fries: Small, 7.2 oz	500	29	57
Regular, 14.4 oz	1000	59	113
Funnel Cake Sticks:			
with Chocolate Sauce, 3.4 oz	300	6	48
with Powdered Sugar, 2.6 oz	210	5	26
with Raspberry Sauce, 3.4 oz	270	5	40
Beverages: *Per Regular Size, 16 fl.oz*			
Lemonade:			
Original	150	0	38
Cherry	210	0	52
Lime	230	0	57

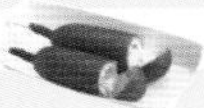
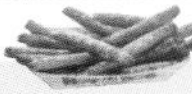
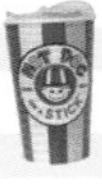

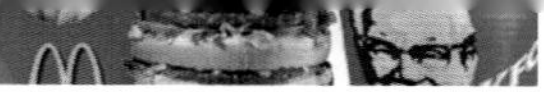

Hungry Howie's Pizza® (Oct '21)

Counts may vary in Florida.

	C	F	Cb
Howie Rolls, average all varieties	625	22	79
Pasta: *Per Regular*			
Baked:			
Orig.; Pasta & Mushrms	450	12	64
Pasta & Meatballs	780	36	70
Chicken Parmesan	740	29	81
Specialty Pizza: *12" Pizza, Per ⅛ Slice*			
Bacon Cheddar Cheeseburger	270	13	25
BBQ Chicken	230	8	29
Buffalo Chicken	210	8	24
Howie Special	210	7	26
Meat Eaters	250	11	25
Works	250	11	26
Veggie	200	6	28
Spicy Chicken Tenders, each	130	7	9
Subs: *Per ½ of Large Sub, with Set Menu Toppings*			
Ham & Cheese	590	23	62
Italian	620	27	62
Steak & Cheese	650	29	62
Turkey Club	840	46	60
Veggie	580	24	69
Salads: *Regular Size, without Dressing*			
Antipasto	400	26	14
Chicken Asiago; Chicken Caesar, av	230	9	15
Garden	90	3	14
Greek	230	11	18
Grilled Chicken	360	19	15
Spicy Chicken	640	36	39
Dressings: *Per 1 oz*			
Caesar	180	18	2
Creamy Italian; Greek, av	115	12	2
Ranch; Thousand Island, av.	140	14	2

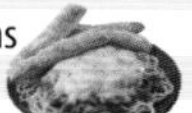

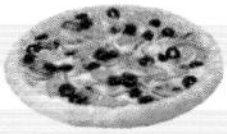

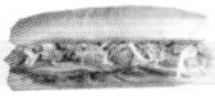

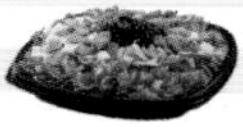

In-N-Out Burger® (Oct '21)

Burgers:	C	F	Cb
Hamburger: with Onion	390	19	39
w/ Mstrd & Ketchup, w/out Spread	310	10	41
Protein Style with Lettuce Wrap, without Bun, with Lettuce	240	17	11
Cheeseburger: with Onion	480	27	39
w/ Mstrd & Ketchup, w/out Spread	400	18	41
Protein Style with Lettuce Wrap, without Bun, with Lettuce	330	25	11
Double Double: with Onion	670	41	39
w/ Mstrd & Ketchup, w/oit Spread	590	32	41
Protein Style with Lettuce Wrap, without Bun, with Lettuce	520	39	11
French Fries, 4.5 oz	370	15	52
Hot Cocoa: 8 fl.oz	130	3	26
with Marshmallows, 8 fl.oz	150	3	32
Shakes: *Per 15 fl.oz*			
Vanilla	570	30	65

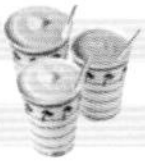

IHOP® (Jun '21)

Pancakes: *With Menu Set Toppings*	C	F	Cb
Cannoli (3)	970	44	125
Double Blueberry (4)	610	16	101
NY Cheesecake (4)	910	35	125
Orig. Buttermilk (3)	430	17	56
Strawberry Banana (4)	650	15	115
Griddle Faves: *With Menu Set Toppings*			
French Toast: Original	740	36	84
Strawberry Banana	840	31	121
Stuffed, Plain	920	40	125
Waffles, Belgian	590	29	69
Crepes: *With Menu Set Toppings*			
Chicken Florentine with Swiss Cheese	790	45	44
German Crepes	610	32	65
Strawberries & Cream	710	29	96
Swedish	600	28	72
Omelettes: *Without Side Choices or Additions*			
Big Steak	830	55	20
Chicken Fajita	910	57	25
Garden	800	61	17
Spicy Poblano	1020	76	30
Spinach & Mushroom	910	71	22
Combos: *With Two B'Milk Pancakes, w/o Sides or Sauce*			
Chicken & Pancakes	880	39	88
Sirloin Tips & Fried Egg	860	42	63
Smokehouse, with Poached Egg	940	68	42
T-Bone Steak (12 oz), w/ Fried Egg	990	45	63
Ultimate Steakburgers: *With Standard Ingredients, without Sides or Dressings*			
Big Brunch	1000	64	58
Cowboy BBQ	950	54	75
The Classic	670	42	41
Sandwiches: *Without additional ingredients, Sides or Dressing*			
BLTA on Sourdough	1160	85	73
Philly Cheese Steak Stacker on Hoagie	800	40	60
Spicy Buffalo Chicken on Brioche	630	31	58
Turkey Cheddar Club on Sourdough	1180	78	66
Entrees: *As Served, without Sides, Dressing or Bread*			
Fried Chicken	980	54	30
Grilled Tilapia	240	10	2
Pot Roast	370	20	15
Smoked Sausage	660	60	9
55+ Lunch: *Without Soup, Salad or Dressing*			
BLT Sandwich, on White Bread	410	28	27
Grilled Cheese S'wich, on Sourdough	630	31	61
Sides: Crispy Breakfast Potatoes	290	13	37
Crispy Potato Pancakes	370	24	35
French Fries	320	15	41
Hash Browns	210	14	19
Onion Rings	530	30	60

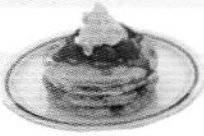

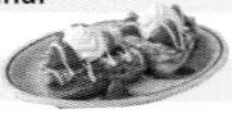

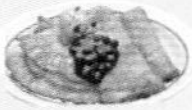

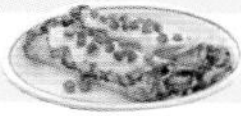

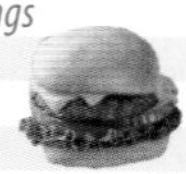

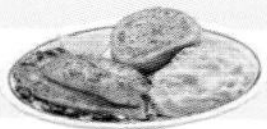

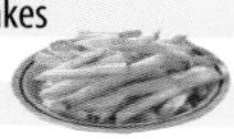

IHOP® cont... (Jun '21)

Bowls: Per Bowl	C	F	Cb
Big Country, w/ Gravy	1020	76	39
New Mexico Chicken, av.	960	47	84
Southwest Chicken, w/ Salsa, av.	1110	80	42
Spicy Poblano Fajita	1060	75	42
Spicy Shredded Beef	900	42	85
The Classic: with Bacon	870	65	22
with Sausage	910	73	30
Burritos:			
Big Coungry, w/ Gravy, av.	1300	85	85
New Mexico Chicken, w/ Salsa, av.	1240	55	129
Southwest Chicken, w/ Salsa, av.	1400	88	86
Spicy Shredded Beef	1180	50	130

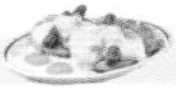
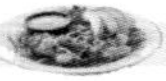
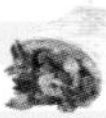

Jack in the Box® (Oct '21)

Sandwiches & Burgers:	C	F	Cb
Bacon Swiss Buttery Jack	890	59	48
Bacon Ultimate Cheeseburger	930	65	32
Classic Buttery Jack	860	58	51
Double Jack	830	58	34
Jumbo Jack	520	33	32
Jumbo Jack Cheeseburger	600	40	33
Quad Bacon Cheesy Jack	950	68	32
Sourdough Jack	700	45	39
Spicy Sriracha Burger	620	45	38
Triple Bacon Cheesy Jack	810	57	32
Ultimate Cheeseburger	840	59	31
Chicken & Fish Sandwiches:			
Chicken Fajita Pita	330	9	35
Chicken Sandwich	510	31	42
H'style Ranch Chicken Club	630	25	69
Jack's Spicy Chicken S'wich	500	25	48
Sourdough Grilled Chicken Club	580	30	38
Chicken: Crispy Strips, 4 pieces	570	26	43
Nuggets, 5 pieces	240	17	13
Teriyaki Bowl	630	6	109
Breakfast:			
Biscuit: Bacon, Egg & Cheese	410	25	26
Sausage, Egg & Cheese	535	38	27
Breakfast Jack: Bacon	380	21	30
Ham	350	18	30
Sausage	485	33	29
Burrito: Meat Lovers, with Salsa	810	51	50
Grand Sausage with Salsa	1070	72	70
Croissants: Sausage	555	39	32
Supreme	450	27	32
Mini Pancakes (8), without syrup	145	2	28
Sandwiches: Extreme Sausage	650	49	29
Grilled Sourdough Swiss	580	34	36
Loaded	705	47	36
Ultimate	520	31	30

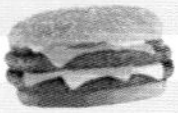
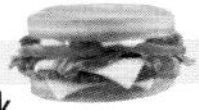
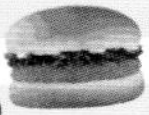
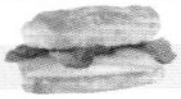
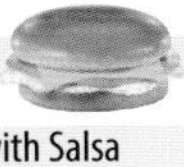
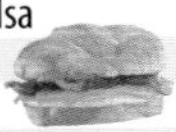
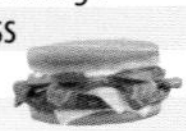

Jack in the Box® cont... (Oct '21)

Munchie Meals: *Includes 2 Tacos, Halfsie Fries & 20 fl.oz Coke*	C	F	Cb
Chick-N-Tater Melt	2030	110	220
Spicy Nacho Chicken S'wich	1530	80	155
Srircha Curly Fry Burger	1715	87	196
Stacked Gr. Cheese Burger	1890	94	213
Snacks & Sides:			
Bacon Cheddar Potato Wedges	650	40	57
Jumbo Egg Roll (1)	210	12	20
Onion Rings (8), 4.2 oz	445	24	52
Stuffed Jalapenos: 3 Pieces	220	12	21
7 Pieces	510	29	49
French Fries: Small	300	14	40
Medium	430	20	58
Large	550	25	75
Seasoned Curly Fries: Small	280	16	30
Medium	430	25	46
Large	480	28	52
Salads: *Without Dressing or Toppings/Croutons*			
Chicken Club: Crispy Chicken Strips	530	30	30
Grilled Chicken	230	8	12
Side Salad	20	0	4
Southwest Chicken:			
Crispy Chicken	510	25	45
Grilled Chicken	340	13	25
Croutons	70	3	9
Dressing: Creamy S'thwest, 1.75 oz	190	19	3
Ranch, 1.75 oz	250	25	5
Low Fat Balsamic Vinaigrette, 1.5 oz	25	1.5	3
Desserts: Mini Churros (5)	350	18	42
Choc. Overload Cake	320	11	53
New York Style Cheesecake	310	17	32
Ice Cream Shakes: *16 fl.oz, with Whipped Topping*			
Chocolate; Strawberry, av	670	24	105
Oreo Cookie	690	28	100
Vanilla	580	23	83

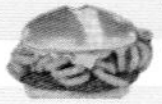
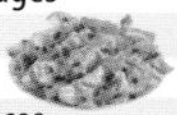
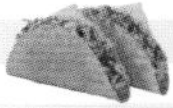
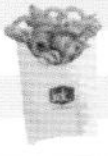
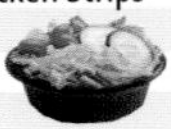
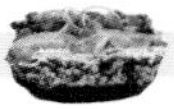
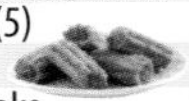
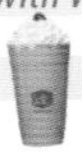

For Complete Nutritional Data ~ see Calorieking.com

Jack's® (Oct '21)

Burgers & Sandwiches:	C	F	Cb
Big Bacon	800	57	36
Big Jack Burger	720	47	43
Cheeseburger; Gr. Chkn S'wch. av	440	20	37
Double Cheeseburger	680	43	38
Hamburger	400	19	38
Chicken: Fried Chkn Breast	670	36	37
Chicken Fingers Snack & Fries, 3 pcs	920	56	77
French Fries, large	380	23	39
Sides: Coleslaw, 4 oz	210	18	13
Mashed Potatoes, 4 oz	140	4	26
Breakfast: Hash Browns, regular	360	25	31
Bacon, Egg & Cheese Biscuit	520	36	32
Big Breakfast Sausage Sandwich	830	60	44

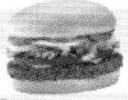
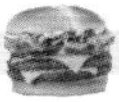
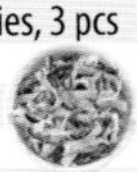

Jamba Juice® (Oct '21)

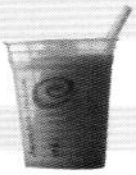
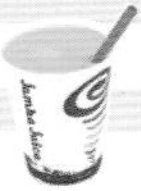
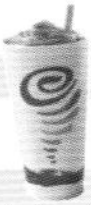
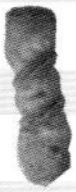
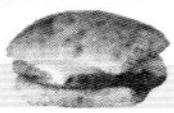
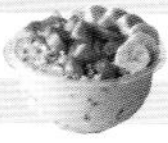

	C	F	Cb
***Freshly Squeezed Juice:** 16 fl.oz*			
Orange Carrot Twist	210	1	48
Purely Carrot	190	1	45
Purely Orange	220	1	52
Veggie Vitality	190	1	44
***Smoothies:** Per 16 fl.oz, Without Boosts or Add Ins*			
Classic: Caribbean Passion	260	1	63
Mango-A-Go-Go	300	1	73
Orange Dream Machine	310	1.5	68
Razzamatazz	270	1	65
Strawberry Surf Rider	250	1.5	60
Strawberries Wild	240	0	57
Watermelon Breeze	300	1	72
Plant-Based: Apple 'n Greens	250	1	58
Greens 'n Ginger	230	1	56
Mega Mango	210	0.5	50
Peach Perfection	210	0	51
Strawberry Whirl	210	0.5	51
Super Blends:			
Acai Super-Antioxidant	330	4	68
PB & Banana Pea Protein	470	22	43
PB & Banana Whey Protein	540	22	51
Whey Protein Berry Workout	300	1	52
Tasty Bites:			
Baked Goods: *Per Item*			
Belgian Waffle	310	15	39
Cheddar Tomato Twist	250	5	41
Savory Pretzel	420	11	69
Breakfast Sandwiches:			
Classic Sausage, Egg & Cheese	320	23	14
Impossible	220	12	16
Breakfast Wrap,			
Turkey Sausage 'n Cheese	320	15	30
Spring Veggie Bake	200	14	8
Steel-Cut Oatmeal: *Without Add-Ons*			
Plain	170	2.5	31
***Energy Bowls:** Per 16 fl.oz without Add-Ons*			
Acai Primo	510	10	101
Chunky Strawberry	580	17	94
Island Pitaya	480	8	102
Vanilla Blue Sky	330	9	62

Jersey Mike's Subs® (Oct '21)

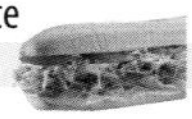
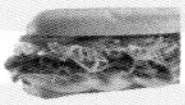
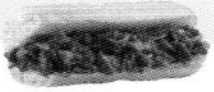
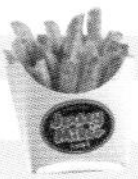
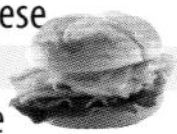
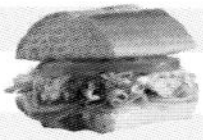
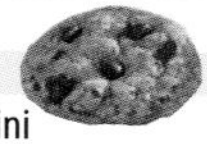

	C	F	Cb
***Cold Subs:** Per Regular, on White Roll, with Standard Menu Components*			
#1 BLT, with Mayo	710	44	59
#2 Jersey Shore Favorite	810	45	63
#3 Ham & Provolone	810	44	62
#5 Super Sub	820	44	64
#6 Roast Beef & Provolone	870	46	60
#7 Turkey & Provolone	780	47	61
#8 Club Sub with Mayonnaise	1120	79	63
#9 Club Supreme w/ Mayonnaise	1120	79	61
#10 Albacore Tuna	1020	71	62
#13 Original Italian	940	55	65
#14 Veggie	920	58	63
***Hot Subs:** Per Reg., on White Roll, with Standard Menu Components*			
#15 Meatball & Cheese	800	39	73
#17: Mike's Philly	710	30	63
#19 BBQ Beef	660	11	81
#20 Grilled Pastrami Reuben	700	30	67
#42 Chipotle Chicken Cheese Steak	930	55	65
#43 Chipotle Cheese Steak	980	61	63
#55 Big Kahuna Chkn Cheese Steak	710	29	67
#56 Big Kahuna Cheese Steak	760	35	64
French Fries: 5 oz	310	19	34
6 oz	370	23	41
***Salad:** Without Dressing*			
Grilled Chicken	800	25	51
Tossed	180	2	39
***Mini Breakfast Subs:** On White Bread, w/ Standard Menu Components, without Ketchup*			
#2: Bacon, Egg & Cheese	490	26	38
#3: Sausage, Egg & Cheese	880	64	38
#4: Ham, Egg & Cheese	500	23	39
#5: Steak, Egg & Cheese	530	23	38
***Kid's:** On White Bun, with Standard Menu Components, without Condiments*			
Ham Sub	230	56	30
Salami Sub	250	10	30
Turkey Sub	230	7	30
Desserts:			
Brownie, regular	500	28	63
Choc. Chip Cookie, mini	180	9	26
Tastykake: Butterscotch Krimpet	320	9	58
Chocolate Cupcake, regular	340	10	59
Cream Filled, regular	390	14	62

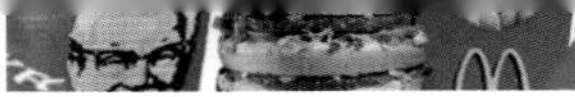

Jimmy John's® (Oct '21)

Original Subs: (8") Figures Based on French Bread w/ Standard Menu Board Toppings	C	F	Cb
#1 Pepe	600	29	50
#2 Big John	500	21	47
#3 Totally Tuna	500	22	51
#4 Turkey Tom	480	19	48
#5 Vito	580	27	51
#6 Veggie	670	39	50
JJBLT	590	32	47
***Favorite Subs :** (8") Figures Based on French Bread. with Standard Menu Set Toppings*			
#7 Spicy East Coast Italian	850	49	53
#8 Billy Club	810	33	73
#9 Italian Night Club	930	46	77
#10 Hunter's Club	830	34	70
#11 Country Club	780	31	74
#12 Beach Club	860	40	74
#13 Jimmy Cubano	720	38	47
#14 Bootlegger Club	680	23	71
#15 Club Tuna	850	42	75
#16 Club Lulu	690	26	71
#17 Ultimate Porker	690	28	72
***Plain Slims:** Figures Based on French Bread without Toppings, Dressing or Mayo*			
Slim 1 Ham & Provolone Cheese	540	13	69
Slim 2 Roast Beef	440	5	66
Slim 3 Tuna Salad	600	23	70
Slim 4 Turkey Breast	420	3	68
Slim 5 Salami Capicola & Cheese	630	23	69
Slim 6 Double Provolone	590	21	68
Sides:			
Jimmy Chips: Average	290	17	33
Thinny	260	11	39
Cookies: Chocolate Chip, 3 oz	410	19	56
Raisin Oatmeal, 3 oz	370	13	57
Jumbo Kosher Dill Pickle, 6.9 oz	20	0	3

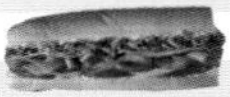
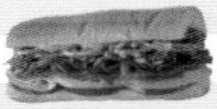
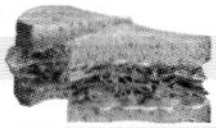
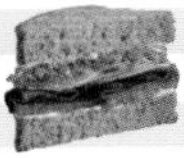
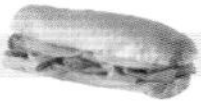
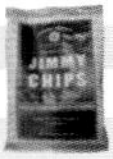

Johnny Rockets® (Oct '21)

Starters:	C	F	Cb
Chili Bowl	620	50	20
Fries: Plain	330	10	50
Bacon Cheese	630	30	60
Cheese	540	30	60
Chili Cheese	820	50	70
Onion Rings	630	30	80
Tots: Plain	740	50	70
Bacon Cheese	1050	70	80
Cheese	960	70	80
Chili Cheese	1230	90	90

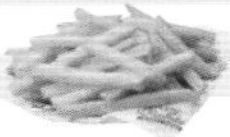
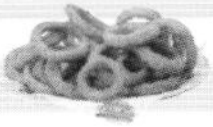

Johnny Rockets® cont... (Oct '21)

***Burgers:** Per Regular Size Bun*	C	F	Cb
Bacon Cheddar:			
Beef Burger	780	50	40
Boca Veggie Burger	680	40	50
Grilled Chicken	720	40	40
Original: Beef Burger	680	40	40
Gardein	640	40	70
Rocket: Beef Burger	690	40	40
Boca Veggie Burger	590	30	50
Turkey	810	60	40
Smokehouse: Beef Burger	800	40	70
Boca Veggie Burger	710	30	80
Gardein Burger	760	40	90
Spicy Houston:			
Beef Burger	640	40	40
Grilled Chicken	580	30	40
Turkey	770	50	40
Chicken, Tenders, BBQ Sauce	670	20	90
Hot Dogs:			
Rocket Dog	480	30	40
Rocket Chili Dog	670	50	40
Philly Cheese Steak, Beef	780	40	60
Melts:			
BBQ Chicken	940	30	100
Tuna on Sourdough	650	40	50
***Sandwiches:** On Sourdough, without substitutions*			
BLT	690	50	50
Fried Chicken Club	910	50	70
Grilled Chicken Club	800	40	50
Grilled Cheddar Cheese	600	40	50
Sourdough Burger Melt	680	40	50
***Salads:** Without Dressing*			
Crispy Chicken Club	420	20	20
Grilled Chicken Club	400	20	10
Garden Salad	150	10	10
***Breakfast:** Standard, without Subsititutions*			
French Toast: 2 slices	620	10	100
3 slices	800	20	130
Pancakes: B'milk (2) w/ Sausage	1020	50	110
Buttermilk (2), with Bacon	700	20	110
Scramblers: Bacon Denver	1130	60	80
Biscuits, Sausage & Gravy	2010	130	120
Cheesy Bacon Lovers	1170	70	80
Philly Cheesesteak	1270	70	80
***Shakes:** Without Malt*			
Banana	830	40	90
Chocolate	910	40	110
Hershey's Chocolate	920	40	110
Oreo Cookies & Cream	1020	50	120
Peanut Butter Banana	1050	60	100

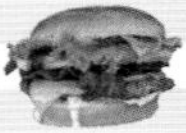
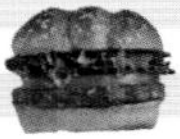
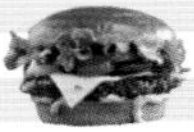
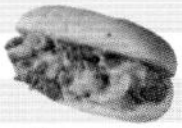
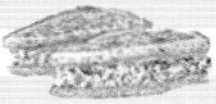
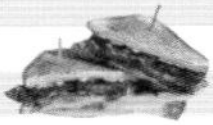
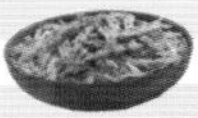
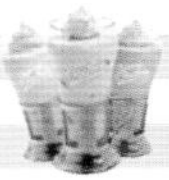

For Complete Menu & Data ~ see CalorieKing.com

KFC® (Oct '21)

Chicken On The Bone: Per Piece	C	F	Cb
Original Recipe: Breast, 6 oz	390	21	11
Drumstick, 1.87 oz	130	8	4
Thigh, 3.7 oz	280	19	8
Whole Wing, 1.5 oz	130	8	3
Extra Crispy: Breast, 6.3 oz	530	35	18
Drumstick, 1.9 oz	170	12	5
Thigh, 3.5 oz	330	23	9
Whole Wing, 1.7 oz	170	13	5
Kentucky Grilled: Breast, 4.6 oz	210	7	0
Drumstick, 1.4 oz	80	4	0
Thigh, 2.5 oz	150	9	0
Whole Wing, 1 oz	70	3	0
Spicy Crispy: Breast, 5.2 oz	350	20	11
Drumstick, 1.6 oz	130	8	5
Thigh, 2.8 oz	270	20	10
Whole Wing, 1.2 oz	120	8	5
Chicken:			
Kentucky Fried Wings: Buffalo, 1.2 oz	100	7	3
Honey BBQ, 1.35 oz	100	6	8
Nashville Hot, 1.2 oz	130	11	4
Unsauced, 1 oz	80	6	3
Nashville Hot:			
Extra Crispy: Breast, 7.4 oz	770	60	21
Drumstick, 2.3 oz	250	21	6
Thigh, 4.72 oz	500	40	11
Grilled:			
Breast, 4.86 oz	260	12	1
Thigh, 2.6 oz	180	12	0
Spicy Crispy:			
Breast, 6 oz	540	40	14
Thigh, 3.3 oz	390	32	12
Popcorn Nuggets: Kids	290	19	19
Large	620	39	39
Famous Bowls & Pot Pie:			
Chicken Pot Pie, 14 oz	720	41	60
Famous Bowl:			
Snack Size	270	14	27
Large	740	35	81
Salads: W/out Dressing or Croutons			
Caesar, Side	40	2	2
House Side Salad	15	0	3
Dressings & Add-Ins:			
Buttermilk Dressing, 1 oz	160	17	1
Creamy Parmesan Caesar, 2 oz	260	26	4
Light Italian, 1 oz	15	0.5	2
Original Ranch Fat Free, 1.5 oz	35	0	8
Croutons, Parmesan Garlic, 1 pouch	60	3	8

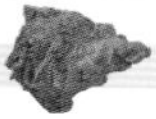
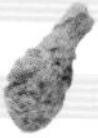
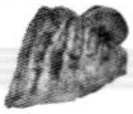
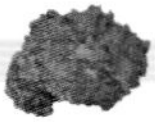
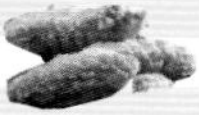
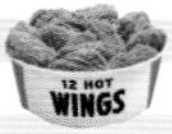

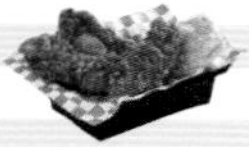
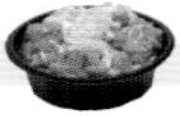
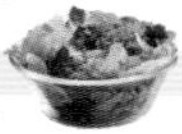

KFC® cont... (Oct '21)

Dipping Sauces & Condiments: Per 0.9 oz Container	C	F	Cb
BBQ Dipping Sauce Cup	45	0	11
Colonel's Buttery Spread	35	4	0
Honey Musard Dipping Sauce	110	9	6
Honey Sauce; Ketchup	30	0	8
KFC Dipping Sauce Cup	90	8	5
Lemon Juice, 0.14 oz	5	0	1
Ranch Dipping Sauce Cup	130	14	2
Strawberry Jam	35	0	9
Sandwiches:			
Chicken Littles: Regular	300	15	27
Buffalo; Honey BBQ, average	315	16	29
Nashville Hot	340	19	27
Colonel's Crispy Sandwich:			
Buffalo	500	27	39
Honey BBQ	510	25	48
Nashville Hot	540	32	40
Crispy Twister	630	34	53
Honey BBQ	350	4	55
Spicy Chicken	620	33	49
Homestyle Sides: Per Individual Portion			
BBQ Baked Beans, 4.25 oz	190	1	34
Biscuit	180	8	22
Coleslaw, 4.2 oz	170	12	14
Corn on the Cob, 2.5 oz	70	0.5	17
Green Beans	25	0	5
Mac. & Cheese, 4.8 oz	140	6	17
Mashed Potatoes, 4.2 oz	110	4	17
Mashed Potatoes with Gravy, 5 oz	130	5	20
Potato Salad	340	28	19
Sweet Kernel Corn, 2.75 oz	70	0.5	16
Kids: Chicken Little, w/ Mac & Cheese, & 1% Choc Milk	700	30	85
Extra Crispy Tenders, with Potato Wedges & 1% Choc Milk	600	22	80
Desserts:			
Apple Turnover, 2.9 oz	230	10	32
Cafe Valley: Choc. Chip Cake, 1 slice	300	15	39
Mini Choc. Chip Cake (1)	300	12	49
Lemon Cake, 1 slice	220	10	30
Chocolate Chip Cookie (1)	120	6	18
Oreo Cookies & Creme Pie	270	13	35
Reese's Peanut Butter Pie, 2.6 oz	300	17	33

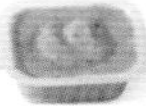
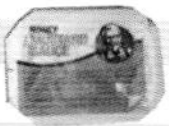
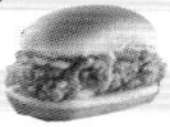
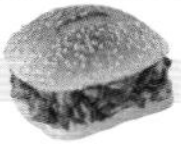
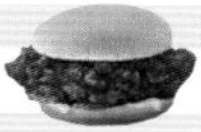

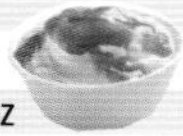
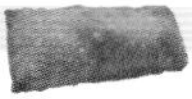
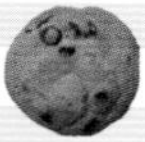

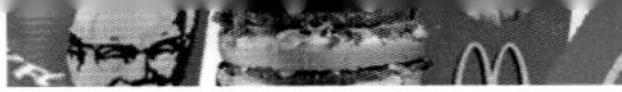

Krispy Kreme® (Oct '21)

Doughnuts:	C	F	Cb
Apple Fritter	350	19	42
Chocolate Iced: Cake	340	19	40
Custard Filled	300	15	37
Glazed	240	11	33
with Sprinkles	260	11	36
Kreme Filling	350	19	41
Cinnamon Apple Filled	270	15	31
Cinnamon Bun	270	16	29
Cinnamon Sugar	190	11	21
Cruller: Glazed Cake	240	15	25
Chocolate Iced Glazed Cake	240	15	25
Double Dark Chocolate	370	20	46
Dulche De Leche	300	16	35
Glazed: Kreme Filling	350	19	40
Lemon Filled	290	15	37
Maple Iced	240	11	34
Sour Cream Cake	300	15	40
Strawberry Iced	240	11	33
Powdered Cake	310	19	32
Powdered Lemon Kreme	290	17	32
Powdered Strawberry Filled	270	15	30
Glazed Doughnut Holes:			
Blueberry Cake; Cake (1)	45	2	7
10 Holes	470	19	69
Original Glazed:			
Regular (1)	45	3	5
10 Holes	430	23	51
Hot Beverages: *Per 12 fl.oz*			
Chocolate	410	12	63
Mocha Latte	300	9	45
Coffee: Cappuccino	120	4	12
Latte wth Whipped Cream:			
Caramel	340	9	52
Mocha	300	9	45
Vanilla Latte	220	5	32
Frozen Coffees: *Per 12 fl.oz with Whipped Cream*			
Caramel Latte	310	14	43
Mocha	310	14	42
Vanilla Latte	300	14	41
Frozen Lemonade Chiller, 12 fl.oz	210	0	54
Iced: *Per 12 fl.oz with Whipped Cream,*			
Caramel Latte	320	10	48
Caramel Mocha	250	10	33
Mocha	280	10	41

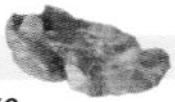
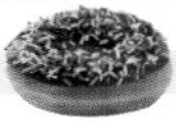
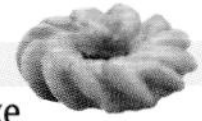
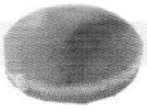
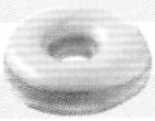
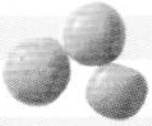
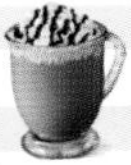
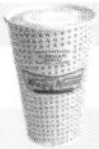
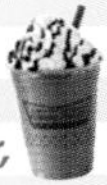
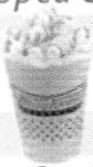

For Complete Menu & Data ~ See CalorieKing.com

Krystal® (Oct '21)

Krystals:	C	F	Cb
Original	130	6	15
with Cheese	150	8	15
Double	190	11	16
with Cheese	240	15	16
Bacon Cheese	190	10	16
Chik, regular	280	16	23
Pups: Chili Cheese Pup	300	20	16
Classic	170	10	14
Corn	290	21	18
Fries:			
French Fries: Small	140	9	14
Medium	240	15	24
Large	300	19	30
Loaded: Chili Cheese Fries	670	47	40
Junk Yard	800	59	42
Nuggets: 4 pieces	240	19	8
10 pieces	600	47	20
Sauce:			
Honey Mustard; Ranch, average	130	12	2
Sweet & Sour/Baby Rays BBQ, av.	50	0	13
Wings, Spicy (12)	1170	90	36
Breakfast:			
3 Egg Plates:			
Eggs, Bacon & Biscuit	480	30	29
Eggs, Sausage & Biscuit	520	36	28
Biscuits: Bacon, Egg & Cheese	380	23	28
Chik	380	21	36
Sausage, Egg & Cheese	410	29	28
Scramblers:			
Original: with Bacon	300	19	17
with Sausage	340	24	16
Low-Carb Scramblers:			
with Bacon	300	23	3
with Sausage	360	34	2
Sides: Grits, bowl	210	5	36
Tots, medium	330	23	28
Dessert, Apple Turnover	290	18	31
Hand-Spun Shakes: *Regular*			
Chocolate	650	18	114
Oreo	650	22	101
Strawberry	560	17	92
Vanilla	510	17	80

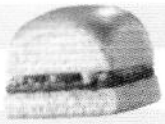
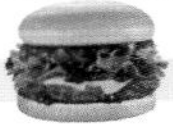
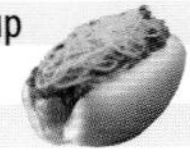
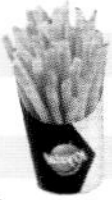
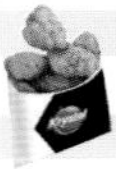
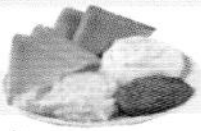
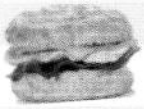
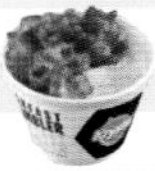
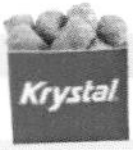

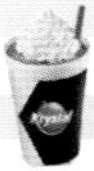

For Complete Menu & Data ~ see CalorieKing.com

LaRosa's Pizzeria® (Oct '21)

Classic Pizzas:	C	F	Cb
Hand Tossed: *Per Slice, 1/8 of 12" Medium Pizza*			
Chicken Bacon Ranch	330	18	29
Double Pepperoni	290	13	30
Hawaiian	280	11	33
Zesty BBQ Chicken	290	10	34
Traditional: *Per Slice, 1/12 of 14" Large Pizza*			
Chicken Bacon Ranch	290	18	18
Double Pepperoni	230	13	19
Hawaiian	240	11	21
Zesty BBQ Chicken	240	11	23
Deluxe Pizzas:			
Hand Tossed: *Per Slice, 1/8 of 14" Large Pizza*			
Buddy	490	24	47
Meat	560	30	46
Original	490	23	47
Veggie	370	12	48
Pan: *Per Slice, 1/8 of 14" Large Pizza*			
Buddy	510	26	47
Meat	580	31	46
Original	500	25	47
Veggie	380	13	48
Plant Based Pizzas: *Per Slice, 1/8 of 12" Medium Pizza*			
Pan Crust: Buffalo Chicken	280	13	30
BBQ Chicken	250	7	35
Deluxe	280	10	32
Pepperoni & Sausage	270	10	31
Hoagies: *With White Bun & Provolone Cheese*			
Baked Meatball & Pasta Sauce	810	36	89
Fried Cod, w/ Tartar Sce & Provolone	820	28	99
Steak w/ Tomato, Onion & Mayo	880	48	71
Pasta Entrees: *Without Bread, Soup or Salad*			
Lasagna, with Meat Sauce	1040	62	77
Ravioli: Cheese, with Pasta Sauce	750	29	89
Meat, with Pasta Sauce	730	26	89
Spaghetti, 3 Meatballs & Pasta Sce	1010	32	146
Ziti, Chicken Alfredo	890	27	112
Salad : *Entree, w/out Dressing or Breadstick*			
Antipasto for One	370	26	14
Crispy Chicken	500	27	36
Grilled Chicken	280	11	11
JoJo BLT	160	11	9
Tossed Garden	160	9	11
Salad Dressings: *Per 2 oz Cup*			
Blue Cheese	280	30	2
Honey French	250	19	18
Italian	320	34	4
Soup: *With 2 Packets Saltine Crackers*			
Baked Onion	220	9	29
Minestrone	120	1.5	24

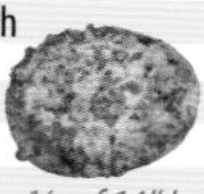
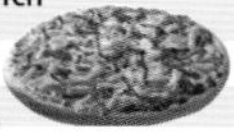
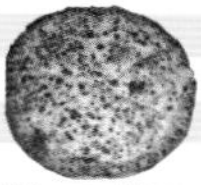
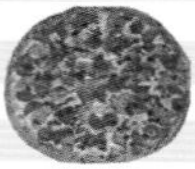
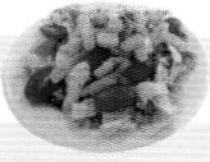

LaRosa's Pizzeria® cont... (Oct '21)

Appetizers:	C	F	Cb
Cheesy Flatbread, w/ Pizza Sauce	1480	88	117
Fried Mozz. Chse Stick w/ Pizza Sce	640	35	46
Garlic Fries, w/ Ranch Dressing	920	65	76
Rondo:			
Pepperoni, with Pizza Sauce	1410	84	115
Spinach, with Pizza Sauce	1290	71	114
Traditional Wings with Sauce: *Without Sauce Cup*			
BBQ (5)	400	23	19
Diablo (5)	470	31	17
Garlic-Romano (5)	610	51	9

La Salsa Fresh Mexican® (Oct '21)

Breakfast:	C	F	Cb
Burritos: Chicken	660	30	56
Steak	700	36	55
Huevos Ranchero Platter:			
Chicken	500	14	59
Chorizo	610	27	61
Steak	550	20	58
Taco	200	10	14
Burritos: *Without Chips*			
Black Beans & Cheese:	720	37	62
with Carnitas	820	41	62
with Grilled Chicken	810	40	63
California Steak, w/ Black Beans	830	39	81
Grande, Black Beans:			
with Carnitas/Chicken, average	750	31	79
with Steak	810	38	80
Pinto Beans & Cheese: no meat	810	37	79
with Carnitas	910	42	79
with Steak	970	49	80
Overstuffed Burrito:			
with Carnitas	860	35	56
with Grilled Chicken	860	32	59
with Steak	980	49	58
Platters:			
Enchiladas:			
Pinto Beans: Carnitas; Chicken, av.	985	53	59
Cheese	850	49	58
Steak	1070	63	59
Taquitos & Quesadillas:			
Pinto Beans: Carnitas; Chicken, av.	1600	76	134
Cheese	1470	72	129
Steak	1660	84	134
Three Pepper Fajita Flour Tortilla:			
Black Beans: Carnitas	700	29	55
Chicken	690	27	58
Steak	820	44	57
Tacos: *Without Chips*			
Baja Grilled Fish	260	12	23
Baja Shrimp	250	9	23
Guadalajara Carnitas	300	17	22

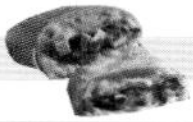
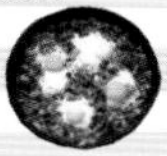
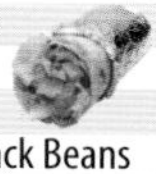
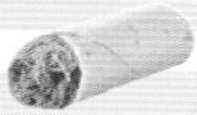
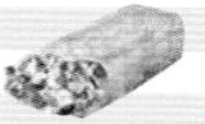
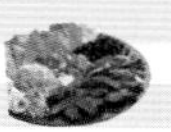
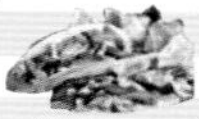

La Salsa Fresh Mex® cont... (Oct '21)

Favorites: Without Chips	C	F	Cb
Classic Quesadillas: Carnitas	980	58	59
Cheese	880	54	59
Chicken	980	57	60
Steak	1040	65	60
Fire Roasted Bowls:			
Black Beans: Carnitas	510	18	54
Chicken	500	16	55
Steak	570	25	55
Nachos:			
Black Beans: with Carnitas	1150	56	93
with Chicken	1150	54	95
with Steak	1210	63	94
Pinto Beans:			
with Carnitas	1190	56	101
with Chicken	1170	54	98
with Steak	1230	63	98
Stuffed Fajita Quesadilla: Carnitas	930	49	59
Cheese	830	45	59
Chicken	930	48	60
Steak	990	57	60

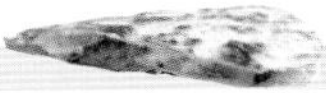
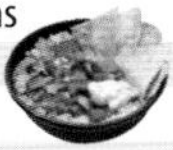
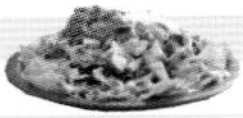
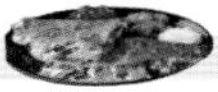

Little Caesars® (Oct '21)

14" Pizza: Per Pizza	C	F	Cb
Classic: Beef, seasoned	275	8	32
Cheese	245	8	31
Italian Sausage	285	11	32
Pepperoni	275	11	31
Deep!Deep! Dish:			
3 Meat Treat; 5 Meat Treat, av.	435	22	40
Hula Hawaiian	335	11	43
Ultimate Supreme	380	16	42
Veggie	340	12	42
***Caesar Wings:** Per 8 Wing*			
BBQ	620	35	32
Buffalo	510	35	3
Garlic Parmesan	670	51	5
Oven Roasted	510	35	3
***Caesar Dips:** Per 1.5 oz Container*			
Buffalo Ranch	230	23	4
Butter Garlic Flavor	370	42	0
Cheezy Jalapeno	210	21	3
Ranch	230	23	4
Bread: Crazy Bread, 1 stick	100	3	16
Italian Cheese Bread	135	6	15
Crazy Sauce, 1 cup	30	0	7

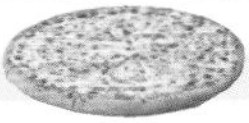
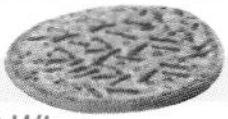
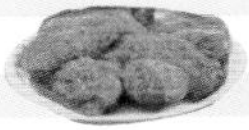
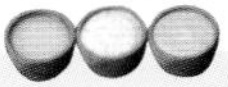
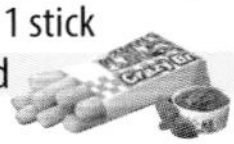

Long John Silver's® (Oct '21)

Sandwiches:	C	F	Cb
Fish	400	16	44
***Seafood:** Without Sides*			
Baked Cod, 1 piece, 6 oz	160	1	1
Battered: Alaskan Cod, 1 piece, 3 oz	190	11	9
Alaskan Pollock,1 piece, 3.2 oz	200	10	16
Cod, 1 piece, 3 oz	190	11	9
Breaded Clam Strips	340	20	35
Lobster Stuffed Crab Cake (1), 2.2 oz	280	15	26
Popcorn Shrimp, 3 oz	210	9	24
Grilled:			
Rice Bowls: Seasoned Salmon	360	8	45
Seasoned Shrimp	360	8	47
Southwest Salmon	420	15	45
Southwest Shrimp	420	16	48
Sweet Salmon	370	9	48
Sweet Chili Shrimp	390	11	51
Tacos: Baja Salmon (1)	210	9	23
Seasoned Shrimp (1)	180	5	23
Southwest Salmon (1)	220	9	23
Sauces & Condiments:			
Dipping Sauces: BBQ, 1 oz	40	0	10
Cocktail; Marinara, av.	20	0	4
Sweet & Sour 1 oz	45	0	12
Other Sauces & Condiments:			
Honey Mustard, 0.4 oz packet	60	6	2
Ketchup, 1oz pouch	30	0	8
Louisiana Hot Sauce, 1 tsp	0	0	0
Tartar Sauce, 0.5 oz packet	40	4	3
Sides: Baked Potato, 12 oz	295	0	67
Battered Onion Rings, 4 oz	480	35	39
Breaded Mozzarella Sticks (3)	370	23	24
Broccoli Cheese Bites, 5 pieces	310	24	18
Brocc. Chse Soup, 1 bowl, 7.4 oz	220	18	8
Clam Chowder, 1 bowl, 8 oz	230	16	16
Cole Slaw, 4 oz	170	11	18
Corn Kernels, 4 oz	160	8	9
Crumblies, 1 oz	170	12	13
Green Beans, 4 oz	25	0	4
Hushpuppies, 2 pcs	150	7	19
Jalapeno Peppers (1)	15	0	2
Macaroni & Cheese, 4 oz	150	6	19
Rice, 5 oz	180	1	37
Fries, 3.7 oz	350	17	44
Dessert: Choc. Chip Cookie (1)	190	11	22
Chocolate Cream Pie, 1 slice	280	17	28
Strawberry Swirl Cheesecake, 1 sl.	320	17	35

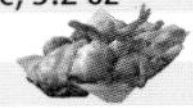
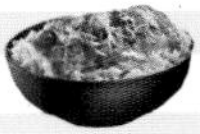
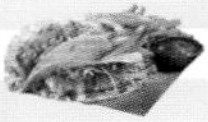
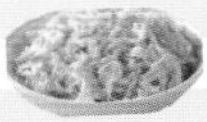
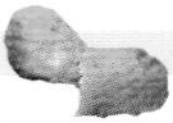
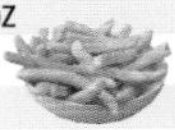

For Complete Menu & Data ~ see CalorieKing.com

Macaroni Grill® (Oct '21)

Antipasti: As Served	C	F	Cb
Baked Prosciutto & Mozzarella	610	36	35
Calamari Fritti	760	55	33
Crispy Brussels Sprouts	370	25	37
Crispy Fresh Mozzarella	820	79	17
Goat Cheese Peppadew Peppers	350	11	56
Mushroom Arancini	610	40	40
Spinach & Artichoke Dip	1100	61	109
Stuffed Mushrooms	510	38	20

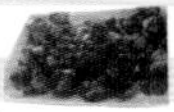

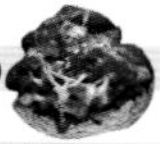

Meals: With Menu Set Sides	C	F	Cb
Carne: Braised Lamb Shank	1390	101	29
Gr. Steak & Potatoes: Rosemary Butt.	1250	94	34
with Oreganata Sauce	1220	85	42
Grilled Pork Chop,			
with Wild Mushroom Risotto	1420	93	48
Porterhouse Steak	1480	115	16
Chicken: Caprese	560	22	40
Carmela's Mix & Match	630	31	66
Marsala	790	32	61
Lunch Portion	670	26	74
Parmesan	1610	92	120
Lunch Portion	960	96	97
Scaloppine	1240	76	83
Lunch Portion	1050	76	59
Pasta: Butternut Tortellaci	980	66	63
Eggplant Parmesan	1340	90	103
Fettuccine Alfredo	1140	56	114
with Chicken	1370	72	117
Lasagna Bolognese	1110	67	69
Mushroom Ravioli	930	66	53
Penne Rustica	1060	52	82
Truffle Mac & Cheese	1060	89	24
Seafood: Grilled Salmon	930	45	82
Lobster Ravioli	920	74	36
Parmesan-Crusted Sole	1180	66	115
Pasta Di Mare	1030	43	101
Shrimp Portofino	1200	78	93
Shrimp Scampi	1180	88	56
Brick Oven Pizza: Per Whole Meal, as Served			
Cheese	1170	41	146
Farmhouse	1350	60	136
Margherita	1140	41	146
Pepperoni	1280	76	143
Kids: Chicken Strips with Fries	1250	73	108
Macaroni & Cheese	540	31	44
Pepperoni Pizza	570	19	70
Spaghetti, with Pomodoro Sauce	290	8	43

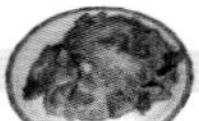

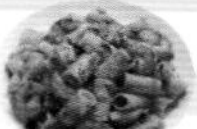

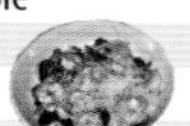

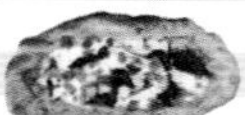

Macaroni Grill® cont... (Oct '21)

Salads: Includes Menu Set Dressing	C	F	Cb
Bibb & Bleu: with Shrimp	590	43	18
with Salmon	830	57	14
Chicken Florentine	1340	94	89
Italian Chopped	4920	34	20
Parmesan Crusted Chicken	1080	48	100
Rosa's Signature Caesar	470	41	14
with Chicken	630	41	15
Dessert: Decadent Choc. Cake	1090	88	79
Lemon Passion	740	45	77
NY Style Cheesecake	690	41	70
Romano's Cannoli	640	32	69
Tiramisu	600	39	54

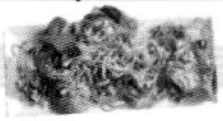

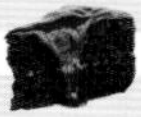

Manhattan Bagel® (Oct '21)

Bagels: Per Bagel	C	F	Cb
Plain; Salt	310	1	64
Honey Wheat	320	1	66
Gourmet: Asiago	340	4	64
Blueberry Glaze	380	1	82
California Power	350	1	64
Signature: Blueberry	320	1	68
Chocolate Chip	300	3	59
Cinnamon Raisin	320	1	67
Egg	310	1	64
Everything; Poppy, average	330	3	65
Pumpernickel	310	1	64
Cream Cheese: Plain; Scallion, av.	120	11	3
Lox, 1.2 oz	110	10	4
Sandwiches:			
Deli: Avocado BLT Thin	480	26	48
BLT on Multigrain Bread	510	34	34
Chicken Salad Croissant	650	44	45
Ham & Swiss on Sesame Bagel	580	17	67
Nova Lox	690	34	71
Roast Beef on Cheddar Roll	550	14	68
Turkey & Cheddar	610	39	37
Signature Lunch Sandwiches:			
Avocado Veg Out	470	14	74
East Side Reuben	630	27	61
Ellis Isl. Hot Pastrami	560	15	67
Manhattan Cheesesteak	660	30	59
Soup (8 oz): Beef Chili	290	15	25
Chicken Noodle	110	4	12
Cream of Broccoli	180	9	19
Minestrone	90	1	15
Breakfast Sandwiches:			
Plain Bagel: Cheese	490	15	65
Bacon & Cheese	540	19	66
Pork Roll & Cheese	720	33	67
Croissant: Bacon & Cheese	650	39	45
Ham & CHeese	650	39	45
Sausage & Cheese	830	60	44

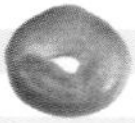

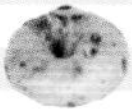

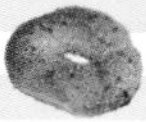

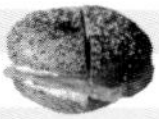

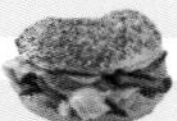

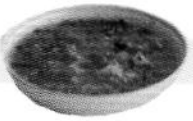

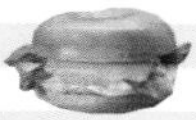

Marie Callender's® (Oct '21)

Appetizers: As Served	C	F	Cb
Crispy Chicken Tenders, 12.9 oz	870	47	72
Crispy Green Beans, 10.5 oz	810	52	75
Mozzarella Sticks, 8.6 oz	690	42	46
Onion Rings	1150	63	129
Burgers and Sandwiches: *With Fries*			
Original Burger	1290	87	84
Albacore Tuna Melt	1430	92	99
Callender's Cheeseburger	1450	99	85
Frisco Chkn Breast On Parm Sourd.	1290	81	95
Meatloaf on Parm. Sourdough	1250	78	96
Roasted Turkey Croissant Club	1450	97	95
Main Meals: *With Menu Set Sides*			
Comfort Classics:			
Braised & Slow Rstd Pot Roast	740	39	39
Chicken & Broccoli Fettuccine	1090	49	98
Crispy Fish & Shrimp Platter	1700	97	143
Home-Style Beef Stroganoff	850	30	99
Home-Style Meatloaf Dinner	610	35	34
Honey Ginger Glazed Salmon	570	30	29
Roasted Turkey Dinner	730	36	65
Shrimp & Chicken Carbonara	1140	50	93
Pies, Chicken Pot Pie, w/out sides	1140	79	70
Savory Skillets:			
Kickin' Chicken Bacon Broccoli	720	37	40
Spicy Beef & Chicken	790	54	27
Thai Shrimp	730	43	52
Salads:			
Cobb without Dressing	570	31	15
Combo Caesar with Caesar Dressing	240	18	9
Honey Mstd Chkn Crunch w/ dressing	950	61	54
Trad. Caesar w/ Caesar Dressing	490	35	28
Sides: Cornbread, w/ Honey Spread	340	21	33
French Fries, 4 oz	380	20	45
Loaded Mashed Potatoes, 6.2 oz	340	23	23
Macaroni & Cheese, 6.4 oz	230	9	26
Tater Tots, 5 oz	330	20	33
Soups: *Per Bowl*			
Chicken Tortilla	230	10	26
Clam Chowder	270	13	22
Hearty Vegetable	90	3	13
Potato Cheese	590	40	49
Breakfast: *With Menu Set Items*			
Classics: Croissant Sandwich	1100	70	76
Calif. Eggs Bened.	830	53	66
Triple Egg Dare Ya	1380	71	132

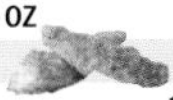
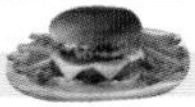
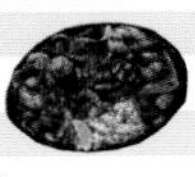
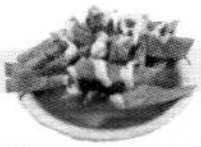
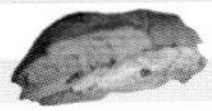

Marie Callender's® cont... (Oct '21)

Breakfast (Cont.): *W/ Set Menu Sides*	C	F	Cb
Griddle Greats: Belgian Waffles	600	19	99
Banana Cream Pie Pancakes	800	28	118
Buttermilk Pancakes (3)	670	28	92
Old Fashioned French Toast	830	31	123
Omelets, w/out Tater Tots: BTA	1210	66	103
Oh My	1340	74	98
Veggie	570	37	23
Quiche: Bacon, 1 sl.	990	79	45
Ham, 1 slice	1030	81	40
Vegetable, 1 slice	990	80	42
Desserts: *Per Slice Unless Indicated*			
NY Style Cheesecake, slice	740	52	58
Pies: Cream Cheese	620	38	63
Banana Cream, with Meringue	510	24	66
Chocolate Cream, with Meringue	570	25	77
Kahlua Cream Cheese	670	36	76

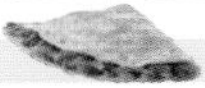
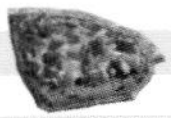

Max & Erma's® (Oct' 21)

Shareables: *As Served*	C	F	Cb
Chicken Fajita Quesadillas	1250	78	80
Knock Out Nachos	1570	100	116
Loaded Tots	1230	90	71
Potato Skins	1970	95	231
Wings with Blue Cheese Dressing:			
Cherry Cola BBQ	1990	120	95
Sweet Chili	1830	120	53
Burgers & Sanwiches: *Without Fries*			
BBQ Pulled Pork Sandwich	760	33	71
Big Ol' Buffalo Chicken Sandwich	1370	71	144
Bodalicious Bacon Burger	1230	83	59
Cola BBQ Bacon Burger	1510	99	94
Garbage Burger, 6 oz	1680	126	61
Reuben Grill Sandwich	1060	58	84
Sauteed Mushrm & Swiss Burger	1200	85	53
Tortilla Burger	1270	84	62
Turkey Avocado Swiss Burger	830	55	35
Salads: *Entrée Size, w/ Dressing, without Breadstick*			
3rd Street	1160	100	41
Grilled Chicken Santa Fe	1090	83	46
Mediterranean Salmon	610	42	16
Village	410	39	13
Garlic Breadstick	160	6	23
Sides: Baked Potato, plain	220	0	51
Creamy Coleslaw	160	12	14
Fresh Fruit Salad	100	0	25
Mashed Potatoes	270	14	32
Seasoned Fries	360	17	49
Steamed Broccoli	30	0.5	6
Tater Tot	320	19	33
Dessert: Banana Cream Pie	790	37	107
Chocolate Cake a la Mode	1600	82	206

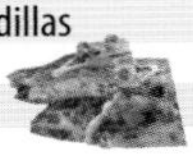
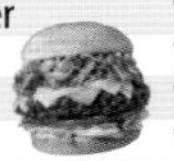
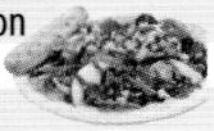
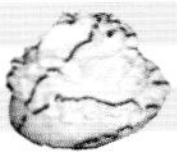

For Complete Menu & Data ~ See CalorieKing.com

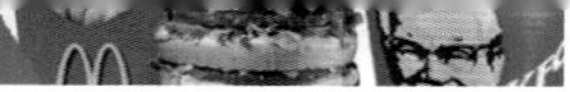

McAlister's Deli® (Oct '21)

Sandwiches: Standard Components	C	F	Cb
Black Angus Club	880	45	74
Four Cheese Melt	750	38	66
French Dip	570	21	44
Grilled Chicken Club	830	35	78
Harvest Chicken Salad	680	44	53
McAlister's Club	820	36	78
Reuben	900	41	76
The Rachel	800	31	77
Giant Spuds: Bl. Angus Roast Beef	1050	35	135
Chipotle Chicken & Bacon	1200	46	139
Spud Max	1070	39	135
Sides: Mac & Cheese	220	12	20
Potato Salad	250	17	22
Steamed Broccoli	80	6	6
Tomato & Cucumber Salad	70	4	6

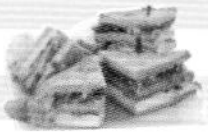
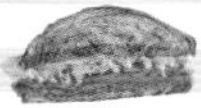
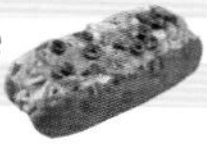

Mellow Mushroom® (Oct '21)

Burger,	C	F	Cb
Ritz Burger	1140	75	60
Calzones: Chicken & Cheese	1340	43	151
Steak & Cheese	1400	50	151
Hoagies, Whole: Chicken & Chse	1100	49	98
Italian	1300	80	88
Meatball	820	29	93
Mushroom Club	1450	77	101
Steak & Cheese	1170	61	96
Tofu	970	49	97
Munchies: Garlic Cheese Bread	830	42	83
Magic M'shrm Soup	350	24	15
Meatball Trio	360	24	11
Roasted Red Potatoes	150	3	27
Spinach & Artichoke Dip	760	44	67
Tomato Bisque	290	22	18
Wings: *Without Extras*			
BBQ (10)	700	35	41
Sweet Thai Chili (10)	780	33	60
Pizzas: With Baked Crust, Per Medium Slice			
Buffalo Chicken	520	31	46
Funky Q Chicken	450	20	51
Kosmic Karma	420	22	47
Salads: Per Regular Size			
Caesar, with Caesar Dressing	840	76	19
Greek, without Dressing	300	17	20
Dressing, Balsamic Vinaigrette, 1 oz	90	8	5
Desserts: Choc Chunk Cookie Sundae, with Triple Choc. Chunk Cookie	990	53	120
Half Baked Brownie Supreme	800	48	83
Oatmeal Raisin Cookie Sundae	870	41	112
PB Cookie Sundae	970	56	102

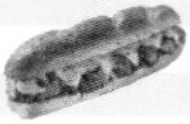
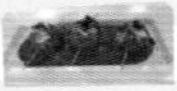
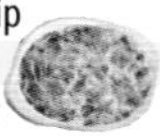
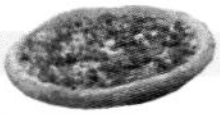

McDonald's® (Oct '21)

Beef Burgers:	C	F	Cb
Big Mac	550	30	45
Cheeseburger: Regular	300	13	32
Double	450	24	34
Hamburger	250	9	31
McDouble	400	20	33
Quarter Pounder: with Cheese	520	26	42
with Cheese Deluxe	630	37	44
with Cheese & Bacon	630	35	43
Dble Quarter Pounder, w/ Cheese	740	42	43
Burger Meal Combos: Includes Medium Fries + Coke			
Big Mac Meal	1080	45	144
Buttermilk Crispy Chicken Sandwich	1130	44	155
Cheeseburger Meal	830	28	131
Double Quarter Pounder with Cheese	1250	55	142
Ten Piece Chicken McNuggets Meal	950	40	124
Quarter Pounder w/ Cheese	1040	40	141
Chicken Sandwiches:			
Crispy Chicken	470	20	45
Deluxe Crispy	530	26	47
McChicken	400	21	39
Spicy Crispy	530	26	47
Deluxe	540	26	48
Filet-O-Fish, regular bun	380	18	39
Chicken McNuggets:			
4 pieces	170	10	10
6 pieces	250	15	15
10 pieces	420	25	25
20 pieces	830	49	51
Sauces: *Per Packet*			
Creamy Ranch	110	12	1
Honey Mustard	50	3	6
Spicy Buffalo	30	3	1
Sweet 'N Sour; Tangy BBQ	50	0	12
Tangy BBQ	40	0	11
Happy Meals: Includes Small Fries, Milk Jug & Apple Slices			
Chicken McNuggets Meal:			
with 4 nuggets	395	17	41
with 6 nuggets	475	22	46
Hamburger Meal	475	16	62
French Fries: Kids, 1.3 oz	110	5	15
Small, 2.6 oz	220	10	29
Medium, 3.9 oz	320	15	43
Large, 5.9 oz	490	23	66
Ketchup, packet	10	0	2

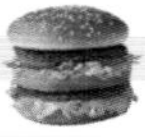
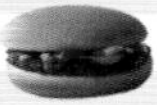
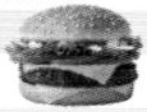
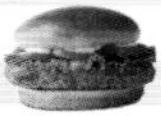
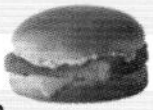
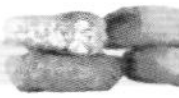

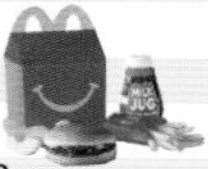
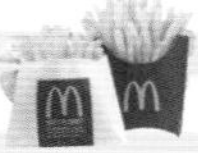

McDonald's® cont... (Oct '21)

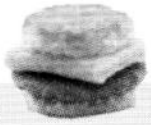
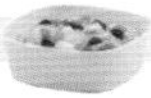
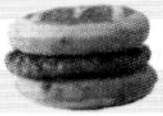
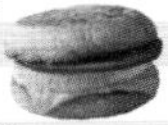
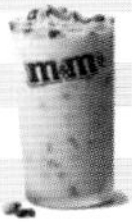

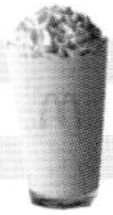
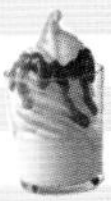
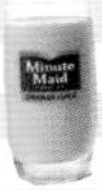
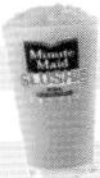

Breakfast:	C	F	Cb
Biscuits: *Regular*			
Bacon, Egg & Cheese	460	26	39
Sausage	460	30	36
Sausage with Egg	530	34	38
Burrito, Sausage	310	17	25
Fruit & Maple Oatmeal, with			
Apples, Cranberries & Light Cream	320	5	64
Hash Brown, 2 oz	140	8	18
Hotcakes & Sausage	770	33	102
McGriddles: Sausage	430	24	41
Sausage, Egg & Cheese	550	33	44
McMuffin: Egg	310	13	30
Sausage & Egg	480	31	30
Snacks, Apple Slices, pkt	15	0	4
Desserts:			
McFlurry's:			
M&M's Candy: Snack	420	14	64
Regular	640	21	96
Oreo Cookies: Snack	340	11	53
Regular	510	16	80
Shakes:			
Chocolate: Small	520	14	85
Medium	620	16	102
Large	830	21	139
Strawberry: Small	530	14	87
Medium	620	16	102
Large	840	21	139
Vanilla: Small	510	13	84
Medium	610	16	101
Large	820	21	138
Sundaes:			
Hot Caramel	330	7	58
Hot Fudge	330	10	51
Vanilla Cone	200	5	33
Beverages:			
Milk: 1% Low Fat Milk Jug	100	2	12
Low Fat, Red. Sugar Choc Milk Jug	130	3	18
Orange Juice: Small	150	0	36
Medium	190	0	45
Large	270	0	65
Pink Lemonade Slushie:			
Small	190	0	53
Medium	250	0	68
Large	350	0	95
Sweet Tea: Small	90	0	21
Medium	110	0	28
Large	160	0	38

McDonald's® cont... (Oct '21)

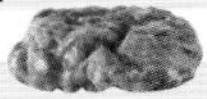
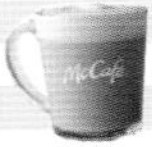
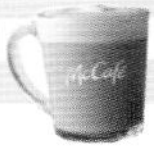
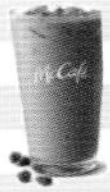
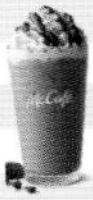
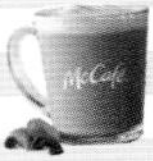

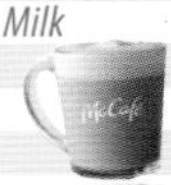
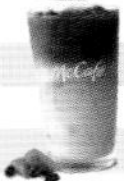

McCafe Food:	C	F	Cb
Bakery: Apple Fritter	510	29	56
Blueberry Muffin	470	21	65
Cinnamon Roll	560	17	92
McCafe Beverages:			
Cappuccino: *With Whole Milk*			
Regular: Small, 16 fl.oz	120	6	9
Medium, 22 fl.oz	160	8	13
Large	210	11	17
Caramel: Small	210	5	35
Medium	260	6	44
Large	340	9	55
French Vanilla: Small	190	5	30
Medium	230	6	37
Large	310	9	47
Frappes: *With Whole Milk & Whipped Cream & Topping*			
Caramel, medium	510	21	72
Mocha, medium	500	20	73
Hot Chocolate: *With Whipped Cream & Toppings*			
Whole Milk: Small	370	14	52
Medium	450	16	63
Iced Coffee: *With Light Cream*			
Regular: Small, 16 fl.oz	140	5	24
Medium, 22 fl.oz	180	7	30
Large, 30 fl.oz	260	9	45
Caramel: Small, 16 fl.oz	140	5	23
Medium, 22 fl.oz	190	7	31
Large, 30 fl.oz	270	9	46
Iced Mocha: *With Whipped Cream & Toppings*			
Small	280	10	39
Medium	320	11	48
Large	450	15	69
Lattes: *With Whole Milk*			
Regular: Small	140	8	12
Medium	190	10	15
Large	250	13	20
Caramel: Small	250	7	38
Medium	320	10	48
Large	400	12	59
French Vanilla: Small	230	7	33
Medium	290	9	42
Large	360	12	51
Macchiato: *W/ Whole Milk*			
Caramel: Small	260	7	41
Medium	320	9	50
Large	400	12	61
Iced Caramel:			
Small	210	6	32
Medium	310	10	45
Large	370	10	58
Smoothies: Mango Pineapple, med.	250	1	57
Strawberry Banana, large	330	1	76

Mimi's Cafe® (Oct '21)

Bakery:	C	F	Cb
Croissants: Just Baked All Butter	360	20	38
Almond	370	20	40
Muffins: Blueberry Crumble	590	30	74
Buttermilk Spice	575	21	85
Carrot Raisin Nut	520	27	64
Chocolate Chip	865	44	105
Breakfast: Without Potatoes			
Benedicts: Eggs, Original	645	39	34
Corned Beef Hash	730	44	46
Smoked Salmon	605	39	33
Add Roasted Potatoes	150	5	23
French Toast Items: *Without Side Options*			
Brioche	595	23	74
Cinnamon Roll	715	29	95
Griddlecakes: *With Eggs, Any Style*			
Berry	1030	38	135
Buttermilk	1025	44	120
3 Egg Omelets: *With Roasted Potatoes*			
Bacon Avocado	920	65	30
Hickory-Smoked Ham & Cheese	675	45	27
Mushroom Bacon & Brie	775	56	28
Smoked Salmon	555	35	24
Malted Berry Waffles:			
with Eggs any style	585	28	61
with Pork Sausage	790	49	61
Lunch & Dinner: Without Side Choices			
Burgers: Brioche Cheeseburger	775	41	56
Hickory Bacon Cheddar	945	50	68
Mushroom & Brie	890	51	51
The French Quarter	1285	90	48
Sandwiches: Croque Monsieur	835	42	62
French Dip	585	14	70
Grilled Chicken Pesto Baguette	920	47	56
Roasted Chicken Croque Monsieur	1090	64	57
Turkey Hummus	560	25	54
West Coast Reuben	1335	72	99
Entrees:			
Beer Battered Fish & Fries	1185	78	79
Coastal Shrimp Pasta	1035	53	99
French Pot Roast	515	32	22
Mimi's Meatloaf	445	25	15
Slow Roasted Turkey	700	29	69
Sides: Broccoli	115	9	5
Coleslaw	250	23	7
French Fries	125	3	22
Garlic Spinach	70	4	4
Mashed Potatoes	130	4	21
Potatoes au Gratin	490	32	32
Roasted Potatoes	150	5	23

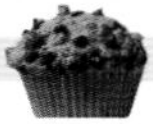
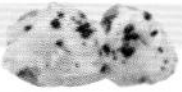
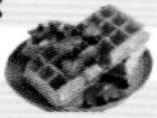
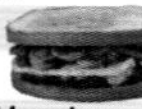
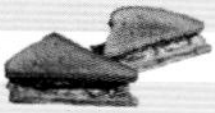
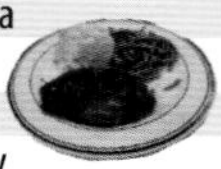
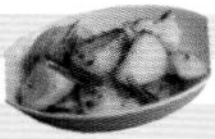

Mr. Goodcents® (Oct '21)

Cold Subs:	C	F	Cb
Per 8" White Bread Sub with Standard Toppings			
Bologna	760	45	64
Centsable	660	33	64
Garden Veggie without Cheese	480	19	67
Goodcents Original	730	43	62
Oven Roasted Chicken Breast	540	19	58
Penny Club	530	19	59
Pepperoni	840	56	58
Tuna Salad	690	37	64
Toasted Sub: Per 8" Wheat Bread Sub with Standard Toppings			
Chicken Bacon Ranch	620	24	55
Meatball	790	35	66
Pasta To Go: Chicken Alfredo	670	31	61
Chicken Tortellini	680	33	57
Pasta with Meatballs	590	19	75
Garlic Bread, 1 pce, 2 4 oz	290	12	44
Soup: Per 16 fl.oz Bowl			
Broccoli Cheese	390	26	28
Chicken Homestyle Noodle	160	5	22
Saltine Crackers for soup bowls	110	2	17

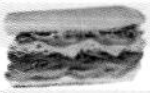
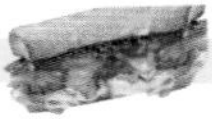
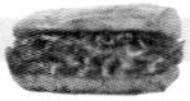
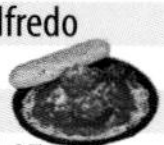

Mr. Hero® (Oct' 21)

7" Subs & Burgers:	C	F	Cb
Burgers: Amazing Ultim. Cheeseburger	454	25	38
Bacon Cheeseburger	450	23	38
Cheeseburger	720	49	44
Romanburger	805	56	46
Romanburger BTE	1005	73	48
Chicken Subs:			
Chicken Bacon Ranch	590	29	43
Chicken Philly	510	22	45
Deli Subs: *Per 7" Sub with Menu Board Toppings*			
Italiano	550	26	54
Original Italian	520	27	50
Tuna 'N Cheese	670	53	45
Turkey	330	3	49
Steak Subs: Hatta Potatta	720	45	53
Sicilian Parm	710	46	40
Sir Racha Bourbon	635	35	48
Zesty Bacon & Swiss	670	41	39
Sides: Per Regular Size			
Coleslaw, 3 oz	130	9	11
Mozzarella Sticks	565	35	43
Onion Petals	545	36	52
Potato Waffers	360	27	29
Kids: Cheeseburger Meal	510	32	43
Nugget Meal	470	33	32
Desserts: Brownie	500	28	63
Funnel Cake Fries, Regular, with Caramel Sauce	285	6	57

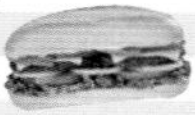
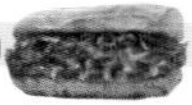
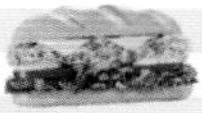
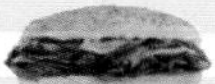
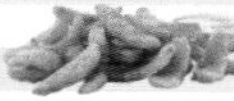
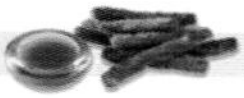

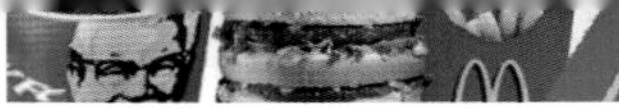

Mrs Fields Cookies® (Oct '21)

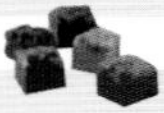
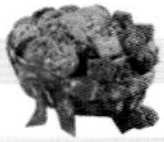
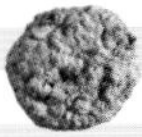
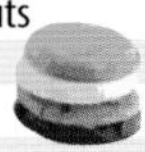
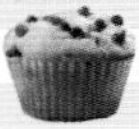

Brownie Bites: Per 3 Bites	C	F	Cb
Butterscotch Blondie	200	8	29
Double Fudge	200	10	27
Toffee Fudge	200	11	26
Bite Size Nibbler Cookies: *Per 3 Cookies*			
Cinnamon Sugar	180	8	25
Debra's Special	160	7	22
Semi-Sweet Chocolate	170	8	23
Triple Chocolate	160	8	22
White Chunk Macadamia	180	9	22
Cake, Chocolate Chip, 3 oz	350	17	45
Cookies: *Per Cookie*			
Cinnamon Sugar	210	8	31
Frosted	270	11	39
Cut Out	280	11	44
Debra's Special	200	9	27
Oatmeal, Raisins & Walnuts	200	9	27
Semi-Sweet Chocolate	210	10	29
Triple Chocolate	210	10	28
White Chunk Macadamia	230	12	28
Muffins: Blueberry	190	9	24
Chocolate Chip	200	10	26

For Complete Nutritional Data ~ see CalorieKing.com

My Favorite Muffin® (Oct '21)

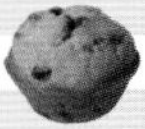
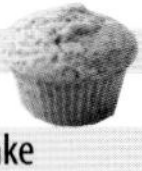
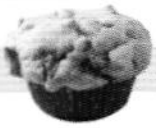

Muffins: Per Large Muffin	C	F	Cb
Blueberry	590	28	78
Boston Cream Pie	740	33	105
Chocolate Chip	790	39	100
Carrot Cake	850	42	112
Deep Dish Apple Pie	560	22	85
Lemon Poppy Seed	670	32	90
NewYork Almond Cheesecake	690	41	74
Pumpkin Spice	600	26	86
Strawberry Cheesecake	580	31	67

Nathan's Famous® (Nov '20)

Burgers:	C	F	Cb
Angus BBQ Bacon Tribeca	740	35	65
Angus NY Attitude	850	54	52
Super Cheeseburger, 5 oz	850	49	49
Cheesesteak, Original Philly, 10.5 oz	600	27	49
Chicken:			
Sandwiches: Battered Chkn S'thern	640	35	51
Grilled Chicken, 8.2 oz	430	17	42
Krispy Chicken, 8.5 oz	600	29	60
Tenders, Krispy,3 pieces, 6.3 oz	520	31	32
Wings, Original Buffalo, 5 pcs	700	62	3

Nathan's Famous® cont... (Nov '20)

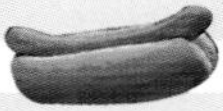
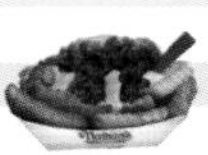

Hot Dogs: With Natural Casings	C	F	Cb
Original, 3.5 oz	290	18	24
Chili, 5.5 oz	410	27	30
Chili Cheese, 6.5 oz	450	29	33
Hot Dog Nuggets, 6 pieces, 3.5 oz	350	27	20
Corn Dog, on a stick, 3.2 oz	360	19	39
Fries: *Per Regular Size*			
Bacon Cheese	720	51	49
Cheese	600	42	48
Chili	660	48	49
Chili Cheese	720	52	53
French Fries	540	39	43
Onion Rings, regular	460	31	39
Salads: Grilled Chicken, 19 oz	300	7	35
Krispy Chicken, 19 oz	500	27	33

New York Fries® ~ *See CalorieKing.com*

Ninety Nine® (Oct '21)

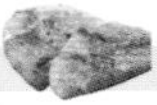
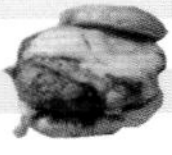
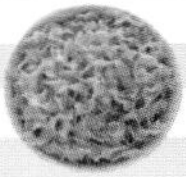

Standout Starters: As Served	C	F	Cb
Boneless Wings & Skins Sampler	1850	123	87
Mozzarella Moons	860	50	66
Outrageous Pot. Skins	1470	102	82
Burgers: *Without Sides*			
Bacon & Cheese	870	43	58
Cheeseburger	750	34	58
Plain Burger	690	28	59
Vermont Cheddar	960	49	64
Sandwiches:: *Without Sides*			
Honey BBQ Chicken Wrap	910	34	100
Spicy Crispy Chicken Sandwich	820	34	92
Entrees: *Without Sides Unless Noted*			
Broiled Sirloin Tips, smothered	730	42	16
Cntry Fried Chkn, Mashed Pot & Bisc.	1240	55	150
Fish & Chips with Fries & Coleslaw	1750	111	130
New England Baked Scallops	680	36	44
Southwest Fajita Bowl with Shrimp	970	56	82
T-Bone Steak,18 oz	900	66	0
Sides: Broccoli Florets	50	0.5	9
Coleslaw	300	25	19
Corn	140	5	26
French Fries, 16 oz	1040	64	107
Pasta with butter	740	28	104
Rice Pilaf	310	8	55
Russet Mashed Potatoes	260	11	36
Petite Treats: Banana Coconut	270	17	27
Mocha Bite	330	20	38
Strawberry & Cream Cake	270	14	35

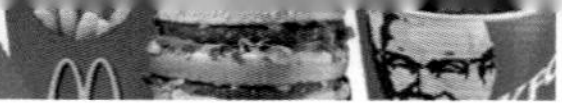

Noodles & Company® (Oct '21)

Asian Noodles: Per Reguar Size	C	F	Cb
Grilled Orange Chicken Lo Mein	**830**	28	103
Japanese Pan Noodles	**640**	12	114
Pad Thai	**1040**	42	143
Spicy Korean Beef Noodles	**880**	34	112
***Bowls:** Per Regular*			
Keto:			
Zucc. Afredo Montamore w/ Gr Chkn	**970**	73	32
Zucchini Pesto with Grilled Chicken	**510**	31	23
Vegetarian: Jap. Pan Noodles w/ Tofu	**870**	26	120
Zucchini Scampi	**350**	23	25
***Classic Noodles:** Regular Size*			
Alfredo MontAmore Parm Chicken	**1410**	84	110
Buttered Noodles	**760**	35	98
Penne Rosa with Parm	**730**	25	104
Pesto Cavatappi with Parm	**760**	32	97
Spaghetti & Meatballs	**980**	48	102
***Macs:** Per Regular Size*			
BBQ Pork Mac	**1210**	47	129
Buffalo Chicken Mac	**1100**	39	128
Gluten Sensitive Pipette Mac	**850**	34	105
Wisconsin Mac & Cheese	**980**	38	119
***Zoodles & Caulifloodles:** Per Regular*			
Cauliflower Rigatoni Fresca w/ Shrimp	**880**	39	102
Zucchini Pesto with Grilled Chicken	**510**	31	23
Zucchini Shrimp Scampi	**410**	24	25
***Salads:** Per Regular , with Dressing*			
Grilled Chicken Caesar	**620**	47	15
Chicken Veracruz	**680**	48	28
The Med, with Chicken	**430**	17	32
***Soup,** regular,*			
Tomato Basil Bisque	**430**	28	37

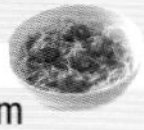
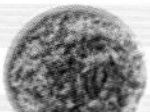
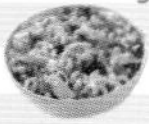
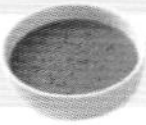

O'Charley's® (Oct '21)

Appetizers: As Served	C	F	Cb
Chicken Tenders, Chipotle	**1160**	40	107
Nashville Deviled Eggs	**720**	61	24
Spicy Jack Cheese Wedges (7)	**720**	48	44
Top Shelf Combo Platter	**1880**	132	74
***Burgers:** Without Sides*			
Better Cheddar Bacon	**1000**	68	49
Classic Cheeseburger	**930**	61	47
***Chicken & Pasta:** Without Sides*			
Chicken Tenders & Fries	**1410**	85	74
Chicken Tender Dinner:			
Buffalo	**1070**	64	31
Nashville Hot	**1260**	87	44
Garlic Shrimp Pasta	**950**	43	104
New Orleans Cajun Chicken Pasta	**1170**	61	99
Peach Chutney Chicken	**470**	8	69
Whisky Chicken Pasta	**1210**	63	108

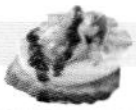
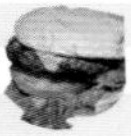
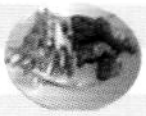

O'Charley's® cont... (Oct '21)

Classic Combos: Without Sides	C	F	Cb
BBQ Ribs & Tenders	**950**	37	84
Steak & Chicken Tenders, 6 oz	**1030**	67	26
Steak & Gr. Atlantic Salmon, 6 oz	**750**	33	5
Steak & Half Rack Baby Back Ribs	**890**	49	48
***Ribs & Steak:** Without Sides*			
Baby Back Ribs: Regular	**1220**	62	95
Carolina Gold	**1220**	62	96
Nashville Hot	**1540**	110	63
BBQ Ribs Platter	**4960**	249	381
Slow Roasted Prime Rib:			
8oz	**830**	70	3
12 oz	**1140**	95	3
16 oz	**1460**	120	4
Steak: Bacon & Bourbon Glazed Filet	**640**	42	28
Filet Mignon, w/ Garlic Butter	**580**	47	1
Grilled Top Sirloin, 6 oz	**270**	18	0
Louisiana Sirloin	**600**	43	3
Ribeye Steak, 10 oz	**720**	56	1
***Sandwiches:** Without Sides Unless Indicated*			
Carolina BBQ Chicken	**650**	22	74
Classic French Dip	**1020**	44	79
Club Sandwich	**950**	85	91
Nashville Hot Chicken, with Fries	**2000**	101	119
***Seafoodl Favorites:** Without Sides Unless Indicated*			
Grilled Blackened Atl. Salmon, 9 oz	**500**	31	3
Grilled Salmon Bowl	**990**	70	44
Hand Battered Fish & Chips	**1420**	92	85
Hand Breaded Catfish, w/ Fries & Slaw	**1720**	124	103
Seafood Platter	**1950**	121	141
Sides: Baked Potato (1)	**200**	1	50
Bacon Smashed Potatoes	**350**	16	44
Broccoli, 5 oz	**110**	8	6
Coleslaw	**200**	15	12
French Fries, 6 oz	**400**	24	40
Loaded Baked Potato, 1 portion	**490**	27	53
Mac & Cheese	**450**	22	47
Seasoned Rice Pilaf, 1 portion	**160**	4	27
Sweet Potato Fries, 1 portion	**280**	19	27
***Salads:** Per Full Salad with Dressing*			
California Chicken	**1020**	67	71
Classic Cobb	**1140**	92	36
Southern Fried Chicken	**1550**	110	48
Southern Pecan Chicken Tender	**1550**	106	95
***Signature Soup:** Per Bowl*			
Chicken Harvest	**210**	13	20
Chicken Tortilla	**190**	7	20
***Desserts:** Per slice*			
Country Apple Pie	**630**	35	77
Double-Crust Cherry Pie	**600**	35	69
French Silk Pie	**580**	43	49
Goo Goo Crunch Pie	**1450**	93	155
Ooey Gooey Caramel Pie	**640**	39	76
Southern Pecan Pie	**730**	45	78

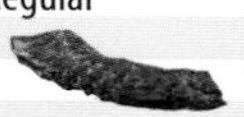
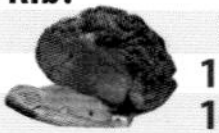
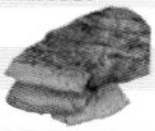
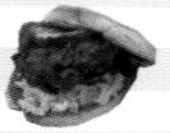
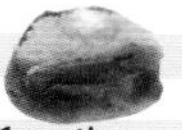
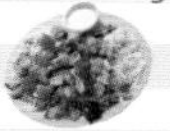
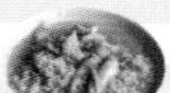
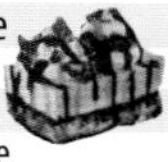

Old Spaghetti Factory® (Oct '21)

Appetizers: As Served	C	F	Cb
Spinach & Artichoke Dip	**640**	46	44
Sicilian Garlic Chse Bread	**1220**	78	97
with Bacon	**1450**	95	97
Entrées, Lunch/Dinner:			
Classics:			
Italian Sausage with Meat Sauce	**980**	38	109
Sicilian Meatballs	**1040**	36	115
Spaghetti: with Marinara Sauce	**570**	7	106
with Rich Meat Sauce	**650**	11	108
with White Clam Sauce	**790**	29	107
Founder's Favorites:			
Baked Lasagna, 17.6 oz	**820**	45	61
Garlic Mizithra, 17 oz	**1360**	85	102
Tenderloin w/ Mizithra & Brocc.	**1260**	87	59
Manager Favorites:			
Marinara: Clam, 15 oz	**690**	18	107
Meat, 15 oz	**600**	8	108
Mushroom, 16.5 oz	**610**	10	109
Signature Pasta:			
Angel Hair Pomodoro, 16.6 oz	**570**	8	98
Fettuccine Alfredo, 13.3 oz	**1090**	72	91
Spinach & Cheese Ravioli, 11 oz	**470**	16	63
Specialty Selections:			
Crab Ravioli	**810**	45	73
Spaghetti Vesuvius	**860**	29	112
Dessert, Tiramisu, 4.5 oz	**295**	14	43

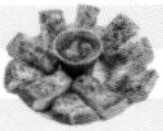
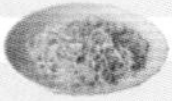
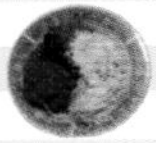
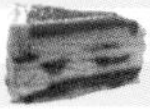

Olive Garden® (Oct '21)

Appetizers:	C	F	Cb
Calamari	**670**	42	48
Fried Mozzarella	**800**	49	57
Sauce: Marinara	**45**	2.5	6
Ranch	**250**	27	2
Lasagna Fritta	**1130**	76	75
Lunch: Fettuccine Alfredo	**650**	45	47
Chicken Parmigiana	**660**	29	65
Eggplant Parmigiana	**660**	32	74
Lasagna Classico	**500**	30	33
Shrimp Scampi	**480**	19	53
Dinner Entrees: Chicken Alfredo	**1570**	95	96
Five Cheese Ziti al Forno	**1220**	71	103
Herb Grilled Salmon w/out Sides	**460**	29	8
Sides: French Fries	**260**	13	32
Steamed Broccoli	**35**	0	7
Desserts: Choc. Brownie Lasagna	**910**	52	144
Black Tie Mousse Cake	**750**	50	76
Chocolate Mousse	**240**	18	18
Tiramisu	**470**	27	54
Warm Italian Donuts witout sauce	**810**	28	119

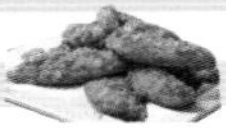
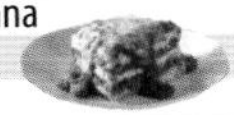

On the Border® (Oct '21)

Appetizers: As Served	C	F	Cb
Border Sampler	**2040**	142	101
Quesadillas:			
Fajita Chicken	**1190**	82	58
Fajita Steak	**1280**	96	55
Stacked Nachos	**2030**	129	145
Classic Burritos: *Without Beans, Rice or Sauce*			
Carnitas	**780**	41	49
Shredded Beef	**750**	37	53
Chimichangas: *Without Beans, Rice or Sauce*			
Carnitas	**960**	57	54
Shredded Chicken Tinga	**800**	45	51
Enchiladas: *Without Bean or Rice*			
Border Queso: Seasoned Beef	**510**	29	35
Shredded Beef	**440**	22	34
Salads: *W/out Dressing*			
Fajita: Chicken	**430**	20	27
Steak	**500**	28	30
Grande Taco Salad: Chkn Tinga	**630**	39	42
Seasoned Ground Beef	**710**	49	40
Dressings: Ranch	**230**	24	2
Smoked Jalapeno Vinaigrette	**120**	10	9
Tacos: *Without Beans or Rice*			
Dos XX Fish Taco w/ Red Chili Sce	**410**	25	34
Shredded chicken Tinga, Crispy	**200**	10	16
Sides: Black Beans	**200**	1	36
Cilantro Lime Rice	**180**	2	37
Corn Tortilla (1)	**60**	0.5	12
Mexican Rice	**220**	6	37
Refried Beans	**220**	7	30

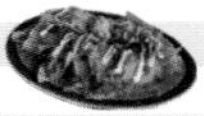
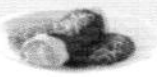
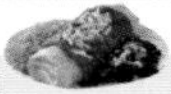
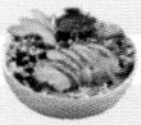
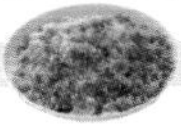

For Complete Nutritional Data ~ see CalorieKing.com

Orange Julius® (Oct '21)

Julius Originals: Per Medium Size	C	F	Cb
Mango Pineapple	**320**	0	78
Orange Julius	**260**	0	65
Pina Colada	**540**	7	117
Strawberry Banana	**460**	7	99
Premium Fruit Smoothies: *Per Medium Size*			
Mango Pineapple	**340**	0	80
Pomegranate Berry Blast	**380**	0	89
Strawberry Banana	**360**	0	85
Strawberry Watermelon Sensation	**340**	1	80
Light Smoothies: *Per Medium Size*			
3 Berry Daylight	**210**	0	51
Berry Pomegranate Twilight	**210**	0	51
Boost, Banana, Small drink	**30**	0	7

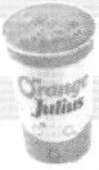
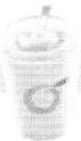
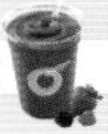

Outback Steakhouse® (Oct '21)

Aussie-Tizers: Per Regular Size, with Selected Dressing/Sauce	C	F	Cb
Aussie Cheese Fries, Large	**1760**	122	115
Bloomin' Onion	**1350**	54	200
Kookaburra Wings, Hot:			
Small	**1050**	89	24
Medium	**1570**	125	44
Seared Peppered Ahi, large	**470**	28	21
Steakhouse Mac & Cheese	**770**	54	47
Three Cheese Steak Dip	**1460**	113	85
Burgers/Sandwiches: Without Sides			
BBQ Chicken & Bacon Sandwich	**670**	30	53
Bloomin' Fried Chicken Sandwich	**700**	32	66
Outback Burger without cheese	**730**	43	47
Prime Rib Sandwich	**1820**	127	94
The Bloomin' Burger	**1030**	60	75
Chicken & Ribs:			
Alice Springs Chicken & Fries, 5 oz	**920**	53	64
Baby Back Ribs & Fries, full rack	**2400**	151	103
Grilled Chickn On The Barbie, 8 oz,	**360**	7	17
with Fresh Mixed Veggies	**520**	17	34
Pork Porterhouse with Mashed Pot.	**670**	35	21
Queensland Chicken & Shrimp Pasta	**1150**	49	93
Signature Steaks: Without Sides			
Melbourne Porterhouse, 22oz	**860**	57	8
Outback Centre Cut Sirloin: 6 oz	**210**	7	0
8 oz	**280**	9	0
Ribeye, 13 oz	**710**	45	0
Victoria's Filet Mignon, 6 oz	**240**	9	0
Straight From The Sea: Without Sides			
Botany Bay: Halibut	**480**	23	7
Mahi	**400**	21	7
Simply Grilled: Halibut	**460**	23	3
Salmon, 10 oz, with Remoulade	**720**	54	3
Toowoomba Samon, 8 oz	**760**	53	7
Big Bowl Salads:			
Aussie Cobb: w/out dressing	**370**	22	18
add Grilled Chicken	**160**	4	0
Brisbane Caesar: with dressing	**410**	34	18
add Grilled Chicken	**160**	4	0
add Grilled Shrimp	**160**	4	2
Steakhouse, with dressing	**930**	65	39
Side Salads: With Dressing			
Caesar	**290**	25	10
House: Base Salad	**140**	8	12
add Blue Cheese Vinaigrette	**260**	23	8
add Caesar Dressing	**200**	21	2
add Honey Mustard	**230**	20	11
add Mustard Vinaigrette	**220**	22	4
add Thousand Island	**250**	25	6

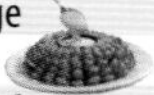
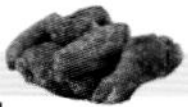
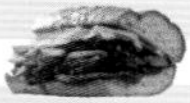
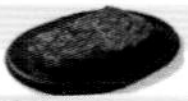
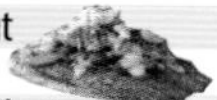
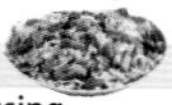
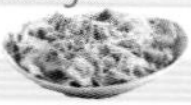
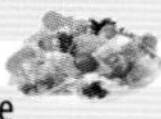

Outback Steakhouse® cont...(Oct '21)

Soups: Per Cup	C	F	Cb
Baked Potato	**300**	19	24
Chicken Tortilla	**260**	17	18
Cream of Broccoli	**200**	14	12
Sides: Aussie Fries	**410**	20	52
Baked Potato with toppings	**440**	17	58
Creamed Spinach	**570**	45	23
Fresh Seasonal Mixed Veggies	**160**	10	17
Grilled Asparagus	**60**	3	6
Homestyle Mashed Potatoes	**240**	15	20
Loaded	**320**	22	22
Steamed Broccoli	**150**	10	14
Steakhouse Mac & Cheese	**850**	51	67
Sweet Potato, with all toppings	**410**	11	72
Kid's Menu: Without Sides or Drink			
Entrees: Boomerang Cheeseburger	**600**	36	40
Chicken Fingers	**480**	25	33
Grilled Cheese-A-Roo	**580**	21	77
Grilled Chicken on the Barbie	**160**	4	0
Joey Sirloin	**180**	6	0
Mac-A-Roo 'N Cheese	**510**	19	65
Desserts: Per Whole Dish			
Chocolate Thunder	**1520**	105	142
NY Style Cheesecake, w/ Choc. Sce	**1080**	73	92
Salted Caramel Cookie Skillet	**860**	40	117
Triple Layer Carrot Cake	**1290**	68	174

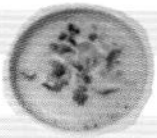
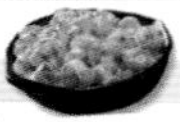
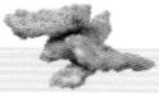
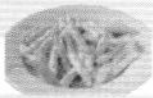

For Complete Menu & Data ~ see CalorieKing.com

Panda Express® (Oct '21)

Appetizers:	C	F	Cb
Chicken Egg Roll (1), 2.75 oz	**200**	10	20
Cream Cheese Rangoon (3), 2.4 oz	**190**	8	24
Veggie Spring Rolls (2), 3.4 oz	**190**	8	27
Entrées:			
Beef: Beijing Beef, 5.6 oz	**470**	26	46
Black Pepper Angus Steak, 5.3 oz	**180**	7	10
Broccoli Beef, 5.4 oz	**150**	7	13
Chicken:			
Black Pepper, 6.3 oz	**280**	19	15
Breast: String Bean, 5.6 oz	**190**	9	13
SweetFire, 5.8 oz	**380**	15	47
Grilled Teriyaki, 6 oz	**300**	13	8
Kung Pao, 6.2 oz	**290**	19	14
Mushroom, 5.7 oz	**220**	14	10
Orange, 5.7 oz	**490**	23	51

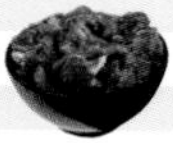
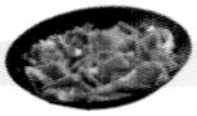

Panda Express® cont... (Oct '21)

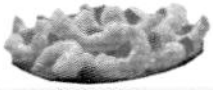

Entrees (Cont):	C	F	Cb
Shrimp:			
Honey Walnut, 3.7 oz	**360**	23	35
Wok Seared Steak & Shrimp, 5.6 oz	**240**	7	21
Vegetables: Eggplant Tofu, 6.1 oz	**340**	24	23
Super Greens, 3.5 oz	**45**	2	5
Sides:			
Chow Mein, 9.4 oz	**510**	20	80
Fried Rice, 9.3 oz	**520**	16	85
Steamed White Rice, 8.1 oz	**380**	0	87
Super Greens, 7 oz	**90**	3	10
Dessert: Choc Chip Chunk Cookie	**160**	7	25
Fortune Cookies, 0.18 oz	**20**	0	5

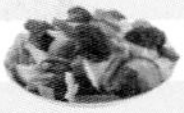

Panera Bread® (Oct '21)

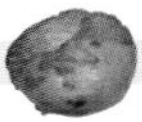

Bagels:	C	F	Cb
Asiago Cheese	**320**	5	55
Cinnamon Crunch	**420**	7	83
Breakfast Sandwiches:			
Avocado, Egg White & Spinach, on Flat Sprouted Grain Bagel	**360**	14	39
Bacon, Egg & Cheese on Tomato Wrap	**450**	24	32
Bacon, Scramb. Egg & Cheese Ciabatta	**450**	20	41
Sausage, Egg & Cheese on Brioche	**540**	32	33
Sandwiches: *Per Full Sandwich*			
Bacon Turkey Bravo on Tomato Basil	**860**	41	75
HClassic Grilled Cheese on White Miche	**860**	48	67
Mediterranean Veggie on Tomato Basil	**540**	12	89
Roasted Turkey & Avocado BLT, on Country Rustic Sourdough	**850**	53	54
Tuna Salad on Black pepper Focaccia	**740**	33	81
Entree:			
Bowls, Baja with Chicken	**740**	35	81
Flatbread Pizza, Cheese	**820**	34	86
Mac & Cheese:			
Small, 1 cup	**470**	31	33
Large, 2 cups	**950**	62	66
Salads: *Full Size, with Dressing, without Bread*			
Asian Sesame w/ Chicken	**410**	21	28
Chicken Caesar	**440**	27	21
Fuji Apple with Chicken	**560**	34	37
Greek	**400**	35	16
S'west Chili Lime Ranch w/ Chicken	**670**	34	57

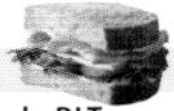

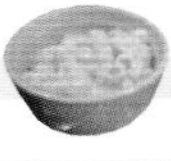

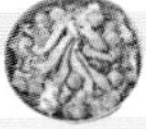

Panera Bread® cont... (Oct '21)

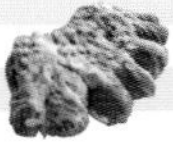

Soups: Per Cup, without Bread	C	F	Cb
Baked Potato	**220**	14	22
Bistro French Onion	**190**	8	21
Broccoli Cheddar	**230**	13	19
Cream of Chicken & Wild Rice	**180**	10	18
Ten Vegetables	**60**	1	10
Vegetarian Creamy Tomato	**230**	14	24
Pastries & Sweets:			
Bear Claw	**500**	23	66
Chocolate Croissant	**380**	22	39
Brownie, (1)	**400**	13	68
Cake, Cinnamon Crumb Coffee, slice	**520**	28	61
Cookie: Kitchen Sink	**800**	44	99
Oatmeal Raisin with Berries (1)	**340**	13	55
Muffin: Choc. Chip	**640**	28	91
Blueberry with Fresh Blueberries	**460**	18	69

Papa Gino's® (Oct '21)

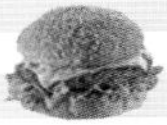

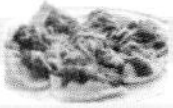

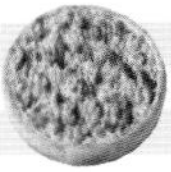

Burgers: Without Fries	C	F	Cb
Cheeseburger	**550**	31	37
Classic Burger	**690**	44	42
Double Cheeseburger	**830**	49	37
Hamburger	**520**	28	36
Entree Pasta: Fettuccine Alfredo	**760**	23	108
Mac & Cheese	**960**	47	85
Penne & Meatballs	**840**	27	126
Ravioli	**530**	13	76
Pizzas:			
Thin Crust: *Per Slice, ⅛ Large Pizza*			
Boss BBQ Chicken	**310**	11	39
Cheese	**230**	7	32
Crispy Buffalo, w/ Blue Cheese	**370**	18	36
Meat Combo	**390**	16	44
Pepperoni	**280**	11	32
Super Veggie	**250**	8	35
Works	**310**	13	33
Subs: *Per Small Sub*			
BLT	**720**	45	60
Chicken Breast Filet	**1050**	51	101
Chicken Parm	**1050**	41	109
Italian	**790**	43	59
Meatball Parmesan	**1140**	69	85
Tuna	**820**	55	58
Turkey	**450**	6	52
Turkey Club	**740**	37	62
Salads: *Without Dressing or Breadstick*			
Caesar	**190**	10	18
Garden	**190**	8	27
Breadstick, Cheese w/ Marinara (1)	**230**	8	30
rench Fries, side, 1 serving	**280**	12	40
Dressings: Blue Cheese	**270**	28	3
Caesar	**200**	22	1
Greek	**210**	24	1

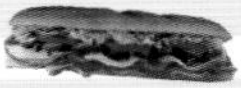

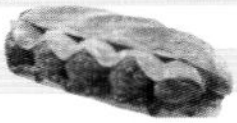

Papa John's® (Oct '21)

Pizzas:	C	F	Cb
Original Crust (14"): *Per ⅛ of Large 14" Pizza*			
BBQ Chicken & Bacon	340	11	45
Cheese	290	10	38
Extra Cheesy Alfredo	320	13	37
Fiery Buffalo Chicken	330	12	38
Garden Fresh	280	9	39
Hawaiian BBQ Chicken	360	11	47
Pepperoni	320	13	38
Pepperoni Sausage & Six Cheese	390	20	36
Sausage	330	14	38
The Works	340	14	39
Papadias: Italian	940	53	76
Meatball Pepperoni	940	49	79
Philly Cheesesteak	810	35	80
Wings: Per 8 Wings, with Dipping Sauce			
BBQ	880	57	20
Honey Chipotle	900	57	27
Spicy Buffalo	840	58	8
Sides:			
Bacon Cheddarsticks, 10"	120	6	11
Chicken Poppers: 5 Poppers	270	10	21
10 Poppers	530	21	42
Breadsticks:			
Regular, 1 X 12"	130	2	24
Cheesesticks, 1 X 10"	90	4	10
Garlic Parmesan, 1 X 12"	160	5	24
Garlic Knots, each	110	4.5	14
Desserts: Chocolate Chip Cookie	190	9	26
Double Chocolate Chip Brownie	240	12	34

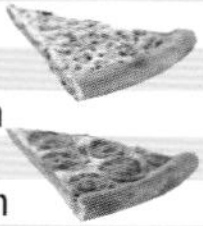
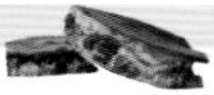
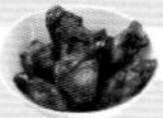
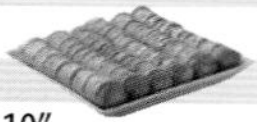
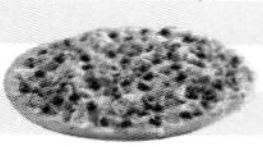

Papa Murphy's® (Oct '21)

Pizzas:	C	F	Cb
Original Crust: *Per 1⁄12 of Family Size Pizza*			
BBQ Chicken	330	13	36
Chicken Garlic	310	14	29
Cowboy	360	18	31
Garden Veggie	260	10	31
Gourmet Vegetarian	300	14	30
Hawaiian	270	9	32
Murphy's Combo	340	17	31
Papa's Favorite	340	17	31
Pepperoni	290	13	29
Rancher	310	14	30
Thai Chicken	330	12	39
Stuffed Pizzas: *Per 1⁄16 of Family Size Pizza*			
5 Meat	440	18	49
Big Murphy	440	18	50
Chicago Style	440	18	49
Chicken and Bacon	420	16	49

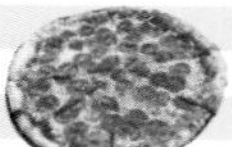
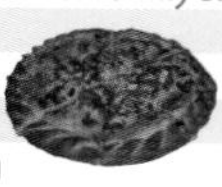
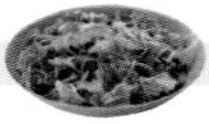

Papa Murphy's® cont... (Oct '21)

Pizzas (Cont):	C	F	Cb
Salads: Per Whole Salad, w/out Dressing or Croutons			
Caesar	100	5	7
Club	270	16	12
Garden	190	11	13
Italian	270	19	11
Mediterranean	320	17	23
Desserts:			
Choc. Chip Cookie, ⅛ slice	170	11	34
Cinnamon Wheel, ⅛ slice	250	7	42
S'mores Dessert Bar	130	7	25

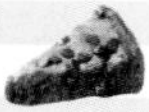
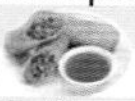

Pei Wei Asian Diner® (Oct '21)

	C	F	Cb
Shareables: Without Sauce			
Crab Wonton (1)	85	5	7
Steamed Veggie & Chicken Dumpling	30	1	4
Trad'nl Edamame, large	320	13	19
Vegetable Spring Rolls (1)	120	6	15
Classic Entrees: Per Regular Size			
Beef & Broccoli	790	49	53
Kung Pao Shrimp	740	50	42
Mongolian Chicken	635	27	39
Orange Chicken	980	50	94
Pei Wei Original Shrimp	790	36	98
Spicy Korean BBQ Steak	780	45	39
Spicy Thai Basil Cashew Chkn	1050	65	47
Teriyaki Tofu	1060	52	104
Thai C'nut Curry Chkn	640	8	42
Thai Dynamite Fried Tofu	890	52	60
Noodle/Rice Bowls:			
Brown Rice, regular	350	3	73
Cauliflower Fried Rice	470	27	41
Dan Dan	990	40	110
Chicken Fried Rice	1105	27	137
Chicken Lo Mein	1170	42	123
Chicken Pad Thai	1490	42	167
Chicken Pad Thai without Tofu	1370	40	161
Drunken Noodles	1160	26	145
Fried Rice, regular	750	20	118
White Rice, regular	400	0	90
Salad Bowls: With Dressing			
Asian Chopped Chicken	660	35	44
Spicy Polynesian Poke Bowl	710	29	88
Soup: Thai Wonton, cup	70	2	17
Thai Wonton, bowl	140	4	43
Dessert: Fudge Brownie	430	22	57
Thai Donuts	500	19	74
Sauce for Donuts, 2 oz	260	6	44

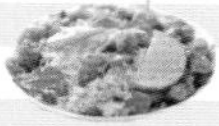
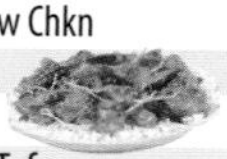
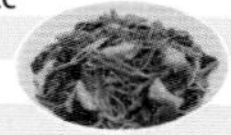
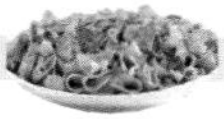
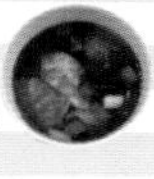
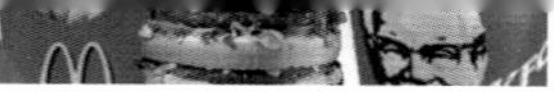

Pepe's Mexican® ~ see CalorieKing.com

Perkins® (Oct '21)

Breakfast: Without Side Choices	C	F	Cb
Classic: Country Fried Steak & Eggs	**740**	45	47
Hearty Man's Combo	**800**	69	11
Magnificent Seven	**720**	39	68
Eggs Benedict	**660**	31	61
Omelets:			
Everything	**550**	40	14
Farmer's	**660**	54	8
Granny's Country	**640**	41	34
Griddle Greats: Belgian Waffle	**410**	21	49
Blueberry Pancakes (3)	**520**	21	73
Buttermilk Pancakes (3)	**490**	21	66
Platters: Belgian Waffle	**570**	33	51
French Toast	**570**	27	53
Potato Pancake	**650**	42	48
Syrups & Toppings:			
Apricot Syrup, 2 oz	**120**	0	30
Glazed Blueberries, 6 oz	**200**	0	51
Glazed Strawberries, 6 oz	**140**	0	36
Pancake/Twinberry Syrup, 2 oz, av.	**130**	0	33
Sugar Free Pancake Syrup, 2 oz	**20**	0	6
(contains sugar alcohol)			
Side Choices: Bacon, 4 slices	**140**	12	0
Blueberry Muffin, with butter	**600**	27	81
Breakfast Potatoes, 5 oz	**280**	17	30
English Muffin, with butter	**180**	6	28
Fresh Cut Fruit, 4 oz	**70**	0	19
Ham, sliced, 3.4 oz	**140**	5	4
Hash Browns, 4.3 oz	**210**	13	22
Oatmeal, with butter blend, 2% Milk & Brown Sugar	**340**	9	57
Sausage Patties (2)	**380**	38	1
Smoked Sausage, 4.1 oz	**380**	34	8
Sticky Bun, with butter	**740**	36	98
Turkey Bacon, 4 slices	**100**	6	0
White Toast (2), with butter	**260**	11	34
Whole Wheat Toast (2), with butter	**260**	8	38
Burgers: *Without Sides*			
BBQ Tangler	**1190**	73	82
Classic Burger	**710**	40	48
Classic Cheeseburger	**870**	54	48
Sandwiches: *Without Sides*			
Chicken Strips Melt, on Sourdough	**1190**	70	88
Country Club Melt, on Sourdough	**940**	52	64
Pot Roast Melt, on Sourdough	**880**	49	63
Reuben Melt, on Rye	**1000**	50	79

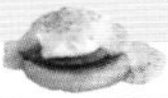
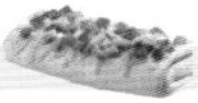
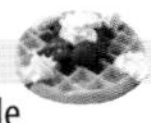
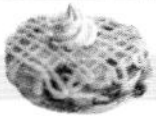
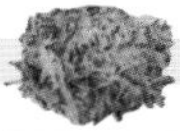
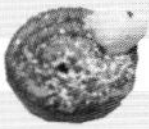
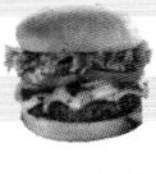

Perkins® cont... (Oct '21)

Lunch & Dinners:	C	F	Cb
Comfort Classics: *Without Sides*			
Chicken Strips	**800**	43	59
Country Fried Steak	**570**	32	45
Fish 'n Chips, with Tartar Sauce	**1290**	85	97
Grilled Garlic Tilapia & Shrimp	**550**	20	57
Grilled Salmon	**430**	29	2
Turkey & Dressing, w/- Cranb. Sce	**430**	20	21
Supper Skillets:			
Hibachi Fried Chicken	**780**	29	103
Hibachi Gr. Shrimp	**610**	20	85
Steak & Pepper	**800**	43	58
Sides: Applesauce	**40**	0	9
Baked Potato,with Lt. Sour Cream	**250**	7	42
Buttered Corn	**120**	4	17
French Fries	**570**	36	56
Green Beans & Bacon	**45**	2.5	4
Herb Rice Pilaf	**270**	6	50
H'style Seasoned Potato	**210**	3	40
Macaroni & Cheese	**300**	9	46
Mashed Potatoes & Gravy	**240**	9	34
Sauteed Spinach	**70**	3.5	4
Tater Tots	**470**	28	47
Soups: *Per Bowl, Includes Crackers*			
Chicken Noodle	**260**	6	37
Loaded Potato; Tomato Basil	**460**	26	46
Salads: *With Set Dressing Unless Indicated*			
Honey Mstrd Chicken Crunch	**980**	63	63
Southwest Avocado	**820**	50	61
55 Plus Lunch/Dinner: *Without Sides*			
Cheeseburger	**640**	34	41
Pork Chop Dinner	**560**	32	8
Pot Roast Dinner	**560**	31	16
Dessert: *As Served*			
Muffins: *Includes Whipped Butter Blend*			
Apple Cinnamon	**580**	27	76
Banana Nut	**740**	41	85
Blueberry	**600**	27	81
Pies: *Per Slice*			
Banana Cream Pie	**650**	43	62
Caramel Apple, 7.2 oz	**500**	22	68
Cherry	**580**	27	75
Chocolate French Silk	**730**	52	63
Southern Pecan, 5.5 oz	**670**	33	86
Wildberry, no sugar added, 7 oz	**470**	27	50

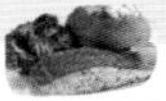
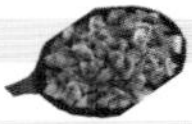
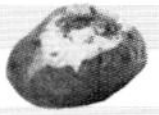
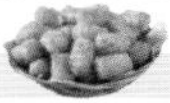
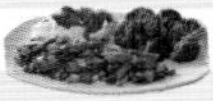
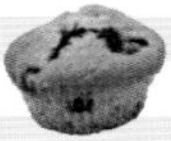
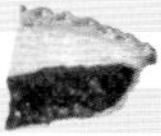

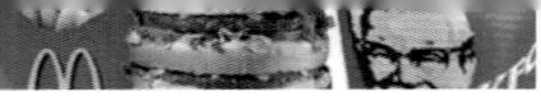

Peter Piper Pizza® (Oct'21)

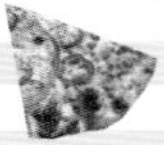
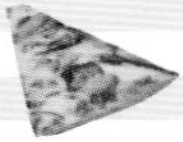
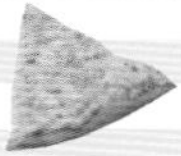
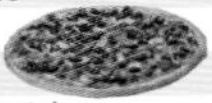
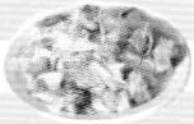
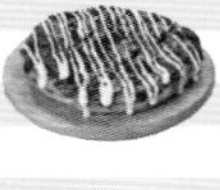

Signature Pizzas:	C	F	Cb
Original Crust: *Per 1/8 of Large 14" Pizza*			
5 Meat Supreme	**360**	15	39
California Veggie	**290**	9	41
Cheese	**320**	11	39
Chicago Classic	**330**	13	40
Hearty Hawaiian	**310**	9	41
New York 3 Cheese w/ Pepperoni	**390**	18	39
Pizza Mexicana	**390**	18	39
Spinach Chkn Alfredo	**350**	15	37
The Werx	**310**	11	40
Veggie Harvest	**300**	9	42
Original Crust: *Per 1/12 of Extra Large 16" Pizza*			
5 Meat Supreme	**350**	16	34
California Veggie	**250**	8	35
Cheese	**280**	10	34
Chicago Classic	**300**	12	35
Hearty Hawaiian	**270**	8	36
New York 3 Cheese w/ Pepperoni	**350**	16	34
Pizza Mexicana	**340**	15	34
Spinach Chkn Alfredo	**310**	14	32
The Werx	**290**	11	34
Veggie Harvest	**260**	8	36
Pasta: With 2 Breadsticks			
Mac & Pepperoni	**1670**	91	168
Meaty Ziti	**1240**	78	79
Spinach Alfredo	**1640**	89	153
Salads: Small Size, without Dressing			
Caesar, with Croutons	**320**	14	35
Chopped Italian	**260**	19	10
Wings & More: Without Sides			
Cheddar Bacon Roll (1)	**350**	18	34
Garlic Cheese Bread, 3.25 oz	**390**	17	45
Handmade Breadsticks, with Marinara Sauce (6)	**1190**	31	199
Loaded Tots	**1280**	102	70
Wings: Bone In (10), without sauce	**1160**	97	0
Boneless, 10 oz, w/out sauce	**880**	58	47
Mango Havanero Boneless, w/ Ranch	**1510**	95	123
Sweet BBQ Wings, Bone In	**1410**	97	63
Dipping Sauces:			
BBQ	**240**	0	60
Buffalo	**120**	9	6
Ranch	**320**	36	2
Sweet Chili	**200**	0	46
Xtra Hot Buffalo	**90**	6	5
Dessert:			
Cinnamon Crunch, small slice	**380**	9	69
Vanilla Soft Serve: Cone	**200**	6	35
Cup	**180**	6	31

P.F. Chang's® (Oct'21)

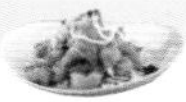
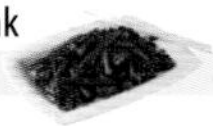
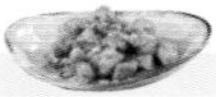
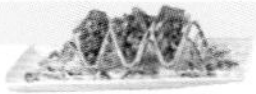
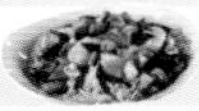
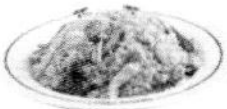
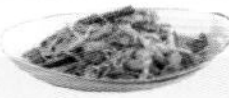
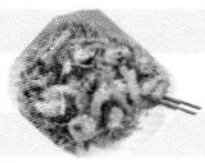

Shareables/Sides:	C	F	Cb
Calamari & Vegetables Tempura	**960**	73	61
Chang's BBQ Pork Spare Ribs (6)	**810**	21	36
Chang's Chicken Lettuce Wraps	**710**	27	77
Chang's Vegetarian Lettuce Wraps	**620**	28	64
Crispy Green Beans	**990**	78	70
Dynamite Shrimp	**640**	48	36
Edamame with Kosher Salt	**400**	17	25
Kung Pao Brussels Sprouts	**720**	42	84
Entrées:			
Beef: *Per Whole Meal*			
Beef with Broccoli	**670**	33	46
Korean Bulgogi Steak	**1370**	58	121
Mongolian	**770**	42	39
Pepper Steak	**640**	36	29
Chicken: *Per Whole Dish, without Rice*			
Chang's Spicy	**840**	33	77
Crispy Honey Chkn	**1120**	60	87
Ginger Chicken with Broccoli	**480**	12	41
Kung Pao	**960**	58	46
Sesame Chicken	**920**	37	82
Sweet & Sour Chicken	**860**	41	86
Seafood: *Per Whole Meal, without Rice*			
Crispy Honey Shrimp	**1020**	55	79
Kung Pao Shrimp	**760**	52	40
Miso Glazed Salmon	**660**	37	30
Oolong Chilean Sea Bass	**560**	35	30
Salt & Pepper Prawns	**500**	22	37
Shrimp with Lobster Sce	**500**	27	22
Vegetarian: *Without Rice*			
Buddha's Feast: Steamed	**260**	4	32
Stir-Fried	**380**	8	53
Noodles & Rice:			
Fried Rice: Combo	**1200**	35	160
with Beef	**1140**	33	155
with Chicken	**1100**	26	159
with Pork	**1190**	37	161
with Shrimp	**1000**	20	154
Lo Mein: Beef	**980**	31	127
Chicken	**950**	24	130
Combo	**1050**	33	132
Pork	**1030**	35	133
Shrimp	**850**	18	126
Vegetables	**760**	13	135
Singapore Street Noodles	**1180**	13	226

P.F. Chang's® cont... (Oct '21)

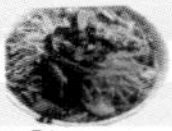
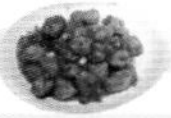
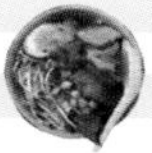
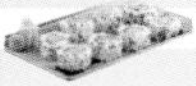
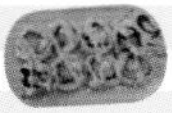
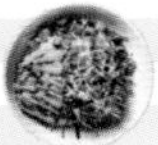

Noodles & Rice (Cont):	C	F	Cb
Pad Thai: Chicken	1320	39	190
Combo	1290	38	190
Shrimp	1270	37	190
Lunch Bowls: *Without Rice*			
Beef & Brocoli	370	19	29
Crispy Honey Chicken	840	42	71
Mongolian Beef	490	28	89
Spicy Chicken	680	27	127
Sides: Brown Rice, 6 oz	190	0	40
Fried Rice	510	15	77
White Rice, 6 oz	220	0	49
Ramen: Braised Pork	210	13	3
Spicy Miso	700	22	106
Tonkotsu	790	34	106
Sushi: California Roll	390	16	53
Kung Pao Dragon Roll	510	23	60
Shrimp Tempura Roll	580	25	69
Spicy Tuna Roll	300	6	43
Salad: Asian Caesar	410	30	22
Mandarin Crunch	750	46	75
Add: Chicken	160	5	4
Salmon	240	16	0
Soup: Egg Drop, bowl	270	7	42
Hot & Sour, bowl	470	12	63
Wonton, bowl	570	17	53
Dessert: Banana Spring Rolls	940	35	149
New York Style Cheese Cake	940	61	80
The Great Wall of Chocolate	1700	71	259
Vietnamese Chocolate Lava Cake	820	48	97

Pita Pit® ~ *See CalorieKing.com*

Pizza Hut® (Oct '21)

All Pizzas are with Standard Ingredients & Sauce

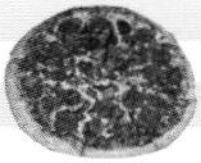
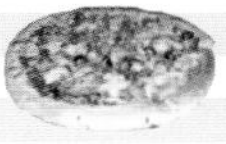

Hand-Tossed Style: *Per ⅛ of Medium 12" Pizza*	C	F	Cb
Buffalo Chicken	200	5	28
Cheese	210	8	26
Meat Lover's	290	15	26
Pepperoni	220	9	25
Pepperoni Lover's	270	13	26
Supreme	240	10	26
Ultimate Cheese Lover's	230	10	25
Veggie Lover's	200	6	27
Original Pan: *Per ⅛ of Medium 12" Pizza*			
Backyard BBQ	270	10	33
Cheese	250	10	28
Meat Lover's	320	17	28
Pepperoni	250	11	28
Pepperoni Lover's	300	15	28
Supreme	270	13	29
Ultimate Cheese Lover's	270	13	27
Veggie Lover's	230	9	29

Pizza Hut® cont..(Oct '21)

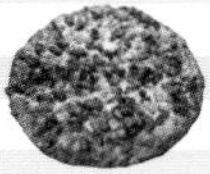
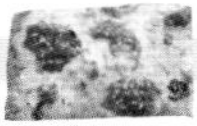
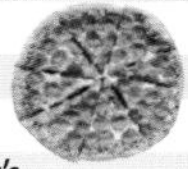
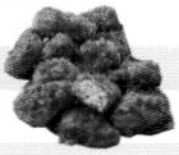
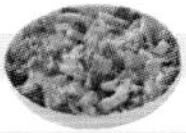

Personal Pan: *Per ¼ of 6" Pizza, with Standard Ingredients & Sauce*	C	F	Cb
Backyard BBQ Chicken	180	6	25
Meat Lover's	210	12	18
Pepperoni	150	7	17
Pepperoni Lover's	180	9	17
Supreme	170	8	18
Ultimate Cheese Lover's	170	8	17
Veggie Lover's	140	5	18
Rectangle Slices: *Per Slice, ⅛ of Pizza*			
Backyard BBQ Chicken	260	9	34
Buffalo Chicken	240	8	32
Cheese	240	9	29
Pepperoni	250	11	28
Veggie Lovers	220	8	30
Thin 'n Crispy: *Per ⅛ of Medium 12" Pizza*			
Backyard BBQ Chicken	210	7	27
Cheese	190	7	22
Chicken-Bacon Parmesan	210	9	21
Meat Lover's	260	14	22
Pepperoni Lover's	260	13	22
Supreme	210	9	23
Ultimate Cheese Lover's	220	10	22
Veggie Lover's	180	6	24
Pastas, Tuscani:			
Creamy Chicken Alfredo, 9.9 oz	990	57	77
Meaty Marinara, 9.6 oz	880	40	88
Sides:			
Saucy Wings: BBQ (1)	60	3.5	2
Buffalo (1)	60	3.5	1
Breadstick (1), without sauce	140	4.5	19
Cheese Stick without sauce	150	4.5	20
Garlic Bread, 1 piece	140	8	15
with Cheese	210	13	16
Salad: *Without Dressing*			
BLT	290	16	29
Chicken Caesar	410	21	30
Chicken Garden	420	19	39
Crispy Chicken Caesar	830	53	60
Zesty Italian	390	23	33
Dressing: Blue Cheese, entree size	450	48	3
Creamy Caesar, entree size	360	37	5
French, entree size	330	23	29
Light Italian Vinaigrette, entree size	150	11	11
Desserts: Fried Apple Pie, no sauce	170	9	22
Triple Choc. Brownie, ⅑ square	230	10	34
Ultimate Chocolate Chip Cookie	190	9	26

Pizza Ranch® (Oct '21)

Pizza:	C	F	Cb
Original Crust: *Per Slice, 1/10 of Medium Pizza*			
Bacon Cheeseburger	**180**	7	20
BBQ Chicken	**170**	5	21
Bronco	**200**	8	20
Buffalo Chicken	**180**	8	18
Chicken Bacon Ranch	**230**	12	19
Macaroni 'N' Cheese	**220**	10	22
Prairie (Veggie)	**180**	6	21
Stampede	**200**	8	21
Sweet Swine	**170**	5	20
Taco Texan	**230**	10	26
Thin Crust: *Per 1/10 Slice of Medium Pizza*			
BBQ Chicken	**130**	5	12
Bronco	**160**	9	10
Mac 'N' Cheese	**180**	10	13
Ranch Wraps: *With Set Sauce or Dressing*			
BBQ Chicken	**1180**	48	129
Caesar Chicken	**1310**	80	93
Chicken Bacon	**1720**	120	95
Sides: Coleslaw	**180**	16	11
Corn	**200**	1	42
Mashed Potatoes & Gravy, 8 oz	**260**	6	41
Ranch Potato Wedges (8)	**520**	14	85
Salads: Chef	**440**	19	11
Chicken Fiesta	**180**	7	11
Garden	**90**	5	9
Taco	**590**	36	51

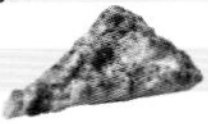
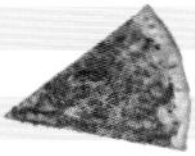
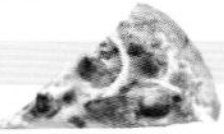
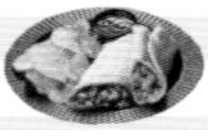
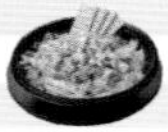

For Complete Menu & Data ~ see CalorieKing.com

Pollo Tropical® ~ *See CalorieKing.com*

Popeye's® (Oct '21)

Chicken Pieces: *Mild & Spicy with Skin*	C	F	Cb
Breast	**380**	20	16
Leg	**160**	9	5
Thigh	**280**	21	7
Wing	**210**	14	8
Nuggets: 6 pieces	**225**	14	15
9 Pieces	**340**	20	23
Tenders: Mild/Spicy, 3 pieces	**445**	21	29
5 pieces	**740**	34	48
Sandwiches & Wraps: *Each*			
Classic Chicken S'wich	**700**	42	50
Loaded Chicken Wrap	**310**	12	35
Spicy Chicken	**700**	42	50
Seafood: Catfish Fillets, 2 pieces	**460**	29	27
Butterfly Shrimp (8)	**420**	25	34
Popcorn Shrimp, 4 oz	**390**	25	28

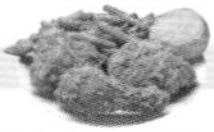
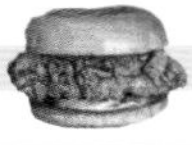

Popeye's® cont... (Oct '21)

Sides:	C	F	Cb
Biscuit	**205**	13	20
Cajun Fries, regular	**270**	14	33
Cajun Rice, regular	**185**	6	24
Cole Slaw, regular	**140**	10	12
Corn on the Cob (1)	**210**	6	34
Mshd Potatoes, w/ Cajun Gravy, reg.	**110**	4	18
Onion Rings, regular	**280**	19	25
Red Beans & Rice, regular	**245**	16	22
Breakfast:			
Biscuits: Bacon	**400**	25	37
Chicken	**490**	26	47
Egg	**510**	29	41
Egg & Sausage	**690**	45	43
Sausage	**540**	36	41
Sausage & Gravy	**510**	33	42
Grits	**370**	5	80
Hash Rounds	**360**	20	41
Desserts:			
Edward's Sliced Pecan Pie, 3.4 oz	**410**	21	52
Mardi Gras Cheesecake, 3 oz	**320**	21	29
Mississippi Mud Cake, 3 oz	**260**	7	50
Sweet Potato Pie 3.4 oz	**350**	19	41

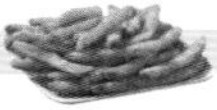
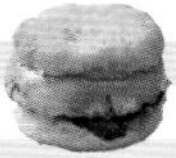
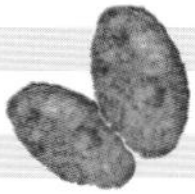

Port of Subs® (Oct '21)

Figures Based on West Coast Outlets	C	F	Cb
Classic Subs: *Per 8" White Sub with Standard Menu Components*			
#1 Ham, Salami, Capicolla, Pepperoni, Provolone	**630**	26	64
#2 Ham & Turkey, Provolone	**530**	14	65
#3 Salami & Turkey, Provolone	**560**	19	65
#4 Ham, Salami, Provolone	**550**	20	63
#5 Smoked Ham, Turkey, Cheddar	**560**	17	65
#6 Vegetarian, 3 Chse	**670**	34	68
#7 Roast Beef, Prov.	**540**	14	61
#8 Turkey, Provolone	**540**	14	66
#10 Rstd Chicken Breast, Provolone	**550**	14	64
#11 Ham, American Cheese	**530**	16	64
#12 Salami, Provolone	**590**	25	63
#13 Peppered Pastrami Turkey, Swiss	**540**	15	65
#15 Salami, Pepperoni, Provolone	**600**	27	63
#16 Chkn, Pepperoni, Pepper Jack	**590**	22	62
#17 Tuna, Provolone	**700**	29	65
#18 Roast Beef, Turkey, Provolone	**540**	14	64

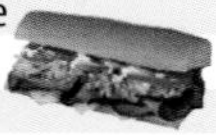

Port of Subs® cont... (Oct '21)

Figures Based on West Coast Outlets

	C	F	Cb
Hot Subs: *Per 8" White Sub with Provolone, without Additional Toppings*			
Melts: Grilled Buffalo Chicken	590	13	60
Grilled Chicken	590	13	60
Grilled Teriyaki Chicken	670	13	77
Pastrami	780	39	64
NY Steak	650	28	59
Ultimate BLT	690	36	61
Flatbreads: *With Provolone without Sauce*			
All American Club	410	17	36
Melts: Pastrami	550	30	37
NY Steak	450	22	33
Pulled Pork	390	13	33
Ultimate BLT	450	25	35
Wraps: *On Wheat Wrap w/ Standard Menu Compnents, without shakers*			
Grilled Chicken Caesar	670	25	60
Pastrami Melt	850	47	62
Ultimate BLT	760	45	59
Fresh Salads: *Standard Components, w/out Dressing or Shakers*			
Caesar; Garden	70	2.5	9
Chef	250	14	13
Grilled Chicken; Gr. Chkn Spinach	280	7	11
Spinach	60	2.5	8
Tuna	350	20	12
Salad Dressings: *Per 2 fl.oz*			
Caesar; Ranch, average	220	22	4
Honey Mustard	260	26	10
Mayo	150	16	0
Sides: *Per Regular, 8 oz*			
Macaroni Salad	520	36	44
Potato Salad	370	20	45
Soup: *Per Small Serving*			
Chicken Buffalo	190	12	13
Chicken Noodle	90	2.5	12
Cream of Broccoli	200	12	17
Tomato Bisque	200	11	19
Breakfast Sub: *With American Cheese & Egg*			
5" White Bread:			
Bacon	450	23	38
Smoked Ham	390	15	39
Turkey Sausage	480	22	38
Flatbread: Bacon	460	25	35
Smoked Ham	400	17	35
Turkey Sausage	490	24	35
Desserts:			
Chocolate Chunk Cookie, 4 oz	500	23	71
Jumbo Brownie	760	36	109
Oatmeal Raisin Cookie, 4 oz	480	20	69
White Choc. Macadamia Nut Cookie	530	26	67

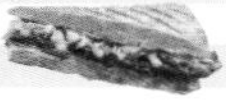
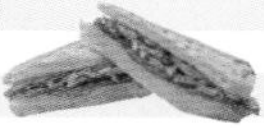
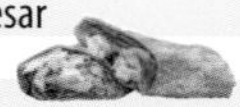
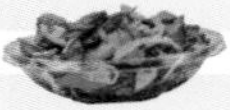
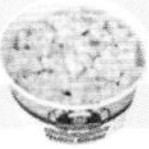
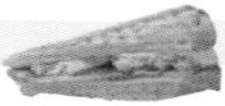
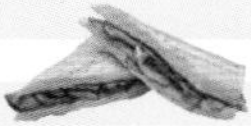

Pret A Manger® (Oct '21)

East Coast Outlets.

	C	F	Cb
Baguettes:			
Caprese	690	35	69
Ham & Cheese	620	23	70
Maine Lobster Roll	700	37	68
Romesco Chicken & Mozzarella	670	29	71
Hot Food: *Per Pack*			
Cauliflower & Chickpea Grain Bowl	410	21	51
Chipotle Chkn Grain Bowl	400	6	67
Chicken Parm	530	22	53
Lobster Mac & Cheese	640	32	58
Spinach & Tomato Mac & Cheese	620	31	59
Pot, Egg & Spinach	160	11	3
Sandwiches: *On Multigrain Bread Unless Indicated*			
Chicken & Bacon	570	29	33
Egg Salad & Arugula	530	32	41
Roasted Turkey, Swiss & Apple	530	25	49
Soups: *Per Small*			
Moroccan Lentil	220	10	25
Tomato Feta	130	7	13
Salads: *Without Dressing*			
Chicken Avocado	340	19	23
Chicken Caesar	260	14	6
Mediterranean Mezze	370	17	46
Salmon & Mango Grain	430	21	41
Wraps:			
Bang Bang Chicken	580	26	65
Crunchy Chipotle Chicken & Avocado	540	26	59
Falafel & Hummus	540	17	86
Green Goodness Roasted Turkey	660	41	55
Breakfast:			
Brioche: Egg & Bacon	510	27	33
Egg & Cheddar	370	17	33
Shakshuka Frittata	300	12	13
Tomato & Mozzarella Croissant	440	29	28
Bakery: *Per Pack*			
Croissants: Almond	370	21	39
Chocolate	350	20	33
Pain au Raisin	390	20	46
Cookies: Chocolate Chunk, 2.5 oz	310	16	42
Harvest, 2.5 oz	280	12	40
Muffin, Blueberry, 4.5 oz	420	16	63
Beverages: *Per 12 fl.oz*			
Chai Latte	190	0	37
Hot Chocolate	370	0	62

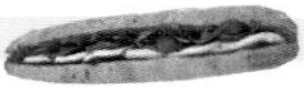
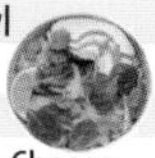
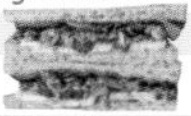
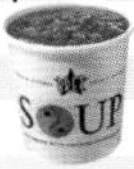

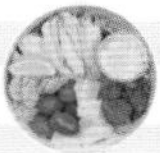
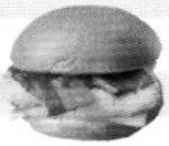
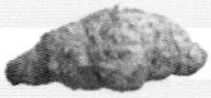
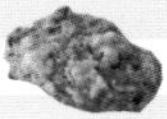

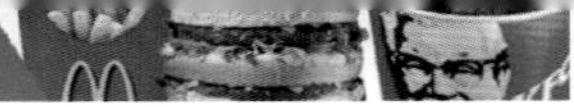

Pretzelmaker® (Oct '21)

Pretzels: Per Small Serving	C	F	Cb
Bites: Salted, 6 oz	500	14	85
Cinn. Sugar, 6 oz	530	14	90
Whole: Plain, 4 oz	310	3	66
Cinnamon Sugar, 5 oz	450	12	79
Garlic, 5 oz	430	12	74
Parmesan, 5 oz	450	15	66
Ranch, 5 oz	440	12	72
Pretzel Dogs: Regular	420	23	31
Mini (8)	430	29	33
Jalapeno (1), 6 oz	450	24	34
Sauces: Per 2 oz			
Caramel	100	1	22
Cheddar/Nacho Cheese, average	80	6	5
Cream Cheese	200	20	2
Pizza Sauce	30	1	6
Vanilla Glaze	170	0	42
Beverages: Per 20 oz Unless Indicated			
Blended Drinks:			
Cool Cappuccino	430	22	58
Mango Madness	500	16	90
Mocha Mania	580	22	94
Power Pomegranate	490	16	86
Strawberry Bananza	500	16	85
Fresh Lemonade: Original, 20 oz	140	0	38
Strawberry; Raspberry, 20 oz, av.	210	0	52

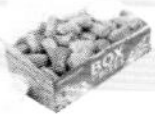
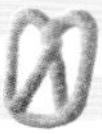
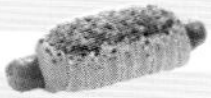
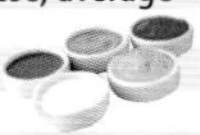
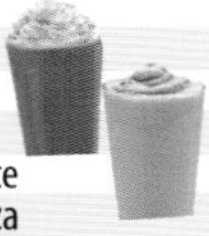

Qdoba® (Oct '21)

Make Your Own Burrito:	C	F	Cb
Meat: Chorizo; Ground Beef, av. 3 oz	180	10	5
Grilled: Adobo Chicken, 3.5 oz	150	9	2
Steak, av., 3.5 oz	230	15	4
Pulled Pork, 3.5 oz	110	4.5	3
Smoked Brisket, 3.5 oz	270	20	3
Other Burrito Fillings:			
Black Beans, 4 oz	140	1	24
Cilantro Lime Rice, 4 oz	190	3	38
Corn Tortilla Strips, 4 oz	560	26	75
Fajita Veggies, 2 oz	35	2	4
Hand Crafted Guac., 4 oz	170	14	10
Pico De Gallo, 2 oz	10	0	3
Pinto Beans, 4 oz	130	1	23
Romaine Lettuce for Salads, 3.5 oz	15	0	3
Salsas, average	20	0	4
Seasoned Brown Rice, 4 oz	170	2	36
Seasoned Potatoes, 2 oz	130	6	17
Shredded Cheese, 1 oz	110	9	1
Shredded Lettuce, 0.25 oz	7	0	1
Sour Cream, 1 oz	50	5	3
Tortillas: Corn, 5.5"	60	1	11
Crispy Taco Shell	60	3	8
Crunchy Flour Tortilla Bowl	390	22	41
Flour Tortilla: 5.5"	70	2	12
10"	210	5	36
12.5"	300	7	52

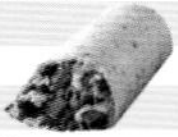
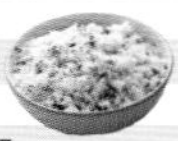
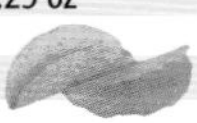
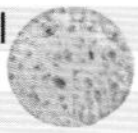

Qdoba® cont...® (Oct '21)

Signature Eats:	C	F	Cb
Bowls: Chicken Protein	610	29	48
Chicken Queso	780	34	75
Impossible Fajita	580	15	85
Burrito, Chicken Cheese	1080	41	127
Quesadills, Steak Fajita	1130	68	72
Street Style Tacos:			
Chicken:			
Corn Tacos (3)	470	22	51
Flour Tacos (3)	520	25	54
Kid's Meals: Burrito	480	15	67
Quesadilla	260	12	25
Taco: with Beef	220	12	11
with Chicken	200	11	11
Beans with Cheese, side	170	3	25
Desserts:			
Chocolate Chunk Cookie, 1.9 oz	260	14	34
Double Chocolate Brownie, 3.1 oz	360	16	52

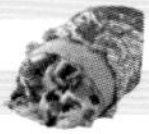
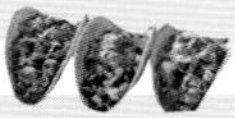
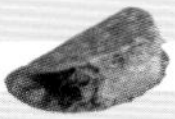

Quiznos Subs® (Oct '21)

Subs: Per 8" Regular Japaleno Cheddar Sub, with Standard Menu Toppings Unless Indicated

Chicken:	C	F	Cb
Baja	800	32	76
Carbonara	890	42	73
Honey Mustard	850	36	80
Mesquite	800	33	73
Southwest Chicken	860	45	73
Classic:			
Italian	890	48	79
Spicy Monterey	600	15	81
Tuna Melt	660	22	76
Turkey Ranch & Swiss	670	25	73
Veggie Guacamole	810	44	81
Steak:			
Black Angus Steak,			
On Rosemary Parmesan	780	27	88
Chipotle Steak & Cheddar	840	44	73
French Dip	760	30	79
Peppercorn Steak	840	42	76
Salads: Per Full Size With Set Dressing			
Apple Harvest	520	29	48
Chef	640	47	14
Italian	700	57	18
Sides:			
Classic Tater Tots	210	11	25
Loaded	320	19	25
Side Salad with Red Wine Vinaigrette	270	26	9

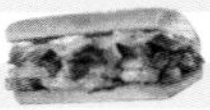
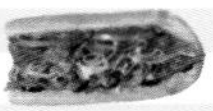
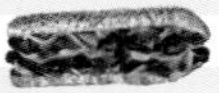
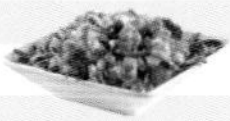
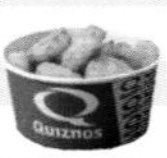

Quiznos Subs® cont... (Oct '21)

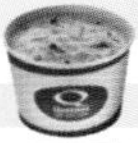
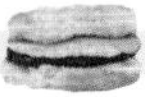
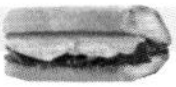

Soups: Per Regular	C	F	Cb
Broccoli Cheese	220	14	18
Chicken Noodle	120	4	14
Chili	290	10	34
Tomato Basil Bisque	290	21	21
Breakfast:			
Biscuit: Egg & Cheddar	460	31	31
Sausage, Egg & Cheddar	630	48	31
Subs:			
Bacon, Egg & Cheddar	370	17	34
Ham, Egg & Cheddar	340	14	36
Sausage, Egg & Cheddar	550	37	35
Desserts: Chocolate Brownie, 3 oz	440	23	56
Chocolate Chunk Cookie, 3 oz	400	18	57
Cinnamon Sugar Cookie, 3 oz	400	17	58
Oatmeal Raisin Cookie, 3 oz	360	12	58

Rally's/Checkers® (Oct '21)

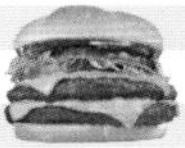
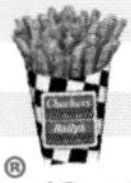

Burgers:	C	F	Cb
Baconzilla	910	62	43
Big Buford	660	39	39
Cheese Champ	430	21	39
Sandwiches: Crispy Fish	530	29	52
Spicy Chicken	340	13	40
Classic Wings: Buffalo, med., 5 pcs	360	23	3
Garlic Parmesan, 5 pcs	510	40	3
Sweet & Smokey BBQ, 5 pieces	430	23	19
Fries: Regular, medium	500	24	63
Chili Cheese Fries	420	25	43
Fully Loaded Fries	870	56	72

Ranch One® (Oct '21)

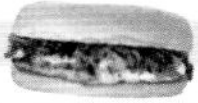
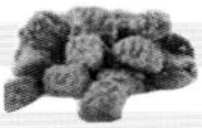
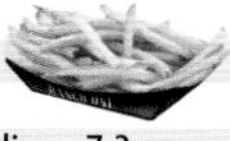

Sandwiches:	C	F	Cb
Chicken & Cheese	390	12	40
Chicken Philly, 9.3 oz	410	13	40
Grilled Classic Chicken, 9.4 oz	680	47	37
Original Crispy Chicken, 11.5 oz	640	31	60
Other Favorites:			
Chicken Fajitas, 10 oz	540	24	53
Chicken Platter, with Rice, 11.9 oz	270	6	28
Popcorn Chicken:			
Small, 5.5 oz	310	10	30
Large, 7.5 oz	420	14	40
Salads: Completed			
Grilled Chicken Caesar, 13.3 oz	430	30	14
Southwest Chicken, 17.5 oz	680	43	44
Fries:			
Medium, 5.8 oz	380	19	43
Large, 10.9 oz	530	27	58
Cheese Fries: Medium, 7.3 oz	490	27	46
Large, 11 oz	760	44	66

Red Hot & Blue® (Oct '21)

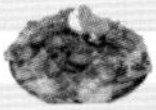
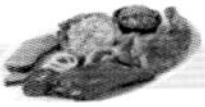
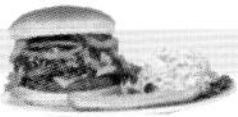
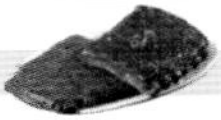
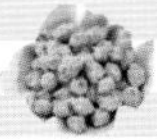
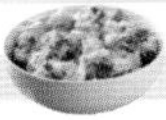

Starters:	C	F	Cb
Catfish Fingers	590	19	75
Nachos, with Chili	1005	51	103
Smokin Buffalo Wings	1045	85	28
BBQ Platters: Five Meat	935	63	15
Delta Double with Memphis Chkn	900	54	12
Pulled Pork	325	21	7
Smoked Sausage	965	68	36
Burgers:			
ALL IN	915	52	46
Classic Blues	665	32	44
Favorite Entrees: Delta Catfish	835	42	57
Delta Surf & Turf	1025	68	38
Southern Fried Chicken Crispers	760	35	50
Rib & Crispers Platter	1060	68	39
Ribs, Full Slab:			
Dry	1870	144	28
Sweet	1895	142	44
Sandwiches:			
Fried Delta Catfish	655	25	71
Grilled Chicken	360	6	40
Sides: BBQ Beans	255	2	48
Collard Greens	50	2	7
Fried Ocra	190	8	29
Mashed Potatoes, with gravy	310	14	44
Memphis Fries, 6 oz	345	19	38
Potato Salad	405	28	33
Sweet Potato	495	0	114
Sweet Potato Fries	375	19	49
Salads: Grilled Chicken Caesar	770	46	47
Southern Fried Chicken	710	31	60
Texas Smokehouse	670	36	36

Red Lobster® (Jun '21)

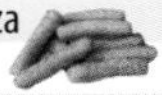
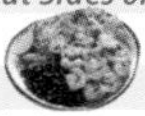
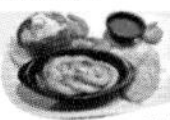

Appetizers: As Served	C	F	Cb
Lobster & Langostino Pizza	700	35	59
Mozzarella Cheesesticks	700	40	56
Parrot Isle Jumbo Cocktail Shrimp	610	39	52
Seafood Stuffed Mushrooms	390	22	18
Signature Jumbo Shrimp Cocktail	130	0	11
Whie Wine & Roasted Garlic Mussels	880	53	67
Lunch Favorites: *Without Sides or Sauces*			
Baja Shrimp Bowl	1130	70	88
Crispy Cod Sandwich	830	46	60
NashvilleHot Chicken Sandwich	1140	69	84
Sailors Platter	1170	78	71
Sesame Soy Salmon Bowl	870	41	80

continued next page...

Red Lobster® cont... (Jun '21)

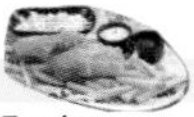
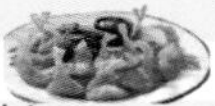
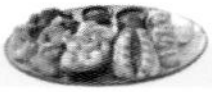
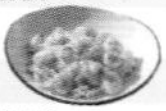
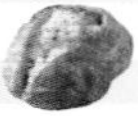
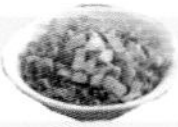
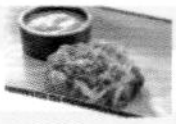
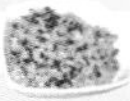
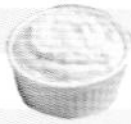
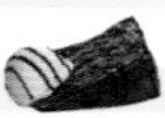

Lunch Classics: Without Sides or Sauces	C	F	Cb
Fish & Chips	1230	65	117
Hand Breaded Chicken Tenders	910	61	30
New Orleans Salmon, full	890	60	9
NY Strip Steak, 12 oz	600	36	3
Parrot Isle Jumbo Coconut Shrimp	1220	76	96
Simply Grilled Garlic Shrimp Skewers	320	10	31
Sirlion Steak, 7 oz	290	13	2
Walt's Favoriet Shrimp	550	24	60
Wild-Caught Snow Crab Legs	440	34	0
Feasts: Without Sides or Sauces			
Admirals Feast	1570	94	121
Bar Harbour Lobster Bake	1100	54	80
Lobster, Shrimp & Salmon	710	50	5
Seaside Shrimp Trio	1500	82	114
Ultimate Feast	1070	68	60
Pastas:			
Garlic Linguini Alfredo:			
with Cajun Chicken	1070	54	83
with Crab	1110	68	75
King Pao Noodles with Chicken	1330	37	182
Lobster Linguini	1120	59	79
Sides:			
Baked Potato, Plain	270	3.5	55
Broccoli	40	0	8
Caesar Side Salad	290	25	12
Cheddar Bay Biscuit	160	10	16
Green Beans	90	6	8
Garden Salad, without dressing	100	5	10
Housemade Crab Cake	370	31	16
Loaded Baked Potato	520	26	57
Mashed Potatoes	190	9	24
Quinoa Rice	160	3	30
Sea Salted Fries	510	20	74
Sauces: 100% Pure Melted Butter	300	33	0
Cocktail Sauce	45	0	11
Sour Cream for Baked Potato	25	2	0
Tartar Sauce	210	21	4
Desserts:			
Brownie Overlboard	1020	57	121
Chocolate Wave	1110	62	134
Key Lime Pie	500	21	70
Vanilla Bean Cheesecake	700	50	60

For Complete Nutritional Data ~ see CalorieKing.com

Red Robin® (Oct '21)

Nutritional Information varies between restaurants. Please refer to Red Robin's website for further information.

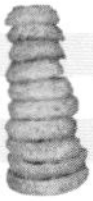
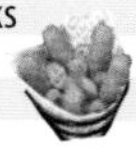
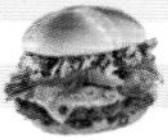
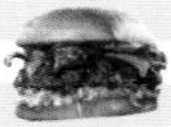
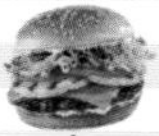
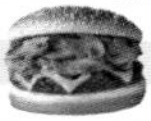
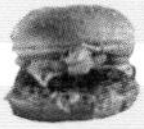
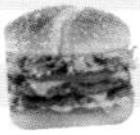
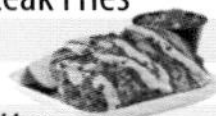

Appetizers:	C	F	Cb
Fried Pickle Nickels	740	50	62
Pretzel Bites	810	40	95
The O-Ring Shorty	910	56	94
Towering Onion Rings	1290	57	179
Jump Starters, without Dressing:			
Cheese Sticks	530	30	40
Fresh Fried Zucchini Sticks	510	43	27
Fried Jalapeono Coins	670	47	55
Fried Pickle Nickels	620	44	49
Sweet Potato Fries	410	14	68
Wings:			
Bone In Bar: with Buzz Sauce	1260	88	26
with Whisky River Sauce	1280	76	58
Boneless: with Buzz Sauce	990	55	71
with Whisky River Sauce	1010	42	103
Burgers: Without Fries or other Options			
Finest: Black & Bleu	850	53	52
Smoke & Pepper	790	40	58
The MadLove	1060	57	71
The Master Cheese	790	45	48
The Southern Charm	1140	67	81
Gourmet: Bacon Cheeseburger	990	67	47
Banzai	950	60	61
Burnin' Love	910	61	56
Guacamole Bacon	920	57	50
Impossible	760	41	68
Keep It Simple, Beef	540	24	46
Monster	1220	77	60
Red Robin Gourmet Cheeseburger	810	47	58
Royal Red Robin	1100	77	48
Sauteed 'Shroom	770	40	53
Scorpion	950	57	67
The Wedgie	540	34	18
Veggie Burger	750	44	69
Whiskey River BBQ	1140	75	73
Tavern Burgers: Big Haystack	920	58	61
Pig Out	790	50	41
The Big Pig Out	1070	70	62
Tavern Double	600	35	33
The Big Tavern	730	43	47
Veggie Vegan Burger,			
with Steamed Broccoli	260	11	34
Entrées:			
Arctic Cod Fish & Steak Fries	1520	89	135
Clucks & Fries	1330	82	104
Buffalo Style	1630	113	106
Ensenada Chkn Platter	390	14	123
One Breast Platter	210	7	8

Red Robin® cont... (Oct '21)

S'wiches & Wraps: Without Sides	C	F	Cb
BLTA Croissant	680	40	49
Caesars Chicken Wrap	820	50	59
Whiskey River BBQ Chicken Wrap	1030	58	81
Soups:			
Chicken Tortilla: Cup	200	9	19
Bowl	390	19	37
Clam Chowder:			
Cup	210	15	12
Bowl	420	31	25
Red's Chili:			
Cup	210	9	18
Bowl	430	18	36
Salads: Without Dressing Unless Indicated			
Avo-Cobb-O	510	26	25
Crispy Chicken Tender	880	50	60
Mighty Caesar, with Caesar Dressing	760	62	20
Simply Grilled Chicken	280	8	19
Southwest	890	61	42
Sides: Bottomless Steak Fries	360	16	49
Onion: Rings	280	1	61
Sauteed	25	1.5	2
Straws	200	14	16
Sauteed Mushrooms	140	7	13
Steamed Broccoli	30	0.5	6
Sweet Potato Fries	460	23	59
Yukon Chips	500	35	41
Zucchini Fries	260	17	23
Desserts: Mountain High Mudd Pie	1360	59	193
Gooey Chocolate Brownie Cake	880	33	139

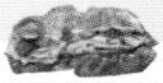
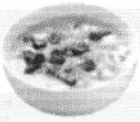
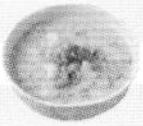
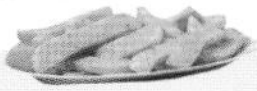
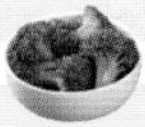

Roly Poly® (Oct '21)

Wraps: Per 6" White Tortilla Unless Indicated	C	F	Cb
Chicken: Basil Cashew Chicken	300	10	30
Chicken Caesar	310	11	30
Chicken Fajita	315	9	28
Santa Fe Chicken	305	11	28
Beef/Ham: Philly Melt	280	11	25
Ranch Roast	320	15	28
Tuna: Classic Tuna Melt	340	17	26
Popeyes Tuna on Wheat	305	10	31
Texas/Thai Hot Tuna, average	300	11	30
Turkey: Applejack	320	12	30
California	330	12	30
Veggie & Cheese:			
California Humer	305	13	32
Nutty Avocado on Wheat Tortilla	265	12	35
Salads: Without Dressing			
Alpine Chef	315	16	13
Chipotle Caesar	520	25	21
Just Veggies	95	0	19
Walnut Spinach	420	33	14

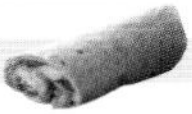
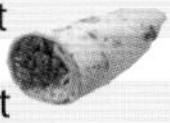
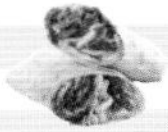
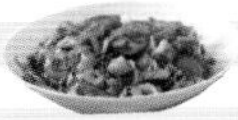

Round Table Pizza® (Oct '21)

Appetizers:	C	F	Cb
Boneless Wings, Oven Roasted:			
with BBQ Sauce (1)	100	2	13
with Buffalo Sauce (1)	90	3.5	8
Garlic Bread: 1 piece	70	3.5	9
with Cheese, 1 piece	110	6	9
Garlic Parmesan Twists, 1 twist	160	5	24
Pizzas: Per 1/12 of Large 14" Pizza			
Original Crust: Cheese	230	10	24
Gourmet Veggie	230	10	25
Guinevere's Garden Delight	220	8	26
Hawaiian	220	8	27
Italian Garlic Supreme	270	14	24
King Arthur Supreme	270	13	26
Maui Zaui Chicken	260	11	28
Montague's All Meat Marvel	290	15	24
Smokehouse Combo, Pepperoni	290	14	27
Triple Play Pepperoni	250	12	24
Pan Crust: BBQ Chicken	320	12	39
Gourmet: Chkn & Garlic	290	10	35
Veggie	280	10	35
Guinevere's Garden Delight	270	9	36
Hawaiian	280	8	37
Hearty Bacon Supreme	330	14	34
King Arthur Supreme	320	13	35
Montague's All Meat Marvel	340	16	35
Pepperoni	300	12	34
Triple Play Pepperoni	310	13	34
Skinny Crust: BBQ Chicken	230	11	22
Cheese	200	9	18
Chicken Garlic Gourmet	220	11	19
Gourmet Veggie	200	10	18
Hawaiian	190	8	20
King Arthur Supreme	230	12	19
Maui Zaui	220	10	21
Pepperoni	210	11	17
Smokehouse Combo, Chicken	240	11	20
West Coast Combo	230	6	17
Sandwiches: Chicken Club	670	27	58
Ham Club	670	30	59
Meatball	750	37	70
RT Pizza Veggie	550	21	62
Turkey: Club	650	27	59
Pesto	710	37	56
Santa Fe	730	40	57

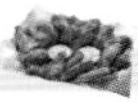
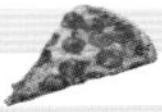
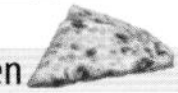
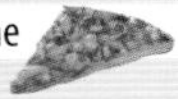
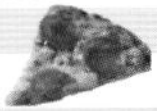
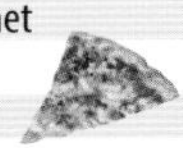
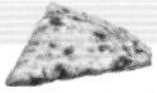
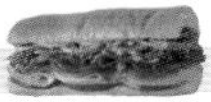
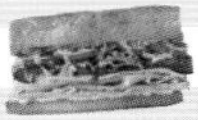

For Complete Nutritional Data ~ see CalorieKing.com

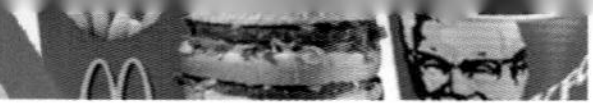

Rubio's Coastal Grill® (Oct '21)

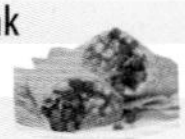
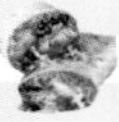

Burritos: Flour Tortilla, As Served	C	F	Cb
Beef: All Natural Steak	930	39	103
California Steak	1120	63	88
Chicken, All Natural	880	34	105
Grilled Seafood:			
Ancho Citrus Shrimp	830	34	103
Beer Battered Fish	940	55	83
Classic Grilled Shrimp	880	35	101
Grilled Wild Alaska Salmon	870	39	93
Grilled Wild Mahi Mahi	830	36	93
Shrimp & Bacon	1010	52	93

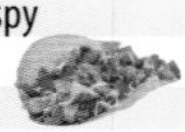
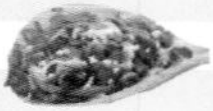

Tacos: With Corn Tortilla Unless Indicated	C	F	Cb
Carnitas: Classic	300	17	22
2 Taco Plate Carnitas	610	33	43
Grilled Gourmet	400	23	23
2 Taco Plate	800	46	46
Chicken: *Per One Taco*			
Blaised & Glazed Crispy	270	16	23
Classic All Natural	250	12	21
Grilled Gourmet	350	19	22
Natural Steak, Grilled: *Per One Taco*			
Classic	270	14	20
Gourmet	370	21	22
Street	120	5	9

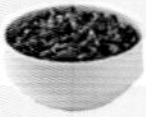
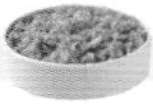

Sides:	C	F	Cb
Black Beans: Regular	100	1.5	15
Large	280	2.5	46
Cauli Rice: Regular	40	2.5	3
Large	120	8	10
Mexican Rice: Reg.	100	1.5	20
Large	270	4	53
No Fried Pinto Beans: Regular	110	1	17
Large	300	2	51
Quinoa & Brown Rice: Regular	80	1	14
Large	210	2.5	39
Tortilla Chips: Regular	210	2.5	43
Large	460	5	96
Salsas, average all varieties	10	0	3

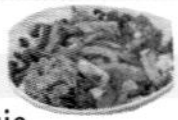
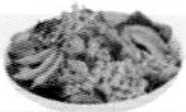

Salad & Bowls: Entrée Size, Includes Dressing	C	F	Cb
Bowls: Cilantro Lime Quinoa	570	27	67
Mexican Street Corn	730	34	93
Salads:			
Balsamic & Grilled Veggie	380	33	22
Keto, with Salmon	610	45	20
Keto, with Steak	610	45	20
Chopped Salad	380	30	19
Keto, with Salmon	500	36	14
Keto, with Steak	500	36	14
Mango Avocado	460	33	39

Ruby Tuesday® (Oct '21)

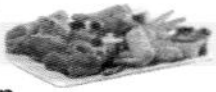

Shareables: As Served	C	F	Cb
Cheddar Cheese Queso & Dip	1290	85	96
Chicken quesadillas	1170	77	43
Classic Sampler	1500	72	152
Spicy Bangin' Shrimp	950	79	41
Spinach Artichoke Dip	1060	64	100

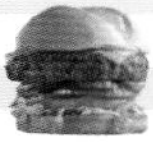

Burgers: Without Fries	C	F	Cb
Bacon Cheeseburger	820	49	37
Classic	670	37	37
Classic Cheeseburger	720	41	38
Hickory Bourbon Bacon	970	56	52
Smokehouse	980	54	63
Turkey	650	37	37

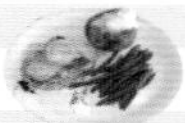

Chicken: Without Sides or Breadstick	C	F	Cb
Asiago Bacon	450	26	11
Fresco	320	19	3
Hickory Bourbon	250	5	18
Smokey Mountain	480	24	17

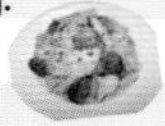

Pasta: As Served	C	F	Cb
Blackened Shrimp & Ssg.	1100	60	94
Chicken & Broccoli	1510	98	103
Parmesan Shrimp	1120	59	101

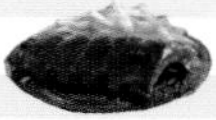
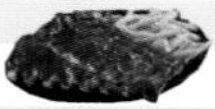
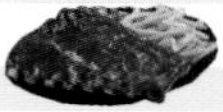

Ribs & Combos: Without Sides or Breadstick	C	F	Cb
Classic BBQ Ribs:			
Half Rack	470	24	21
Full Rack	940	47	42
Hickory Bourbon:			
Half Rack	570	24	42
Full Rack	1140	47	84
Nashville Hot:			
Half Rack	580	42	9
Full Rack	1170	84	17
Texas Dusted Ribs: Half Rack	590	35	24
Full Rack	1100	69	30

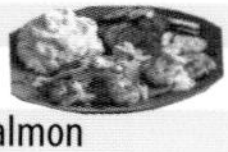

Seafood: Without Sides or Breadstick	C	F	Cb
Blackened Tilapia	200	7	2
Grilled Salmon	330	22	0
Hickory Bourbon Salmon	410	22	18
New Orleans Seafood	320	14	6

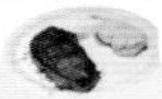

Steak: Without Sides Or Breadstick	C	F	Cb
Asiago Sirloin, 6 oz, w/ Gr. Shrimp	470	30	7
Hickory B'rbon Bacon Sirloin, 6 oz	290	10	14
Ribeye, 12 oz	730	56	0
Top Sirloin, 6 oz	290	17	2

Ruby Tuesday® cont... (Oct '21)

Soup:	C	F	Cb
Broccoli Cheese	290	20	20
Chicken Corn Chowder	310	19	22
Roasted Tomato	380	22	36
Sandwiches: *On Brioche Bun Without French Fries*			
Crispy Chicken: Classic	710	32	68
with Pimento	1130	72	73
Spicy	1060	69	73
with Pimentos	1480	109	78
Grilled Chicken	540	22	36
Sliders:			
Bacon Cheeseburger: with Fries	830	45	72
with Tatet Tots	780	43	66
Classic Cheeseburger: with Fries	790	42	72
with Tater Tots	740	40	66
Sides:			
Baked Potato			
Buttered Corn	230	14	26
Cauliflower Au Gratin	400	32	14
French Fries	420	21	53
Grilled Zucchini	20	0.5	3
Loaded: Baked Potato	600	31	48
Tater Tots			
Mac'N Cheese	480	27	43
Mashed Potatoes	220	11	27
Onion Rings	340	19	37
Rice Pilaf	190	3	33
Roasted Baby Bellas	100	6	6
Steamed Broccoli	60	3.5	5
Sweet Potato Fries	370	20	46
Tater Tots	365	16	45
White Rice	190	1	40
Salads: *With Dressing*			
Caesar: Crispy Chkn	890	59	50
Grilled Chicken	780	50	37
Hickory Bourbon: Crispy Chicken	990	64	41
Grilled Chicken	760	46	27
Desserts: *As Served*			
Apple Crumble Skillet	620	30	79
Cake: Chocolate Tall	1310	63	172
Chocolate Lava	620	33	77
Pineapple Upside Down	500	19	74
Chocolate Chip Cookie Skillet	1350	71	174
New York Cheesecake	780	74	96

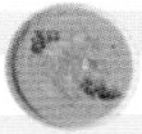
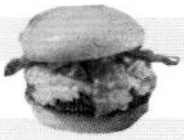
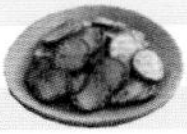
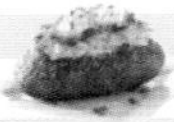
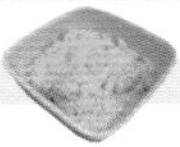
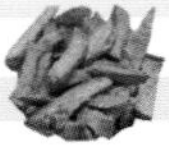
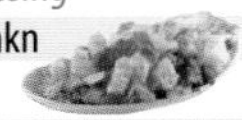
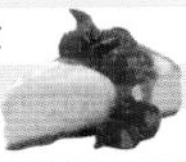

For Complete Menu ~ see CalorieKing.com

Runza® (Oct '21)

Burgers:	C	F	Cb
¼ Lb: BBQ Bacon & Swiss	530	32	26
Bacon Cheeseburger	490	28	23
Cheeseburger	430	22	23
French Onion	490	29	26
Hamburger	350	18	21
Spicy Jack	570	38	23
Swiss Cheese Mushroom	480	29	24
Chicken Sandwiches:			
BBQ Grilled	400	11	40
Buffalo Grilled	360	11	37
Spicy Jack Grilled	530	28	26
Wraps: Buffalo Jr.	330	17	32
Ranch Jr.	330	17	31
Chicken Strips, 2 pieces	220	12	14
Runza Sandwiches: Original	530	20	67
Cheese Runza	590	25	69
Original Vegetarian	530	9	94
Spicy Jack Runza	750	41	69
SW Black Bean Vegetarian	470	12	76
Swiss Cheese Mushroom Runza	620	28	68
Sides: Chili	290	11	26
French Fries: Small	210	9	28
Medium	300	13	40
Large	440	19	59
French Onion Dip	100	7	6
Frings, Medium	320	17	39
Onion Rings: Medium	320	19	35
Large	550	31	58
Salads: *Without Dressing*			
Side	20	0	4
Southwest Chicken Salad, w/ Salsa	360	18	32
Sweet Berry Chicken	400	20	20
Dressings: Honey Mustard	200	18	9
SW Ranch	220	24	4
Soups: *Per Bowl*			
Boston Clam Chowder	280	15	29
Broccoli Cheese	240	16	20
Chicken Tortilla	150	6	16
Potato Bacon	260	14	30
Kids: *Without Beverage*			
Chicken Strip Meal w/ Small Fries	430	21	42
Junior: Cheeseburger, plain	260	13	18
Hamburger, plain	200	9	16
Swiss Cheese Mushroom Burger	300	17	17
Desserts:			
Chocolate Chip Cookie	370	18	53
Choc./Vanilla Ice Crm Cones	210	6	32
Shake, Cappuccino, regular	490	12	82
Sundaes: Caramel; Chocolate	300	7	51
Turtle	360	13	53

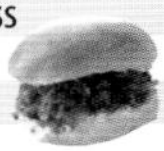
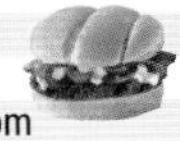
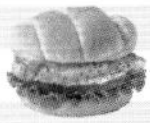
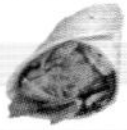
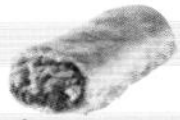
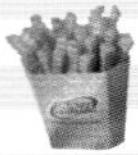
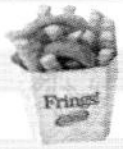

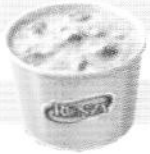
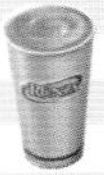

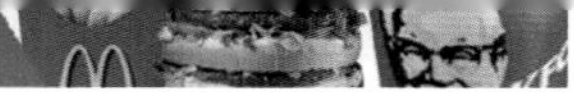

7-Eleven® (Sept '18)

	C	F	Cb
Breakfast Sandwiches: *Please visit Stores for latest menu items and nutritional information*			
Biscuits:			
Sausage, 3.3 oz	330	22	28
Spicy Chicken, 4.5 oz	270	14	30
Croissants:			
Sausage, Egg & Cheese, 4.7 oz	450	32	23
English Muffin:			
Egg, Bacon & Chse, 4.5 oz	300	14	28
Egg, Cheese & Sausage, 5 oz	390	25	24
Salads: *Per Container*			
Balsamic Garden Salad, with Chicken, 6.5 oz	170	9	18
BLT, 8 oz	270	18	12
Caprese Salad, 4.5 oz	150	11	7
Chicken Caesar, 7.5 oz	390	28	17
Chicken Caesar Pasta Salad, 9 oz	540	24	61
Kale & Quinoa Salad, 6 oz	300	18	30
Mediterranean Pasta Salad, 8.5 oz	490	29	49
Side, 5 oz	30	0	7
Sandwiches/Melts:			
Chicken, Bacon Ranch Melt, 7.4 oz	560	22	56
Chicken Salad Sandwich, 6.6 oz	470	21	49
Double Cheeseburger, with American Cheese, 9.6 oz	800	54	35
Egg Salad Sandwich, 6.8 oz	480	24	50
Go!Smart Turkey Sandwich	300	2.5	48
Grilled Chicken Sandwich, w/ Honey Mustard BBQ Sauce, 6 oz	340	10	39
Italian Melt, 7.8 oz	610	39	38
Southwest Turkey Sandwich, 8 oz	560	28	48
Steak & Cheese Melt, 7.8 oz	680	35	57
Sides:			
Hash Brown (1), 2 oz	100	5	12
Potato Wedges (6), 0.7 oz	240	4.5	27
Taquitos,			
Chicken & Monterey Jack, (2), 5.3 oz	330	12	44
Drinks: Cappuccino, 8 fl.oz	180	4	36
Caramel Macchiato, 8 fl.oz	190	5	34
Cuban Coffee, with milk, 8 fl.oz	200	7	34
French Vanilla Cappuccino, 8 fl.oz	190	6	34
Skinny, 8 fl.oz	140	4.5	30
Hot Chocolate, 8 fl.oz	170	2.5	37
Peppermint Mocha, 8 fl.oz	180	4	36
Pumpkin Spice Late, 8 fl.oz	190	6	35
Slurpees, average all flavors:			
12 oz cup	95	0	26
22 oz cup	175	0	44
28 oz cup	220	0	56
Sugar Free, 12 oz cup	30	0	9

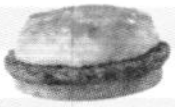
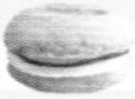
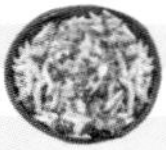
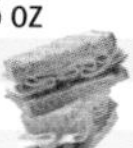
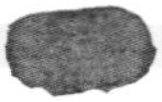
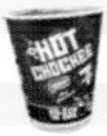

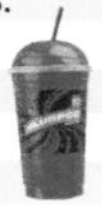

Saladworks® (Oct '21)

	C	F	Cb
Paninis:			
Buffalo Chicken	870	36	85
Caprese	940	47	94
Chicken Parmesan	870	32	93
Turkey Melt	1020	49	90
Sandwiches: *With Menu Set Ingredients*			
Avocado BLT on Rustic White Bread	680	32	76
Turkey Bacon 'n Ranch, on Wheatberry Bread	760	38	70
Wraps: *With Flour Wrap & Menu Set Ingredients*			
Asian Crspy Chkn w/ Swt Sesame Drsng	750	22	117
Avocado Cobb, w/ T. Island Dressing	900	49	68
Bentley with Green Goddess Drssng	810	41	62
Buffalo Bleu w/ Blue Cheese Drssng	750	37	65
Farmers Market w/ Bals. Vinaigrette	800	38	80
Grilled Chicken Caesar w/ Caesar Dr.	610	20	81
Rstd Turkey with Ranch	800	33	90
Smokey BBQ Crispy Chkn with Ranch	830	40	97
Sophie's Salad with Lt. Vinaigrette	780	26	105
Salads: *W/out Dressing or Bread*			
Asian Crispy Chicken	350	9	57
Avocado Cobb	450	28	15
Bently	350	18	11
Buffalo Bleu	290	13	16
Classic Greek	250	13	12
Grilled Chicken: Caesar	390	19	28
Mediterranean	230	10	16
Farmers Market	350	16	28
Roasted Turkey Club	340	9	40
Smokey BBQ Crispy Chicken	370	16	47
Sophie's	430	18	48
Soups: *Per Medium Serve, without Bread Roll*			
Baked Potato	340	24	28
Broccoli Cheddar	280	19	18
Chicken Noodle	180	5	18
Chicken Poblano	350	21	26
Chicken Tortilla	270	14	19
Lasagna w/ Turkey Ssg	230	11	21
Lobster Bisque	470	39	21
New England Clam Chowder	370	27	22

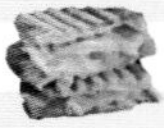
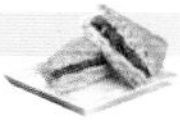
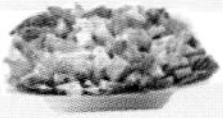
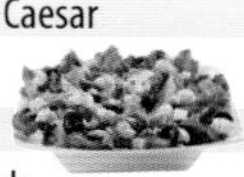
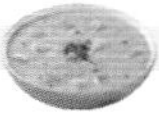
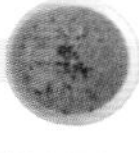

Sandella's® (Oct '21)

Grilled Flatbread:	C	F	Cb
BBQ Cheese	430	9	67
Bacon & Cheddar	630	34	54
Chicken Fajita	500	18	52
Chicken Parmesan	560	20	55
El Paso	710	19	97
Ham & Cheddar	570	25	51
Meatball	630	29	56
Olympian	480	26	53
Pesto & Peppers	530	27	52
Philly Style	450	10	54
Spinach & Artichoke	610	33	54
Thai Chicken	630	24	66
Tomato Bacon	580	26	58
***Paninis:** With Standard Toppings*			
Americana	580	25	54
Arizona Chicken	660	23	78
BBQ Chicken	490	2	92
Beef Fajita	630	27	58
Bistro Ham & Brie	560	19	70
Brazilian Beef, without cheese	500	6	86
Genoa	730	37	53
Napoli Chicken	440	17	49
Pastrami Melt	670	33	55
Philly Cheese	590	25	55
Spinach & Bacon	610	29	65
Toasted Caprese	380	14	50
***Quesadillas:** With Standard Toppings*			
Barbecue	570	18	66
Beef Fajita	570	22	55
Buffalo Chicken	510	20	49
Thai Veggie	570	27	60
***Salads:** With ½ Flatbread, without Dressing*			
Apple Walnut	370	13	60
Napa Valley	770	60	54
Panzanella	190	3	36
Siesta	310	15	44
Thai Chicken	330	13	35
***Rice Bowls:** Includes Flatbread & Standard Toppings*			
Asian Chicken & Broccoli	680	3	138
Mesquite BBQ	930	21	140
Southwest Veggie	810	20	126
Thai Peanut Saute	680	16	116
***Wraps:** With Standard Toppings*			
California Turkey	410	10	55
Greek Salad	370	13	55
Nut & Honey	800	32	116
Seven Layer	570	23	66
Swiss Salad	500	20	62
Texas Beef	420	10	58
The Russian	400	7	60
Veggie & Cheese	450	19	52

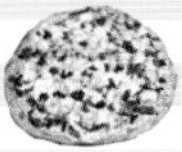
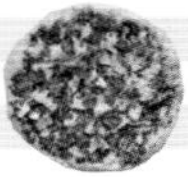
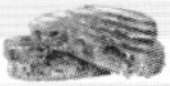
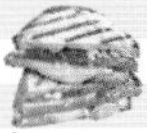
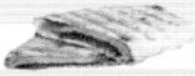
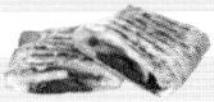
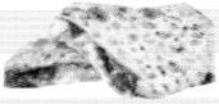
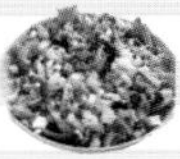
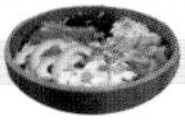
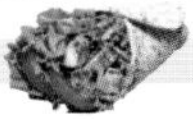

Sarku Japan® (Oct '21)

Bento Box:	C	F	Cb
Fried Rice: Beef	830	32	98
Chicken	820	35	95
Shrimp	750	27	96
D'Lite Meals, Vegetables:			
with Fried Rice	430	10	79
with Noodles	640	14	109
with Steamed Rice	410	6	83
***Teriyaki Meals:** With Steamed Rice*			
Beef	580	16	80
Beef & Shrimp	690	21	85
Chicken	640	24	79
Chicken & Shrimp	750	29	85
Shrimp	530	12	80
Sushi Rolls: California	330	8	57
Chicken Teriyaki	360	11	53
Dancing Eel	430	13	61
Green Dragon	650	35	71
Philadelphia	430	18	49
Rainbow	360	7	51
Rock & Roll	550	21	66
Salmon	220	5	33
Tuna	190	0	33
Sauce, Teriyaki, 1.5 oz	45	0	9
Sides: Chicken Egg Roll	160	6	21
Dumplings (6)	260	12	29
Edamame	170	7	11
Miso Soup	50	2	6
Seaweed Salad	70	2	13
Shrimp Tempura (3)	390	30	23
Vegetable Spring Roll	190	9	15

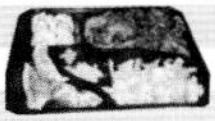
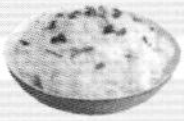
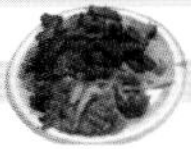
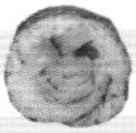
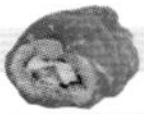
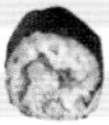
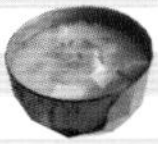

Schlotzsky's® (Oct '21)

***Sandwiches:** Per Medium*	C	F	Cb
Angus Beef & Cheese	780	30	81
Beef Bacon Smokecheesy	810	43	77
Chicken Bacon Smokecheesy	860	31	80
Corned Beef Reuben	700	26	77
Deluxe Original	980	47	81
Fiesta Chicken	810	31	78
French Dip	670	22	59
Fresh Veggie	500	14	74
Ham & Cheese, Original	730	25	81
Pastrami Stacker	740	31	81
Smoked Turkey Breast	500	6	80
The Original	780	34	78
The Tuscan	850	41	79
Turkey Bacon Club	770	30	81
Turkey Original	820	33	81

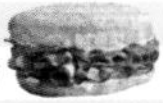
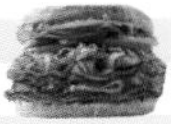
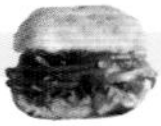
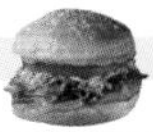

continued next page...

Schlotzsky's® cont... (Oct '21)

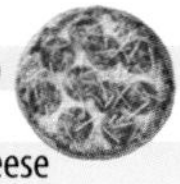
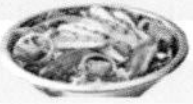
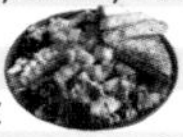
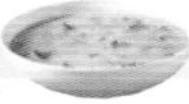
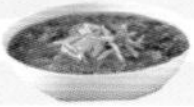
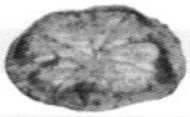
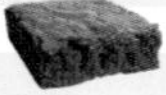
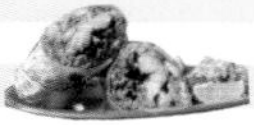
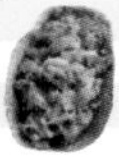

	C	F	Cb
Pizzas: *Per 10" Pizza*			
BBQ Chicken & Jalapeno	970	22	148
Double Cheese	990	34	125
Pepperoni & Double Cheese	1170	48	127
Fresh Veggie	950	30	128
Salad Wraps: *With Wheat Tortilla, without Dressing*			
Chicken Caesar	350	10	37
Southwest Chicken	340	11	34
The Orchard	440	13	56
Turkey Avocado Cobb	370	13	41
Salads: *Large, without Dressing*			
Chicken Caesar	410	14	29
Southwest Chicken	410	15	24
The Orchard	600	19	69
Turkey Avocado Cobb	460	18	36
Dressing: Blue Cheese; Caesar, 3 oz	460	48	4
Italian, 3 oz	410	43	3
Ranch, 3 oz	340	34	4
Thousand Island, 3 oz	360	36	16
Soup: *Per 10 oz Bowl*			
Broccoli Cheese	185	12	14
Chicken & Wild Rice	280	14	25
Chicken & Drumpling	145	4.5	15
Loaded Baked Potato	385	31	29
Timberline Chili	380	21	27
Tomato Basil	320	26	21
Chips:			
Baked: Lays Regular	140	4	26
Other varieties, average	230	14	24
Kidz Meals: *Without Cookie or Drink*			
Cheese Pizza	480	16	63
Ham & Cheese S'wich	410	15	48
Pepperoni Pizza	570	23	63
Turkey & Cheese Swwich	410	15	49
Desserts:			
Brownie (1)	500	28	62
Cookies: Chocolate Chunk (1)	370	18	52
Sugar (1)	390	20	48
Breakfast: *Per Whole Burrito/Sandwich*			
Burritos: Bacon	460	22	41
Ham	490	21	44
Sausage	570	31	41
Veggie	430	19	44
Sandwiches: Bacon; Veggie	500	21	51
Ham	530	22	50
Sausage	650	32	49
Tacos: Bacon; Ham, average	250	14	18
Sausage	290	17	18
Veggie	220	10	21
Sides:			
Hash Brown, 1 piece	60	5	8
Mixed Fruit, 1 scoop	20	0	6

Second Cup® ~ *see CalorieKing.com*

Shake Shack® (Oct '21)

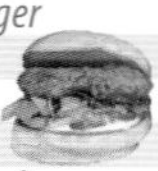
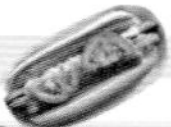
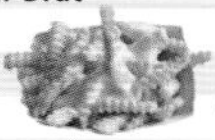
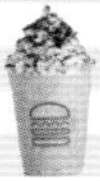

	C	F	Cb
Burgers: *Per Single Burger*			
Bacon Cheeseburger	500	29	25
Cheeseburger	440	24	25
Crackle Shack	580	37	25
Green Chile Cheddar Shack	470	26	28
Hamburger	370	18	24
Lockhart Link	780	56	27
Shackburger	500	30	26
Shack Stack	770	45	50
SmokeShack	610	39	28
Veggie Shack: Regular	530	27	56
Vegan Style	390	22	50
Chicken: Bites (6)	300	19	15
Chick'N Shack	550	31	34
Flat-Top Dogs:			
Garden Dog	180	3	27
Hot Dog	350	22	25
Shackmeister Cheddar Brat	690	51	33
Fries: Bacon Cheese	840	52	65
Cheese	710	44	64
Double Down	1910	49	164
Regular	470	22	63
Floats, Creamsicle; Purple Cow, av.	450	15	77
Shakes: *Without Whipped Cream*			
Chocolate	750	45	76
Cookies & Cream	850	44	98
Vanilla	680	36	72
Add On, Whipped Cream	70	5	5
Breakfast:			
Single Sandwiches: Bacon	400	23	25
Egg & Cheese	530	32	28
Sausage	340	19	25

Shakey's® (Oct '21)

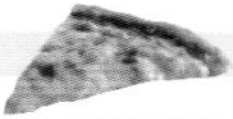

	C	F	Cb
Pizzas: *Per Slice, 1/10 Medium Size 12" Pizza*			
Big Island: Pan Crust	210	6	30
Thin Crust	160	6	19
California Pizzarito: Pan Crust	265	12	30
Thin Crust	215	11	19
Cheese: Pan Crust	190	5	30
Thin Crust	135	5	17
Firehouse: Pan Crust	280	13	30
Thin Crust	230	12	20
Garden Veggie: Pan Crust	205	6	30
Thin Crust	150	6	19
Rustic Garlic Chicken: Pan Crust	215	6	30
Thin Crust	160	6	18
Shakey's Special: Pan Crust	255	11	30
Thin Crust	200	10	18
Texas BBQ Chicken: Pan Crust	220	6	32
Thin Crust	165	5	20
Ultimate Meat: Pan Crust	310	15	30
Thin Crust	260	14	20

Shakey's® cont... (Oct '21)

Golden Fried Chicken: Per Piece	C	F	Cb
Breast	360	11	16
Leg	175	10	6
Thigh	350	24	9
Wing	130	9	4
Rice: Per ½ Cup			
Mexican Fiesta	100	0	22
Pilaf	120	3	22
Sides & Extras: Enchilada	180	2	37
Garlic Bread, 1 piece	180	4	30
Macaroni & Cheese, 1 cup	350	17	33
Mashed Potatoes, ½ cup	65	1	13
Mojo Potatoes, 5 pieces	215	11	25
Penne Rigate	200	1	42
Pepperoni Pizza Twists	215	8	29

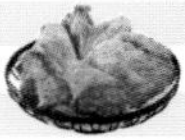
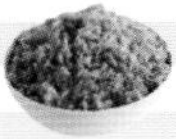
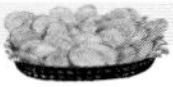

Shari's® (Oct '21)

Breakfast: As Served	C	F	Cb
Bacon & Eggs without extras	290	22	1
Buttermilk Pancakes	800	27	123
Country Sausage Benedict	1470	102	90
Double Smoked Sausage & Egg	450	32	6
French Toast, Traditional	960	62	82
Meat Lover's Skillet	1100	86	38
Sausage & Eggs Only	630	57	1
Shari's Sampler	1610	105	116
Ultimate Country Fried Steak	1060	72	67
Waffle	340	14	48
Lunch: Without Side Choices			
Chicken Strips	340	18	23
Salads: *Entrée Size, with Dressing*			
Caesar	460	40	15
Northwest Steak	890	50	65
Rustic Tuscan Chicken	510	32	21
Sandwiches: *Per Whole Sandwich*			
BLT on Texas Toast	540	26	51
Cajun Chicken Avocado Club	1360	74	115
Cuban on Ciabatta Roll	680	30	60
Grilled Ham & Four Cheese Melt, on Sourdough	1140	68	78
Hot Turkey on Whole Wheat	1040	31	129
Prime Rib Dip on French Roll	680	33	63
Traditional Club	1310	72	114
Dinner: With Menu Set Sides			
Beer Battered Fish & Chips	1600	119	104
Chopped Steak	930	50	50
Country Fried Steak	1010	63	83
Grilled Lemon Chicken	450	17	17
Slow Roasted Turkey	980	50	109
Wild Alaskan Salmon, grilled	470	28	19

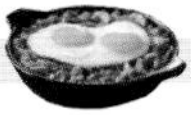
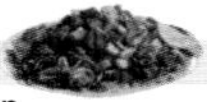
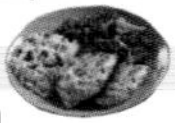

Shari's® cont... (Oct '21)

Sides, Add-Ons:	C	F	Cb
Baked Potato: Plain	210	5	37
with Sour Cream & Butter	330	18	38
Broccoli	130	11	7
Coleslaw	140	10	11
French Fries	490	32	48
Loaded Baked Potato	330	15	38
Loaded Mashed Potatoes	410	21	42
Rice Pilaf	90	5	10
Shrimp Skewer	90	1	1
Stuffed Hash Browns	420	28	32
Tater Tots	370	26	33
Desserts:			
Pies:			
Banana Cream Dream	450	26	48
Chocolate Cream Supreme	510	30	54
Creamy Caramel Pecan Crunch	730	49	67
Peanut Butter Chocolate Silk	620	45	51
Tropical Coconut Cream	580	37	63

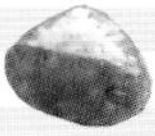
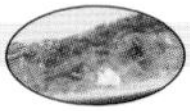
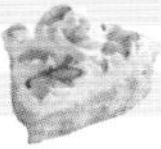

Sheetz® (Oct '21)

Breakfast Sandwiches:	C	F	Cb
Dreamy Bacon Croissant	400	25	28
Twisted BLT	710	42	53
Walker Breakfast Ranger	550	23	58
Burgerz: Big Mozz	670	33	57
Boss Bacon	790	56	35
Cowboy	730	39	56
Twisted Swiss	760	45	50
Hot Dogs: With Standard Hot Dog			
BLT	450	28	33
Junkyard	340	16	38
Philly	360	19	39
Shmokehouse	390	20	40
Mac & Cheese Platter: Boom Chicka	650	39	43
Meatball	750	49	38
Morning	650	43	43
Sandwichez:			
Deli: Boom Boom BLT	820	46	52
Ciabatta Bing	620	34	54
Garden of Eatin	470	18	59
Grilled Chicken Breast: Big Mozz	600	19	60
Carolina Slaw	500	17	47
Twisted Brunch	800	42	54
Shwingz: with BBQ Sauce (6)	540	28	39
with Boom Boom Sauce	700	55	20
with Garlic Parmesan Sauce	660	50	18
with Spicy Asian Sauce	540	30	37

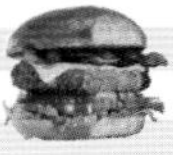
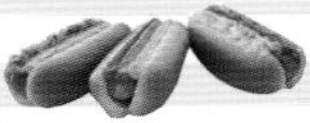
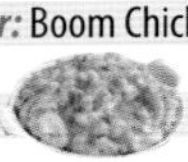
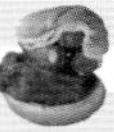

continued next page...

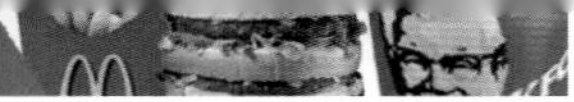

Sheetz® cont... (Oct '21)

Subz: Per Half	C	F	Cb
Big Philly Sub, on Pretzel Sub	590	19	71
Cali Turkey on Flatbread	780	43	55
Southwest Veggie, on White Roll	470	20	61
Sidez:			
Coleslaw	250	11	35
Crispy Chicken Stripz, w/out sauce:			
3 pieces	330	11	39
5 pieces	550	18	65
Fryz, without sauce, 1 cup	390	13	64
Hard Cooked Egg, 1.5 oz	70	4.5	0
Jalapeno Poppers, without Sauce	330	18	35
Loaded Fryz, without toppings	600	20	97
Mac & Cheese, without toppings	320	18	28
Onion Rings, without sauce, 1 cup	470	27	52
Popcorn Chicken, without Sauce:			
Regular	300	14	28
Large	610	28	55
***Beverages:** With 2% Milk & Chocolate Sauce*			
Caramel Hot Chocolate	700	23	109
Hot Chocolate	730	22	118

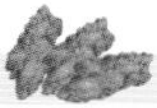
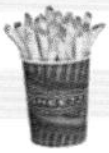
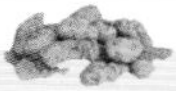

Sizzler® (Oct '21)

Menus May Vary. Please Check Your Local Outlet For Menu Choices And Further Nutritional Information.

Burgers & Sandwiches:	C	F	Cb
Classic ⅓ lb Burger	830	57	44
Mega Bacon Burger	940	61	49
Smokey Bacon Burger	950	5	47
***Entrees:** Without Sides, Condiments, Dipping Sauce or Optional Accompaniments*			
Chicken: *Small Plate*			
Italian Herb Chicken	230	6	1
Malibu Chicken	680	60	14
Combo Nation:			
Classic Steak Trio	1270	89	48
Steak & Jumbo Crispy Shrimp (8)	720	32	47
Steak & Lobster	720	51	2
Steak & Malibu Chicken	920	73	14
Ribs:			
BBQ: 6 bones	1870	145	32
3 Bones & BBQ Chicken, 7 oz	1170	70	34

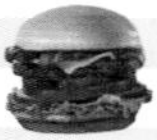
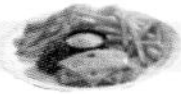
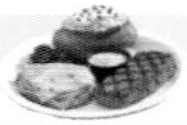
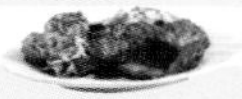

Sizzler® cont... (Oct '21)

Entrees (Cont):	C	F	Cb
Seafood: Grilled Salmon, 6 oz	370	23	3
Cilantro Lime Barramundi	470	17	37
Jumbo Shrimp Skewers (2)	440	15	29
Steaks:			
New York Strip, 12 oz	830	61	2
Ribeye, 14 oz	1100	88	3
Tri-Tip Sirloin, 8 oz	340	16	0.5
Steak Toppings: Grilled Onions	80	6	7
Sauteed Button Mushrooms	180	17	5
Sides: Cheese Toast	290	19	22
Cilantro Lime Rice	150	0	31
Garlic Mashed Potatoes	200	3.5	39
Rice Pilaf	170	3.5	31
Salted Baked Potato	510	30	55
Loaded	760	57	55
Street Fries	500	31	52
Vegetable Medley	80	4.5	8
Yeast Roll	190	7	29

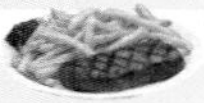
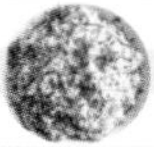
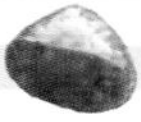

Skyline Chili® (Oct '21)

Burritos:	C	F	Cb
Chili Deluxe	610	33	38
Original	610	31	54
Coneys/Sandwiches:			
Coneys: Cheese, w/ onions & mstrd	350	23	25
Coney, plain	220	13	22
Sandwiches: Chili Cheese, with onions & mustard	290	17	24
Chili, with onions & mustard	180	8	23
Ways:			
Chili Spaghetti with Onion:			
Small	200	10	26
Regular	410	19	52
Large	540	25	70
Bowls: Black Beans & Rice	400	14	48
Chili	200	12	0
Loaded Chili	480	28	20
Steamed Potatoes:			
3-Way Potato	620	26	65
Cheddar Potato	630	33	65
Sour Cream Potato	460	19	65
***Salads:** Without Dressing*			
Buffalo Chicken	220	11	12
Greek	210	12	17
Fries: Chili Cheese	840	53	61
Regular Fries	430	24	51

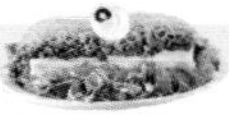
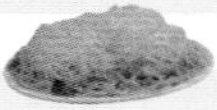
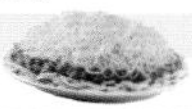
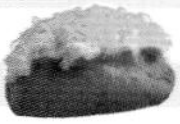
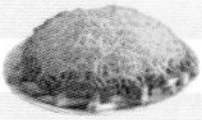

Smoothie King® (Jun '21)

Fruit Smoothies: Per 20 oz, with Standard Menu Components	C	F	Cb
Be Well Blends: *Without Turbinado*			
Blueberry Heaven	270	1	57
Vegan:			
Dark Chocolate Banana	350	1.5	80
Pineapple Spinach	360	5	75
Get Fit Blends:			
High Intensity: Chocolate Cinnamon	410	14	45
Veggie Mango	390	13	43
Keto Champ: Berry	440	30	17
Chocolate with Stevia	430	30	16
Coffee	410	30	12
Original High Protein:			
Banana	340	12	36
Chocolate	400	12	45
Pineapple	320	12	30
Peanut Power Plus: With Turbinado			
Chocolate	690	22	111
Strawberry	680	22	109
The Activator: Chocolate	210	2.5	21
Blueberry Strawberry	260	0	37
Coffee	240	2.5	26
Pineapple	290	0	48
Strawberry Banana	180	0	21
The Hulk: With Turbinado			
Chocolate	750	30	112
Strawberry	890	32	147
Stay Slim Blends:			
Metabolism Boost:			
Banana Passionfruit	250	2	44
Mango Ginger	270	2	48
Slim-N-Trim: With Stevia			
Chocolate	220	2	37
Strawberry	160	2	26
Vanilla	180	2	33
The Shredder:Strawberry	310	1	44
Vanilla	230	2	15
Take A Break Blends: *With Turbinado*			
Angel Food	340	0	84
Banana Boat	470	5	99
Caribbean Way	390	0	98
Coffe D-Lite: Mocha	360	5	61
Vanilla	270	5	43
Passion Passport	410	0	102
Pineapple Surf	420	1	98

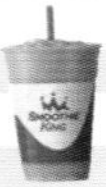
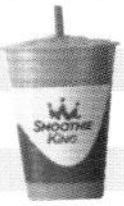
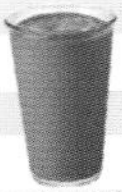
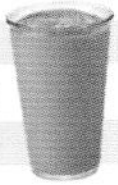
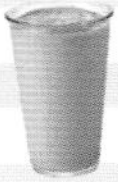
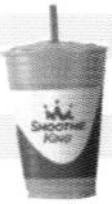

Snappy Tomato® (Oct '21)

Snappetizers:	C	F	Cb
Bone In Wings (6)	460	34	4
Flatbread, medium, ⅙ flatbread	270	12	33
Wedge Fries, plain	220	10	28
Hoagies: Chicken Ranch	910	44	75
Grilled Chicken	640	15	70
Ham & Cheese	570	15	71
Italian Combo	650	23	69
Steak & Cheese	760	35	73
Veggie Melt	490	11	74
Pasta, Plain Spaghetti/Rigatoni, av.	350	1.5	70
Toppings: Bacon	120	8	1
Beef; Black or Green Olives, av.	50	3.5	2
Cheese	90	7	1
Chicken	120	2.5	1
Pepperoni	140	10	0
Peppers	5	0	1
Sausage	80	6	1
Tomatoes	5	0	1
Sauce: Ranch	570	60	8
Snappy	80	2	8
Salads: Crispy Chkn, w/o dressing	280	9	24
Garden, without dressing	90	4.5	11
Grilled Chicken, w/out dressing	160	2.5	10
Dessert: Cinnabread, med., ⅙ slice	350	13	57
Raspberry Cinnabread, ⅙ slice	370	13	62

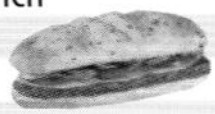
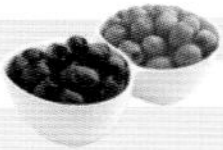

Sonic Drive-In® (Oct '21)

Burgers:	C	F	Cb
Bacon Cheeseburger, with Mayo	860	54	54
Double	1140	77	52
Cheeseburger w/ Mayo & Ketchup	720	42	52
Double	1070	71	54
Jalap. Dble Chseburger, w/ Mstrd	1030	65	55
Jr. Burger	340	17	32
Veggie Burger w/ Mayo & Ketchup	500	17	70
Chicken:			
Sandwiches: Classic Crispy Chicken	550	30	48
Classic Grilled Chkn	470	22	39
Boneless Wings: *6 Pieces*			
Asian Sweet Chili	470	24	32
Honey BBQ	470	24	33
Buffalo	440	28	17
Jumbo Popcorn: Small	330	19	24
Medium	490	28	36
Large	750	43	55
Tenders: Crispy, 3 pieces	260	12	16
5 pieces	430	20	27
Coneys: Chili Cheese	470	29	34
Footlong Quarter Pound	790	49	55

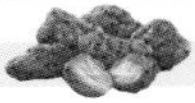
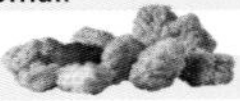
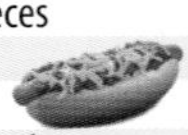

continued next page....

Sonic Drive-In® cont... (Oct '21)

6" Hot Dogs:

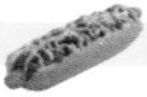

	C	F	Cb
All American Dog	410	21	41
Cheesy Bacon Pretzel	430	29	27
Chicago Dog; New Yoork, average	400	22	38

Breakfast:

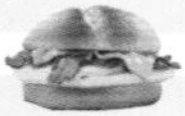

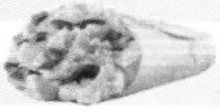

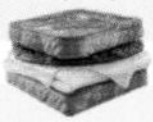

	C	F	Cb
Bagel Sandwich:			
Bacon	660	29	68
Sausage	770	41	68
Biscuit Sandwich: Bacon	570	30	40
Ham	510	32	53
Brioche Sandwich: Bacon	530	30	38
Ham	470	22	40
Burrito: Bacon	470	25	35
Ham	440	20	38
Supersonic	610	35	49
Cinnasnacks, w/out Frosting (3)	380	22	38
Croissonic: Bacon	560	37	31
Ham	490	29	33
French Toast Sticks, w/o syrup (4)	480	25	54
Toaster: Ham	540	22	54
Sausage	720	43	52

Sides: Medium

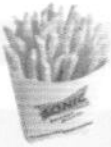

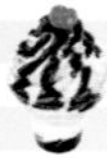

	C	F	Cb
Chedd 'R' Peppers (6)	490	48	56
Fries	290	13	38
with Cheese	380	22	39
with Chili & Cheese	450	26	42
Onion rings	580	29	74
Ice Cream Sundaes: Caramel	490	22	58
Chocolate; Strawb, av.	435	22	51
Hot Fudge	520	26	65
Add Ons: Peanuts	40	3.5	2
Whipped Topping	70	5	5

Classic Shakes: Per Medium

	C	F	Cb
Caramel	830	41	97
Chocolate	810	43	95
Fresh Banana	850	41	108
Hot Fudge	940	48	113
Peanut Butter	940	59	87
Strawberry	790	41	92
Vanilla	820	45	89

Master Shakes: Per Medium

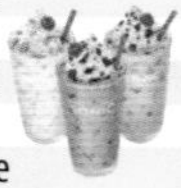

	C	F	Cb
Cheesecake	840	43	101
Oreo Cheesecake	1030	51	131
Oreo Chocolate	1000	51	125
Oreo Peanut Butter	1130	66	116
Strawberry Cheesecake	890	43	112

Sonic Blast: Per Medium

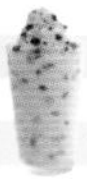

	C	F	Cb
Butterfingers Pieces	980	48	118
Choc. Chip Cookie Dough	920	45	118
M&M's Minis Choc. Candy	1060	54	127
Oreo Pieces	860	44	103
Reese's Peanut Butter Cups	990	55	110
Snickers Bars	890	46	103

Sonic Drive-In® cont... (Oct '21)

All Natural Lemonade:

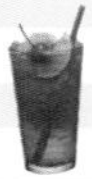

	C	F	Cb
Small	160	0	42
Medium	270	0	69
Large	400	0	105
Limeade Slush: Small	190	0	53
Medium	280	0	74
Large	430	0	116

Cold Brew Iced Coffee: Per Medium

	C	F	Cb
Original	260	13	32
French Vanilla	300	13	42

For Complete Nutritional Data ~ see CalorieKing.com

Southern Tsunami® (Jun '21)

Appetizers:

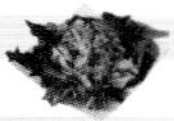

	C	F	Cb
Calamari Salad, 4 oz	140	1	15
Edamame, 3 oz	120	4.5	10
Grilled Dumplings, Shrimp, pkg	320	12	43
Seabreeze Salad, 4 oz	90	2.5	17

Bowls:

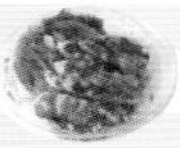

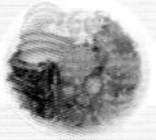

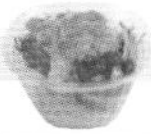

	C	F	Cb
Chirashi: *With White Rice*			
Chicken	790	26	117
Kani Kama	780	25	124
Salmon, Tuna	810	29	115
Hawaiian Poke: *With White Rice*			
Tuna	660	18	96
Tuna, Salmon	710	24	96
Tuna, Salmon, Albacore	690	21	96
Ramen Noodle Salad, with Sesame Dressing	630	40	58

Rolls: With White Rice

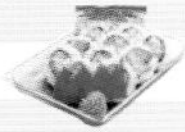

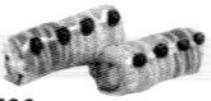

	C	F	Cb
Classic Rolls: Calif. & Inari, 4 pcs	210	4	40
Cream Cheese: Imit. Crab, 15 pcs	530	15	83
Salmon, 15 pieces	580	22	76
Crunchy Shrimp, 6 pieces	250	9	35
Hawaiian, 5 pieces	240	9	34
Inari, 10 oz	510	8	97
Ocean Crab, 6 pieces	180	4	31
Hybrid:			
Berry Roll, 9 oz	400	13	64
Blueberry Roll, 5 pieces	240	9	29
Crunchy Tempura Roll, 10 oz	460	16	69
Done Deal Roll, 10.8 oz	520	22	64
Dynamite Roll, 5 pieces	290	10	34
Happy Mango Roll, Eel, 10 oz	490	18	69
Spicy Mango Roll, Unakaba, 9.9 oz	440	23	51

Southern Tsunami® cont... (Jun '21)

One Roll: *With White Rice*	C	F	Cb
California, 10 pieces	310	6	58
California Salad Roll, 10 pieces	340	9	57
Cream Cheese Roll:			
Imit. Crab, 10 pcs	360	10	57
Salmon, 10 pieces	400	15	53
Crunchy CA Roll, 10 pieces	510	24	65
Crunchy Dragon:			
Orange, 10 pieces	620	34	62
Red, 10 pieces	570	27	62
White, 10 pieces	550	25	70
Crunchy Shrimp Tempura, 10 pcs	580	27	74
Dragon, 10 pieces	480	22	65
Eel, 10 pieces	360	8	58
Rainbow Roll:			
Albacore, Salmon, Tuna, 10 pcs	450	13	59
Salmon, Shrimp, Tuna, 10 pcs	440	13	57
Wraps: Berry , 4 pcs	80	3	12
Califormia, 4 pieces	120	6	13
Smoked Salmon Roll, 3.5 oz	160	10	11
Spicy California Wrap, 4 pieces	150	10	13
Spicy Chkn Roll, 3.5 oz	120	6	11
Spicy Salmon, 4 pieces	140	9	11
Summer Roll 2, 1 piece, 3.5 oz	90	3	14
Teriyaki Chicken Roll, 1 piece, 3.5 oz	100	3	14
Vegetable Wrap, 4 pieces	80	4	11

Starbucks® (Oct '21)

Please Check Instore Nutritional Information for Milk Varieties and Added Extas

Brewed Coffee: With 2% Milk Only	C	F	Cb
Caffe Misto: Short, 8 fl.oz	50	2	5
Tall, 12 fl.oz	80	3	8
Grande, 16 fl.oz	110	4	10
Venti, 20 fl.oz	130	5	13
Hot Drinks:			
Chocolate: *W/- 2% Milk , Drizzle, Sauce & Whipped Cream*			
Kid's or Short, 8 fl.oz	190	9	21
Tall, 12 fl.oz	280	12	32
Grande, 16 fl.oz	370	16	43
Venti, 20 fl.oz	450	18	54
White Chocolate: *W/- 2% Milk , Drizzle, Sauce & Wh. Cream*			
Kid's or Short, 8 fl.oz	240	11	28
Tall, 12 fl.oz	350	15	41
Grande, 16 fl.oz	440	19	55
Venti, 20 fl.oz	540	22	69

Starbucks® cont... (Oct '21)

Steamers:	C	F	Cb
Cinnamon Dolce Creme: *W/- 2% Milk, Sprinkles, Whipped Cream & Syrup*			
Tall, 12 fl.oz	280	12	33
Grande, 16 fl.oz	360	15	44
Venti, 20 fl.oz	430	17	54
Vanilla Creme: *With 2% Milk, Whipped Cream & Syrup*			
Tall, 12 fl.oz	280	12	34
Grande, 16 fl.oz	350	14	44
Venti, 20 fl.oz	430	16	55
Hot Espresso Beverages: *With 2%*			
Caffe Latte: *Without Toppings or Extras*			
Short, 8 fl.oz	100	3.5	10
Tall, 12 fl.oz	150	6	15
Grande, 16 fl.oz	190	7	19
Venti, 20 fl.oz	250	9	24
Caffe Mocha: *With Whipped Cream & Syrup*			
Short, 8 fl.oz	200	9	22
Tall, 12 fl.oz	290	13	33
Grande, 16 fl.oz	370	15	43
Venti, 20 fl.oz	450	18	54
Cappuccino: *Without Toppings or Extras*			
Short, 8 fl.oz	70	2.5	7
Tall, 12 fl.oz	100	4	10
Grande, 16 fl.oz	140	5	14
Venti, 20 fl.oz	200	8	20
Caramel Macchiato: *With Drizzle & Syrup*			
Short, 8 fl.oz	120	4	16
Tall, 12 fl.oz	190	6	26
Grande, 16 fl.oz	250	7	35
Venti, 20 fl.oz	310	9	44
Cinn. Dolce Latte: *W/ Toppings, Wh. Cream & Syrup*			
Short, 8 fl.oz	190	9	22
Tall, 12 fl.oz	270	12	33
Grande, 16 fl.oz	340	14	43
Venti, 20 fl.oz	420	16	54
Honey Almondmilk Flat White: *Without Toppings*			
Short, 8 fl.oz	80	3.5	15
Tall, 12 fl.oz	120	4	22
Grande, 16 fl.oz	170	5	30
Venti, 20 fl.oz	210	7	38
Cold Brew: *With Honey Syrup, without Extras*			
Honey Almondmilk:			
Tall, 12 fl.oz	30	0.5	6
Grande, 16 fl.oz	50	0.5	11
Venti, 20 fl.oz	80	1	17
Trenta, 30 fl.oz	100	1	22
Iced Espresso: *With 2% Milk, w/out Toppings or Cream*			
Caffe Latte: Tall, 12 fl.oz	100	3.5	10
Grande, 16 fl.oz	130	4.5	13
Venti, 20 fl.oz	180	6	18

continued next page...

Starbucks® cont... (Oct '21)

Frappuccino Blended Coffee: *Per 16 fl.oz Grande w/ Whole Milk, & Whipped Cream*

	C	F	Cb
Caffe Vanilla	400	14	65
Caramel	380	16	55
Java Chip	440	18	65
Mocha	370	15	54
White Chocolate Mocha	420	17	61

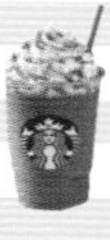

Frappuccino Blended Creme: *Per 16 fl.oz Grande, with Whole Milk and Whipped Cream*

	C	F	Cb
Chai	340	6	46
Double Chocolaty Chip	410	20	51
Vanilla Bean	380	16	53
White Chocolate	380	18	49

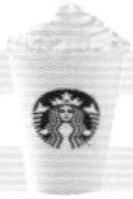

Refreshers: *Per 16 oz Grande*

	C	F	Cb
Mango Dragonfruit	90	0	21
Pink Drink	140	2.5	27
Strawberry Acai	90	0	23
Violet Drink	110	3	22

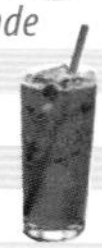

Teas: *Per 16 fl.oz Grande*

	C	F	Cb
Hot Tea: Honey Citrus Mint	130	0	32
Lattes: *With 2% Milk & Standard Ingredients*			
Chai	240	4.5	45
London Fog Latte	180	4	29
Matcha Tea Latte	240	7	34
Royal English B'fast, sweetened	150	4	21
Iced Tea: Green Tea Lemonade	50	0	12
Latte: Chai	240	4	44
London Fog	140	2.5	25

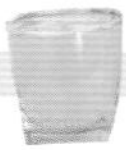

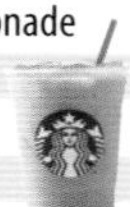

Breakfast:

	C	F	Cb
Sandwiches:			
Bacon, Gouda & Egg/Artisan Roll	360	18	35
Impossible/Arisanal Sesame Ciabatta	420	22	36
Wrap, Spinach, Feta & Egg White	290	8	34
Oatmeal: Classic	160	2.5	28
Hearty Blueberry	220	2.5	43
Overnight Grains,			
Strawberry	300	16	35
Parfait, Berry Trio	240	3	39

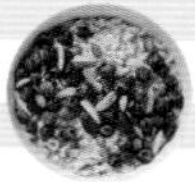

Sandwiches:

	C	F	Cb
Paninis: Chicken & Bacon	600	25	65
Ham & Swiss	480	23	41
Turkey & Pesto	550	21	53
Tomato & Mozzarella	370	14	42
Sandwich, Grilled Cheese	520	27	47
Yogurt, Siggi's 0% fat, Vailla, 5.3 oz	110	0	12

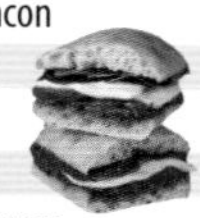

Starbucks® cont... (Oct '21)

Bakery: *Each*

	C	F	Cb
Bagels: Everything	290	3	57
Sprouted Grain	330	6	57
Brownie, Double Chocolate, 3.67 oz	480	28	55
Cake, Red Velvet, 4.12 oz slice	410	16	60
Cookie, Cinnamon Coffee, 3.85 oz	330	15	43
Croissants: Almond	420	25	40
Butter	260	15	27
Chocolate	340	20	38
Danish, Cheese, 2.82 oz	290	14	33
Dessert Bar,			
Marshmallow Dream, gluten free	230	5	44
Muffin, Blueberry, 3.5 oz	320	14	49

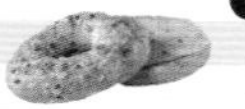

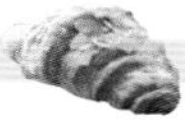

Bottled Drinks ~ See Page 37

Steak Escape® (Oct '21)

Cheesesteaks: *Per Regular Size*

	C	F	Cb
Bourbon & Bacon	1100	64	89
Grand Escape	690	28	66
Original Philly	710	30	68
Sriracha	790	34	73

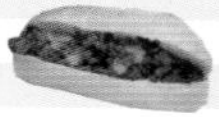

Sandwiches: *Per Regular Size*

	C	F	Cb
Chicken Bacon Club	980	58	62
Crispy Buffalo Chicken	1020	48	90
Grandest Chicken	680	22	65
Regin Cajun	700	27	50
Simply Chicken	550	13	60

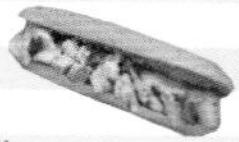

Subs: *Per Regular Size*

	C	F	Cb
Black & Bleu	740	37	65
Cubano	910	47	66
Delerious Dagwood	1180	76	62
Hangover	890	39	76
Italian Hottie	920	48	66

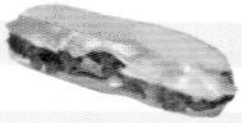

Wraps:

	C	F	Cb
Bourbon & Bacon	1010	63	80
Smokin BBQ	700	32	68
Steakhouse Sirloin	950	63	65
Fries: Buffalo Chicken; Cajun Bleu	950	60	83
Loaded Cheese & Bacon, small	920	63	79
Naked, regular	650	34	78
Sriracha Steak	900	53	87
Potatoes: Bourbon & Bacon	1020	54	101
Delerious Dagwood	1100	66	74
Simply Chicken	460	4	72
Triple Cheesesteak	910	45	78
Salads: Bourbon & Bacon	720	54	33
Cubano	530	38	10
Hangover	630	29	50
Sriracha Cheesesteak	410	24	17

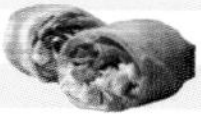

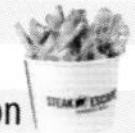

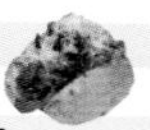

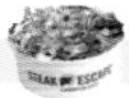

For Complete Nutritional Data ~ see CalorieKing.com

Steak 'n Shake® (Oct '21)

Steakburgers: Without Fries	C	F	Cb
Bacon Lovers	870	55	34
Bacon 'n Cheese: Single	460	26	29
Double	600	38	29
Triple	1030	74	32
Garlic Double	730	50	33
Jalapeno Crunch	690	43	39
Portobello & Swiss	740	50	36
Royale	750	49	33
Single Burger with Cheese	390	20	32
The Original: Double	460	26	33
with Cheese	530	32	32
Western BBQ 'N Bacon	790	43	54
Chili: 3-way	710	21	98
5-way	1160	57	103
Chili Deluxe: Bowl	1000	56	71
Cup	500	28	36
Chili Mac: Regular	1200	61	112
Supreme	1410	78	114
Melts: Frisco	960	66	51
Veggie, with Portobellos	620	45	44
Sandwiches: Fish	470	19	18
Grilled Cheese	620	43	41
Grilled Chicken	360	7	37
Spicy Chicken	480	16	48
Steak Franks:			
Chili Cheese Frank	710	44	46
Steak Frank	390	23	32
Salad, Garden, without dressing	310	19	18
Fries: *Per Regular*			
Reg.; Cajun; Parm. & Garlic Herb, av.	450	24	54
Cheese Fries	590	35	63
Chili Cheese Fries	760	39	83
Sides: Baked Beans	310	0	64
Coleslaw	160	11	13
Onion Rings, medium	330	17	39
Breakfast:			
Breakfast Bowl with Hash Browns	460	42	11
Bagel Sandwich: with Bacon	450	16	53
with Sausage	690	37	53
Banana Pancakes	970	16	189
Biscuits: Bacon	380	25	33
Bacon, Egg & Cheese	520	35	34
Sausage, Egg & Chse	760	56	34
Hash Browns, Shredded	300	28	15
Milk Shakes: *Per Regular*			
Banana	700	17	126
Birthday Cake	840	26	136
Reese's Choc. Peanut Butter	980	47	118
White Chocolate	630	18	105

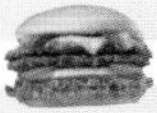
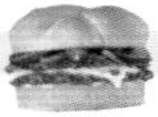
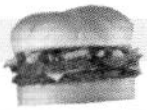
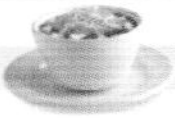
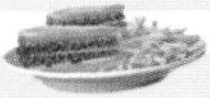
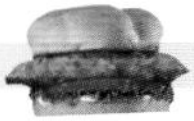
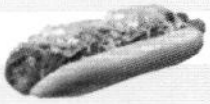
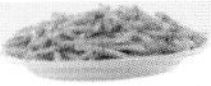
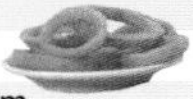
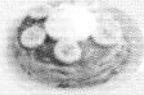
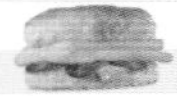

Subway® (Oct '21)

Sandwiches On 6" 9-Grain Sub: *With lettuce, tomatoes, onions, green peppers & cucumber. Without any condiments*

	C	F	Cb
BBQ Chicken	300	3.5	49
Black Forest Ham	270	4	41
Buffalo Chicken	330	11	39
Chicken Bacon Ranch	500	25	39
Melt	550	28	38
Chkn Mango Curry	300	7	42
Chicken Tikka	270	4.5	38
Chicken Vindaloo	310	8	41
Cold Cut Combo	280	10	38
Italian BMT	360	16	39
Meatball Marinara	400	17	46
Melt	520	28	49
Oven Roasted Turkey	270	3	41
Paneer Tikka	550	29	47
Spicy Italian	420	24	39
Steak & Cheese	320	10	37
Melt	500	28	39
Sweet Onion Chicken Teriyaki	330	4	52
Tuna	430	25	37
Melt	570	37	35
The Bacon Tatum	440	24	37
The DrayPotle Steak	390	17	38
Veggie Delite	190	2	39
Paninis: *With Standard Menu Board Components*			
Chicken Pesto	590	21	61
Wraps: *With Standard Menu Board Components*			
All American Club	550	20	57
Black Forest Ham	440	12	57
Buffalo Chicken	550	19	55
Cold Cut Combo	530	24	54
Italian BMT	680	36	57
Meatball Marinara	770	39	75
Oven Roasted Turkey	440	10	56
Spicy Italian	810	52	57
Tuna	820	54	52
Veggie Delite	330	8	56

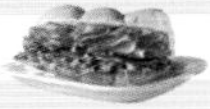
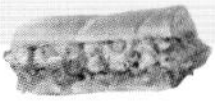
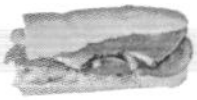
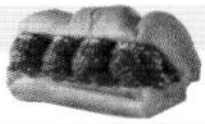
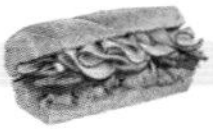
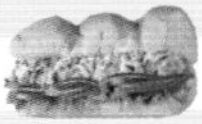
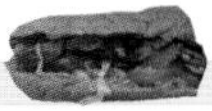
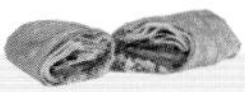
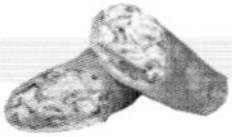
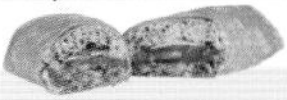
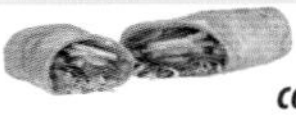

continued next page...

Subway® cont... (Oct '21)

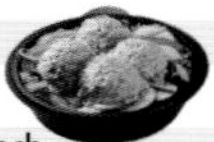
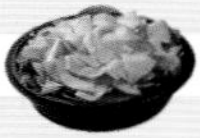
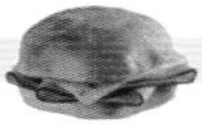
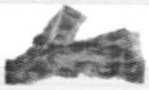
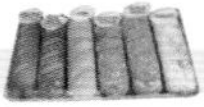
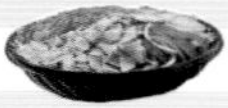
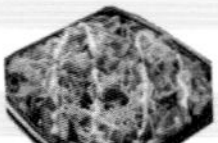
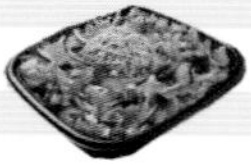
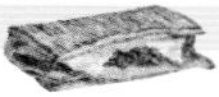

Protein Bowls:	C	F	Cb
American Club	**420**	24	14
BLT	**340**	23	10
Chicken & Bacon Ranch	**600**	40	12
Meatball Marinara	**520**	32	33
Pizza Sub	**610**	48	18
Steak Club	**440**	26	12
Sweet Onion Teriyaki	**300**	5	33
Turkey Italiano	**570**	42	14
***Sliders:** With Menu Set Components*			
Ham & Jack	**130**	3.5	18
Little Cheesesteak	**160**	7	19
Little Turkey	**180**	9	17
***Sandwich Extras:** For 6" Sandwiches*			
Bacon Strips, 0.5 oz	**80**	7	1
Bread: Artisan Flatbread	**230**	4	43
Artisan Italian	**160**	2	34
Hearty Multigrain	**190**	2	36
Italian Herbs & Cheese	**200**	4	36
Spinach or Tomato Basil Wrap	**290**	8	49
Cheese: American, 0.4 oz	**40**	4	1
Average other varieties, 0,.5 oz	**50**	4	0
***Salads:** With Menu Set Ingredients, without Dressing*			
All American Club	**440**	23	23
Black Forest Ham	**120**	3	12
Buffalo Chicken	**220**	11	12
Chicken & Bacon Ranch	**460**	33	13
Cold Cut Combo	**160**	9	10
Italian BMT	**240**	15	12
Meatball Marinara	**290**	17	22
Oven Roasted Turkey	**110**	2	11
Rotisserie Style Chicken	**150**	5	10
Spicy Italian	**300**	23	12
Steak & Cheese	**210**	3	30
Tuna	**310**	24	10
Turkey Italiano	**290**	20	13
Veggie Delite	**50**	1	9
Breakfast:			
Flatbread Sandwich:			
Bacon, Egg & Cheese	**710**	42	48
Black Forest Ham, Egg & Chse	**670**	38	49
Egg & Cheese	**640**	37	48
Steak, Egg & Chse	**700**	40	49

Swiss Chalet® (Oct '21)

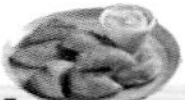
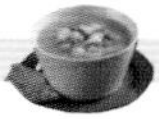
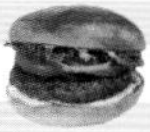
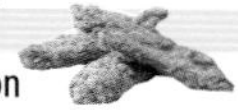
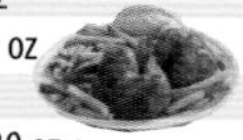
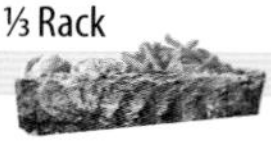

Canadian Outlets	C	F	Cb
Starters:			
Cheese Perogies, 9.45 oz	**510**	15	80
Chicken Spring Rolls, 8 oz	**460**	10	63
Caesar Salad: no protein, 5 oz	**340**	6	14
with Bacon	**400**	11	14
Rotisserie Chicken Soup with crackers:			
Cup	**110**	3	13
Bowl	**200**	6	20
Wings: 5 pieces	**530**	42	10
15 pieces	**1070**	74	20
***Burgers:** With Mayo, Without Sides*			
Classic Hamburger	**600**	29	49
Veggie Burger	**420**	12	53
Main Menu:			
Chicken Strips: 3 pieces	**620**	26	65
5 pieces	**930**	43	88
Poutine: with Bacon	**1730**	111	112
with Crispy Chicken	**1590**	98	126
Rotisserie Chicken: *W/ Dinner Roll & Chalet Sauce*			
¼ Dark Meat Chicken, 11.4 oz	**480**	18	31
¼ White Meat Chicken, 12.9 oz	**520**	16	31
½ Chicken, 22 oz	**1060**	45	31
Double Leg, 16.9 oz	**950**	53	31
Pot Pie, 17.9 oz	**840**	38	78
Whole Chicken, 30 oz	**1510**	66	31
Sandwiches/Wraps:			
Hot Rotisserie Chicken: Bun	**570**	19	48
Sandwich	**510**	9	58
Rotisserie Chicken Club Wrap	**720**	34	55
Southern Canuck	**710**	23	71
Wings, without Sides or Sauce:			
5 pieces with Dinner Roll	**570**	29	45
10 pieces	**740**	50	19
***Ribs:** With Dinner Roll & Coleslaw*			
BBQ Side Ribs: ⅓ Rack	**700**	33	63
½ Rack	**930**	45	72
Full Rack	**1360**	71	87
BBQ Back Ribs: ½ Rack	**820**	40	59
Full Rack	**1270**	62	87
***Entree Salads:** As Served*			
Caesar: without protein	**690**	12	27
with Crispy Chicken & Bacon	**1340**	51	62
with Rotisserie Chicken	**920**	22	27
with Rotisserie Chicken & Bacon	**1110**	36	28

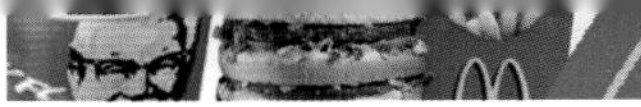

Swiss Chalet® cont... (Oct '21)

Sides: Per Serving	C	F	Cb
Baked Potato w/ Sour Crm & Onions	410	11	73
Creamy Mashed Potatoes w/ Gravy	200	4	42
Garden Salad without dressing	30	0.2	6
Garlic Green Beans	230	19	13
Market Vegetables, 8 oz	60	0.5	12
Poutine	800	47	76
with Rotisserie Chicken	940	51	76
Seasoned Rice Pilaf	630	13	119
Sweet Potato Fries	840	50	97
Fries: Fresh Cut, 8 oz	550	30	68
Harvey's, 8 oz	630	26	96
+Sauce: Chalet Dipping, 4 oz	25	0.5	5
Plum, 2 oz	120	0	27
Smoky BBQ, 2 oz	110	0	24
Wing: Hot, 2.25 oz	80	5	10
Mild, 2.45 oz	120	23	25
Medium, 2.4 oz	100	4	16
Desserts/Pies: Slice			
Apple Pie, 4.2 oz	290	12	45
Cheesecake w/ Strawb Syrup, 6.8 oz	550	22	77
Coconut Cream Pie, 5.4 oz	420	24	47
Lemon Meringue Pie, 4.5 oz	290	8	53
Pecan Pie, 4.5 oz	490	24	66
Super Sundae, 4.5 oz	340	21	67

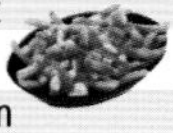
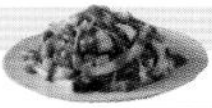
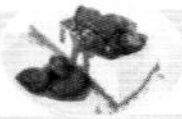

Taco Bell® (Oct '21)

Burritos:	C	F	Cb
Bean	350	9	54
Beefy 5-Layer	490	18	63
Black Bean Loaded Taco Fries	570	27	68
Chili Cheese, regional	370	17	40
Loaded Taco Fries	590	30	63
Quesarito: Beef	650	33	67
Chicken; Steak, av.	625	29	66
Supreme: Beef	390	14	51
Chicken; Steak	370	11	49
Loaded Taco Fries: Regular	560	36	49
Black Bean	550	32	55
Nachos:			
Nachos BellGrande: Beef	740	38	82
Chicken	720	35	81
Steak	720	36	81
Nacho Fries	320	18	35

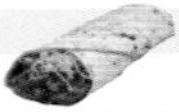
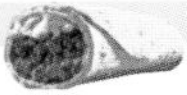
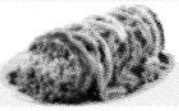
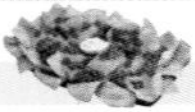

Taco Bell® cont... (Oct '21)

Power Bowls:	C	F	Cb
Chicken	470	19	50
Steak	480	20	51
Veggie	430	17	57
Quesadillas:			
Chicken	510	26	38
Steak	520	27	38
Tacos:			
Chalupa Supreme: Beef	350	18	33
Chicken	330	15	31
Steak	330	16	32
Cheesy Gordita Crunch	500	28	41
Crunchy: Beef	170	9	13
Taco Supreme	190	11	15
Nacho Cheese Doritos:			
Locos Taco	170	9	13
Locos Taco Supreme	190	11	15
Soft: Grilled Chicken	160	5	16
Seasoned Beef	180	9	17
Supreme Soft: Chicken	180	7	18
Seasoned Beef	210	10	20
Sides: Regular Size			
Black Beans & Rice	170	4	31
Black Beans	50	1	8
Cheesy Fiesta Potatoes	230	12	28
Breakfast:			
Crunchwrap:			
Bacon & Egg	670	41	50
Marinated Steak	660	38	51
Sausage Crumbles	610	37	50
Cheesy Toasted Burrito:			
Bacon & Egg	350	16	36
Fiesta Potato	340	17	36
Grande Toasted Burrito:			
Bacon & Eggs	560	30	49
Marinated Steak	560	28	50
Sausage Crumbles	560	31	49
Hash Brown Toasted Burrito:			
Bacon & Eggs	570	33	49
Marinated Steak	570	30	50
Sausage Crumbles	570	34	49
Sweets: Cinnabon Delights:			
2 Pack	160	9	17
12 Pack (serves 4)	930	53	104
Freeze, Wild Strawb. Lemonade, 16 fl.oz	180	0	49

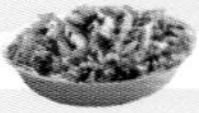
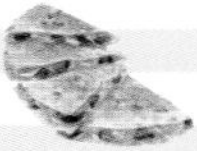
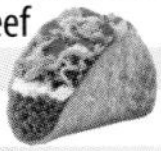
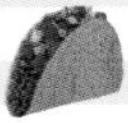
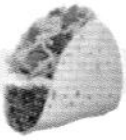
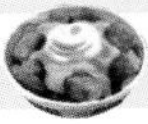
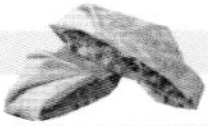
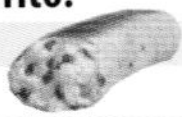
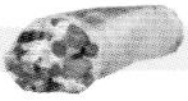
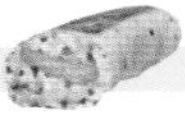
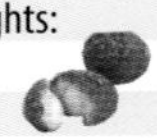

Note: Nutritional Information varies from state to state. Please refer to Taco Bell's Website

Taco Cabana® (Oct '21)

Burritos: *Includes Flour Tortilla, Rice, Refried Beans, Romaine, Meat, Shredded Cheese, Pico de Gallo & Sour Cream*

	C	F	Cb
Beef Cabana	720	29	79
Brisket Canana	790	40	76
Chicken Cabana	770	30	81
Flame Grilled Chicken Fajita	730	26	79
Steak	750	31	79

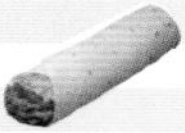

Bowls: *Includes Shell, Rice, Lettuce, Meat, Shredded Cheese, Pico de Gallo & Sour Cream*

	C	F	Cb
Beef; Chicken Fajita, average	715	35	64
Brisket	780	48	60
Shredded Chicken	760	37	66
Steak	740	39	63

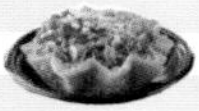

	C	F	Cb
Enchiladas: Beef (1)	200	11	14
Cheese (1)	320	23	13
Chicken (1)	280	13	21
Flautas, Chicken (3)	360	12	40

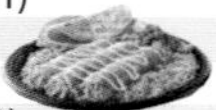

Quesadillas: *Small, with Lettuce, Guac. & Sour Cream*

	C	F	Cb
Brisket	920	63	51
Cheese	770	50	51
Flame-Gr. Chkn Fajita	840	52	52
Steak	850	55	52

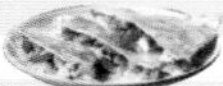

Tacos:

	C	F	Cb
Crispy: Beef	180	8	15
Shredded Chicken	200	9	16
Soft: Bean & Cheese	300	14	31
Beef, ground	210	9	21
Black Bean	220	5	38
Brisket	280	13	31
Carne Guisada	210	8	20
Flame Grilled Chicken Fajita	210	6	21
Shredded Chicken	240	9	23
Steak	220	9	21
Street, Beef (3)	460	25	40

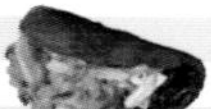

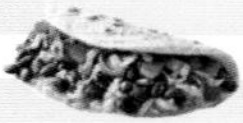

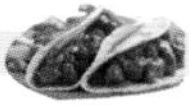

Salads: *Includes Shell, Lettuce, Meat, Shredded Cheese, Pico de Gallo & Sour Cream*

	C	F	Cb
Beef, ground	570	34	37
Chicken, shredded	610	35	39
Flame Grilled Chicken Fajita	570	31	36
Steak	600	36	36

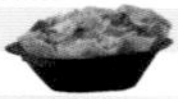

	C	F	Cb
Sides & Add-Ons: Black Beans	240	2	42
Borracho Beans, reg.	290	6	40
Chips & Queso, 4 oz	490	28	50
Chips & Guac, 4 oz	490	30	51
Guacamole, 3 oz	110	9	7
Queso, 3 oz	110	8	5
Refried Beans with Cheese, reg	530	29	49
Rice, regular	310	6	58
Salsa, all flavors, 1 oz	5	0	1
Sour Cream, 3 oz	160	15	3
Table Tortillas, Corn, 0.9 oz	60	1	13

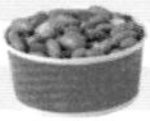

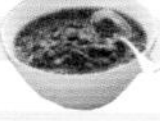

Taco Del Mar® (Oct '21)

Burritos: *Includes Flour Tortilla, Rice, Refr. Beans, Protein, Cheese, Pico de Gallo & Sour Crm*

	C	F	Cb
Regular: Chicken	910	31	115
Ground Beef	950	37	116
Pork	900	31	115
Shredded Beef	910	31	116
Steak	870	27	117
Vegan with guac., without sour cream, cheese or meat	680	15	115
Veggie with guac., without meat	840	29	119

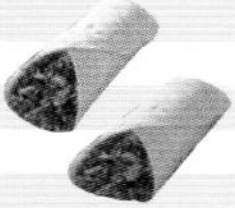

Burrito Bowls: *Per Regular Bowl, with Rice, Refried Beans, Protein, Cheese, Pico de Gallo & Sour Cream*

	C	F	Cb
Beef, shredded	600	24	64
Chicken	600	24	63
Pork	590	24	63
Steak	560	20	65
Vegan, with guacamole, without meat, cheese or sour cream	370	8	63
Veggie with addeed guacamole	530	22	67

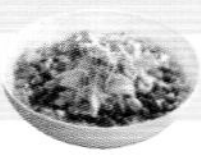

Nachos: *Includes Chips, Refried Beans, Protein, Cheese, Pico de Gallo, Guacamole & Sour Cream*

	C	F	Cb
Beef: Ground	1210	78	90
Shredded	1160	71	90
Cheese	1040	66	88
Chicken; Pork, av.	1160	72	89
Fish	1200	74	100
Steak	1130	68	91

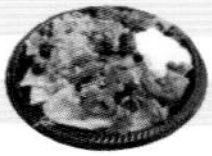

Enchilada Taco Platters: *Per 1 Corn/1 Flour Tortilla, Protein, Cheese, Rice, Ench. Sce. Refr. Beans, Lettuce, Pico de Gallo, Guacamole &, Sour Cream*

	C	F	Cb
Cheese	830	33	107
Chicken	870	31	107
Fish	1030	48	120
Ground Beef	910	38	108
Pork	860	31	106
Steak	830	28	109

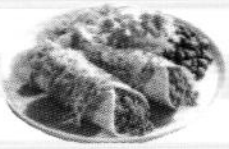

Quesadillas: *Includes Flour Tortilla, Meat, Cheese & Pico*

	C	F	Cb
Cheese	590	29	57
Chicken	720	35	58
Fish	750	37	69
Ground Beef	760	41	59
Pork; Shredded Beef, average	705	34	58
Steak	680	31	60

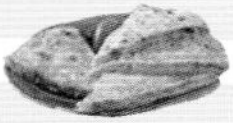

Taco Salads: *Includes Shell, Cheese, Refried Beans, Lettuce, Meat, Sour Cream & Pico de Gallo*

	C	F	Cb
Chicken	710	38	59
Fish	730	41	70
Ground Beef	750	45	60
Pork	690	38	58
Steak	670	35	61

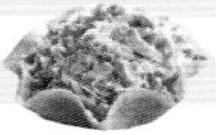

Note: Nutritional Information varies from state to state. Please refer to Taco Del Mar Website

Taco John's® (Oct '21)

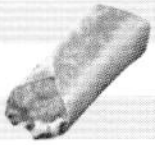
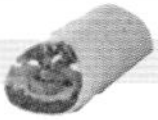
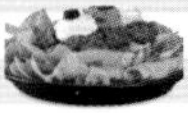
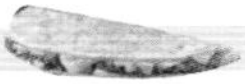
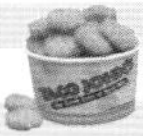
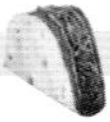
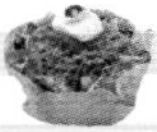
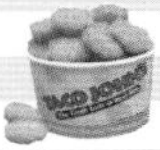
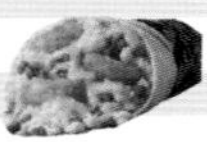

Burritos:	C	F	Cb
Bean, 6.6 oz	**360**	10	54
Combination, 6.6 oz	**400**	15	48
Grilled Beef, 9.75 oz	**740**	45	54
Grilled Chicken, 8.7 oz	**600**	29	52
Meat & Potato: Beef, 8.35 oz	**510**	24	59
Chicken, 8.35 oz	**480**	19	58
Sirloin Steak	**520**	23	58
Super, Beef, 8.85 oz	**440**	18	51
Super Nachos:			
Beef, 12.62 oz	**800**	43	82
Sirloin Steak, 13.1 oz	**810**	42	81
Quesadillas:			
Cheese, 5.7 oz	**480**	26	41
Chicken, 8.8 oz	**570**	27	50
Super Potato Oles, reg., 16.86 oz	**1090**	67	98
Tacos: Crispy Beef, 3.25 oz	**170**	10	11
Softshell Taco: Beef, 4 oz	**210**	10	21
Chicken, 4 oz	**180**	5	20
Single Street: Chkn, 3.25	**170**	6	17
Sirloin Steak, 3.25	**180**	8	17
Stuffed Gr. Beef, 6.6 oz	**450**	21	47
Taco Bravo Beef, 6.5 oz	**320**	13	36
Salads: Without Dressing			
Beef Taco Salad	**540**	33	45
Chicken Taco Salad	**500**	27	44
Crunchy Chicken	**630**	36	58
Sides:			
Black Beans & Rice, 6 oz	**200**	3	36
Chips & Nachos, 5 oz	**380**	20	45
Potato Oles: Small	**480**	27	52
Medium	**670**	38	73
Large	**860**	49	94
Refried Beans, 9.5 oz	**320**	7	45
Side Salad, without dressing 3.2 oz	**40**	3	3
Condiments: Guacamole, 2.5 oz			
Bacon Ranch Dressing, 1.5 oz	**120**	9	10
House Dressing, 1.5 oz	**70**	7	2
Nacho Cheese Sauce, 3 oz	**110**	9	5
Pico de Gallo, 1 oz	**10**	0	2
Salsa, average 1 oz	**7**	0	1
Sour Cream, 2.5 oz	**140**	13	4
Breakfast:			
Burritos: Bacon & Potato, 7.7 oz	**540**	25	57
Bacon Scrambler, 8.7 oz	**550**	25	59
Sausage Scrambler, 8.7 oz	**650**	33	60
Potato Ole Scrambler, Ssg, 116.8 oz	**1190**	79	88
Desserts: Churro Bites, 2.7 oz	**280**	13	37
Mexican Donut Bites, 3.2 oz	**290**	12	47

Taco Mayo® (Oct '21)

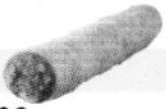
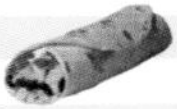
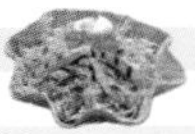
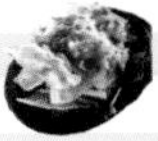
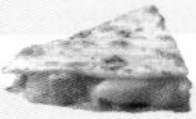
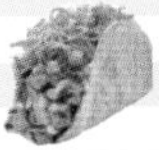
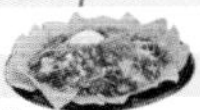
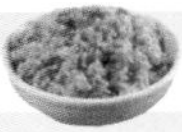
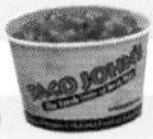

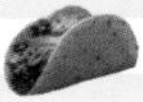

Burritos:	C	F	Cb
Bean	**450**	14	63
Chicken Burrito Supreme	**420**	19	40
Double Smothered Dble Queso:			
Beef	**930**	43	88
Chicken	**850**	39	83
Mexicali Gr. Chicken	**635**	38	48
Super: Regular	**525**	21	56
Beef	**525**	21	56
Mexicali Bowls: Chipotle Chicken	**1225**	71	91
Insalata Little Big	**275**	16	14
Mexicali Little Big	**450**	18	41
Queso Chicken	**1035**	48	92
Nachos:			
Classic: Beef Supreme	**790**	38	81
Cheese	**370**	20	44
Chicken Supreme	**710**	34	77
Ultimate Grande	**990**	51	93
Quesadillas: Beef Melt	**655**	35	45
Chicken Melt	**575**	30	41
Chicken Platter	**690**	40	45
Tacos: Crispy Beef	**160**	9	10
Fish	**280**	13	27
Soft Taco: Beef	**230**	10	19
Chicken	**185**	8	16
Taco Burger	**360**	15	32
Tamale Ole	**715**	38	64
Salads: As Per Menu Description			
Beef	**665**	33	55
Chicken	**445**	26	31
Sides: Cheddar & Chips	**555**	31	62
Guacamole	**185**	16	11
Guacamole & Chips	**575**	35	63
Mexicali Rice	**180**	9	17
Mixed Fruit Cup	**60**	0	16
Queso & Chips	**575**	30	62
Potato Locos, small	**400**	25	37
Refried Beans	**225**	4	34
Kids Meals:			
Burritos: with Fruit Cup	**505**	14	78
with Potato Loco	**845**	39	99
Quesadillas: with Fruit Cup	**270**	12	31
with Potato Loco	**605**	37	52
Tacos:			
Crispy: Beef with Fruit Cup	**220**	8	29
with Potato Loco	**560**	33	50
Soft: Beef w/ Fruit Cup	**290**	10	35
with Potato Loco	**630**	36	56

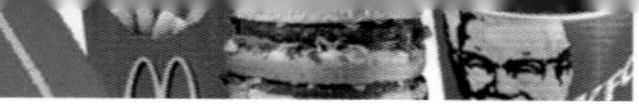

Taco Time® (Oct '21)

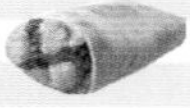
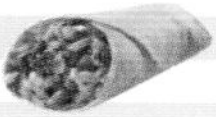
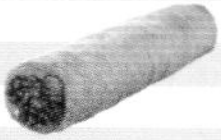
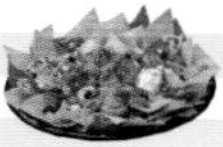
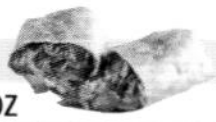
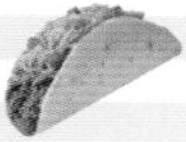
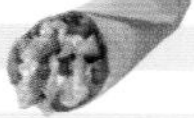
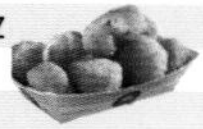
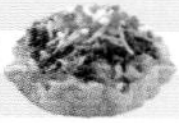
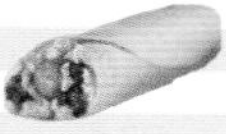
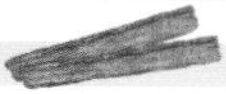

Burritos:	C	F	Cb
5 Alarm	420	15	58
Chicken B.L.T.	600	31	46
Sweet Pork	550	18	72
Big Juan: Chicken	590	16	79
Seasoned Beef	650	22	83
Casita: Chicken	450	16	44
Seasoned Beef	510	22	48
Crisp Burrito:			
Chicken	380	17	39
Meat	390	17	43
Pinto Bean	380	13	53
Soft Burrito: Pinto Bean	380	10	56
Seasoned Beef	420	16	46
Veggie	440	17	60
Nachos: Original	900	39	91
Chicken	970	39	92
Seasoned Beef	1020	45	96
Optionals:			
Green Chili Pork Carnita: Burrito	460	18	43
Chimichanga	590	21	65
Enchiladas	340	12	26
Soup, Enchilada, 8 oz	130	0.5	20
Quesadillas: Cheese	450	23	39
Chicken	520	24	42
Tacos:			
Soft Tacos: Chicken	360	10	42
Junior	300	13	29
Pork	440	16	43
Super Soft Tacos: Chicken	500	16	61
Pork	590	21	62
Seasoned Beef	560	21	65
Fries:			
Mexi: Small, 3.2 oz	190	12	19
Regular, 4.7 oz	300	19	29
Stuffed: Small, 4.5 oz	320	20	29
Regular, 6.6 oz	460	28	42
Salads:			
Fiesta, Chicken, 12.3 oz	340	11	37
Taco: Chicken, 8 oz	310	14	26
Seasoned Beef, 7.5 oz	360	19	28
Breakfast:			
Burritos: *Regular Size*			
Bacon & Egg	450	20	48
Egg & Cheese	370	16	40
Enchilada	450	20	46
Sausage & Egg	560	30	48
Ultimate	760	48	50
Quesadilla	300	17	18
Taters & Gravy, regular	410	27	36
Churros: Plain	210	16	15
Bavarian Cream	320	8	54
Cinnamon Crustos	320	5	64

TCBY® (Oct '21)

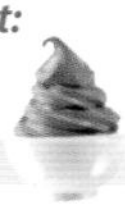
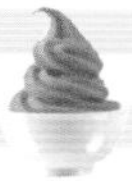
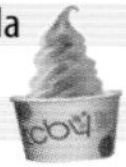

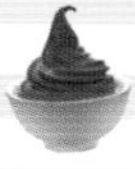
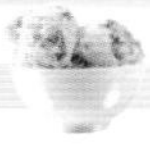
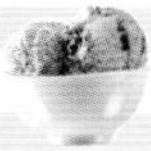
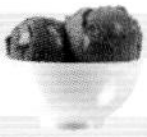
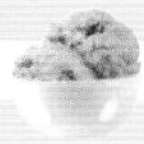

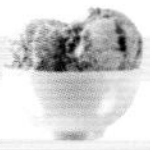

Soft Serve Frozen Yogurt:	C	F	Cb
Per ½ Cup, 4 fl.oz			
Dairy Free/Sorbet:			
Chocolate Almond	100	1	28
Coconut	125	5	18
Kiwi Strawberry Sorbet	90	0	22
Mango Sorbet	95	0	24
Orange Sorbet	90	0	23
Watermelon Sorbet	100	0	25
No Sugar Added, av. all flavors	63	0	18
Super Fro Yo: Bananas Foster	90	0	23
Cake Batter; Golden Vanilla	105	2	22
Chocolate	100	2	22
Dutch Chocolate	95	0	23
Graham Cracker	105	2	25
Greek Honey Vanilla	100	0	20
New York Cheesecake	115	2	23
Old Fashioned Vanilla	90	0	23
Peppermint	140	2	22
White Chocolate Mousse	120	2	24
Hand-Scooped Frozen Yogurt:			
Dairy Free, Psychedelic Sorbet	130	0	33
Gluten Free:			
Butter Pecan: Kid's, 4 fl.oz	220	10	27
Small, 6.4 fl.oz	350	16	43
Regular, 12.8 fl.oz	705	32	86
Chocolate Chocolate:			
Kid's, 4 fl.oz	120	2.5	20
Small, 6.4 fl.oz	190	4	38
Regular, 12.8 fl.oz	385	8	76
Peanut Butter Delight:			
Kid's, 4 fl.oz	250	13	30
Small, 6.4 fl.oz	400	21	48
Regular, 12.8 fl.oz	800	42	96
Pralines & Cream: Kid's 4 fl.oz	210	6	27
Small, 6.4 fl.oz	335	10	43
Regular, 12.8 fl oz	670	19	86
Vanilla Bean:			
Kid's, 4 fl.oz	170	5	27
Small, 6.4 fl.oz	270	7	43
Regular, 12.8 fl.oz	545	14	86
Other Flavors:			
Cookies & Cream:			
Kid's, 4 fl.oz	200	6	32
Small, 6.4 fl.oz	320	10	51
Regular, 12.8 fl.oz	640	19	102

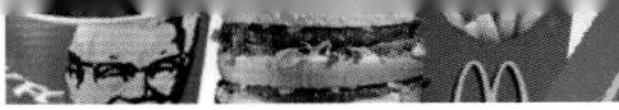

TGI Friday's® (Oct '21)

Appetizers/Snacks:	C	F	Cb
Chips & Salsa	240	10	29
Giant Onion Rings with BBQ Ranch	1120	52	146
Loaded Potato Skins, with Ranch Sour Cream	2120	92	283
Mozzarella Sticks, with Marinara	840	52	54
Pan Seared Potstickers, with Szechuan Sauce	590	25	72
Philly Cheesesteak Egg Rolls, with Beer Cheese Sauce	1070	61	82
Spinach Artichoke Dip	760	55	43
***Burgers:** With Regular Bun, without Sides*			
Bacon Cheeseburger	840	54	47
Beyond Meat Cheesebgr	860	52	52
Cheeseburger	770	52	41
Signat. Whiskey-Glazed	1140	56	117
Green Style: Beyond Cheeeseburger	580	40	16
Spicy Reaper	590	48	10
Chicken & Seafood:			
Crispy: Chicken Tenders, with Slaw, Fries & Honey Mustard	1030	67	74
Fried Shrimp, with Fries, Coleslaw & Cocktail Sauce	820	45	82
Parmesan Crusted Chicken, with Mashed Pot. & Lemon Butter Sce	920	41	55
Simply Gr. Salmon, Broccoli, Jasmine Rice & Lemon Buter	830	41	81
***Pasta:** Full Order, Fried*			
Cajun Shrimp & Chicken, with Breadstick	1390	60	132
Chicken & Broccoli Chseee Tortelloni with Breadscick	1850	110	140
Chicken Parmesan, w/ Breadstick	1630	75	161
***Ribs:** With Coleslaw & Seasoned Fries*			
Apple Butter: Half Rack	770	53	50
Full Rack	1150	81	66
Whiskey Glazed: Half Rack	1070	53	127
Full Rack	1620	81	185
***Sandwiches:** Without Sides*			
Bacon Ranch Chicken	690	31	47
Buffalo Fried Chicken	920	55	66
Southern Fried Chicken	920	55	65
Whiskey Glazed Chicken	1160	56	107
***Sizzling:** With Mashed Potatoes*			
Chicken & Shrimp	1030	71	41
Chicken & Cheese	930	60	37
Whiskey-Glazed Flat Iron Steak	1470	78	127

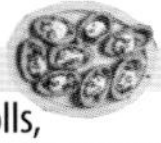

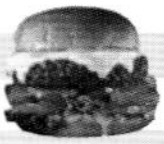

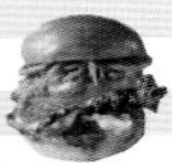

TGI Friday's® cont... (Oct '21)

***Steaks:** With Mashed Potatoes & Lemon Butter Broccoli*	C	F	Cb
NY Strip: with Parm Butter	740	34	36
with Whiskey Glaze	890	30	85
Sirloin:			
with Parm. Butter	440	21	36
withWhiskey-Glaze	540	17	71
Salads:			
Caesar: with Grilled Chicken	790	59	21
without Protein	600	54	19
Million $ Cobb: Gr Chkn & Ranch	1000	75	21
without Protein	820	70	19
Soups: French Onion	590	18	84
New England Clam Chowder	500	30	45
Tomato Basil	300	24	20
White Cheddar Broccoli Cheese	290	20	18
Sides: Cheddar Mac & Cheese	530	28	49
Coleslaw	150	11	13
Fruit cup	50	0	13
Giant Onion Rings with Ranch	510	26	61
Jasmine Rice	370	10	63
Lemon Butter Broccoli	90	5	11
Mashed Potatoes	130	4	23
Seasoned Fries	230	15	21
***Desserts:** Per Whole Dish*			
Brownie Obsession	1180	58	154
Oreo Madness	540	23	79
Red Velvet Cake	1560	82	191

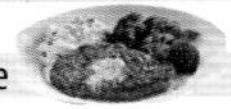

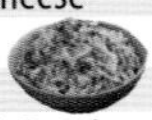

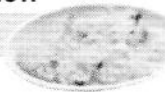

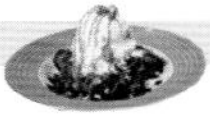

Thundercloud Subs® (Oct '21)

***Subs:** Small, w/ Standard Toppings*	C	F	Cb
Classic: BLT	405	20	36
Genoa Salami	280	7	35
Roast Beef	290	4	35
Smoked Chicken	270	4	35
Turkey	255	4	36
Signature Subs:			
Club	445	19	38
California Club	475	23	40
NY Italian	540	30	37
Office Favorite	790	39	71
Texas Tuna	675	44	39
Veggie Delite, with Hummus	385	19	52

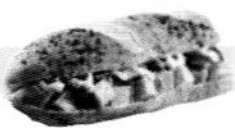

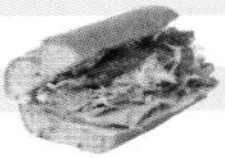

T.J. Cinnamons® (Oct '21)

Bakery:	C	F	Cb
Orig. Gourmet Cinn. Roll, 7.8 oz	840	42	106
Pecan Stick Bun, 8.3 oz	940	49	111

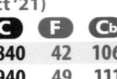

Tim Hortons® (Oct'21)

Breakfast:	C	F	Cb
Bagel BELT	560	24	62
Biscuit Sandwich:			
Angus Steak & Egg	400	20	34
Bacon, Egg & Cheese	420	23	33
Sausage, Egg & Cheese	530	34	33
Turkey Sausage, Egg & Cheese	350	16	31
Grilled Breakfast Wrap: Farmer's	680	42	54
Steak & Cheddar	440	21	40
Oatmeal, with Mixed Berries, reg.	210	3	44
Hash Brown, 1.9 oz	130	7	16
Lunch:			
Chili, regular	480	27	26
Pasta, Mac & Cheese	490	27	48
Soup: *Per Regular Size*			
Broccoli Cheddar	270	15	23
Chicken Noodle Soup	160	2	30
Hearty Vegetable Soup	110	0.5	20
Potato Bacon Cheddar Soup	380	23	31
Roasted Red Pepper & Gouda	310	20	24
Turkey & Wild Rice	180	2	35
Wraps:			
Grilled Chicken Fajita	430	19	39
Steak Fajita	430	20	40
Sides,			
Kettle Cooked Potato Chips, 1.4 oz	220	14	22
Cookies: Chocolate Chunk	210	9	32
Oatmeal Raisin Spice	210	8	32
Peanut Butter	250	15	24
White Chocolate Macadamia	220	11	29
Donuts: Apple Fritter	290	8	48
Chocolate Dip	190	7	29
Football	230	8	34
Maple Dip	190	6	29
Old Fashion Dip	250	11	33
Vanilla Dip with Sprinkles	270	9	45
Muffins: Chocolate Caramel	410	15	64
Wild Blueberry	340	11	57
Whole Grain Pecan Banana Bread	350	11	60
Timbits: Apple Fritter (1)	50	2	9
Chocolate Glazed (1)	70	3	10
Honey Dip (1)	45	1	8
Old Fashioned Glazed (1)	70	3	10
Sour Cream Glazed (1)	90	5	12
Salted Caramel (1)	70	3	11

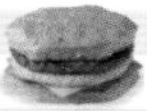
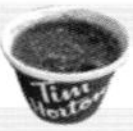

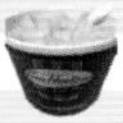
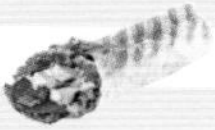
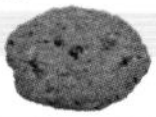
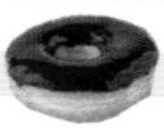
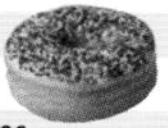
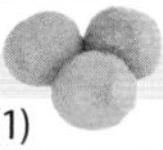

Tim Hortons® cont... (Oct'21)

Beverages:	C	F	Cb
Hot: Cappuccino, 15 fl.oz	100	0	15
Mocha Latte, 15 fl.oz	230	7	32
Iced: Coffee, cream & Sugar, 20 fl.oz	110	7	11
Latte, 20 fl.oz	240	7	35
Mocha Latte, 20 fl.oz	390	9	68

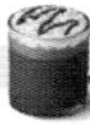
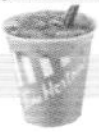

Togo's® (Oct'21)

California Outlet ~ Please check local outlet for menu items and nutritional information

	C	F	Cb
Cold Sandwiches: *Per Regular 6", with Menu Set Components on White Bread*			
#2: Ham & Swiss	690	28	70
#3:Turkey & Cheddar	800	39	68
#4: Turkey, Salami & Cheddar	980	56	68
#5: Turkey & Cranbery	650	18	86
#7: Roast Beef	710	21	67
#8: Roast Beef & Turkey	880	40	69
#16: The Italian	880	47	70
#20: Albacore Tuna	670	27	72
#23: Salami & Provolone	1020	61	68
Hot Sandwiches: *Per Regular 6", with Menu Set Components on White Bread*			
#1: Chicken & Cheddar	930	51	71
#6: Meatball	890	40	81
#9: Pastrami	740	34	73
#32: Pepperjack Melt	1010	59	73
Wraps: *Per Whole 12" Spinach Tortilla Wrap, with Menu Set Components*			
Asian Chicken	650	28	70
Bacon Ranch Chicken	680	33	55
Cali Veggie	810	49	63
Chicken Caesar	570	21	62
Greek Veggie	760	45	78
Santa Fe Chicken	710	34	69
Salads: *Per Full Salad, with Dressing*			
Asian Chicken	670	43	44
Chicken Caesar	450	26	22
Farmer's Market	480	39	26
Santa Fe Chicken	780	55	37
Soups: *Per 10 oz*			
Broccoli Cheddar	220	14	16
Chicken Noodle	120	4	15
Chicken Tortilla	160	5	20
Chili	240	8	23
Clam Chowder	200	9	23
Garden Vegetable	120	5	18
Brownie, Choc. Chunk, 3 oz	440	23	56
Cookies: Choc. Chunk, 3 oz	410	21	54
Oatmeal Raisin, 3 oz	370	13	58
Peanut Butter, 3 oz	430	24	49

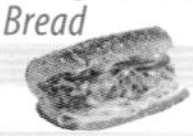
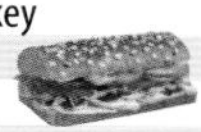
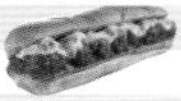
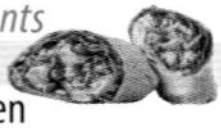
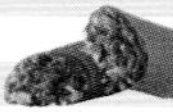
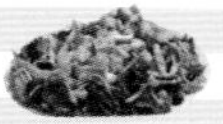
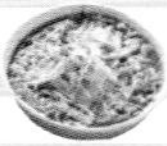
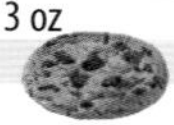

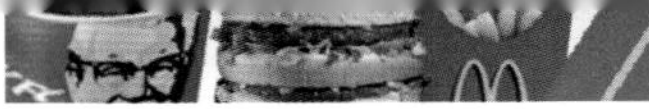

Tropical Smoothie Cafe® (Oct '21)

Menu & Nutrition Differ from Outlets to Outlet. Please Check Instore.

	C	F	Cb
Breakfast:			
All American Omelet Wrap	430	20	37
Peanut Butter Crunch Flatbread	590	24	77
Southwest Omelet Wrap	580	36	38
Flatbreads:			
Chicken Bacon Ranch	500	23	44
Chicken Pesto	430	16	43
Chipotle Chicken Club	490	24	42
Quesadillas: Santa Fe Chicken	600	28	50
Three Cheese Chicken	550	27	41
Sandwiches:			
Chicken Caprese	660	26	62
with Bacon	720	31	62
Turkey Bacon Ranch	560	20	59
Ultimate Club	620	27	59
Toasted Wraps: *In Flour Tortilla*			
Baja Chicken	640	24	67
Buffalo Chicken	510	21	44
Caribbean Jerk Chkn	590	17	74
Hummus Veggie	710	36	80
Supergreen Caesar Chicken	600	31	42
Thai Chicken	500	15	62
Classic Smoothies: *Per 24 oz with Turbinado*			
Bahama Mama	510	4	117
Beach Bum	550	4	131
Blimey Limey	480	0	119
Blueberry Bliss	340	5	86
Island Green	410	0	102
Lean Machine	490	0	124
Mango Magic	400	0	98
Mocha Madness	540	4	124
Paradise Point	430	0	110
Peanut Paradise with Pea	740	17	107
Peanut Butter Cup	710	19	129
Sunrise Sunset	400	0	97

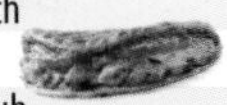
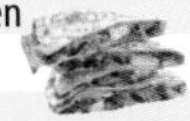
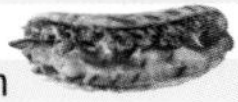
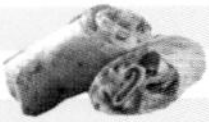
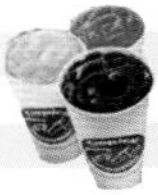
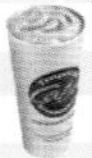

Tubby's® (Oct '21)

Subs: *Per Regular 8" Sub, with Standard Ingredients, without Added Sauce or Dressing*

	C	F	Cb
Deli-Subs:			
Ham & Cheese	540	11	78
Turkey Breast & Cheese	550	10	77
Turkey Club	630	17	77
Grilled Burger Subs:			
Cheeseburger Italiano	790	35	78
Pizza Burger	810	36	81
Taco	960	44	89

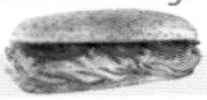
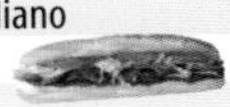

Tubby's® cont... (Oct '21)

Subs (Cont): *Per Reg. 8" Sub, with Standard Ingredients, without Added Sauce or Dressing*

	C	F	Cb
Grilled Chicken Subs: Gr. Chicken	450	5	75
Chicken & Broccoli	550	11	78
Chicken & Cheddar	540	11	75
Crispy Chicken	730	30	87
Grilled Steak Subs:			
Loaded Steak	650	18	82
Mushroom, Steak & Cheese	620	17	77
Pepper Steak & Cheese	630	17	77
Steak & Cheese	620	17	76
Specialty Subs: BLT	570	21	72
Cold Veggie	490	10	86
Tuna	570	11	76
Sides: Breaded Mushrooms	410	22	47
French Fries	390	24	39
Mac & Cheese Bites	510	37	34
Mozzarella Sticks	490	26	42
Seasoned Fries	370	28	30

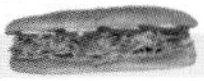
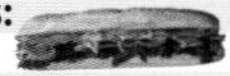
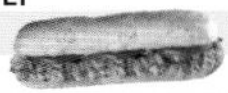
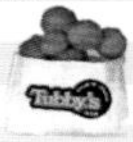

Uno Pizzeria & Grill® (Oct '21)

	C	F	Cb
Appetizers: *Per Whole Dish*			
Mozzarella Sticks	1090	57	107
Muchos Nachos	1700	71	199
Shrimp & Crab Dip	1160	84	66
Burgers: *Without Friess*			
Bacon Cheddar	1350	99	35
Cheddar Burger	1110	81	35
Classic Beyond	560	32	42
Entrees:			
Chicken: *Without Sides or Breadstick*			
Chicken Tender Platter with Fries	1600	106	88
Lemon Herb Chicken Skewers	440	28	2
Mediterranean Chicken	560	21	43
Pasta: *With Housemade Bread*			
Chicken Spinoccoli	1260	62	105
Regular Mac & Cheese	1740	103	140
Shrimp Scampi	1190	54	128
Steak & Seafood: *Without Sides or Breadstick*			
Grilled Shrimp & Sirloin	690	45	1
Lemon Basil Salmon	490	38	0
Sirloin, 10 oz	560	37	0
Sirloin Steak Tips	470	20	4
Deep Dish Individual Pizza: *Per Slice, ⅙ Pizza*			
Chicago Classic	360	26	19
Numero Uno	300	19	20
Prima Pepperoni	280	15	18
Sides: French Fries, 7.5 oz	450	33	35
Loaded Mashed Potatoes	420	26	37
Red Bliss Mashed Potatoes	280	14	36
Steamed Broccoli	70	6	5
Sweet Potato Fries	430	25	47
Dessert: Awesome Chocolate Cake	1740	79	241
Uno Deep Dish Sundae	1520	74	206

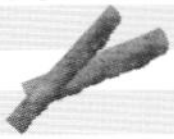
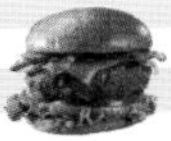
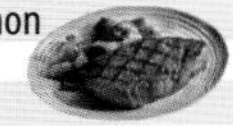
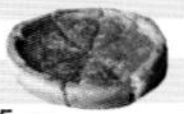

Villa Italian Kitchen® (Oct '21)

Pizzas: Per Slice	C	F	Cb
Neapolitan: Buffalo	770	46	52
Deluxe	530	22	55
Sausage & Pepperoni	550	25	53
Stuffed: Baked Ziti	845	33	97
Spinach & Mushroom	735	33	79
Entrees:			
Chicken Pasta Primavera, 16 oz	505	20	58
Fettuccini Alfredo, 14 oz	765	38	85
Mac & Cheese, 14 oz	725	54	39
Pasta Primavera, 16 oz	495	21	66
Spaghetti & Meatballs, 18 oz	840	28	112
Sides: Caesar Salad, 4 oz	90	5	9
Garlic Roll	260	10	34
Garden Salad, 3 oz	15	0	3
Greek Salad, 6 oz	125	10	7
Roasted Potatoes, 6 oz	210	12	24
Sauteed Vegetables, 6oz	85	6	6

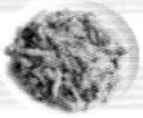
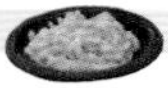
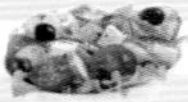

Vocelli Pizza® (Oct '21)

Pizzas:

Artisan: *Per 1/8 of Medium Pizza, with Menu Set Components*	C	F	Cb
BBQ Chicken	290	10	35
Chicken Carbonara	270	11	27
Chicken Pesto	260	10	27
Deluxe	260	11	29
Hawaiian	280	11	29
Meat Magnifico	290	13	28
Philly Steak	270	12	28
Quattro Cheese	260	10	27
Spring Veggie	220	7	29
Linguini Pasta: *Single Serving*			
Chicken Alfredo	1200	54	129
Chicken Parmesan	960	26	144
Chicken Pesto	1230	57	128
House Baked Subs: On Italian Bread			
Buffalo Chicken	950	39	86
Chicken Parmesan	990	39	105
Meatball	1170	55	103
Salads: Per Regular Size, without Dressing			
Chicken Caesar	180	4	14
Mediterranean	230	11	22
Tuscan Grilled Chicken	320	13	22
Desserts: Cannoli	150	7	17
Chocolate Cake	320	14	46
Double Fudge Chunk Brownie	500	28	62

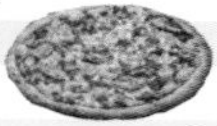
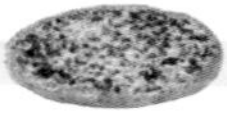
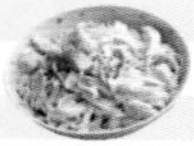
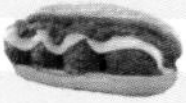
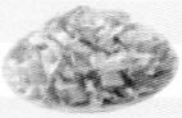
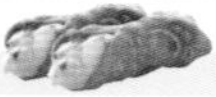

Wahoo's Fish Taco® (Oct '21)

Banzai Bowls: With White Rice & Black Beans	C	F	Cb
Blackened: Chicken	720	14	104
Fish	675	9	104
Carne Asada	795	24	102
Carnitas	890	26	105
Salmon	705	14	102
Burritos: With Brown Rice & White Beans			
Outer Reef: Blackened Chicken	765	32	79
Blackened Fish	725	28	79
Mushroom	700	32	81
Shrimp	705	28	79
Tofu	715	30	81
Side Kicks: Soft Corn Tortillas (3)	145	2	29
Flour Tortilla (1)	300	11	46
Shredder Sandwiches: With White Rice & White Beans			
Blackened or Charbroiled:			
Chicken, average	1045	36	140
Fish, average	1000	32	140
Carne Asada	1110	44	140
Wahoo Salads: Banzai Veggie	415	24	35
Carne Asada	690	48	22
Chicken, Blackened/Charbroiled, av.	540	32	22
Salmon	550	32	22
Shrimp	460	26	24
Tofu	540	31	30
Soup, Chicken Tortilla	130	6	11

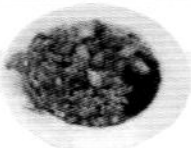
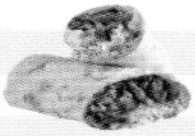
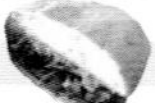
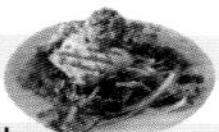

For Complete Nutritional Data ~ see CalorieKing.com

WAWA® (Oct '21)

Breakfast Sizzlis:	C	F	Cb
Bagels: Bacon, Egg & Cheese	430	21	42
Dble Bacon Dble Cheese	560	31	43
Pork Roll, Egg & Cheese	440	22	41
Sausage, Egg & Cheese	540	32	41
Biscuit, Sausage, Egg & Cheese	690	47	47
Bowls: *W/ Starndard Components,, w/o Toppings or Extras*			
Chipotle Beyond Sausage Patty	690	51	14
Egg Omelet	120	9	3
Multigrain Toast Beyond Sausage Patty	360	12	49
Pancake & Beyond Sausage	410	17	52
Pancake & Turkey Sausage	390	14	52
Burritos: *With Egg Omelet & CHeddar Cheese, without Toppings or Extras*			
Bacon	540	29	45
Beyon Sausage Patty	540	29	46
Quesadillas: *With Standard Components, No Extras*			
Black Bean & Egg Omelet	740	43	60
Chipotle Bacon Egg Omelet	760	47	48
Garlic Smoked Turkey & Egg Omelet	730	44	51
S'wich, Spinach, Tomato Egg Omelet on Multigrain Bread	390	13	53

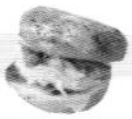
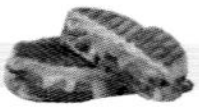

WAWA® cont... (Oct '21)

Hot Hoagies: On Classic Roll, without Cheese, Toppings or Spread	C	F	Cb
Beef Steak	620	21	68
Beyond Meatball	710	24	71
Chicken Steak	530	11	68
Meatball	1070	60	95
***Quesadillas:** Without Toppings*			
BBQ Chicken & Cheddar Cheese	590	21	62
Beef with Cheddar Cheese	560	28	44
***Soups:** Per Medium Serving without Toppings*			
Baked Potato w/ith Cheddar & Bacon	400	27	26
Broccoli Cheddar Soup	280	21	14
Chicken Noodle	180	6	21
New Eng. Clam Chowder	310	20	23
Tomato Soup	330	22	28
***Sides:** Per Medium*			
Beyond Meatball	280	14	12
Buffalo Mac & Cheese	520	27	49
Mashed Potatoes	470	27	47
Meatballs in a Cup	480	38	20
Rice & Beans	270	4	49
Rice	240	0	52
Bakery: Apple Fritter	640	26	96
Chocolate Croissant	400	22	45
Muffins: Banana Nut	580	30	69
Blueberry	560	28	70
Coffee Cake	650	34	80
***Hot Beverages:** Per 16 oz, without Extras*			
Hot Cappuccino, with 2% milk	130	5	13
Mocha Latte, with 2% milk	350	6	64

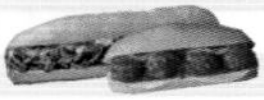
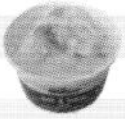
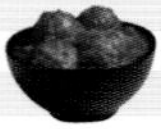
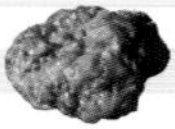
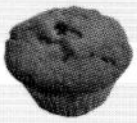

Wendy's® (Oct '21)

Breakfast:	C	F	Cb
Biscuits: Baconator	730	50	37
Bacon, Egg & Cheese	420	27	28
Honey Butter Chicken	500	29	44
Sausage, Egg & Cheese	610	45	29
Croissants: Bacon, Egg & Swiss	410	23	34
Maple Bacon Chicken	560	30	51
Sausage, Egg & Swiss	600	41	34
Hamburgers:			
Baconator	960	66	36
Big Bacon Classic: Single	650	41	37
Double	910	62	37
Bourbon Bacon Cheeseburger:			
Single	710	41	51
Double	970	62	51
Triple	1280	86	52
Daves: Single	590	37	37
Double	860	57	37
Triple	1160	81	38
Jr.: Bacon Cheeseburger	370	23	26
Cheeseburger Deluxe	340	20	27
Son of Baconator	630	40	36

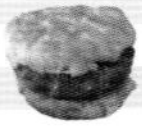
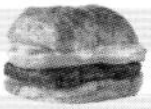
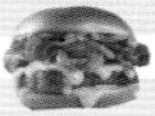
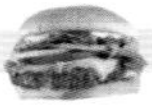
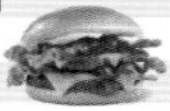

Wendy's® cont... (Oct '21)

Hamburgers (Cont):	C	F	Cb
Pretzel Bacon Pub: Double	1180	79	53
Triple	1520	106	54
Cheeseburger	840	52	53
Sandwiches:			
Asiago Ranch Chicken Club	630	31	50
Classic: Chicken	490	21	49
Jalapeno Popper	600	28	51
Crispy: Chicken	340	17	33
Chicken BLT	420	23	35
Grilled: Asiago Ranch Chicken Club	490	21	34
Chicken	350	8	35
Jalapeno Popper	460	18	35
Pretzel Bacon Pub	700	33	53
Spicy: Asiago Ranch Chkn Club	630	30	52
Chicken	500	19	51
Pretzel Bacon Pub	840	42	71
Crispy Chicken Nuggets: 4 pieces	180	12	9
6 pieces	270	17	14
Spicy Chicken Nuggets: 4 pcs	190	12	9
6 pieces	280	18	13
***Dipping Sauces:** Per 1 oz*			
Barbecue	45	0	11
Buttermilk Ranch	120	12	2
Creamy Sriracha	120	12	3
Honey Mustard	90	7	7
Sweet & Sour	45	0	12
***Fresh-Made Salads:** Full Size with Menu Set Dressing*			
Apple Pecan Grilled Chicken	550	26	42
Parmesan Caesar Chicken	440	28	7
Southwest Avocado Chicken	560	39	16
Taco	690	34	68
Sides:			
Apple Bites	35	0	8
Baconator Fries	470	27	43
Baked Potatoes: Plain	270	0	61
Bacon Cheese	440	13	64
Cheese	450	14	65
Chili & Cheese	500	14	74
Sour Cream & Chives	310	3	63
Cheese Fries	450	27	40
Chili: Small	240	11	22
Large	340	15	31
Chili Cheese Fries	530	28	53
Natural Cut French Fries: Jr.	220	10	28
Small, 4 oz	270	13	36
Medium, 5 oz	360	17	47
Large, 6.5 oz	480	23	63
Pub Fries	480	28	44
Frosty:			
Chocolate; Vanilla, av: Small	345	9	57
Medium	460	12	77
Large	580	15	96

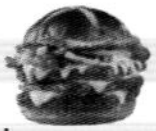
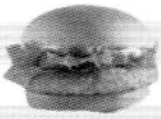
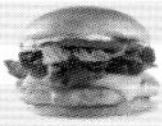
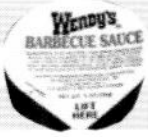

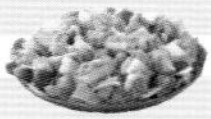
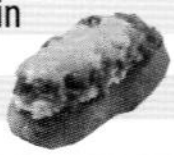
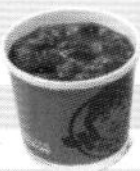
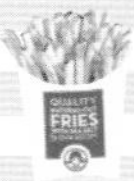

For Complete Nutritional Data ~ see CalorieKing.com

Whataburger® (Oct '21)

Burgers & Sandwiches:	C	F	Cb
Whataburger:			
#1 Original	590	25	62
#2 Double Meat	830	44	62
#3 Triple Meat	1070	63	62
#4 Jalapeno & Cheese	680	32	63
#5 Bacon & Cheese	750	37	62
#6 Double Meat Jr.	420	20	37
#7 Whataburger Jr.	310	11	36
All Time Favorites:			
Honey BBQ Chicken Strip Sandwich	890	42	87
Mushroom Swiss Burger	1110	70	61
Patty Melt	940	61	45
Sweet & Spicy Bacon Burger	1080	62	69
Whatachick'n:			
Bites: 6 pieces	390	19	25
9 pieces	580	28	37
Grilled Chicken Sandwich with Mayo	470	20	42
Strips, 3 pieces	460	27	30
French Fries: Small	270	14	34
Medium	400	21	51
Large	530	28	68
Onion Rings: Medium	300	17	32
Large	450	25	49
Salad: Without Dressing			
Apple & Cranberry Grilled Chicken	380	12	38
Cobb with Spicy Chicken	550	32	21
Breakfast:			
Buttermilk Biscuit:			
with Bacon	490	31	35
with Sausage	640	44	35
Honey Butter Chicken	580	36	52
Jalap. Cheddar Biscuit w/- Bacon	370	23	31
Taquitos: *With American Cheese*			
Bacon	400	23	29
Potato	440	25	28
Sausage	420	26	28
Desserts:			
Chocolate Chunk Cookie	230	11	31
Hot Apple Pie, 3 oz	270	14	34
Malts: Chocolate, 20 fl.oz	590	13	110
Vanilla, 20 fl.oz	540	14	94
Shake, Chocolate, 20 fl.oz	560	14	102

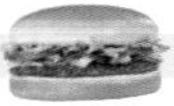
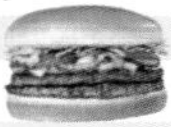
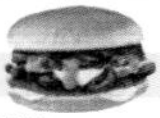
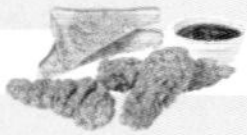
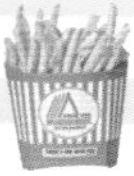
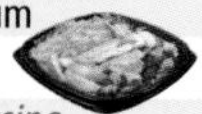
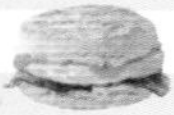
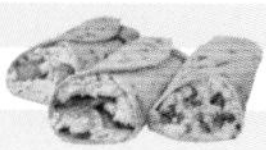
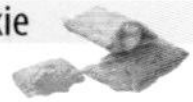
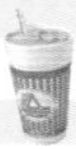

White Castle® (Oct '21)

Note: Nutritional Information varies from state to state. Please check instore	C	F	Cb
Sliders:			
Bacon Cheese	220	14	15
Cheese	170	9	16
Crispy Chicken & Waffles	350	18	36
Crispy Chicken Breast with Cheese	230	10	22
Chicken Ring with Cheese	200	10	18
Double Original	250	13	24
Double Smoked Cheddar Cheese	320	19	26
Impossible with Smoked Cheddar	230	13	17
without Cheese	190	10	16
Fish, plain	320	20	25
Jalapeno Cheese	170	9	16
Panko Surf & Turf with Cheese	550	36	34
Surf & Turf with Cheese	520	36	31
The Original	140	7	16
Veggie: with Ranch	320	23	23
with Honey Mustard	210	10	27
Sides: Chicken Rings, 3 piece	160	10	6
Clam Strips, medium	410	34	9
Fish Nibblers: Small	320	16	28
Medium	590	29	51
Mozzarella Cheese Sticks (3)	460	33	26
Onion Chips, medium	930	65	73
Onion Rings, small, 5 oz	480	33	40
Fries:			
Cheese Fries	400	27	35
Clam Strips, medium	410	34	9
French Fries, medium	600	39	57
Loaded Fries, 5.7 oz	460	38	20
Mozzarella Cheese Sticks (5)	760	55	40
Onion rings, small	480	33	40
Breakfast: With Cheddar Cheese			
B'Fast Sliders: Bacon, Egg & Cheese	260	17	15
Bologna, Egg & Cheese	350	24	17
Egg & Jalapeno Cheese	210	13	15
Sausage, Egg & Chse	350	26	15
Original Slider, with Egg & Cheese	270	18	16
Toasted Sandwiches:			
Bacon, Egg & Chse	380	23	29
Egg & Cheese	270	13	29
Sausage, Egg & Chse	420	27	29
Waffle Sliders:			
with Bacon, Egg & Cheese	390	26	27
with Sausage, Egg & Cheese	490	36	28
Hash Round Nibblers:			
Small	360	28	25
Medium	600	46	42
Dessert:			
On A Stick: Fudge Dipped Brownie	250	12	33
Fudge Dipped Cheesecake	180	10	21

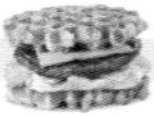
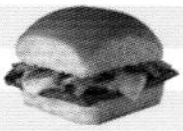
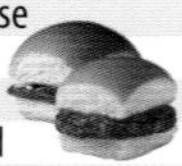
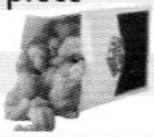
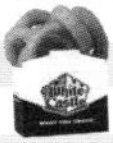
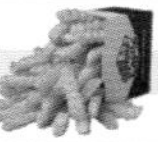
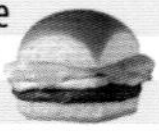
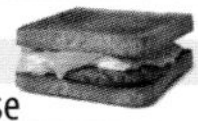
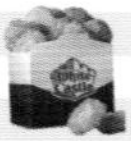

Wienerschnitzel® (Oct '21)

Hot Dogs: On Hot Dog Bun	C	F	Cb
Original:			
Chicago Dog	330	15	37
Chili Dog	300	15	30
Chili Cheese Dog	350	20	30
Junkyard Dog	430	24	42
Kraut Dog	280	14	29
Mustard Dog	280	14	28
Texas BBQ Dog	510	32	36
Hot Dog Substitute, add to any Original Dog:			
All Beef Dog	100	10	1
Polish Sausage	140	12	2
Pretzel Bun Substitute, add to Orig.	80	0	15
Burgers:			
Cheeseburger	390	13	41
Double	770	45	30
Chili Cheeseburger	450	24	27
Double	570	24	42
Corn Dog	230	13	21
Sandwich, Polish Sausage	500	34	36
Sides: Per Regular			
Chili Cheese Fries	530	29	53
Bacon Ranch	630	39	54
Thousand Island	710	45	60
French Fries: Small	310	16	38
Medium	440	23	54
Large	750	39	92
Breakfast:			
Biscuits: Egg, Bacon, Cheese	420	20	28
Egg, Sausage, Cheese	580	39	40
Biscuit & Gravy	390	21	42
Burritos:			
Chili Cheese Egg	350	14	39
Egg, Bacon, Cheese	420	20	38
Egg, Sausage, Cheese	510	29	42
Croissant:			
Egg, Bacon & Cheese	530	31	40
Egg, Sausage & Cheese	620	40	44
Hash Brown Po'Taters	330	23	28
Desserts:			
Classic Banana Split	670	17	129
Cones: With Sprinkles	240	9	40
Chocolate Dipped	350	21	40
Freezee,			
Oreo; M&M, Reese's, av.	630	25	99
Shakes, Chocolate with Oreo	880	31	151
Sundaes:			
Caramel; Choc; Hot Fudge, av.	395	15	64
Strawberry	370	14	59

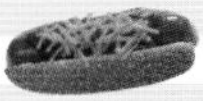
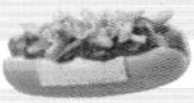
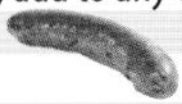
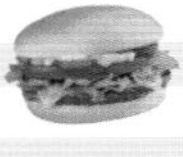
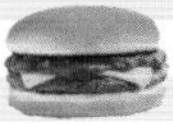
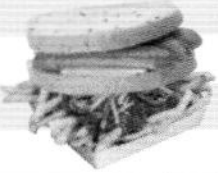
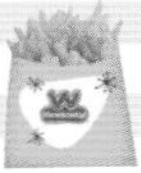
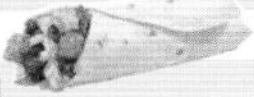
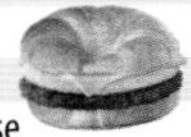
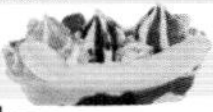
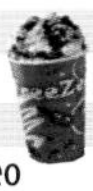

Winchell's® (Oct '21)

Donuts: Per Donut	C	F	Cb
Buttermillk Bars, Choc Iced/Glazed	420	19	61
Cake Donuts: Choc., Choc Iced	210	9	33
Chocolate, Plain	170	9	22
White: Cherry Iced	270	12	40
Maple Iced; Orange Iced	270	12	40
French, Cherry Iced; choc Iced; Glazed	270	14	32
Holes: Chocolate Sprinkles (1)	140	6	21
Cinnamon Crumb (1)	130	5	22
Glazed (1)	90	5	12
Jelly Filled:			
Apple with Cinnamon Crumb	370	15	53
Raspberry with Glaze	390	13	61
Strawberry with Sugar	380	13	60
Old Fashioned, Glazed; Maple Iced	410	17	60
Raised Ring: Chocolate Iced	270	10	41
Coconut	240	12	30
Fanch: Apple Fritter	600	23	93
Bear Claw (1)	700	38	75
Butterfly (1)	530	23	75
Cinnamon Roll (1)	630	31	80

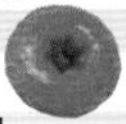
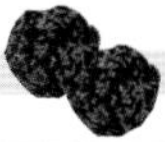
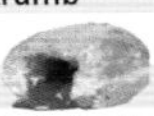
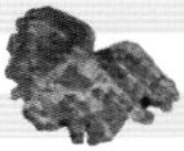

WingStreet (Oct '21)

Chicken: Without Dipping Sauce	C	F	Cb
Bone Out Wings: *Per Wing*			
Buffalo, Mild	90	4	10
Garlic Parmesan	130	9	6
Hawaiian Teriyaki	90	4	9
Honey BBQ	100	4	11
Lemon Pepper; Naked; Ranch Rub	80	4	6
Nashville Hot	90	5	9
Smoky Garlic	110	6	9
Traditional Bone In Wings: *Per Wing*			
Buffalo, Mild	100	5	5
Garlic Parmesan	140	11	0.5
Hawaiian Teriyaki	100	5	4
Honey BBQ	110	5	7
Lemon Pepper; Naked; Ranch Rub	80	5	0.5
Nashville Hot	100	5	4
Smoky Garlic	120	8	3
Rubs & Sauce: Average for Bone In/Bone Out wings			
Buffalo	17	0	4
Garlic Parmesan	55	6	0
Honey BBQ; Hawaiian Teriyaki, av.	20	0	4
Rubs, all varieties	0	0	0
Smokey Garlic	40	2	4

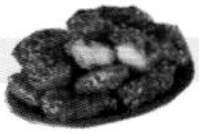
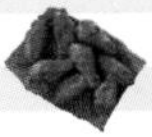
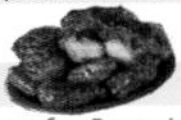

Yard House® (Oct'21)

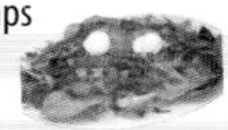
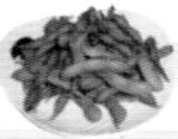
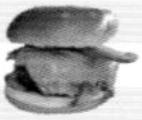
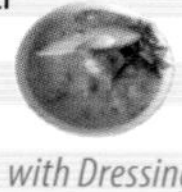

	C	F	Cb
Appetizers: With Sides & Sauce			
Ahi Sashimi	470	30	22
Chicken Lettuce Wraps	770	37	74
Chicken Nachos	2600	164	165
Fried Calamari	990	70	55
Poke Nachos	870	59	51
Snacks:			
Guacamole & Chips	800	53	77
Hot Spicy Edamame	490	36	29
Sweet Potato Fries	650	26	98
Truffle Fries	500	24	63
Grilled Burgers: Without Fries			
BBQ Bacon Cheddar Burger	1280	84	64
Classic Cheeseburger	990	65	47
Kurobuta Pork Burger	1050	63	62
Fries, 1 Serving	360	14	52
House Favorites: As Served			
Braised Short Rib Ravioli	1000	49	80
Chicken Bowl	470	15	47
Maui Pineapple Chicken	1240	27	151
Spicy Jambalaya Pasta, large	1370	73	104
Pizza: Margherita	1070	46	119
The Carnivore	1520	81	111
Seafood: With Sides & Sauce			
Beer-Battered Fish & Chips	1580	107	96
Lobster Bisque Agnolotti	890	47	80
Soups: Per Bowl			
Chicken Tortilla	1220	93	63
Clam Chowder	480	35	29
Salads: Full Entree Size, with Dressing			
Cobb with Chicken	1090	80	25
Kale & Romaine Caesar with Shrimp	770	51	35
Dessert: Mini Cheesecake Brulee	400	24	43
Bread Pudding with Creme Anglaise	810	38	101
Carrot Cake	460	20	65

For Complete Nutritional Data ~ see CalorieKing.com

Yoshinoya® (Oct'21)

	C	F	Cb
Appetizers:			
Clam Chowder, 8 oz	180	12	16
Spring Rolls (2)	280	12	27
Regular Bowls: With White Rice & Mixed & Vegetables			
Grilled: Habanero Chicken	620	11	90
Tilapia	640	27	74
Sweet Chili Shrimp	710	18	112
Kid's Meal: With white Rice & Mixed Veggies			
Original Beef	280	0	61
Orange Chicken	410	11	62
Dessert: Cheesecake	240	13	25
Chocolate Chip Cookie (1)	170	7	26
Flan	270	9	38

Zaxby's® (Oct'21)

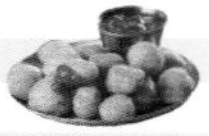
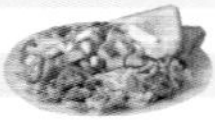

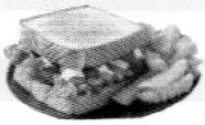
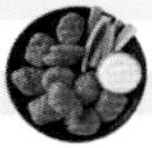
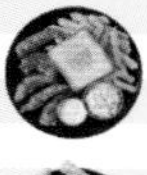
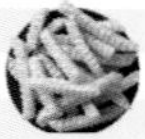
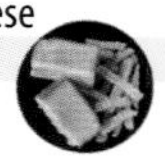

	C	F	Cb
Zappertizers:			
Fried Cheddar Bites, w/ Marinara Sauce	790	50	55
Spicy Fried Mushrooms w/ Ranch Sce	520	41	31
Zalads: With Texas Toast, Without Dressing			
Blackened Blue	530	24	34
Buffalo Blue	680	35	48
Fried Cobb Zalad	820	47	47
Fried House Zalad	700	38	46
Grilled: Grilled Cobb Zalad	700	36	35
Grilled House Zalad	580	27	35
Dressings: Per 1.25 oz Serving			
Blue Cheese	180	19	2
Caesar	90	9	2
Honey Mustard	150	14	6
Mediterranean	140	13	4
Ranch	160	16	1
Thousand Island	230	23	3
Most Popular:			
Boneless Wings & Things	1480	88	109
Buffalo Boneless Wings & Things	1490	90	107
Buffalo Chicken Finger Plate (4)	1220	68	100
Chicken Finger Plate (4)	1190	66	101
Traditional Wings & Things	1530	96	90
Sandwich Meals: With Menu Set Components			
Cajun Club	940	45	82
Grilled Chicken	880	40	82
Kickin' Chicken	1070	55	102
Nibblerz	1280	63	132
Zaxby's Club	1150	62	101
Wings & Fingers:			
Boneless Wings (5):			
Insane	340	17	25
Sweet & Spicy	390	17	36
Teriyaki	370	16	32
Traditional Wings (5): BBQ	440	24	17
HHM	480	33	8
Tongue Torch	400	24	5
Chicken Fingers (5): Original	530	26	23
Wimpy	520	22	29
Sides:			
Crinkle Fries: Basket	850	46	99
Regular	330	14	47
Texas Toast:			
1 Slice, 1.5 oz	150	7	19
Basket, 4.5 oz	450	21	57
Kidz Meals: Kiddie Cheese	730	35	86
Kiddie Finger	700	39	61
Kidz Nibbler	630	29	76

Zero Sub's® ~ *see CalorieKing.com*

Notes on Cholesterol

- **Cholesterol** is a white waxy substance produced mainly by our liver. It is also found in animal food products. Plant foods have no cholesterol.
- **Cholesterol is essential to life.** It is a structural part of every body cell wall and is the building block for vitamin D, sex hormones, and bile acids which help in the digestion of dietary fats. **Cholesterol is also vital for a healthy brain** (which contains some 20% of total body cholesterol).
- **The body makes sufficient cholesterol** for its needs and does not rely on cholesterol in the diet. Dietary fats have a major influence on blood cholesterol levels. (See next page)
- **A high blood cholesterol level increases** the risk of atherosclerosis - the thickening of arteries that can reduce or block blood flow to the heart, brain, eyes, kidneys, sex organs and other body parts.

  This in turn increases the risk of heart attack, stroke, blindness, kidney failure, impotence and other blood circulatory problems.

  Other risk factors which increase the risk of atherosclerosis include high blood pressure, smoking, obesity and uncontrolled diabetes.

HEART ATTACK WARNING SIGNALS

Many victims die before reaching the hospital by ignoring warning signals and delaying medical help.

Symptoms vary and commonly include:

- **Chest pain,** vice-like squeezing or burning sensation in center of the chest or between the shoulder blades, or in the mid-back. Pain may even feel like severe indigestion.
- **Pain** may be felt in the arms, shoulders, neck or jaw.
- **Shortness of breath** often occurs with or before chest discomfort.
- **Other signs,** with or without pain, include a cold sweat, nausea or light-headedness.

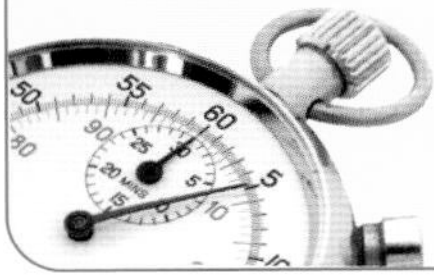

If you experience any of the above symptoms call IMMEDIATELY for medical help. Every minute counts.

***Call 9-1-1** or your emergency number*

BLOOD CHOLESTEROL

CHECK YOUR RISK!

Total Cholesterol Level (mg/dl)		Risk of Heart Attack
240 and above	~	High Risk
200 - 239	~	Borderline/High
Below 200	~	Desirable

- **Know your cholesterol level, particularly if there is a family history of heart disease or stroke. If your level is high, see your doctor.**
- **All adults should have their cholesterol, HDL and triglycerides tested at least every 5 years.**

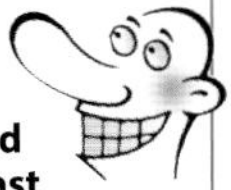

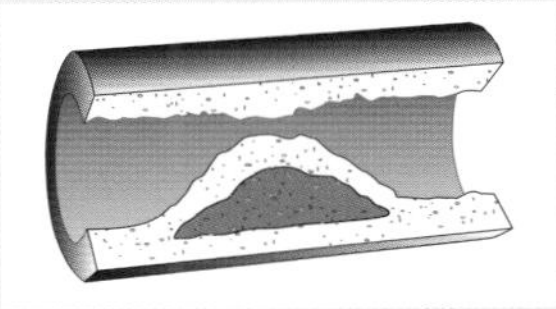

▲ **Atherosclerosis can clog arteries and impede blood flow to the heart or other body organs.**

▼ **A thrombus (blood clot) can form on unstable, festering athero-sclerotic plaque and rapidly block blood flow. A heart attack or stroke can result.**

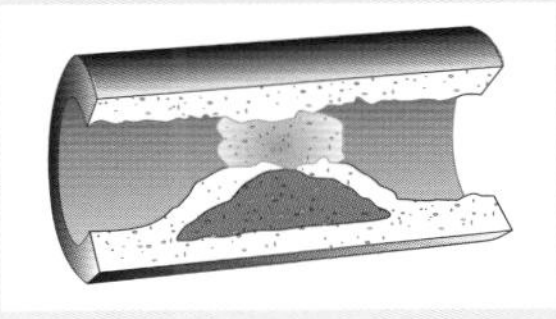

Fats & Cholesterol Guide

The amount and type of dietary fat has the greatest influence on blood cholesterol levels.

Fats in food are a mixture of 3 basic types: saturated, monounsaturated, and polyunsaturated. Animal fats are mainly saturated while plant oils and fish oils are mainly mono- and polyunsaturated.

Saturated fats have subgroups known as long-chain, medium-chain, and short-chain fats. Most of the long chain fats raise blood cholesterol, and increase the risk of blood clots and thrombosis leading to artery blockage.

Long-chain saturated fats are found mainly in full-cream milk, cheese, butter, cream, fatty meats and sausages, and processed foods.

Medium-chain fats (MCT) have little effect on LDL-cholesterol but may raise "good" HDL.
Note: Coconut oil *has some MCT but is mainly saturated fat – so limit use.*

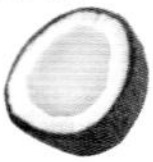

Monounsaturated fats tend to more selectively lower 'bad' LDL cholesterol and maintain the protective 'good' HDL cholesterol in the bloodstream – but only if they replace saturated fats in the diet. Foods rich in monounsaturates include canola and olive oils, canola margarine, peanuts, and avocados.

Polyunsaturated fats consist of two main classes. **Omega-6** polyunsaturates tend to lower blood cholesterol. Rich sources include safflower, sunflower and corn oils.

Omega-3 polyunsaturated fats can lower blood cholesterol; significantly lower blood triglycerides; and reduce the rise of thrombosis, heart arrythmmia, and artery spasm.

Best practical omega-3 sources include canola oil and margarine, soybean oil and fish.

A balanced intake of the two omega classes is important for optimal health. For most Americans, slightly increasing omega-3 intake would help attain a more ideal balance.

Trans fats from hydrogenated vegetable oils and shortenings should also be avoided. They are common in commercial baked and fried food products such as cakes, muffins, pastries, doughnuts, fried snacks and french fries.

DIETARY FATS COMPARISON

Saturated Fat | Monounsaturated Fat

Polyunsaturated Fats:
Linoleic (Omega-6) | Alpha-Linolenic (Omega-3)

OILS	PERCENTAGE CONTENT			
CANOLA OIL	7	63	20	10
LINSEED/FLAX OIL	9	19	17	55
SAFFLOWER OIL	9	14	77	
GRAPESEED OIL	10	22	68	
SUNFLOWER OIL	11	23	66	
CORN OIL	14	32	52	2
OLIVE OIL	14	76	10	
SOYBEAN OIL	15	23	54	8
PEANUT OIL	19	45	34	2
COTTONSEED OIL	26	16	58	
PALM OIL	51	39	10	

SPREADS & FATS
Saturated Fat includes 'Trans Fats' | WATER CONTENT

SPREADS & FATS					
LIGHT MARGARINE	14	14	21	51	
CANOLA MARGARINE	18	45	12	6	19
POLYUNSATURATED MARG	24	20	36	20	
BUTTER	57	18	2	24	
LARD	41	47	12		
BEEF FAT	44	37	4	15	

GOOD SOURCES OF OMEGA-3 FATS

Plant Sources	Omega-3 Fats (Grams)
Canola Oil, 1 Tbsp, ½ fl.oz	1.5g
Flaxseed Oil, 1 Tbsp	8g
Soybean Oil, 1 Tbsp	1.2g
Canola Margarine, 1 Tbsp, ½ oz	1g
Soybeans, cooked, ½ cup, 4 oz	0.5g
Walnuts, ½ oz	0.5g

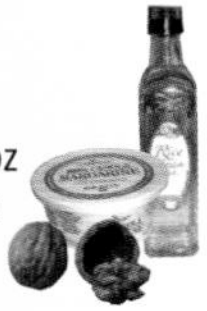

FISH - *Per 4 oz Serving*

High Content: Salmon (Chinook), Tuna, — 3g
Trout (Lake), Sardines, Herring, Mackerel — 3g

Medium Content:
Salmon, (Pink/Red/Coho), 4 oz — 2g

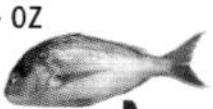

Fair Content: *Per 4 oz Serving*
Bass, Catfish, Cod, Grouper, Hake, Halibut, Kingfish, Perch, Pollock, Shark, Trout (Rainbow), Tuna, Crab, Oysters, Blue Mussels, Shrimp, Squid } 0.5-1g

How Much Is Needed?

As little as 1-2 grams daily of omega-3 fats may benefit general health. High doses of fish-oil supplements should only be taken as directed by your Healthcare provider.

Dietary Cholesterol

Cholesterol in food varies in its effect on blood cholesterol level (BCL) from person to person. Much depends on the amount and type of fat and fiber eaten at the same meal.

Any elevating effect of dietary cholesterol on BCL is more likely to occur when the diet is high in saturated fat. Little elevation, if any, generally occurs when dietary fats are balanced in favor of mono- and poly-unsaturated fats (including omega-3 fats).

Example: While fish does contain cholesterol, the omega-3 fats can prevent any increase in BCL. Conversely, a meal containing no cholesterol but rich in saturated fat may result in a significant increase in BCL - as well as impairing artery wall functions.

Consequently, the need to be overly concerned about dietary cholesterol is being de-emphasized in favor of simply limiting total fat, saturated fat, and trans fat in particular – and substituting unsaturated fats (including omega-3 fats).

Note: Persons with familial (genetic) hyper-cholesterolemia should limit cholesterol; and ideally follow a plant-based diet.

The liver usually cuts back its own cholesterol production in response to cholesterol in the diet. Many people can consume high-cholesterol foods without concern.

However, it is difficult to identify just who is at risk - the so-called 'hyper-responders'. Because over 50% of Americans have a BCL above ideal levels, it may be prudent to limit cholesterol intake to less than 300mg daily, as well as to adopt a heart-healthy diet.

This limitation still allows the inclusion of most foods that are regularly eaten – even the overly maligned egg.

Avocados (like all plant foods) contain no cholesterol. Their fats are mainly monounsaturated and can lower blood cholesterol.

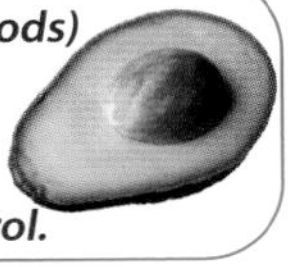

CHOLESTEROL COUNTER

Cholesterol is found only in foods of animal origin. Plant foods contain no cholesterol.

	Cholesterol mg
Meat - Average all types:	
Lean Meat, cooked, 120g	100
Fatty Meat, cooked, 120g	100
Fat, thick strip, 60g	40

Note: While lean meat and fat have similar amounts of cholesterol, choose lean meat to limit fat intake.

	Cholesterol mg
Chicken/Turkey, average, 120g	100
Organ Meats: Liver, fried, 4 oz	500
Brains, beef, pan fried, 3 oz	1700
Sausages: Frankfurter, 40g	25
Salami, 2 slices, 55g	40
Bacon: 3 slices, cooked, 30g	20
Fish: Fish fillets, average, ckd, 120g	70
Tuna/Salmon, canned, 100g	50
Scallops, 9 medium, 3 oz	30
Prawns, raw, 100g	110
Oysters, raw, 6 medium, 85g	45
Crayfish, Crab, cooked, 100g	70
Eggs (Chicken), 1 large	210
1 medium	180
Egg White, *Scramblers*	0
Milk/Yoghurt: Whole, 1 cup, 250ml	30
Light/low-fat Milk (1%), 1 cup	10
Skim/Non-fat, 1 cup	10
Soy Milk, Tofu, Tempeh	0
Cheese: Natural/Hard/Cream, 30g	30
Cottage, low-fat, 2 Tbsp, 40g	5
Cream Cheese, 30g	25
Fats: Butter, 1 Tbsp, 20g	45
Margarine, Oils (vegetable)	0
Mayonnaise, 1 Tbsp	10
Cream: Heavy, whipping, 2 Tbsp, 40g	40
Light/Sour, 2 Tbsp	10
Ice Cream: Full-fat (10-11%), 100ml/50g	20
Low-fat (less than 4%), 50g	5
Fruit, Vegetables, Avocados	0
Nuts, Seeds, Grains	0
Coffee, Tea, Beer, Wine	0

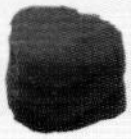
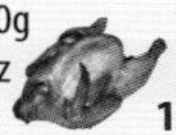
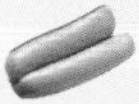
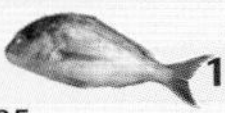

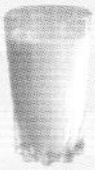
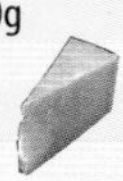
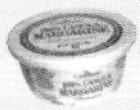
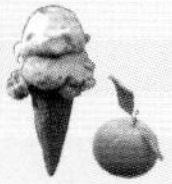

For Comprehensive Food Listings ~ see www.CalorieKing.com

DIETARY TIPS TO LOWER BLOOD CHOLESTEROL

1. **Maintain a healthy weight.**
If overweight, lose weight with a sensible, low-fat meal plan and daily exercise.

2. **Reduce saturated fat intake by:**

(a) eating less dairy fat. Choose low-fat or fat-reduced milk, yogurt, soy drinks, and cheese.

(b) replacing saturated fats with whole foods rich in monounsaturated and polyunsaturated fats – such as fish, nuts, seeds, avocado and olives.

Limit vegetable oils but choose mainly extra virgin olive oil and black seed oil. Avoid frying which can oxidize fats and harm health.

(c) eating less fat from meat and poultry. Choose lean cuts of meat and skinless chicken. Go easy on lunch meats, salami and fatty sausages.

Eat more fish, particularly higher fat fish such as salmon, herring, albacore tuna and sardines. They contain omega-3 fats that benefit the heart and all body cells.

(d) eating less saturated and trans fats from baked and fried fast-foods. Avoid deep-fried foods. Avoid donuts, cakes, pastries and cookies unless made with healthier fats and oils.

3. **Increase your soluble fiber intake.**
Foods rich in soluble fiber include beans, lentils, chickpeas, hummus, nuts, seeds, psyllium-seed husks and psyllium-fiber supplements. Oat bran, rice bran and barley are also good sources; as are fruit, vegetables, nopales (cactus leaves) and avocados. *(See Fiber Guide - Page 264-269)*

4. **Eat more soy bean foods such as:**
soy drinks, tofu, tempeh (cultured soy beans), soy flour, soy vegetarian foods and edamame (fresh green soybeans).

Soy protein in place of animal protein can significantly decrease high blood cholesterol levels, LDL cholesterol and blood triglycerides while maintaining 'good' HDL cholesterol.

5. **Eat more fruit, vegetables, and whole grains** in place of high-fat foods. Aim for 2 fruits and 5 servings of vegetables per day. They also contain valuable antioxidants. The fat of avocados (and most nuts) is mainly unsaturated and can lower blood cholesterol levels.

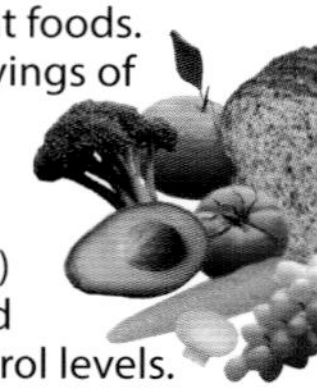

6. **Limit cholesterol to 300mg per day.**
(Extra Notes ~ See Previous Page)

7. **Avoid brewed unfiltered coffee**
(espresso; plunger-style). Several cups per day may raise blood cholesterol. Filtered coffee is fine.

8. **Spread your food intake over the day.**
Have 3-4 smaller meals per day rather than just 1-2 very large meals. Nibbling, versus gorging, favors lower blood cholesterol.
Eat most food during the day and less at night.

ALCOHOL – WINE

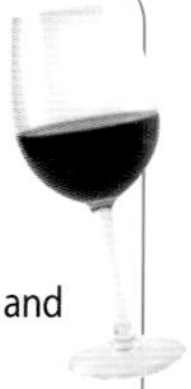

Alcohol is a mixed bag. Moderate amounts of 1-2 drinks daily appear to reduce the risk of heart attack and ischemic stroke in older persons.

However, larger amounts increase the risk of high blood pressure, obesity, heart failure and hemorrhagic stroke, and can aggravate hypertriglyceridemia: as well as many other health hazards. *(See Alcohol Guide – Page 23)*

The speculative benefits of moderate alcohol intake have been overstated in the media.
The overriding harmful effects of excess alcohol do not allow its recommendation for any aspects of health promotion.

Fruit, Vegetables & Tea Also Protect:

Red wine and red grapes (more so than white) contain antioxidants which may help protect cholesterol in the blood from becoming oxidized.

Most fruits, vegetables, whole-grains, nuts and tea also contain protective antioxidants.

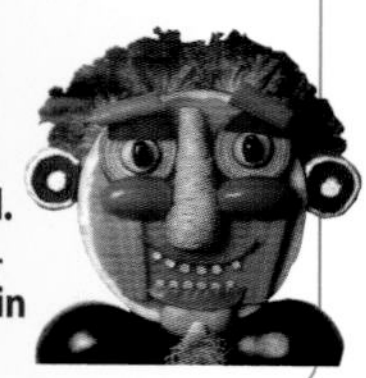

Fats in the diet affect more than blood cholesterol levels. They can also strongly influence blood clot formation and thrombosis, as well as blood flow and ultimate oxygen delivery to body parts and organs. While advanced atherosclerosis can impede blood flow to the heart and other organs, it is thrombosis (complete blockage by blood clots) or arterial spasm which commonly results in a heart attack or stroke.

Plant and fish oils rich in omega-3 fats lessen the risk of blood clots, thrombus formation, and artery spasm by reducing platelet stickiness and adhesion to artery walls. This also reduces inflammation of the artery wall lining. This in turn reduces the risk of atherosclerotic plaque becoming unstable and reactive.

Omega-3 fats also improve blood flow by reducing blood viscosity and increasing the flexibility of red blood cells that need to flex and twist on themselves in order to squeeze through tiny narrow capillaries often half their diameter.

A diet high in saturated fats (longer chain) has the opposite effect by stiffening red blood cell membranes and increasing blood viscosity, thereby hindering blood flow.

Stiff red blood cells may also form aggregates that resemble coin stacks. In narrow blood vessels, this further impedes blood flow and impairs oxygen release through the much-lessened surface area of red blood cell membranes exposed to blood.

Note: Smoking, lack of exercise, and stress can have similar adverse effects on thrombosis, red blood cell flexibility, and blood flow.

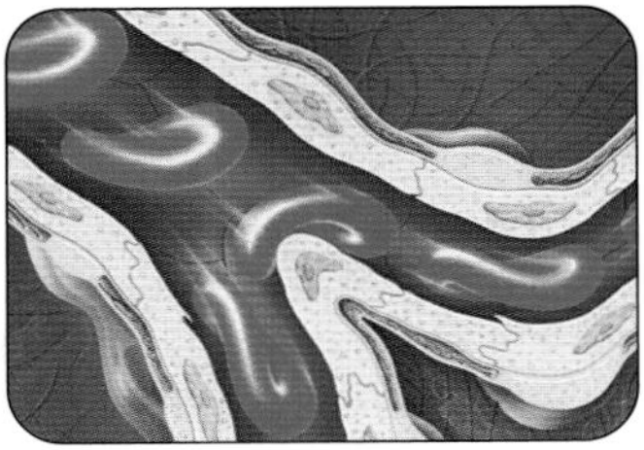

▲ *Picture of Healthy Blood Flow*

Flexible red blood cells twist and slide through tiny capillaries - often half the diameter of red blood cells.

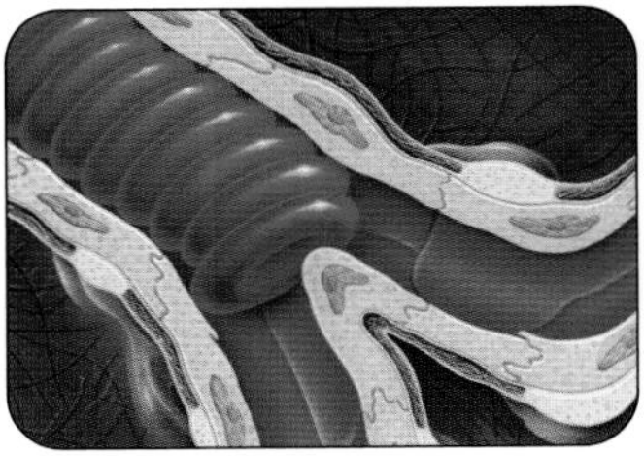

▲ *A Not-So-Healthy Picture!*

Red blood cells have lost their flexibility and ability to twist and slip through capillaries. They are stacked up, thereby impeding blood flow.

A diet high in saturated fats can contribute to this picture - as can smoking, lack of exercise, and stress.

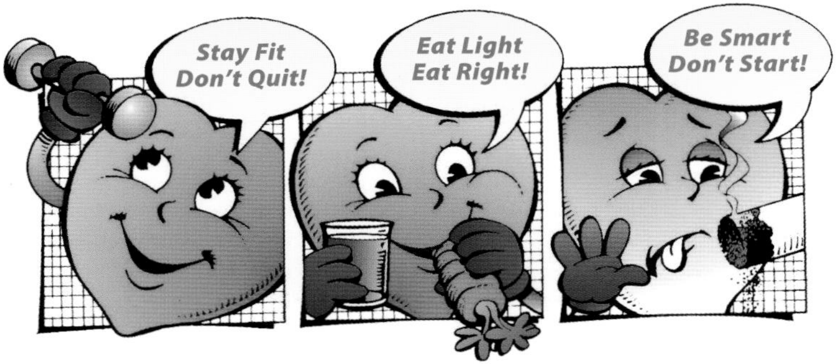
Stay Fit
Don't Quit!
Eat Light
Eat Right!
Be Smart
Don't Start!

Fiber Guide

Introduction

Fiber

Fiber is the general term for those parts of plant food that we cannot digest (although bacteria in the large bowel partly digests fiber through fermentation). It is not found in foods of animal origin (meats, dairy products).

Fiber promotes intestinal health, bowel regularity, can benefit diabetes and blood cholesterol levels, and may help prevent colon cancer. High-fiber foods also assist weight control.

Most Americans don't eat enough fiber – less than 20 grams/day – instead of a healthier 25 to 35 grams/day.

A fiber-rich diet assists the growth of friendly gut microbes that can benefit our metabolism, weight and blood glucose levels – as well as hunger, mood and our immune system.

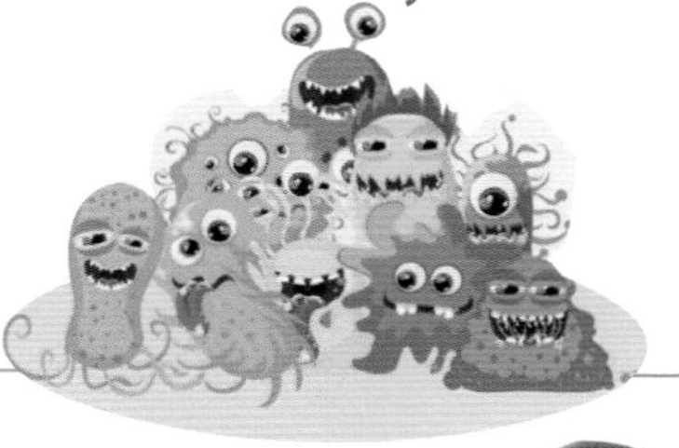

Types of Fiber

Plant foods contain a mixture of different fibers in varying proportions. Insoluble and soluble fiber categories are based on their solubility in water. All types of fiber are beneficial to the body.

- Insoluble fibers (cellulose, hemi-celluloses, lignin) make up the structural parts of plant cell walls.

  Best food sources are wheat bran, corn bran, rice bran, wholegrain cereals and breads, beans and peas, nuts, seeds, and the skins of fruits and vegetables.

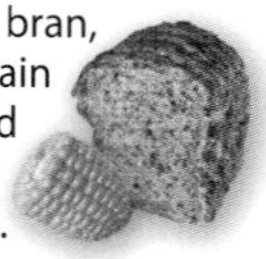

These fibers absorb many times their own weight in water. They create a soft bulk and hasten the passage of waste products through the intestines.

They promote bowel regularity, and aid in the prevention and treatment of uncomplicated forms of **constipation, diverticulosis and hemorrhoids.**

The risk of colon cancer may also be reduced by fiber's diluting effect on potentially harmful substances.

- Soluble fibers **(pectin, gums, mucilages)** are found mainly within plant cells, soy milk (whole bean) and products.

Best Sources of Soluble Fiber:

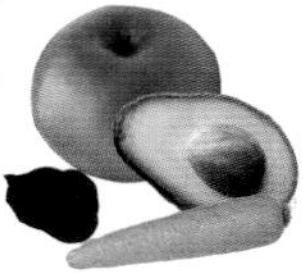

Fruits and vegetables, oat bran, barley, beans and peas, prunes, psyllium and flax seed.

These fibers form a gel which slows both stomach emptying and the absorption of sugars from the intestines. **This helps to control blood sugar levels.**

Weight control is also aided by the slower emptying of the stomach and the feeling of **fullness provided by soluble fiber.**

Soluble fiber can also lower blood cholesterol by binding bile acids and excreting them. More body cholesterol must then be broken down to supply bile acids for emulsification of dietary fats. **Rice bran, while not high in soluble fiber, can also lower blood cholesterol.**

- Resistant starch is that part of starchy foods (approx. 10%) which is tightly bound by fiber and resists normal digestion. Friendly bacteria in the large bowel ferment and change the resistant starch into short-chain fatty acids, which are important to bowel health and may protect against colon cancer.

Starchy foods include bread, cereals, rice, pasta, potatoes and legumes.

Fiber & Weight Control

Fiber can assist weight control in several ways. Fiber-rich foods such as fresh fruit and vegetables, potatoes and wholegrain bread contain few calories for their large volume (due to their low-fat, high-water content).

Their bulk fills the stomach and satisfies the appetite much sooner than fiber-depleted foods. The extra chewing time also contributes to satiety, and gives the stomach time to register a feeling of fullness. Excessive calories are less likely to be consumed.

Fiber-depleted foods and drinks are more concentrated in calories; e.g. fats, sugar, candy, soft drinks, fruit juices, alcohol. They require little or no chewing. Large amounts with excessive calories can be consumed before the appetite is satisfied.

Example: Whereas one fresh apple might satisfy the appetite, an apple juice drink with the equivalent sugars and calories of 2-3 apples only minimally satisfies the appetite. (See illustration below.)

High-fiber foods fill the stomach. Fewer calories are consumed.

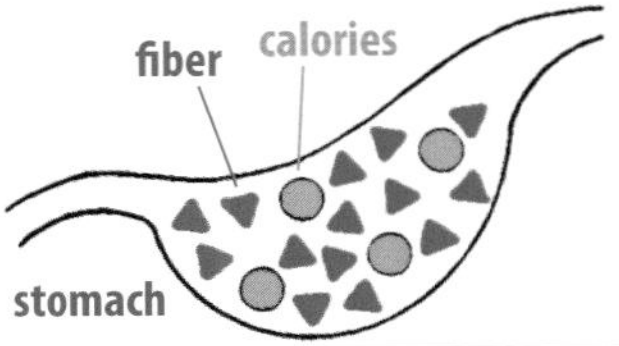

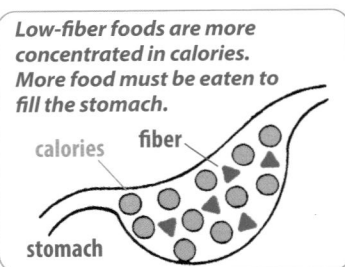

Low-fiber foods are more concentrated in calories. More food must be eaten to fill the stomach.

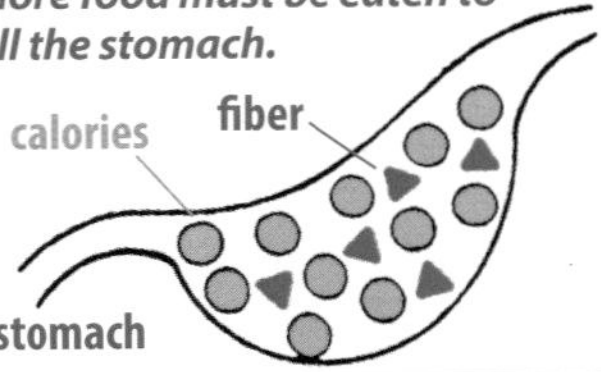

EFFECTS OF REMOVING FIBER FROM FOOD

2-3 pieces of fresh fruit produces 1 glass of fruit juice. The removal of fiber concentrates the sugars and calories.

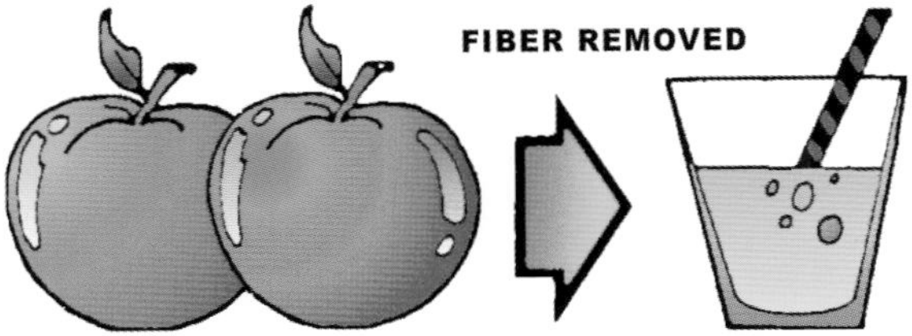

FRESH FRUIT	(Comparison)	FRUIT JUICE
Higher Fiber	↔	Negligible Fiber
Low Calorie Density	↔	High Calorie Density
Long Eating Time	↔	No Eating Time (Drink)
Satisfies Hunger	↔	Does Not Satisfy Hunger
Sugars Slowly Absorbed	↔	Sugars More Quickly Absorbed
Less Insulin Required	↔	More Insulin Required
Supports Gut Microbes	↔	Fewer Benefits to Microbes

Constipation

Constipation can reasonably be defined as a failure to have a bowel movement at least every second day – and just as importantly, without straining or pain.

Typically, constipated stools are too hard, too narrow and too small.

The **main cause** is simply a lack of dietary fiber. Other contributing factors include insufficient fluids, too little exercise, emotional stress, gastrointestinal disease, lack of proper dentition to chew high-fiber foods, and some medications (e.g. some antacids, antidepressants, pain medications).

Note: Check with your doctor to rule out any underlying medical problem – especially if you have a change in bowel habits in middle-age or later years.

DESIRABLE FIBER INTAKE

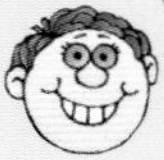

Adults: 25-35gm per day
Children (under 18): Age + 5gm
Example: 6-year old (6 + 5)= 11gm

SAMPLE FOOD QUANTITIES
For 35 Grams of Fiber/Day

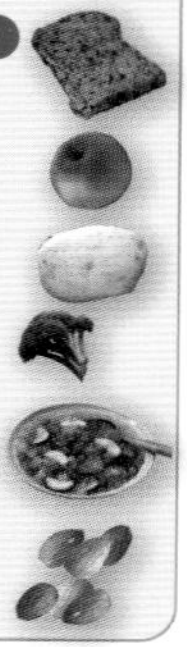

		Fiber
	Breakfast Cereal (higher-fiber)	5g
plus	4 slices wholegrain Bread	6g
plus	3 servings fresh Fruit	9g
plus	1 medium Potato (w. skin)	4g
or	1 cup Brown Rice	
or	½ cup wholegrain Pasta	
plus	3-4 servings Veggies/Salad	6g
plus	1 cup Bean Soup	5g
or	¼ cup Baked/Soy Beans	
or	½ cup Corn/Peas/Lentils	
or	1¼ oz Almonds (natural)	
or	3 medium Figs	

HINTS TO INCREASE FIBER AND AVOID CONSTIPATION

1. **Breakfast is an important** contributor to daily fiber intake. Eat high-fiber breakfast cereals (bran-based cereals, oatmeal etc.). Add 1-2 tablespoons of unprocessed bran.

   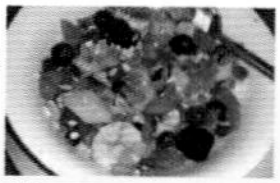

   Dried fruits, chopped nuts, soy grits, and seeds are also excellent additions to cereals.

   Note: A gradual increase in fiber will prevent bloating, gas or pain. People intolerant to bran may benefit from psyllium-based fiber supplements and cereals.
2. **Drink adequate water daily.** Fiber works by absorbing many times its own weight in water.
3. **Eat wholegrain breads,** or fiber-enriched breads. They have over double the fiber of regular white bread.

   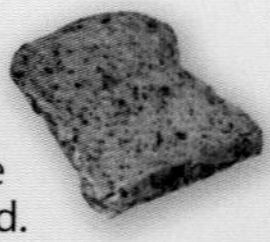
4. **Enjoy fruit as fresh fruit** with skin rather than as fruit juice. Enjoy wholegrain pasta, barley, brown rice, nuts and seeds.
5. **Eat more vegetables,** salads and legumes – especially cooked beans, lentils, potatoes with skins, avocado, broccoli, brussels sprouts, cabbage, carrots, celery, and peas.

   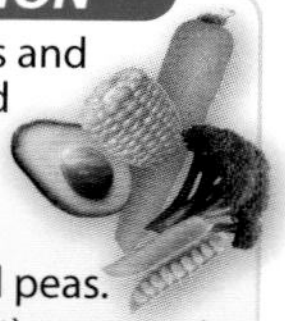
6. **Add bran** (barley/rice/wheat) or soy grits to soups, casseroles, yogurt, desserts, cookies, cakes. Also use whole-meal flour or soy flour in place of white flour. Use nuts, seeds, and ground linseed.
7. **Snack** on fresh or dried fruits, carrot or celery sticks, popcorn, nuts or seeds, wholegrain crackers, high-fiber bars (low-fat). Limit amounts if overweight.
8. **Exercise regularly** to strengthen abdominal muscles and stimulate the gut. Keep up water intake, especially in warm weather.
9. **Avoid** indiscriminate and regular use of harsh laxatives. They can overstimulate the intestinal muscles and may make normal bowel activity impossible. It may take several weeks to restore normal bowel function.

FOODS WITH ZERO FIBER

- **Dairy Products (Milk, Cheese, etc.)**
- **Meats, Poultry, Fish, Eggs**
- **Fats/Oils, Sugar/Syrups**

(Only foods of plant origin contain fiber.)

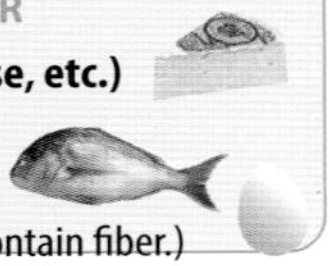

Fiber ~ Fiber (grams)

Breakfast Cereals

	Fiber
General Mills:	
Basic 4, 1 cup, 2 oz	3
Cheerios (Honey Nut; Multigrain), 1⅓ cups, 1 oz	4
Chex, Rice, cup	2
Cinnamon Toast Crunch, 1 cup, 1.4 oz	2
Fiber One, Original Bran, ⅔ cups, 1.4 oz	18
Kix, 1½ cups, 1.4 oz	3
Lucky Charms, 1 cup, 1.3 oz	2
Oatmeal Crisp Almond, 1 cup, 2 oz	6
Raisin Nut Bran, ¾ cup, 1.7 oz	6
Total, Whole Grain, 0.875 oz	2
Trix, 1¼ cups, 1.4 oz	1
Wheat Chex, 1 cup, 2 oz	8
Wheaties, 1 cup, 1.26 oz	4
Kellogg's:	
All-Bran, Buds, ½ cup, 1.58 oz	17
Corn Flakes, 1½ cups, 1.4 oz	1
Frosted Flakes, 1 cuo, 1.4 oz	0.5
Frosted Mini Wheats, 2 oz	6
Krave, Chocolate, 1 pkg, 1.87 oz	3
Raisin Bran, 1 cup, 2 oz	7
Rice Krispies, 1½ cups, 1.4 oz	0
Special K, 1 cup, 1.4 oz	3
Kashi: Organic	
7 Whole Grain Puffs, 1½ cups, 1.4 oz	4
7 Whole Grain Flakes, 1¼ cups, 2.2 oz	7
Blueberry Clusters, 1 cup, 1.9 oz	3
GO: Rise, Original, 1¼ cuos, 2 oz	13
Go Defy, Crunch, ¾ cup, 1.9 oz	9
Honey Toasted Oat, 1 cup, 1.4 oz	5
Strawberry Fields, 1 cup, 1.95 oz	3
Warm Cinnamon Oat, 1 cup, 1.4 oz	5
Whole Wheat Biscuits, 31 pieces, 2.1 oz	7

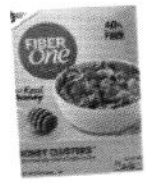

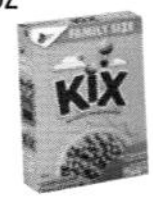

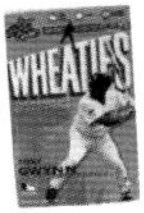

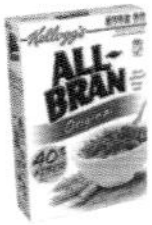

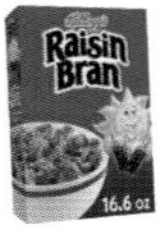

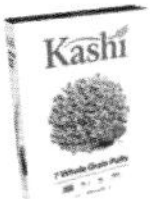

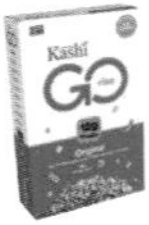

Breakfast Cereals (Cont)

	Fiber
Quaker:	
Corn Crunch, 1 cup, 1.3 oz	5
Life, Original, 1 cup, 1.45 oz	3
Oatmeal Squares, Cinnamon, 1 cup, 1.9 oz	5
Muesli, Raisin Date Almond, ½ cup, 1.8 oz	5
Multigrain Flakes, Honey Vanilla, ¾ cup, 2.2 oz	3
Quisp, 1¼ cups, 1.45 oz	0.5
Real Medleys, Multigrain, Cherry, ¾ cup, 1.9 oz	4
Simply Granola, Oats, Honey, Raisins & Alm., 2.4 oz	7
Post:	
Alpha Bits, 1 cup, 1 oz	2
Better Oats, Maple & Br. Sugar, 1 oz pouch	3
Bran Flakes, 1 cup, 1.34 oz	7
Dunkin', Mocha Latte, 1⅓ cups, 1.34 oz	0
Grape Nuts, Original, ½ cup, 2 oz	7
Great Grains, Blueberry Morning, 1 cup, 2 oz	4
Honey Bunches of Oats, Vanilla, 1 cup, 0.95 oz	4
Raisin Bran, 1¼ cups, 2.1 oz	9
Shredded Wheat, Original, Spoon, 1⅓ cups, 2 oz	8

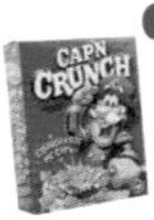

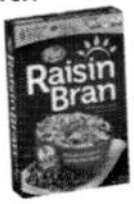

Brans & Supplements, Metamucil

	Fiber
Oat Bran: 1 Tbsp (level)	1
⅓ cup, (5⅓ Tbsp), 1 oz	5
Rice Bran, raw. ⅓ cup, 1 oz	6
Wheat Bran, Unprocessed:	
Raw, 1 Tbsp	1.5
2 Tbsp (level), ¼ oz	3
¼ cup, (4 Tbsp), ½ oz	6
Wheat Germ, Raw, ¼ cup, 1 oz	4
Psyllium Seed Husks, 2 Tbsp	8
Fibersure, 1 heaping tsp	5
Metamucil: Orange, 1 rnd Tbsp, 11g	3
Fiber Wafers (2)	6

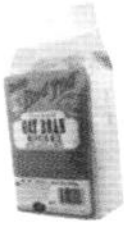
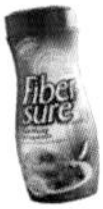

Hot Cereals, Oatmeal

	Fiber
Bulgur (Cracked Wheat), ckd, 1 cup	8
Corn/Hominy Grits, dry, 3 Tbsp, 1 oz	0.5
Cream of Wheat, cooked, 1 oz	1
Oatmeal, cooked ⅔ cup	3

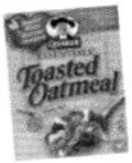

Breads & Crackers

	Fiber
Bread: White, 1 slice, 1 oz	0.6
Whole-wheat, 1 slice, 1 oz	1.5
Wholegrain, 1 slice, 1 oz	2
Rye, Pumpernickel, 1 oz	1.5
Bagel/Roll/Bun, 1 medium, 2 oz	1.5
Pita, whole wheat, 6.5" pocket	4.5
Crackers: Graham, average, 2	0.4
Saltine, 4 crackers	0.4
Crispbreads, average, 2	4
Matzo, 1 board, 1 oz	1
Rice Cakes, average, 1 cake	0.3
Tortilla: Regular, 6"	0.5
Whole-wheat, 6"	1.3

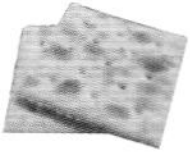

Barley, Pasta, Rice & Flours

	Fiber
Barley, pearled, raw, 1/4 cup, 1.7 oz	8
Rice:	
White, cooked, 1 cup	0.6
Brown, cooked, 1 cup	3.5
Rice-A-Roni, average, 1 cup, prepared	1.5
Spaghetti/Noodles: Cooked, 1 cup	2
Whole-Wheat, cooked, 1 cup	4
Flour: Wheat, All-purpose, 1 cup, 4.5 oz	3.5
Whole-Wheat, 1 cup, 4.5 oz	15
Cornmeal, stone ground, 1 cup, 4.5 oz	13
Carob Flour, 1 cup, 3.5 oz	41
Hemp Wholemeal Flour, 1 cup, 3.5 oz	41
Rye Flour, 1 cup, 3.5 oz	15
Soy Flour: Defatted, 1 cup, 3.5 oz	17
Full-fat, raw, 1 cup, 3 oz	8
Soy Meal, defatted, 1 cup, 4.5 oz	14

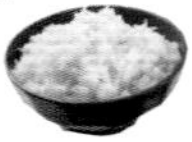
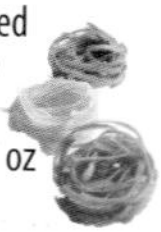
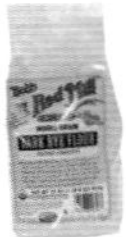

Frozen Entrees & Dinners

	Fiber
***Average All Brands**: Per Serving*	
Beans/Chili base, average	6-10
Potato/Pasta base, average	4-6
Vegetable base, average	3
Meat/Chicken base, average	2-3
Pizzas, 1/4 large, average	3
Vegetarian Soy Burgers, 1 pattie	4

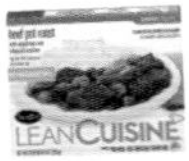

Soups

	Fiber
Chicken Noodle, 1 cup	0.5
Tomato Soup, average, 1 cup	0.5
Vegetable Soup, average, 1 cup	3
***Health Valley:** Per 1 Cup*	
Chicken & Rice	1
Minestrone	6
Split Pea	13
Tomato	5
Vegetable	4
Progresso, Tomato	6

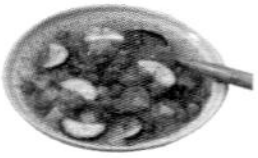
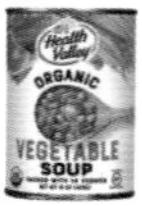

Fast Foods & Restaurants

	Fiber
Hamburgers: Small, average	1.5
Large/Whopper, average	2.5
Hot Dog, Regular	1.5
French Fries: Small serving, 2.5 oz	2.5
Regular/Medium, 3.5 oz	3.5
Chicken Nuggets, 6 pack	0.5
Chicken Sandwich, average	2
Taco, average	4
Sundaes, Shakes, Soft Drinks	0
Arby's, Classic Roast Beef Sandwich	2
Burger King: Whopper	2
Impossible Whopper	4
Del Taco, Beyond 8 Layer Burrito	9
Denny's: House Salad, no dressing	3
Bacon Avocado Cheeseburger	5
Club Sandwich	8
Super Bird Sandwich	2
Domino's: 12" Thin Crust, 1 slice	0.5
12" Handmade Pan Crust, 1 slice	0.5
12" Deluxe, Hand Tossed, 1 slice	1
McDonald's: Big Mac	3
Hamburger	1
Egg McMuffin	2
Quarter Pounder with Cheese	2
***Pizza Hut:** Per 1 Slice, Medium*	
Original Pan Pizza: Cheese, Pepp.	2
Supreme	2
Thin 'n Crispy, Supreme	2
Hand-Tossed, average all varieties	2
Subway: 6" 9 Grain Honey Oat Roll	4
6" 9 Grain Wheat Roll	4
Habanero Wrap	2
Taco Bell: Bean Burrito, vegan	11
Power Menu Bowl, Veggie	10

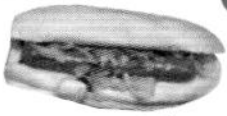
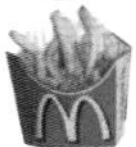
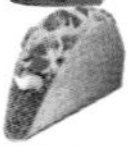
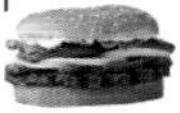
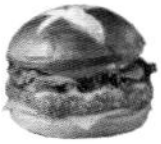
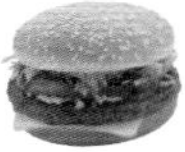
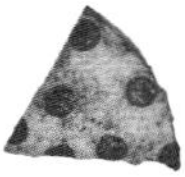
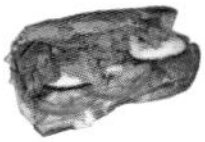

Cakes, Cookies, Snack Bars

	Fiber
Apple/Fruit Pie, 1 serving, 4 oz	2
Cake: With plain flour, 1 serving, 3.4 oz	1.5
With whole-wheat flour, 1 serving	3
Carrot Cake, 4 oz	4
Cookies, oatmeal, (3 small/1 large)	1
Donuts, medium, 1.7 oz	0.7
Fruit Cake, 1 serving, 1.5 oz	2
Fig Bars, 1 cookie, 0.5 oz	0.7
Muffins, Oat Bran (2 small, 1 large), 4 oz	5
Granola Bars, average, 1 bar	2
Atkins Advantage Bars, av.	7
Clif Bars, 2.5 oz	4
Fiber One (Gen. Mills):	
Oats & Chocolate, 0.8 oz	9
Other Bars, 0.8oz	6
Fiber Plus, Chewy, 1.27 oz	9
Health Valley, Cereal Bars	0.5
Luna Bars, avg., 1.7 oz	3
Special K, Chocolate Protein Meal Bar, 1.6 oz	3

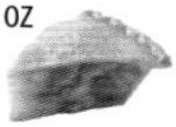
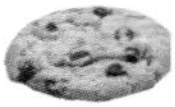
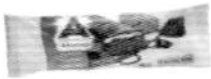
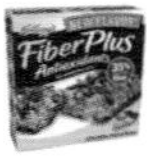

Chocolate, Chips, Popcorn

Food	Fiber
Cheese Balls/Curls/Twists	1
Chocolate, Hard Candy, 1 oz	0
Chocolate with nuts/fruit, 2 oz bar	1.5
Mars Bar, 1.8 oz	1
Potato Chips; corn chips, 1 oz	1
Popcorn, 3 cups	3
Pretzels, Twists (6)	1

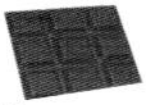

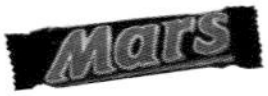

Nuts, Seeds

Food	Fiber
Almonds: Natural, 25 nuts, 1 oz	3.5
Blanched (skins removed), 1 oz	3
Cashews, Filberts, Pecans, 1 oz	1.7
Hepm Seeds, 3 Tbsp, 1 oz	9
Peanuts, Mixed Nuts, Coconut, 1 oz	2.5
Peanut Butter, 2 Tbsp, 1 oz	2
Pistachio Nuts, dried, shelled, 1 oz	3
Walnuts, Black/English, dried, 1 oz	2
Seeds: Amaranth, 2½ Tbsp, 1 oz	3.5
Flax Seeds, 3 Tbsp, 1 oz	7
Psyllium Seed Husks, 5 Tbsp, 1 oz	20
Quinoa Seeds, 3 Tbsp, 1 oz	1.7
Sesame Seeds, whole, 1 oz	3.4
Sesame Butter/Tahini, 2 Tbsp, 1.1 oz	1.4
Sunflower Kernels, ¼ cup, 1 oz	3.8

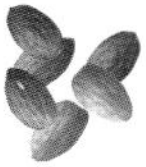

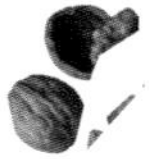

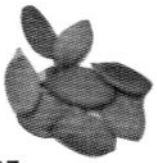

Fruit – Fresh

Food	Fiber
Apples: 1 medium, 5½ oz (whole)	
with skin + core	3.7
with skin, no core	3.2
without skin, no core	1.7
Apricots, 2 medium, 4 oz	1.5
Avocado, average, ½ medium	6
Banana, 1 medium, 6 oz (w. skin)	3
Blueberries, raw, ½ cup, 2.5 oz	1.7
Cherries, sweet, raw, 8 fruits, 1.6 oz	1
Grapefruit, average, ½ fruit, 10 oz	1.4
Grapes, 1 medium bunch, seedless, 7 oz	2
Kiwifruit, 1 medium, 2.7 oz	2.3
Mango, 1 medium, 11 oz (whole)	1.6
Melons, Cantaloupe, 4 oz (edible)	1
Nectarine, 1 medium, 4 oz	1.9
Olives, average all types, 7 jumbo, 2 oz	1.5
Oranges, 1 medium (7-8 oz w. skin)	
5½ oz (peeled)	3.8
Passionfruit, 2 medium, 2.5 oz	5
Peaches, 1 large, 6 oz	2
Pears, raw, 1 medium, 6 oz	4.5
Pineapple, 1 slice, 3 oz	1.2
Plums, 2 medium, 6 oz	1.8
Strawberries, 6 medium/3 large, 2 oz	1
Watermelon, 4 oz (edible)	0.5

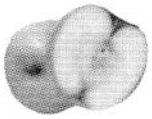

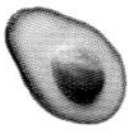

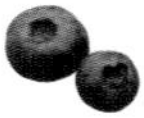

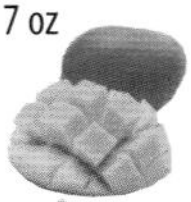

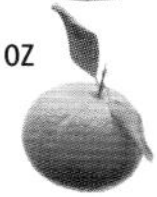

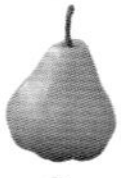

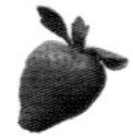

Fruit – Dried, Juice

Food	Fiber
Dried Fruit: Apricots, 8 halves, 1 oz	2.2
Dates (3 med); Raisins (2 Tbsp), 1 oz	1.5
Figs, 3 medium, 1½ oz	5
Prunes, 4 medium, 1 oz	2
Fruit Juice: Orange/Apple etc, 1 glass	<0.5
Prune Juice, 5 oz	1.4
Carrot Juice, 8 oz	1.8

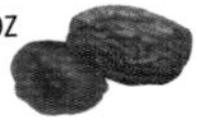

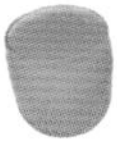

Vegetables

Food	Fiber
Asparagus, 4 medium spears	1.3
Bean Sprouts, ½ cup, 2 oz	1
Beans: Snap/Green, ½ cup, 2 oz	2
Baked Beans in Tom Sce, ½ c, 4.5 oz	5
Dried Beans, cooked, average, ½ cup	7
Beets, ckd, slices, ½ cup, 3 oz	1.7
Broccoli, cooked, ½ cup, 3 oz	2.4
Brussels Sprouts, ckd, ½ cup, 3 oz	3.5
Cabbage: White, ckd, ½ cup, 2.5 oz	1
Red, ckd, ½ cup, 2.5 oz	2
Carrots, 1 medium (7½"), ½ cup, 3 oz	2.5
Cauliflower, cooked, 3 flowerets, 2 oz	1.5
Celery, raw, diced, 1 cup, 3.5 oz	1.6
Chickpeas (Garbanzos), ckd, ½ c., 3 oz	6.5
Corn: Kernels, cooked, ½ cup, 2½ oz	2.5
Corn on the Cob, 1 ear, 5 oz	4
Cucumber/Lettuce/Mushrooms, 2 oz	0.5
Eggplant, raw, sliced, ½ cup, 1.5 oz	2
Lentils, cooked, ½ cup, 3.5 oz	8
Mixed Vegetables, frozen, cooked, ½ cup	3
Onions: Raw, 1 medium, 4 oz	1.5
Spring Onions, chop., ¼ cup, 1 oz	0.7
Peas: Green, raw, ½ cup, 2.5 oz	3.7
Cowpeas (Black-eyed), ckd, ½ cup	10
Split Peas, cooked, ½ cup, 3.5 oz	8
Peppers, sweet, raw, 1 large, 6 oz	3
Potatoes: 1 medium, with skin, 5 oz	4
1 medium, without skin	2.5
½ cup mashed, 3.5 oz	1.5
French Fries, small, 2.6 oz	3
Spinach, cooked, ½ cup, 3 oz	2.2
Squash: Summer, cooked, ½ cup, 3 oz	2.5
Winter, cooked, ½ cup, 3.5 oz	2.4
Tomatoes: 1 medium, 4.5 oz	1.5
Tomato Sauce, 1 cup	0.3
Soybean Products: Miso, ½ c., 5 oz	7.4
Tempeh, cooked, 1 piece, 3 oz	2
Tofu, ½ cup, 4.4 oz	0.4

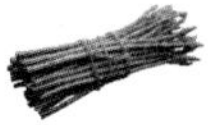

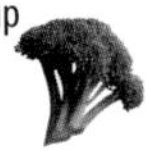

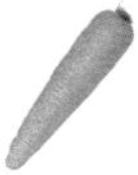

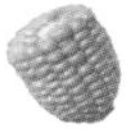

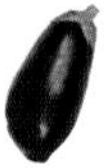

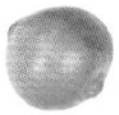

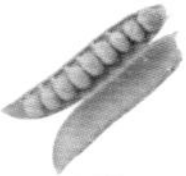

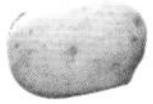

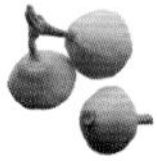

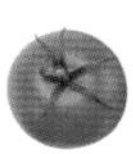

Salads:

Food	Fiber
Side Salad, average	1
Bean Salad, ½ cup	5
Coleslaw, ½ cup	1
Potato Salad, ½ cup	2

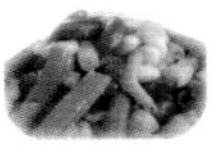

Protein Guide

General Notes

- **Protein has many important body functions.** It builds and repairs muscle, and is the basis of our body's organs, hormones, enzymes, and antibodies to fight infection.
- **Protein is also an emergency fuel** in the absence of sufficient carbohydrate and fats. For this reason, weight loss should be gradual so as to preserve protein levels in muscle, the heart and other body organs.
- **It is easy to obtain sufficient protein,** even if vegetarian. **Plant proteins are not inferior to animal proteins.** In fact, eating more soy and other plant proteins, and less animal protein, may help to build stronger bones and prevent osteoporosis, and may help to control blood cholesterol levels.
- **When changing to a vegetarian diet,** include legume beans (soy, chickpeas etc.), lentils, nuts, seeds, tofu, tempeh; as well as wholegrain cereals and flours. Also try nutritional yeast flakes, and plant-based meat substitutes (*Beyond Meat; Impossible* burgers). Dairy products (lower fat) and eggs can enhance nutrient intake.

Protein & Muscle

- Although muscles are built of protein, protein is not a special fuel for working muscle cells – carbohydrates and fats are.
- In fact, a diet high in protein (and fat) and low in carbohydrate can significantly reduce the performance of endurance sports athletes. **Carbohydrates** are the best fuel for muscles exercised for long periods.
- Any **extra protein** required by athletes and body-builders can easily be obtained from the extra food eaten to satisfy hunger and energy needs.
- Remember, **excessive protein** intake will not build bigger muscles. Any excess is converted and stored as fat. Excess protein can also strain the kidneys, which excrete the waste products of protein metabolism.

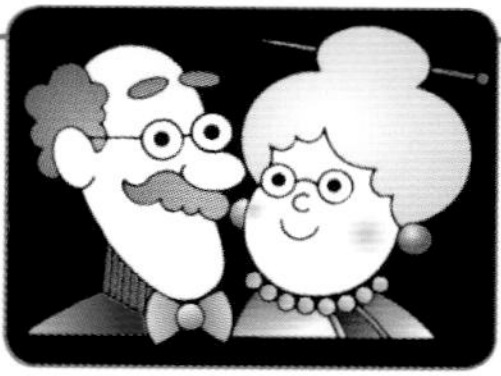

Elderly people (and dieters) must eat sufficient food to ensure adequate protein intake.

Inadequate protein leads to a drop in immune response with greater susceptibility to illness and infections. Muscle strength and muscle mass also drop.

Protein needs are easily met with sensible eating. Athletes who eat enough food for their energy needs can obtain sufficient protein.

RECOMMENDED DAILY PROTEIN INTAKE ~ HEALTHY RANGE ~

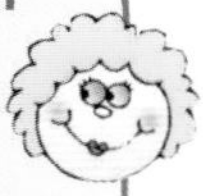

(Lower figure is RDA)

		PROTEIN
Children:	1-3 yrs	13g-26g
	4-8 yrs	19g-38g
	9-13 yrs	34g-64g
Males:	14-18 yrs	52g-120g
	19+	56g-120g
Females:	14+	46g-110g
Pregnancy:		71g-120g
Breastfeeding:		71g-120g

Note: On lower-calorie diets, aim for higher amounts of protein within the Healthy Range.

Pro ~ **Protein (grams)**

Meats, Sausages

	Pro
Bacon, 3 medium slices	6
Ground Beef Patty, lean, cooked, 3 oz	21
Ham: Luncheon, 2 slices, $1\frac{1}{2}$ oz	7
Roasted, 2 pieces, 3 oz	18
Lamb chop, broiled, 3 oz	22
Liver, cooked, 3 oz	23
Pastrami, 3 slices, $1\frac{3}{4}$ oz	10
Pork, cooked, lean, 3 oz	24
Roast Beef, lean, 2 slices, 3 oz	24
Sausages: Bologna, 2 sl., 2 oz	7
Braunschweiger, 2 sl., 2 oz	8
Pork link, thick, 2 oz	6
Frankfurter, $1\frac{1}{3}$ oz	5
Salami, hard, 3 slices, 1 oz	7
Steak: Average all cuts, lean (no fat)	
Small (4 oz raw/3 oz cooked)	23
Medium (6 oz raw/$4\frac{1}{4}$ oz cooked)	34
Large (10 oz raw/$7\frac{1}{4}$ oz cooked)	57

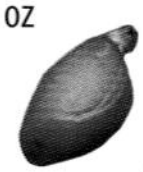
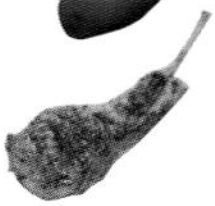
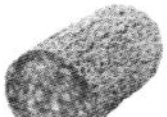
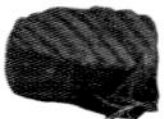

Meat Substitutes (Vegan)

	Pro
Beyond Meat: Beef/Burger, 4 oz	20
Sausages, 2 patties, 2 oz	11
Impossible, 4 oz Patty	19
Vegetarian Patties, av., 4 oz	13

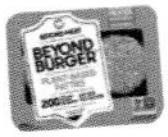

Chicken/Turkey: *Without Skin*

	Pro
Chicken, cooked: Breast, Roasted, 4 oz	36
Leg/Thigh,Roasted, 2 oz	14
$\frac{1}{2}$ Whole Chicken	60
Drumstick, Rstd, 1 med., 3 oz	13
Turkey: Light meat, cooked, 3 oz	28
Dark meat, lean, 3 oz	24

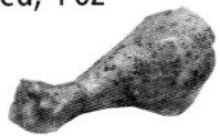

Fish

	Pro
Fresh Fish: *Per 4 oz, cooked*	
Cod, Flounder/Sole, Pollock	28
Catfish, Haddock, Halibut, M/Mahi	28
Ocean Perch, Swordfish, Orange Roughy	28
Canned Fish: Tuna, av., 3 oz	25
Salmon, pink, 3 oz	17
Salmon, red, 3 oz	17
Sardines, 3 whole (3"), $1\frac{1}{4}$ oz	9
Shellfish: Crabmeat, 3 oz	17.5
Clams, raw, 4 large/9 sml, 3 oz	11
Crayfish, cooked, 3 oz	20
Lobster, cooked, 3 oz	17
Oysters, raw, 6 medium, 3 oz	7
Scallops, 2 lge/5 small, 1 oz	5
Shrimp, raw, 6 large, $1\frac{1}{2}$ oz	8.5
Fish Products: Fish Sticks, 4 sticks	10
Fish Portions, in batter, 4 oz	13
Gefilte Fish, 1 medium ball, 2 oz	8

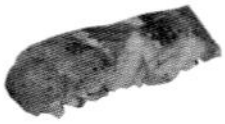
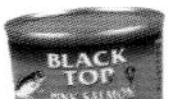

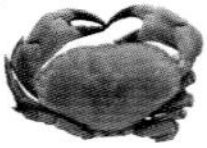
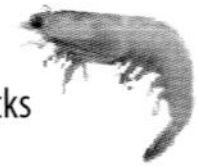

Eggs

	Pro
1 Large Egg, whole	6
Egg Yolk	3
Egg White	3
Omelet: Plain, 2 eggs	13
Ham & cheese	17
Egg Substitutes, (liquid):	
Egg Beaters, $\frac{1}{4}$ cup, 2 oz	4.5
Better 'n Eggs/Scramblers, $\frac{1}{4}$ cup, 2 oz	6

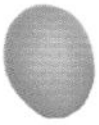
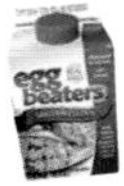

Milk, Yogurt, Ice Cream

	Pro
Milk: Whole: 2%, 1 cup	8
Low-Fat (1%); Fat-Free, 1 cup	8.5
Chocolate Milk, 1 cup	8
Thick Shake: Chocolate, 10 oz	9
Vanilla, 10 oz	11
Soymilk, (fortified), average, 1 cup	7
Soy Dream, Enriched, shelf-stable, 1 cup	7
Yogurt, average all brands:	
Plain, 6 oz	8
Fruit flavors, 6 oz	7
Chobani, Greek, Plain, 6 oz	14
Soy, fruit flavors, 6 oz	7
Ice Cream: Rich, $\frac{1}{2}$ cup	2
Regular, Vanilla, $\frac{1}{2}$ cup	2.5
Sherbet, $\frac{1}{2}$ cup	1
Custard, baked, $\frac{1}{2}$ cup	7

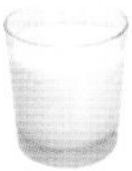
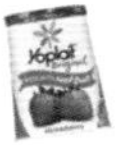

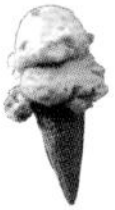

Cheese

	Pro
Hard Cheeses, average, 1 oz	7
Cottage Cheese, $\frac{1}{2}$ cup	13
Cream Cheese, avg., 1 oz	2
Ricotta, part skim, $\frac{1}{2}$ cup	14

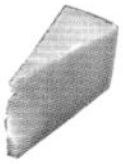

Bread, Bagels, Biscuits

	Pro
Bread: *With enriched flour*	
1 slice, 1 oz	2
4 thin slices, 4 oz	8
4 thick slices, 6 oz	12
Bagel, plain 2 oz	6
Biscuits, 1 oz	2
Pita Bread, 1 pita, $1\frac{1}{2}$ oz	4
Pumpernickel, 1 slice, 1 oz	3

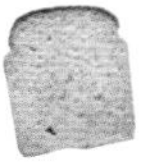
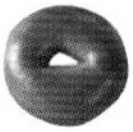

Infant/Baby Foods

	Pro
Infant Formula Milk:	
Enfamil/Gerber/Similac,	
Regular/Low Iron , 5 fl.oz	2.2
Isomil/Nursoy/ProSobee,	3
Baby Cereals: *Average all brands*	
Dry, 4 Tbsp, $\frac{1}{2}$ oz	1
Jars, with fruit, $4\frac{1}{2}$ oz	1

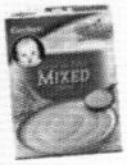

Breakfast Cereals

Hot Cereals ~ *Cooked:*

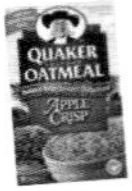

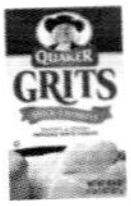

	Pro
Bulgur, cooked, 1 cup, 5 oz	9
Oatmeal: Reg., non-fortified, 1 cup	6
Instant, fortified, avg., 1 pkt	4
Quaker, all flavors, 1/2 cup	5
Corn/Hominy Grits: 1 cup	3
Quaker: Reg., 3 Tbsp, 1 oz	3
Instant White, 1 packet	2
Cream of Wheat, 1 cup	4

Brands ~ *Ready-To-Eat*

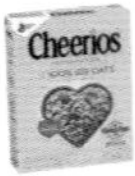

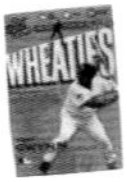

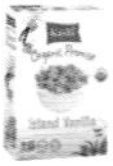

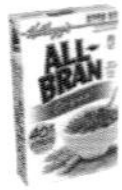

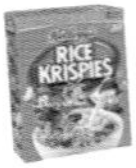

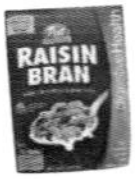

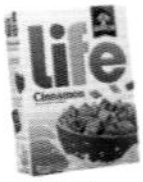

	Pro
***General Mills*:**	
Cheerios, Original, 1¼ cups, 1.4 oz	5
Chex, Corn, 1¼ cups, 1.4 oz	3
Kix, Original,1½ cupss, 1.4 oz	3
Lucky Charms, Original, 3/4 cup, 1 oz	2
Total, Raisin Bran, 1¼ cups, 2.3 oz	4
Wheaties, 1 cup, 1.3 oz	3
Kashi:	
7 Whole Grain Flakes, 1¼ cups, 2.1 oz	7
GO: Love, Chocolate Crunch, ¾ cup, 1.83 oz	10
Rise, Original, 1¼ cups, 2 oz	12
Honey Toasted Oat, 1 cup, 1.41 oz	4
Super Loops, 1 cup, 1.35 oz	4
Warm Cinnamon Oat, 1 cup, 1.41 oz	4
Whole Wheat Biscuits, Autumn, 2 oz	7
Kellogg's:	
All-Bran, Original, 1.83 oz pkg	6
Apple Jacks, Original, 1⅓ cups, 1.4 oz	2
Corn Flakes, 1½ cups, 1.41 oz	3
Product 19, 1 cup, 1 oz	3
Rice Krispies, 1 1/4 cup, 1.2 oz	2
Special K: Original, 1.27 oz	7
Granola, Touch of Honey, ½ cup, 1.83 oz	6
Prottein, 1⅓ cups, 2 oz	15
***Post*:**	
Grape Nuts, Original, 1/2 cup, 2 oz	6
Raisin Bran, 1¼ cups, 2.1 oz	5
***Quaker*:**	
Corn Bran Crunch, 1 cup, 1.35 oz	2
Life, Vanilla, 1 cup, 1.45 oz	4
Multigrain Flakes, Honey Vanilla, ¾ cup, 2.2 oz	7
Simply Granola, Oats, Honey & Alm., ⅔ cup, 2.2 oz	7

Brans & Wheatgerm

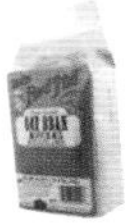

	Pro
Oat Bran, raw, 1 Tbsp	2
Rice Bran, raw, 2 Tbsp	1
Wheat Bran, unprocessed, 2 T.	1
Wheat Germ, 2 Tbsp, 1/2 oz	4

Grains & Flours, Yeast

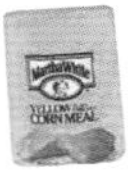

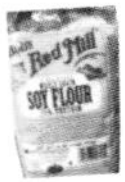

	Pro
Amaranth grain, cooked, 1/2 cup, 4.5 oz	5
Barley, 1/2 cup, 3.2 oz	12
Buckwheat Flour, Whole-groat, 1 cup	15
Carob Flour, 1 cup, 3.6 oz	5
Corn Flour, 1 cup, 4 oz	11
Corn Meal, 1 cup, 4 1/2 oz	8
Flour: White, 1 cup, 5.6 oz	9
Wholegrain, 1 cup, 4¼ oz	16
Hemp Wholemeal Flour, 1 cup, 3.5 oz	30
Millet, wholegrain, 1 cup, 3½ oz	12
Quinoa, raw, ⅓ cup, 1.5 oz	6
Rye Flour: Dark, 1 cup, 4 1/2 oz	18
Light, 1 cup, 3 1/2 oz	9
Soy Flour, full fat, 1 cup, 3 oz	29
Yeast: Brewers, 2 Tbsp, 1/2 oz	8
Nutritional Yeast Flakes *(Red Star),* 1 heaping Tbsp, 1/2 oz	8

Rice, Spaghetti, Macaroni

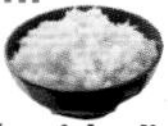

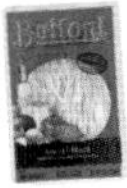

	Pro
Rice: Brown/White, average 1 cup cooked, 6 1/2 oz	5
Spaghetti/Macaroni/Noodles (enriched):	
Cooked, 1 cup, 4 1/2 oz	7
Canned: in Tomato Sce, 1/2 cup	2
with Meatballs, 1 cup, 8 oz	10
Macaroni & Cheese, 1 cup, 9 oz	8

Soups

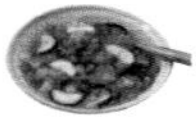

	Pro
With Noodles/Vegetables, 1 cup	3
With Meat/Beans/Peas, 1 cup	8

Fruit

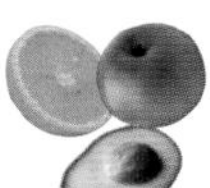

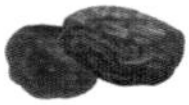

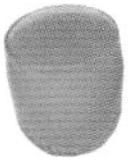

	Pro
Fresh/Canned:	
Average, all types, 1 medium/2 small fruit	1
Avocado, 1/2 medium	2
Dried Fruit: Apricots, 8 halves, 1 oz	1
Dates, 6 dates, 2 oz	1.5
Figs, 4 medium figs, 2 oz	2
Prunes, 5 medium, 1 1/2 oz	1
Raisins, 1 oz	1
Fruit Juice: Average, 1 cup	0.5
Prune Juice, 6 fl.oz	1
Tomato Juice, 1 cup, 8 fl.oz	1.5

Vegetables

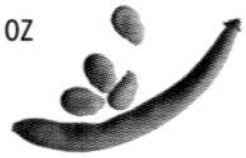
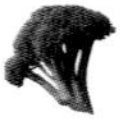
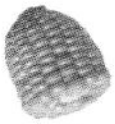
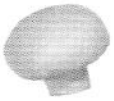
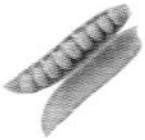
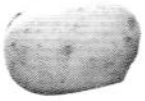
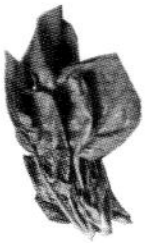

	Pro
Beans: Snap/green, 1/2 cup, 2 oz	1
Dried: Average all types, cooked, 1/2 cup	7
Baked Beans, 1/2 cup 4 1/2 oz	5
Bean Sprouts, mung, 1 c., 4 oz	3
Broccoli, raw, 1/2 cup, 1 1/2 oz	1.5
Cabbage; Cauliflower, raw, 1 c. 3 oz	1.5
Chickpeas, cooked, ½ cup, 3 oz	8
Corn: Raw, 1/2 cup kernels, 3 oz	2.5
1 ear trimmed to 3 1/2"	2
Lentils, cooked, 1/2 cup 3 1/2 oz	9
Mushrooms, raw, 1/2 c., sliced	1
Peas: Green, raw, 1/2 c., 2 1/2 oz	4
Split Peas, cooked, 1 cup, 7 oz	16
Potatoes: *Cooked:*	
1 medium, with skin, 5 oz	3.3
without skin, 4 oz	2.3
French Fries, small, 2.6 oz	2
Potato Salad, 1/2 cup, 4 oz	3.5
Pumpkin, 1/2 cup mashed, 4.3 oz	1
Seaweed, kelp, 1 oz	<1
Spinach, cooked, 1/2 cup, 3 oz	2.7
Squash, ckd, all types, 1/2 cup	1
Tomatoes, 1 medium, 4 1/2 oz	1
Vegetables, mixed, ckd, 1 cup	2.5
Soybeans, cooked, 1/2 cup, 3 oz	14

Tofu, Tempeh, Miso

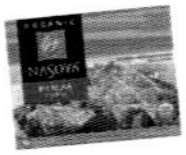

	Pro
Tofu, raw, firm, 1/2 cup, 4 1/2 oz	10
Tempeh, 1/2 cup, 3 oz	16
Miso, 1/2 cup, 5 oz	16
Miso Soup, 1 cup	3
Soybean Protein *(TVP)*, 1 oz	18

Cakes, Pastries, Pies

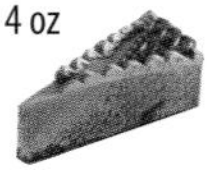
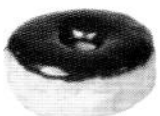
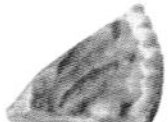

	Pro
Banana Nut Bread, 4 oz	6
Carrot w. cream cheese frosting, 4 oz	4
Cheesecake, 1 piece, 4 oz	6
Chocolate, 1 piece, 2 oz	2
Fruitcake, 1 piece, 3 oz	4
Croissant, plain, small, 2 oz	5
Danish Pastry, 1 pastry, 2 1/4 oz	4
Donuts, average, 2 oz	4
Muffins, average, 1 med., 1 1/2 oz	3
Pancakes, 4" diam., two, 2 oz	4
Pies: Fruit, 1 piece, 5 1/2 oz	4
Pecan, 1 piece, 5 oz	7
Puddings, average, 1/2 cup, 4 1/2 oz	4
Waffles, 1 large, 2 1/2 oz	7

Peanut Butter

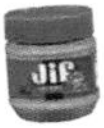

	Pro
Regular: 2 Tbsp, 1.1 oz	8
Peter Pan Plus, 2 Tbsp, 1.1 oz	8

Sugar, Honey, Jam

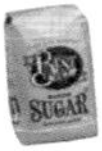

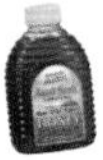

	Pro
Sugar: White	0
Brown, 1 Tbsp	0
Molasses: Light/Med., 1 Tbsp	0
Blackstrap, 1 Tbsp, 3/4 oz	0
Corn Syrup, 1 Tbsp, 3/4 oz	0
Honey, Jams, Jelly	0

Candy, Chocolate, Carob

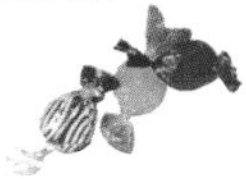

	Pro
Candy, sugar-based	0
Chocolate: Plain, 2 oz bar	4
with nuts, 2 oz bar	6
Carob, plain, 2 oz	6

Cookies, Crackers, Chips

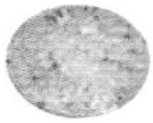

	Pro
Cookies, average, 4 cookies	2
Crackers, Graham, 2 1/2" sq., (2)	1
Rice Cakes, average, one	1
Corn/Potato Chips, 1 oz	2

Nuts:

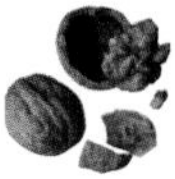

	Pro
Almonds, shelled, 20-25 nuts	6
Brazil Nuts, 7-8 medium nuts, 1 oz	4
Cashews, 12-16 nuts, 1 oz	5
Hemp Seeds, 3 tbsp, 1 oz	9
Macadamias, 1 oz	2
Peanuts, dry rsted, 40 nuts, 1 oz	6
Pecans, 24 halves, 1 oz	2
Walnuts, 15 halves, 1 oz	4

Seeds:

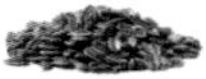

	Pro
Chia Seeds, raw, 2 Tbsp, 1.1 oz	5
Flax Seeds, 3 Tbsp, 1 oz	6
Sesame Seeds, dry, 1 Tbsp	2
Pumpkin Kernels, dry, hulled, 1 oz	7
Sunflower Seeds, dried, hulled, 1 oz	6

Granola & Food/Protein Bars

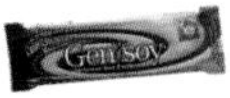

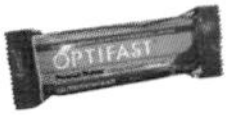

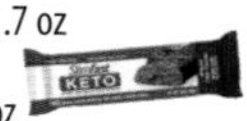

	Pro
Granola Bars, average, 1 bar, 2 oz	2
Bariatrix, Proti-Bars (1), 1.4 oz	15
Cliff, Builder's Protein, av., 1 bar	20
GeniSoy, Protein Bars, 1.6 oz	15
Jenny Craig, Bars, av., 1 oz	10
Luna Protein, av., 1 bar	12
Met-Rx, "Big 100", av., 3.5 oz	31
Myoplex 30, all flavors, 3 oz	30
Optifast 800, all flavors, 1.72 oz	14
PowerBar, Protein Plus	20
Slim-Fast: Protein Meal Bars, 1.7 oz	10
Keto Meal Bar, 1.48 oz	7
Special K: Keto Meal Bars, 2.2 oz	7
Protein Meal Bars, 1.5 oz	7

High Protein Drinks & Powders

	Pro
Atkins, Shakes, 11 fl.oz	15
Bob's Red Mill, Protein Powders:	
Chia Protein, 1/3 cup, 1.45 oz	20
Pea Protein, ¼ cup, 1oz	21
Soy Protein, ¼ cup, 0.75 oz	17
Whey/Hemp Protein, ¼ cup, 0.75 oz	15
Boost, High Protein, 8 fl.oz bottle	20
Plus Protein Shake, 8 fl oz	14
Carnation, B'fast Essentials, 11 fl.oz	10
Ensure, Plus, 8 fl.oz bottle	13
Gatorade, Protein Recovery Shake, 11 oz	20
GNC, Lean Shake, 14 fl oz	25
Hemp Protein Powder, ¼ cup, 1 oz	14
Met-Rx Meal Replacement, RTD:	
High Protein; 51, 15 fl.oz	51
Myoplex, Original Nutrition Shake, 1 pkt	42
Optifast 800, prepared, 8 fl oz	16
Premier Protein, Chocolate, 11 fl.oz	20
Pure Protein Shake, 11 fl.oz	35
Slim-Fast Shakes: Keto, 11 fl.oz	8
Advanced Energy, 11 fl.oz	20
Special K, Protein Shakes, 10 fl.oz	15
Weider, Mass 1000, 4 scoops, 7 oz	34
Pumpkin Protein Powder, 2 Tbsp, ½ oz	9
Whey Protein Powder: 100%, plain, 1 oz	24
Choc Flavor, 1 scoop, 0.8 oz	18

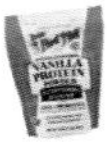
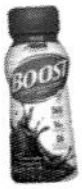

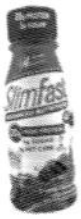

Coffee, Tea, Soda

	Pro
Coffee, Coffee Substitutes, 1 cup, 8 fl.oz	0
Coffee, with 2 oz milk, 1 cup, 8 fl.oz	2
Caffe latte, large, 16 fl.oz	12
Cappuccino, large, 16 fl.oz	8
Frappuccino, average, 16 fl.oz	6
Hot Chocolate, with milk, 1 cup, 8 fl.oz	8
Soft Drinks/Soda, Tea, all types	0

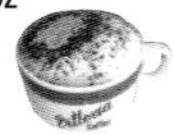
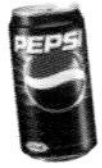

Beer, Wine, Spirits

	Pro
Beer, 12 fl.oz	1
Wines, red/white, 1 glass	0
Spirits/Liquor	0

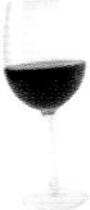

Fast-Foods/Burgers

	Pro
Pancakes, average all outlets, 3	8
Shakes, Chocolate, 16 fl.oz	12
Sundaes, Average all outlets	7
Arby's:	
Buffalo Chicken Slider	12
Buttermilk Crispy Chicken S'wich	24
Classic Roast Beef Sandwich	23
Fire-Roasted Philly	34
Burger King: Cheeseburger	15
Double Bacon Cheeseburger	24
Double Stacker King	61
Impossible Whopper	25
Whopper Sandwich	28

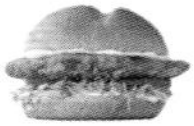
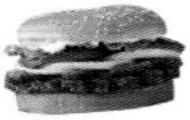

Fast Foods/Burgers (Cont)

	Pro
Carl's Jr: Beyond Famous Star with Cheese	33
Charbroiled Chicken Club Sandwich	44
Famous Star Burger with Cheese	28
Super Star Burger with Cheese	48
Del Taco: Beyond 8 Layer Burrito	27
Beyond Avocado Taco	12
Beyond Taco	19
Epic Beyond Original Mex	44
Domino's Pizza: *Hand Tossed (12")*	
Buffalo Chicken, 1 slice	12
Honolulu Hawaiian, 1 slice	10
Ultimate Pepperoni, 1 slice	11
KFC: Original Breast	39
Extra Crispy Chicken Tender	19
Kentucky Grilled, Breast	38
McDonald's: Big Mac	25
Buttermilk Crispy Chicken S'wch	27
Cheeseburger	15
Chicken McNuggets (4)	9
Filet-O-Fish	16
Hamburger	12
Quarter Pounder with Cheese	30
French Fries: Small, 2.5 oz	3
Large, 5.4 oz	7
Shakes, medium	14
Breakfast: Egg McMuffin	17
Bacon, Egg & Cheese McGriddles	18
Sausage Burrito	13
Sausage McMuffin with Egg	21
Pizza Hut: *Per Medium, 1 slice, 1/8 Pizza*	
Thin 'n Crispy, Supreme	10
Pan Pizzas, Hawaiian Chicken	11
Hand Tossed: Pepperoni Lover's	12
Ultimate Cheese Lover's	11
Red Robin, Veggie Burger	24
Subway: *6" Subs with standard toppings, no oil*	
Black Forest Ham	15
Meatball Marinara	20
Spicy Italian	20
Subway Club	20
Turkey Breast	15
Taco Bell: Bean Burrito, vegan	13
Burrito Supreme, Beef	16
Cheesy Gordita Crunch	21
Chicken Chalupa	16
Grilled Soft Beef Taco	9
Steak Chalupa	15
Wendy's:	
Grilled Asiago Ranch Chkn Club	42
Dave's Double Burger	49
Homestyle Chicken Sandwich	27
Jr Cheeseburger	19
White Castle, Impossible Burger w/o Chse Slider	9

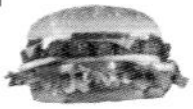
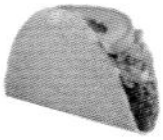
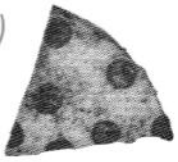
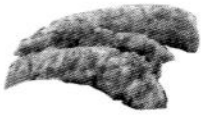
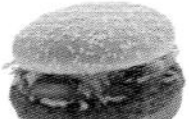
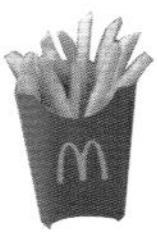
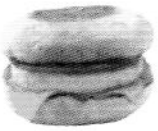
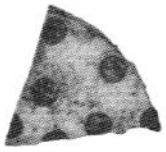
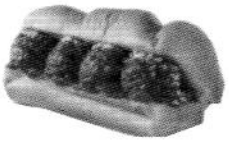
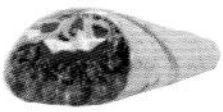
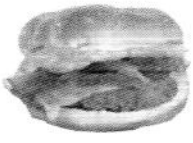

High Blood Pressure

Many American adults have hypertension (high blood pressure), and are unaware of it. It is generally symptomless, so **have your blood pressure checked annually** – particularly if it runs in the family.

Untreated hypertension overworks the heart, damages arteries and promotes atherosclerosis. This in turn greatly increases the risk of heart disease, stroke, blindness, kidney disease and impotence. The earlier hypertension is detected, the sooner it can be brought under control.

BLOOD PRESSURE CLASSIFICATION

For Adults Age 18 & Older ~ Not Acutely ill or on Medication (American Heart Association)

	DIASTOLIC		SYSTOLIC
Normal ➤	Below 80	and	Below 120
Prehypertension ➤	80-89	or	120-139
Hypertension:			
Stage 1 ➤	90-99	or	140-159
Stage 2 ➤	100 or more	or	160 or more

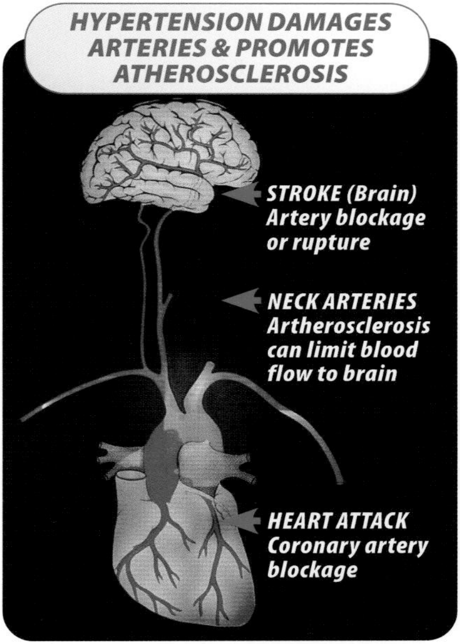

Treating Hypertension

Prehypertension (in the chart above) means you don't have high blood pressure now but are likely to develop it in the future.

You can take steps to lessen the risk by adopting healthy lifestyle habits such as:

- reducing sodium intake
- eating adequate fruit and vegetables
- losing weight if overweight
- limiting alcohol to 2 drinks or less daily
- quitting smoking
- exercising regularly, managing stress.

Stage 1 hypertension can often be treated with the above lifestyle changes.

Stage 2 hypertension usually requires drug therapy. However, salt restriction, abstaining from alcohol, and the above lifestyle changes will improve the success of drug therapy, and enable smaller drug doses to be prescribed.

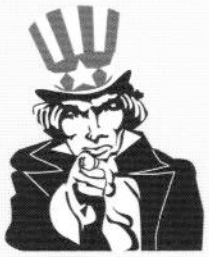

STROKE KNOW THE WARNING SIGNS

Stroke is a medical emergency!
If you notice one or more of these signs, call 9-1-1 or your doctor immediately.

These signs may be signalling a possible stroke or transient ischemic attack:

- **Sudden weakness** or numbness in your face, arm, or leg on one side of your body.
- **Sudden confusion,** trouble speaking or understanding. Slurred speech.
- **Sudden trouble seeing,** in one or both eyes
- **Sudden trouble walking,** dizziness, loss of balance or coordination.
- **Sudden severe headache** - 'a bolt out of the blue' – with no apparent cause.

Extra Info: www.stroke.org

Salt & Sodium

- **Sodium is a mineral element** most commonly found in salt (sodium chloride). It also occurs naturally in much smaller amounts in animal and plant foods, and water – normally sufficient for our needs without having to add salt to our diet.
- **Sodium is required** for nerve and muscle function, as well as to balance the amount of fluid in our tissues and blood. Sodium acts like a sponge to attract and hold fluids in body tissues.
- **Excess sodium** can cause water retention, and increase the risk of developing hypertension. Very high salt intake may also increase the risk of stomach cancer.
- **Too little sodium** may cause low blood pressure (hypotension), and decrease blood flow to the heart, brain and kidneys – especially during exercise. (A certain blood volume is required to sustain the blood pressure needed for adequate blood flow in the capillaries).

Salt-Sensitive Persons

- **Normally, our kidneys** excrete excess dietary sodium. The thirst we feel after a salty meal is the body calling for water to dilute the sodium, and enable the kidneys to flush out excess sodium.
- **However, 'salt - sensitive'** persons (up to 70% of adults) tend to retain excess sodium (above approximately 3000mg daily) instead of excreting it. Such persons are more likely to develop hypertension and would benefit most from sodium restriction. Assume you are susceptible if there is a family history of hypertension.
- **Although not everyone will benefit, all Americans are being asked to moderate their salt and sodium intake** as a public health measure – particularly because so many do not know whether or not they have hypertension, and also because we do not know just who is salt-sensitive.

SAFE SODIUM LEVELS

The American Heart Association recommends a **maximum sodium intake of 1500mg per day** for adults with normal blood pressure.

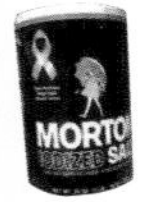

Persons with hypertension and kidney ailments are usually restricted to as little as **1000mg sodium per day**. Your doctor will discuss the correct sodium level for you.

FINDING HIDDEN SODIUM

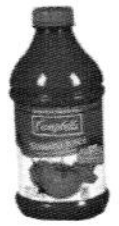

On average, **less than one third of our sodium intake comes from the salt shaker.**
The rest is hidden in processed foods that have salt added during manufacture.

Sodium compounds added to food or medicinals can also contribute significant sodium.

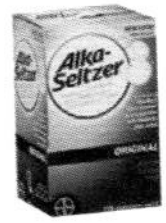

Sodium bicarbonate in particular is widely used in antacid tablets (such as *Alka Seltzer*) and powders. Sodium bicarbonate contains 27% sodium by weight. Each gram has 270mg of sodium. Large amounts of sodium can be unwittingly consumed – up to 600mg per tablet. (See Antacids ~ Page 280)

Example: 2 *Alka-Seltzer* Tablets = 1000mg sodium

Other sodium compounds include monosodium glutamate (MSG), sodium ascorbate, sodium nitrite, and sodium citrate.

POTASSIUM BALANCES SODIUM

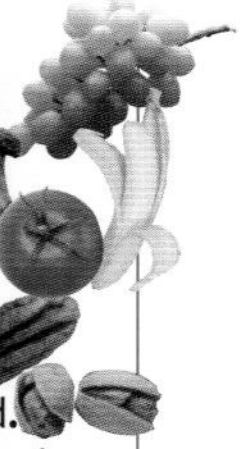

Potassium helps to balance sodium by helping the kidneys to excrete excess sodium.
Fruit and vegetables are rich sources of potassium - another reason to ensure you have your 5-7 servings every day.

Nuts also provide potassium as well as magnesium and other heart-healthy nutrients and anti-oxidants. Eat them unsalted.

Note: This info is only for people with normal kidney function. Also not for persons on potassium-sparing diuretics.

ALCOHOL DANGER

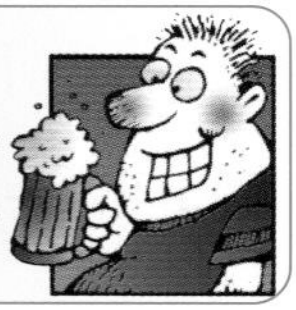

Excessive alcohol intake contributes to hypertension. Susceptible persons should avoid or limit alcohol intake to 1-2 drinks per day.

> **Sodium accounts for only 40% of the weight of salt (sodium chloride). Examples:**
> **1 gram (1000mg) Salt has 400mg Sodium**
> **1 teaspoon (5g) Salt has 2000mg Sodium**

HINTS TO REDUCE SODIUM

- **Cut down use of the salt shaker.** Start with an easy 50% cut in sodium by using Lite Salt (*Morton*) or *Cardia* Salt. Then gradually cut back until you can leave the salt shaker off the table. Sea salt is still high in sodium.
- **Use fresh herbs,** and salt-free seasonings to add flavor to food.
- **Choose low-sodium,** sodium-free, and reduced-sodium products in place of regular, salted products.
- **Check food labels for sodium levels.** FDA Guidelines for sodium descriptors are:
  - **Reduced Sodium:** At least 25% less sodium than the original product
  - **Low Sodium:** 140 mg or less/serving
  - **Very Low Sodium:** 35mg or less/serving
  - **Sodium Free:** Less than 5mg/serving
  - **No Salt Added:** Made without the salt normally added, but still contains the sodium that is a natural part of the food
- **Use reduced-sodium breads,** butter and margarine. Regular varieties are considered high in sodium in view of their significant contribution to our diet.
- **Go easy on salty condiments and sauces** such as ketchup, mustard, soy sauce, spaghetti sauces, and salad dressings. Use low-sodium varieties.
- **Limit pizzas and salty fast-foods.** Check the *CalorieKing.com* food database.
- **Avoid salty snack foods** such as potato chips, corn chips, salted nuts, pretzels and cheesy-flavored snacks. **Choose unsalted** popcorn, nuts or seeds. Eat more fruit.
- **Don't salt children's food** to your taste.
- **Avoid antacids with** sodium bicarbonate (such as *Alka-Seltzer*). They are high in sodium. Look for low-sodium alternatives.

FOODS HIGH IN SODIUM

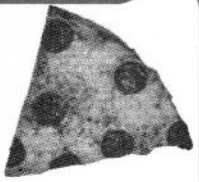
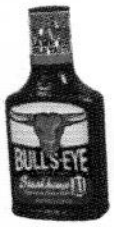

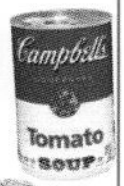

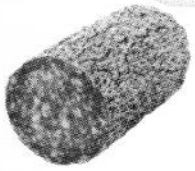
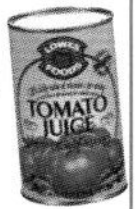

- Bread (4 slices/day), Bagels, Biscuits
- Cheese, Butter, Margarine
- Pickles, Sauerkraut, Olives
- Condiments, Sauces
- Salad Dressings
- Canned vegetables/salads/beans
- Deli Salads (with dressing)
- Frozen/Packaged Meals/Entrees
- Soups: Canned/dry; bouillon cubes
- Meats: Ham, bacon, sausage, luncheon meats, smoked meats
- Canned Fish (in brine/salt)
- Sea Salt, Garlic/Celery Salt
- Snack Foods (potato chips, pretzels)
- Tomato Juice (Canned), V8 Vegetable Juice
- Fast Foods: Pizza, Burgers, Chicken
- *Alka-Seltzer* Antacid

MODERATE SODIUM

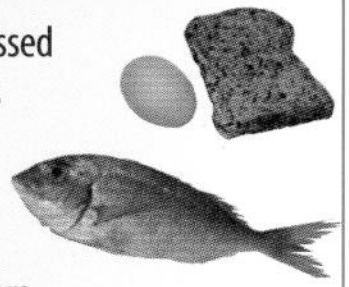

- Meat, Fish, Poultry - Unprocessed
- Milk, Yogurt, Soy Drinks, Eggs
- Peanut Butter
- Breakfast Cereals (less than 200mg/serving)
- Chocolate Candy, Fruit/Nut Bars
- *Reduced Sodium & Low Sodium* Products

FOODS LOW IN SODIUM

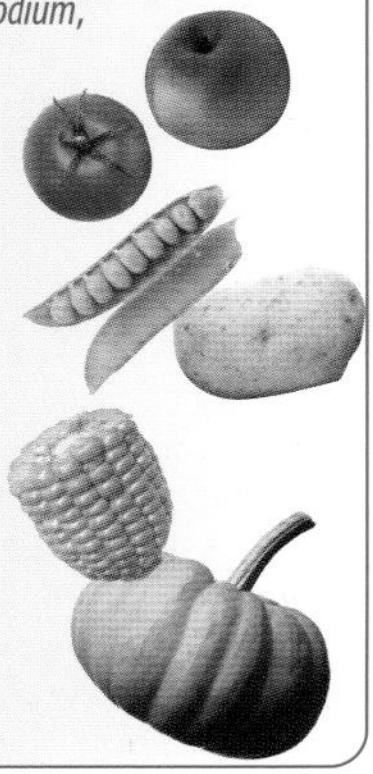

- Products labelled *Very Low Sodium*, or *Sodium Free*
- Bread (No Salt Added)
- Fresh fruits and vegetables
- Canned and Dried Fruits
- Potatoes, Rice, Pasta
- Dried Beans & Lentils, Tofu
- Nuts & Seeds (unsalted)
- Corn & Popcorn (unsalted)
- Pepper, Spices, Herbs
- Jam, Honey, Syrup
- Candy, Gum
- Hard & Jelly Candy
- Coffee, Tea, Alcohol
- Fresh Fruit Juices, Water

Sodium Counter

The American Heart Association recommends a sodium intake of less than 1500mg/day

Milk & Dairy Products

	Sodium
Milk: Whole/lowfat/skim, average	
1 glass, 8 fl.oz	120
Whole, low sodium, 1 cup	5
Choc Milk, 1 cup	130
Soy Milk, 8 fl.oz	30
Buttermilk, cultured, 8 fl.oz	250
Dry/Powder, skim, 1/4 cup, 1 oz	110
Yogurt, with fruit average, 8 oz	130
Cheese: Bleu, 1 oz	330
Cottage Cheese, Creamed, ½ cup, 4 oz	450
Kraft: American, Singles, 1 sl., 0.7 oz	240
American, Deli Deluxe, 2 slices, 0.9 oz	400
Philadelphia Cream Cheese, Tub, Orig.,1.1 oz	125
Parmesan, 1 oz	435
Ricotta Cheese, ½ cup, 4 oz	110
Swiss, Shredded Natural, 1oz	55
Triple Cheddar, 1 oz	170

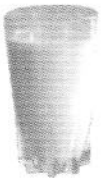
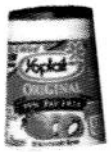

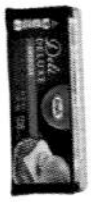

Ice Cream, Frozen Yogurt

Ice Cream, average, 1/2 cup	50
Frozen Yogurt, 1/2 cup	50

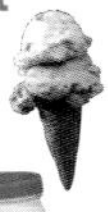

Fats/Oils

Butter/Margarine:	
Regular, 2 Tbsp, 1 oz	230
Unsalted, reg., 2 Tbsp, 1 oz	5
Mayonnaise, avg., 2 Tbsp, 1 oz	160
Oils/Lard/Drippings	0
Cream, average, 1 Tbsp	5
Coffee-Mate: Powdered, Original, 1 tsp	5
Liquid, all flavors	0-5

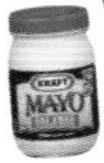

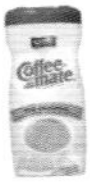

Eggs

Whole, 1 large	70
Omelet: 2 egg, plain	220
With 1 oz Cheddar Cheese	400
Egg Beaters: Original, 3 Tbsp	90
Flavors, average, 3 Tbsp	140

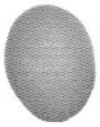
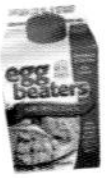

Meats

Meat, average all types, cooked	
Beef/Lamb/Veal/Pork, 4 oz	80
Corned Beef, cooked, 3 oz	800
Bacon, cooked, 2 slices, 0.5 oz	270
Ham, 3 oz	1100

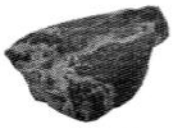
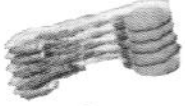

Meat Substitutes (Vegan)

Beyond Meat: Beef/Burger, 4 oz	350
Sausage, cooked, 1 link	500

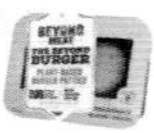

Sodium ~ Sodium (mg)

Sausages & Deli Meats

	Sodium
Bologna, 1 oz	280
Frankfurter, 2 oz	640
Ham, chopped, 0.8 oz slice	290
Liverwurst (Braunschweiger), 1 oz	320
Pepperoni, 5 slices, 1 oz	570
Salami: Cooked, 1 oz	350
dry/hard, 1 oz	600
Sausage, 1 oz link	220
Pork, 2 oz patty	260
Spam: Classic, 2 oz	790
25% Less Sodium, 2 oz	580
Turkey Roll, 1 oz	160

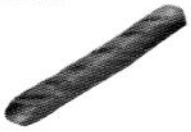
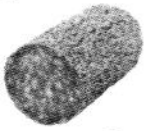
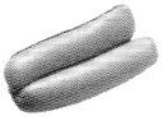
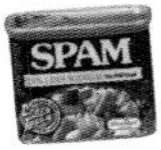

Chicken & Turkey

Chicken/Turkey, cooked, unsalted, 4 oz	80
Stuffing Mixes, average., ½ cup	500

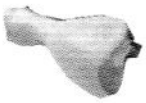

Fish:

Fresh Fish: average, plain	
Cooked, 4 oz, without bone	60
Broiled w. butter, 4 oz	150
Breaded & fried, 4 oz	320
Fish fillets, batter-dipped 3 oz	350
Fish sticks, 1 oz stick	160
Gefilte Fish, with broth, 1 pce, 1.5 oz	220
Herring, pickled, 2 pces, 1 oz	260
Lobster, meat only, 4 oz	180
Oysters, fresh, 6 med., 3 oz	95
Salmon: Canned, 3 oz	460
No Salt Added, 3 oz	65
Smoked fish, average, 3 oz	650
Tuna: Canned, drained, 3 oz	160
Light, drained, 3 oz	200
No Added Salt, 3 oz	40
Spicy Flavored, 5 oz	260

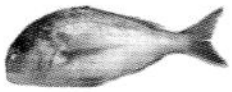
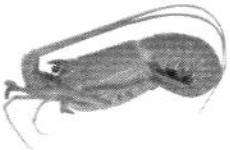
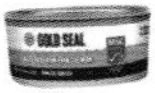

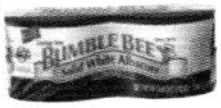

Entrees & Meals

Frozen Meals, average	600-1300
Lean Cuisine, Favorites	500-800
Stouffer's, Meat Lovers Lasagna	750
Dinners, average	900-1200
Side Dishes, average	400-600
Pizza, frozen, 1/4 large, 6 oz	800-1200
Microwave, Cup Meals	900-1200
Cup Noodles, average	1050-1280

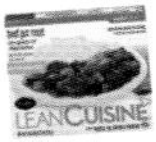

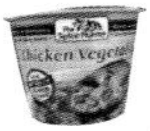

Soups

	Sodium
Condensed: Average, 1 cup, 8 oz	800-1000
Low Sodium, average	70
Chicken Noodle, average, 1 cup	900
Bouillon Cube, average	950
Top Ramen Noodle Soup, 3 oz pkg, av.	1600
Soup Cups, average	850
Soup Mixes, average, 1 cup	900

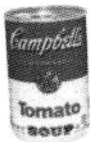

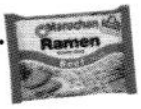

Condiments, Sauces, Dressings

	Sodium
A-1 Sauce, 1 Tbsp	280
Barbecue Sauce, 1 Tbsp	130
Bragg's Liquid Aminos, 1 tsp	350
Chili Sauce, 1 Tbsp	230
Ketchup: Tomato, 1 Tbsp	180
Low Sodium, 1 Tbsp	20
Mayonnaise, 1 Tbsp	80
Mustard, 1 tsp	70
Pizza Sauce, 1/2 cup	700
Salad Dressings, 2 Tbsp, 1 oz	160-400
Spaghetti Sauce, 1/2 cup	500
Soy Sauce: 1 Tbsp	900
Lite, 1 Tbsp	600
Sweet & Sour, 1/2 cup	250
Tabasco, 1 tsp	25
Vinegar, Lemon Juice	0
Worcestershire, 1 Tbsp	65
Tomato: Sauce, 1 cup	1200
Paste/Puree (salted), 1/2 cup	1000
No Salt Added, 1/2 cup	75

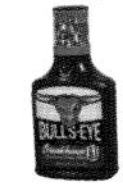

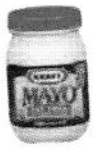

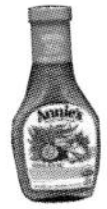

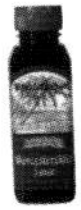

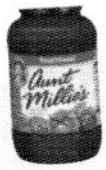

Salt & Salt Substitutes

	Sodium
Table Salt: 1 teaspoon, 6g	2400
Single Serve package, 1 g	400
Cardia Salt, 1 teaspoon	1080
Lite Salt, 1 teaspoon, 6g	1200
Morton, No Salt Substitute, 1 tsp	5
Garlic/Onion/Seasoned Salt, 1 tsp, 4g	1350
Garlic/Seasoned Salt 1 teaspoon, 4g	1300
Sea Salt, 1 teaspoon, 5g	2250

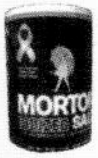

Seasonings, Herbs & Spices

	Sodium
Baking Powder, 1 tsp, 3g	340
Baking Soda (Sodium bicarb), 1 tsp, 3g	810
Accent, Flavor Enhancer, ¼ tsp	160
Chili Powder, 1 tsp, 3g	25
Curry Powder	0
Lemon Pepper 1 tsp	340
Meat Tenderizer, 1 tsp, 5g	1750
MSG (Monosodium Glutamate), 5g	500
Mrs Dash, Blends/Marinades	0
Old Bay: Seasoning, 1 tsp, 2.4 oz	560
Seasoning, Less Sodium, 1 tsp, 2.4 oz	360
Pepper, Mustard (dry), 1 tsp	1
Yeast, Nutritional, 1 Tbsp	10

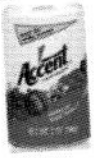

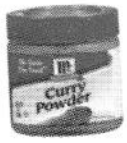

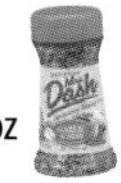

Breakfast Cereals

	Sodium
Kellogg's:	
All-Bran, Original, ⅔ cup, 1 oz	95
Special K, Original, 1¼ cups, 1.4 oz	270
Corn Flakes, 1½ cup,s 1 oz	300
Raisin Bran, 1 cup, 2 oz	200
Quaker:	
Corn Crunch, 1 cup, 1.3 oz	220
Multigrain Flakes, av., ¾ c., 2.2 oz	40
Real Medleys, ⅔ cup, 1.83 oz	15-45
Simply Granola, average, 1/2 cup	30-35
General Mills, Total, 1 cup, 1.4 oz	190
Oatmeal: Regular, 3/4 cup	1
Quaker, Instant Maple & Brown Sugar (1 pkt)	260

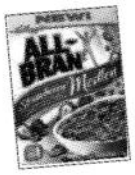

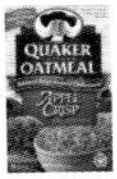

Breads, Bagels, Crackers

	Sodium
Bread: Thin Slice, average 1 oz	140
Thick Slice, 1.5 oz	210
Low Sodium, 1 oz	10
Bagels: Plain, medium, 2 oz	200
Large, take-out, average, 4 oz	550
Panera Bread, 3.8 oz	410
Biscuits, average, 1 oz	180
Bun/Roll: 1 medium, 1.5 oz	200
Large, 4 oz	560
Crackers: Saltine, 2 crackers	70
Low Salt, 2	25
Graham, 2 regular	50
Croissant, Plain, average, 2 oz	280
Rice Cakes, average	25
Ritz Crackers, Hint of Salt, 1 oz	60
RyVita, Original Crispbread, 2 slices	30

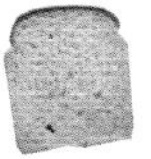

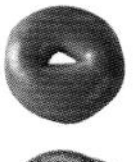

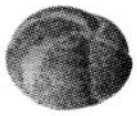

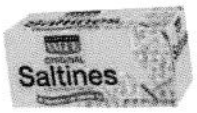

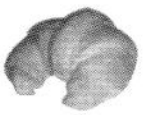

Cookies, Cakes, Desserts

	Sodium
Cookies: Average, 2-3 cookies, 1 oz	100
Average, 1 cookie, 2.5 oz	180
Baked Custard, 1/2 cup	100
Brownie, 1.5 oz	130
Carrot Cake, 8 oz	650
Cheesecake, 7 oz	350
Cinnamon Sweet Roll, 2 oz	250
Danish, Apple/Fruit	250
Donut, average	150
Muffins: 1 medium, 2 oz	150
1 extra large, 4 oz	300
Pancakes, (4"), x 3	360
Fruit Pies, average, 7 oz	600
Pudding: Average, 1/2 cup	160
Jell-O Instant Pudding Mix, 1/4 pkg	350
Waffles: Home-made, 7", 2.5 oz	350
Frozen: Average, 1.2 oz	260
Aunt Jemima, Homestyle, 3 pancakes	460

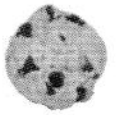

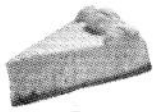

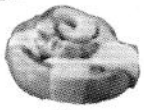

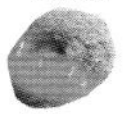

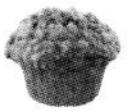

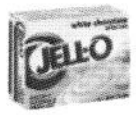

Sodium Counter

Fruit & Juices

	Sodium
Fresh Fruit, average all types, 1 serving	1
Dried/Canned Fruit, ½ cup	1
Fruit Juice: Fresh, squeezed, 6 fl.oz	1
Commercial, aver., 6 fl.oz	20
Tomato Juice *(Campbell's)*, 8 fl.oz	680
Low Sodium (No Salt Added), 8 fl.oz	140
V8 Vegetable *(Campbell's)*:	
11.5 fl.oz bottle	920
Low Sodium, 5.5 fl.oz can	95

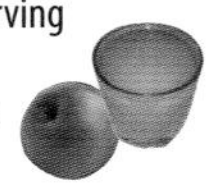
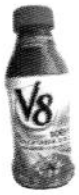

Vegetables

	Sodium
Fresh/Frozen (No Salt Added): Per ½ Cup	
Asparagus, Bean Sprouts, Corn	3
Beets, Carrots, Celery, ½ cup	40
Broccoli, Cabbage, Cauliflower	10
Cucumber, Green Beans, Mushroom, Okra	3
Onions, Peas, Potato, Pumpkin, Squash	3
Peppers, Hot Chili, raw, each	3
Spinach, Turnips, ½ cup, cooked	40
Tomato, 1 medium, 5 oz	10
Canned: Asparagus, 4 spears	300
Beans, baked in tomato sauce	450
Beets, ½ cup, 3 oz	240
Corn Kernels, ½ cup, 3 oz	190
Creamed, ½ cup, 4.5 oz	330
Mushrooms w. butter sce, 2oz	550
Peas, ½ cup, 3 oz	250
Sauerkraut, ½ cup, 4 oz	750

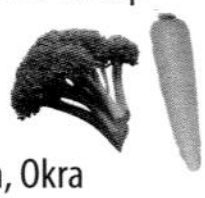
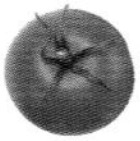
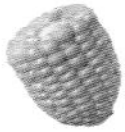
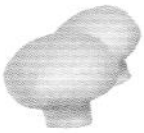

Pickles, Olives

	Sodium
Olives: pickled: Green, 1 large	90
Ripe/black, 1 large	40
Pickles: Bread & Butter, 4 slices, 1 oz	200
Dill, 1 pickle, 2.5oz	900
Sweet, 1 gherkin, 0.5 oz	130

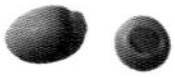
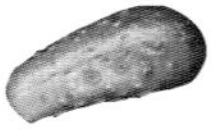

Soybean Products

	Sodium
Miso (Soy Paste), ¼ c., 2.5 oz	2500
Soybean Protein Isolate, 1 oz	280
Tempeh, Natural, ½ cup, 3 oz	5
Tofu, average, ½ cup, 4 oz	5

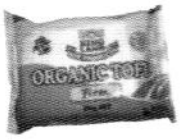

Jam, Honey, Syrups

	Sodium
Jam/Jelly, 1 Tbsp	2
Honey/Maple Syrup, 1 Tbsp	1
Log Cabin, Maple Syrup, 2 Tbsp, 1 fl.oz	55
Syrup, Lite, 2 Tbsp, 1 fl.oz	95

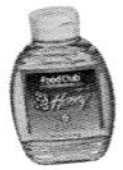

Peanut Butter

	Sodium
Peanut Butter: Regular, 2 Tbsp, 0.5 oz	190
Jif, Low Sodium, 2 Tbsp	65
Trader Joe's, Unsalted, 2 Tbsp	0

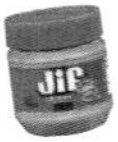

Snacks, Nuts

	Sodium
Cheese Balls/Curls, 1 oz	280
Cheetos, Cheddar Popcorn, 1 oz	260
Corn/Tortilla Chips: average, 1 oz	220
Fritos, Lightly Salted, 1 oz	80
Granola bars, average, 1 bar	80
Nuts: Plain, unsalted, 1 oz	1
Lightly salted, 1 oz	80
Salted or Honey Roasted, 1 oz	160
Popcorn: Plain (unsalted), 1 cup	1
Flavored, average, 1 cup	60
Salt added, 1 cup	180
Potato Chips: Plain, 1 oz	160
Lay's, Lightly Salted, 1 oz	65
Flavored, average, 1 oz	200
Pretzels: Regular, 3, 1 oz	450
Soft, salted, large	1000

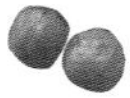
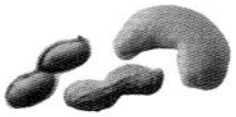
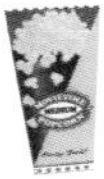
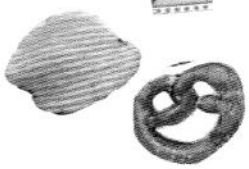
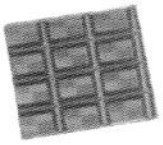

Candy, Chocolate

	Sodium
Chocolate, milk, 1 oz	30
Fudge, chocolate, 1 oz	55
Candy Bars, average, 1.5 oz	60
Hard Candy, 1 oz	10
Licorice, 1 oz	30

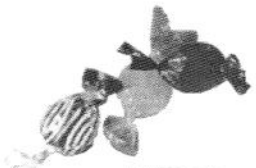

Beverages, Alcohol

	Sodium
Coffee or Tea, 1 cup	1
Cocoa: Dry, plain, 1 Tbsp	0
Mix, average, 1 envelope	120
Quik, 2 tsp	35
Soft Drinks, average, 8 fl.oz	20
Mineral Water: Perrier, 8 fl.oz	5
Gatorade, Thirst Quencher, 8 fl.oz	110
Red Bull: 8.4 fl.oz can	105
Sugar Free, 8.4 fl.oz	105
Water, Average, 1 cup, 8 fl.oz	5
Alcohol: Beer, average, 12 fl.oz	15
Wines, average, 4 fl.oz	10
Spirits (distilled), 1.5 fl.oz	1

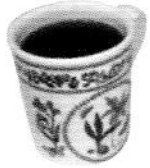
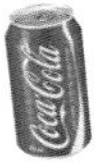

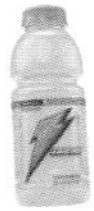

Antacids ~ Alka-Seltzer

Alka-Seltzer: *Per Tablet*	Sodium
Original; Heartburn	570
Extra Strength	590
Lemon Lime	500
Gold	310
Alka-Mints, chewable	0
Bromo Seltzer, ¾ capful	760
Picot, 1 packet, 5g	670
Rolaids, All types	0
Tums, Regular/Extra Strength	0

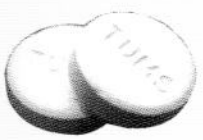

Cold & Flu ~ Alka-Seltzer Plus

	Sodium
Effervescents, average, 1 tablet	480
Fast Crystal Packs; Liquid Gels	0

Fast-Foods & Restaurants

Burger King:

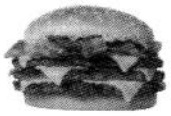
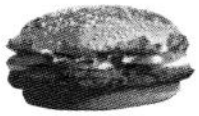

	Sodium
Bacon Double Cheeseburger	670
Cheeseburger	560
Double Stacker King	1871
Hamburger	385
Whoppers: Original	980
Triple with Cheesse	1475
Whopper Jr.	390
Impossible Whopper	1080
Chicken Sandwich, Original	1170
Sides: French Fries, medium, salted	570
Onion Rings, medium	1315
Breakfast, Ham, Egg & Cheese Croissan'wich	1000

Carl's Jr.:

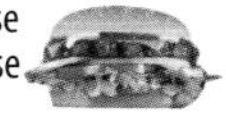

	Sodium
Burgers: Famous Star w/ Cheese	1270
Beyond Famous Star w/ Cheese	1600
The Big Carl	1380

Denny's:

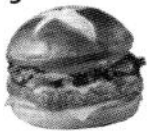
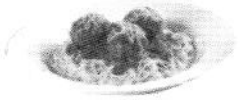
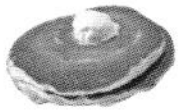

	Sodium
Burgers: Bacon Avocado Cheeseburger	1650
Slamburger	1780
Sandwiches: Club	2060
Mega Philly Cheese Melt	2120
Dinner: Brooklyn Spaghetti & Meatballs	2510
Premium Chicken Tenders	2360
Sides: Broccoli	110
Seasoned Fries	1110
Red-Skinned Potatoes	580
Breakfast: BlueberyPancakes (2)	1400
Moons Over My Hammy Omelette, w/ Hash	2200
Santa Fe Skillet	1700
Sides: Hash Browns, 1 serving	360
Sausages (2)	300

Jack In The Box:

	Sodium
Burgers: Bacon Ultimate Cheeseburger	1590
Jumbo Jack	580
Jumbo Jack Cheeseburger	990
Sandwiches: H'style Ranch Chicken Club	1869
Sourdough Grilled Chicken Club	1500

KFC:

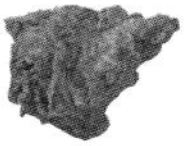
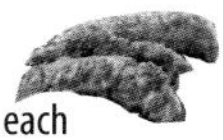
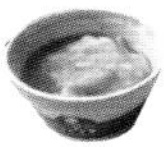

	Sodium
Chicken Breast: Original	1190
Extra Crispy	1150
Kentucky Grilled	710
Popcorn Nuggets, Large	1820
Sandwich, Crispy Twister	1260
Tenders, Extra Crispy Tenders, each	610
Wings, Nashville HotSpicy Crispy (1)	450
Sides: Macaroni & Cheese	590
Mashed Potatoes with Gravy	520
Potato Wedges	700

Fast-Foods & Restaurants

McDonalds:

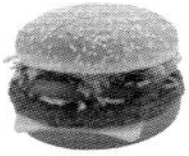

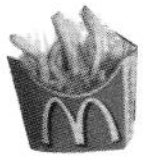
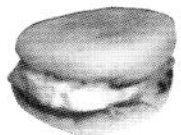

	Sodium
Burgers: Big Mac	1010
Cheeseburger	720
Double	1180
Hamburger	510
Quarter Pounder with Cheese	1150
Chicken McNuggets, 4 pieces	330
McChicken, Sandwich	560
French Fries: Small, 2.6 oz	180
Medium, 3.9 oz	260
Large, 5.9 oz	400
Ketchup, 1 package, 10g	90
Breakfast: Egg McMuffin	760
Big Breakfast	1490
Hash Browns, 2 oz	310
Hotcakes & Sausage	880
Sausage Burrito	800
Sausage McGriddles	990
Desserts/Shakes: Hot Fudge Sundae	180
Strawberry Banana Smoothie, medium	50

Pizza Hut:

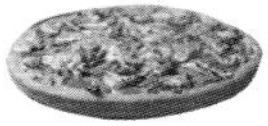

	Sodium
Original Pan Pizza: *Per Slice, Medium 12"*	
Meat Lovers	660
Cheese	450
Pepperoni Lover's	580
Supreme	500

Subway: *On 9 Grain Wheat Bread*

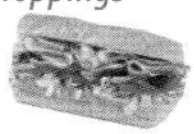
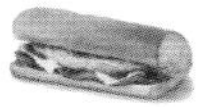

	Sodium
6" Sandwiches: *With Set Menu Toppings*	
Chicken Bacon Ranch Melt	1100
Meatball Marinara	1040
Spicy Italian	1240
6" Breakfast Flatbread S'wich: *With Set Menu Toppings*	
Bacon, Egg & Cheese	1200
Black Forest Ham, Egg & Chse	1180
Egg & Cheese	950
Steak, Egg & Cheese	1270

Taco Bell:

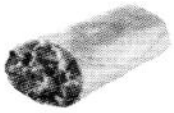
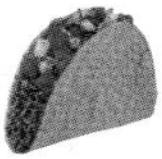

	Sodium
Burritos: Beefy 5-Layer	1250
Supreme, Chicken	1110
Chalupa Supreme, Chicken/Steak, av	545
Nachos: BellGrande, Chicken	1050
Steak	1030
Specialties, Cheese Quesadillas	990
Tacos: Soft Chicken	450
Crunchy Supreme	340

FAST-FOODS INDEX
~ PAGE 175 ~

FAST-FOODS INDEX
~ PAGE 175 ~

FAST-FOODS INDEX
~ PAGE 175 ~

Notes

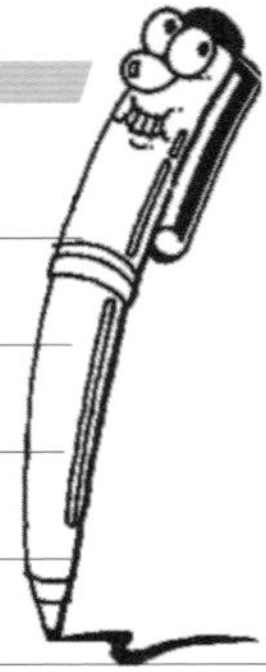

THE UNICORN'S SECRET COLLECTION

THE UNICORN'S SECRET COLLECTION

Moonsilver

The Silver Thread

The Silver Bracelet

The Mountains of the Moon

by Kathleen Duey
illustrated by Omar Rayyan

ALADDIN PAPERBACKS
New York London Toronto Sydney

For all the daydreamers . . .

This 2006 edition created exclusively for Barnes & Noble, Inc. by arrangement with Simon & Schuster Children's Publishing Division.

ISBN-13: 978-0-7607-8593-5
ISBN-10: 0-7607-8593-7

Printed and bound in the United States of America

1 3 5 7 9 10 8 6 4 2

This book is a work of fiction. Any references to historical events, real people, or real locales are used fictitiously. Other names, characters, places, and incidents are the product of the author's imagination, and any resemblance to actual events or locales or persons, living or dead, is entirely coincidental.

THE UNICORN'S SECRET

Moonsilver

✦ CHAPTER ONE

Heart Avamir was tired.

Everyone else had gone home.

It would be dark soon.

The stiff wheat stubble had scraped her hands bloody. There were long scratches on her bare feet.

Heart smiled. Her sack was half full. The harvesters had hurried through the fields this year, missing more grain than usual.

Lord Dunraven wouldn't like the gleaners finding so much fallen grain. But the people of Ash Grove were happy. They would have more bread this winter.

Lord Dunraven didn't need their little bit of gleaned wheat.

He owned every wheat field, every barley field, every hillside.

He owned the forest on the other side of the Blue River. The bridge that crossed the Blue River and the road that led to Derrytown belonged to him, too. Lord Dunraven owned towns and villages.

He owned everything.

Old Simon cleared his throat and spat. "What's that?" he asked, pointing.

Heart faced the sunset. Something was moving at the far end of the field, near the edge of a grove of old oak trees.

"A deer?" she replied.

"Looks like a cow," Simon said.

Heart squinted. "I can't tell." The animal was moving farther into the deep shadows.

"Whose cow would be out for wolves to find?" Simon asked. He tied up their wheat sacks with twine he kept in his pockets.

"I'll go see," Heart said.

Simon nodded. "Hurry back. No playing."

Heart glanced at Simon's angular face and thin gray hair. She wished that he loved her. But she knew he didn't.

Simon Pratt was not her father, after all. Nor was he an uncle or a grandfather or any kind of family.

Five years before, Simon had found her sleeping in the high grass by the Blue River. He had come upon her that morning the way someone stumbles across a nest of quail eggs.

Simon told her all about it. He'd been gathering firewood among the cottonwood trees by the river. She had been wrapped in a beautiful blanket, her hair knotted and tangled.

"Can you see what it is?" Simon shouted now.

Startled from her thoughts, Heart whirled around.

"Not yet!" she shouted over her shoulder. Whatever the animal was, it was deep in the dappled shade now.

Walking slowly toward the edge of the woods,

Heart tried to recall something, anything, from *before* the morning Simon had awakened her in the tall grass.

She couldn't.

She never could.

Her first memory was this:

Her eyes had flown open and her breath had come quicker than a startled rabbit. And Simon had been there, leaning over her, with his sharp-nosed face, his dark eyes and dark clothes.

And that was it.

Heart could remember everything back to that instant, perfectly. But then her memories just *ended*.

Simon had called her "Girl" for weeks. He had not named her. Ruth Oakes had done that. But he had fed her. She was alive. She knew she should be grateful.

But all the other children in Ash Grove knew their parents. They knew their grandparents and their great-grandparents. They didn't trust her. They wouldn't play with her, or even talk to her.

"What is it?" Simon called. "Why can't you see?"

Startled again, Heart stopped, peering into the dusky shade under the oak trees.

"It's a horse!" she called back, surprised. No one in Ash Grove owned horses, except Tin Blackaby. "A mare!"

"Then it's Blackaby's," Simon called. "Leave it alone!"

Heart nodded. She felt sorry for the horse.

Blackaby was Lord Dunraven's steward. He counted out crops and chicks and sheep and corn. He weighed out the peppers and onions people raised to sell to the Derrytown merchants. He told people how much they had to give to Lord Dunraven and how little they could keep. He was not kind. He worked his men and his horses hard.

"Blackaby's men will come," Simon shouted. "They'll think we're trying to steal it."

"Wait," Heart pleaded. "This isn't Tin Blackaby's horse."

"You're sure?" Simon shouted.

"Yes!" Heart called back. She could see the mare better now. It was white. She'd never seen a white horse in Tin Blackaby's corrals.

Coming close, Heart saw the mare's coat was rough, mud-speckled. She was thin, too, her ribs jutting out.

Her tail was full of river burrs.

"Easy, now," Heart said softly. The mare lifted her head and turned. Heart could see scars on her face. The biggest one crossed her forehead, a curved band of stretched, dark skin.

"How did you survive that wound?" Heart whispered.

The mare lowered her head and came forward. Heart could smell her grass-sweet breath. The horse brushed Heart's cheek with her warm muzzle. Heart closed her eyes at the gentle touch.

"Catch it!" Simon shouted. "Use your belt!"

Heart opened her eyes and did as she was told. She untied her rough rope belt. The mare stood quietly. Then she lowered her head and let Heart slip the loop over her ears.

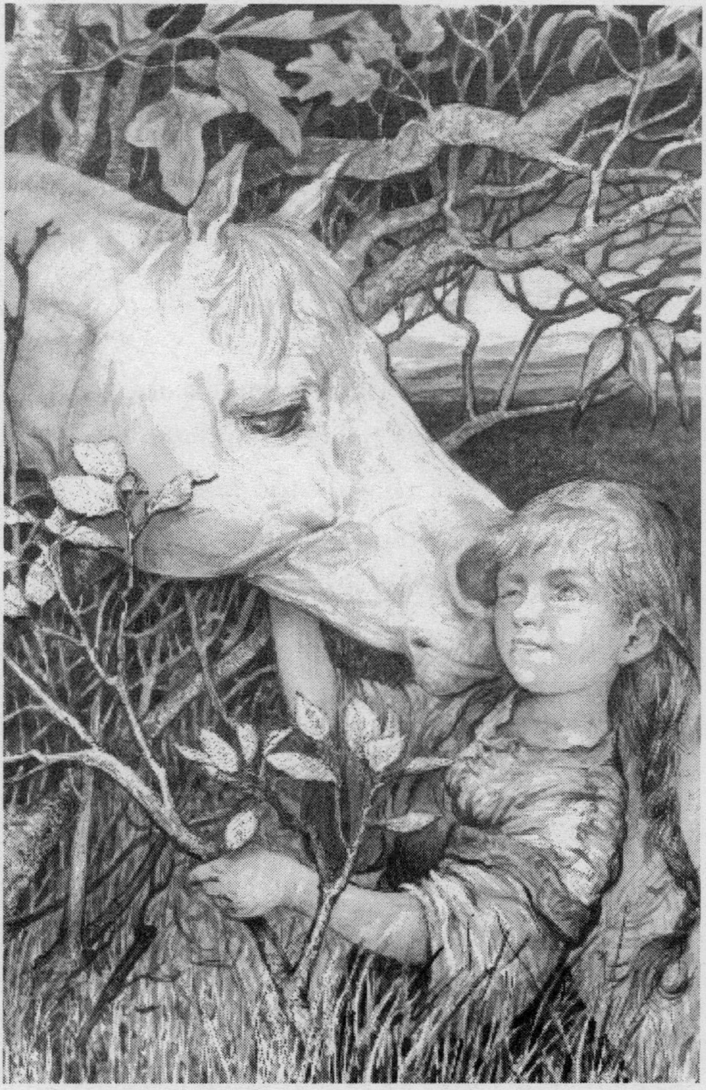

"Good girl!" Simon shouted. Heart glanced back. He was flapping his arms at her. He looked like a crow.

Heart tugged gently at the rope. The mare stepped forward, limping. Heart saw dark, dried blood on her foreleg.

"You're hurt," Heart said.

The mare touched Heart's cheek once more. Then she lowered her head. Heart held the rope loosely, careful not to walk too fast.

"Hurry along!" Simon shouted.

Heart pretended not to hear him. This mare needed rest and good forage. She needed care.

"Well, well," Simon said, rubbing his hands together.

As Heart got closer, she saw his eager expression fade.

"It's all scarred up," he growled. "And bone thin. Best to sell it to the knacker—before it dies. They pay less for dead."

Heart swallowed hard.

The knacker killed old animals and boiled the

meat for tallow. Candle makers and soap makers bought barrels of the smelly fat.

Heart shivered. "She's just hurt and starved."

Simon puffed out his cheeks. He was thinking it over. Heart held her breath. The mare stood behind her, still as stone.

"Bring it along then," Simon said.

The mare nudged Heart gently from behind. They followed Simon out of the field and up the slope to the road.

✦ CHAPTER TWO

Simon kept glancing back, motioning for Heart to catch up.

But the mare's limp was worse now that they were headed up the long hill on River Road.

Simon frowned over his shoulder. "Come on now, girl, come on!"

"I'm trying," Heart answered. "I'm tired, Simon."

She didn't want him to notice how lame the mare really was. He'd decide to go by the knacker's tonight after all. She could smell the stink of the tallow works as they passed Crosswater Street.

"Hurry," Simon kept insisting.

"I am," Heart said, without changing pace. But, as if she could understand human speech, the mare limped along a little faster. Her clopping hooves scuffed up puffs of late-summer dust.

It was good they had worked so late, Heart thought. No one else was on the road.

Simon glanced back. "You are sure it isn't Blackaby's horse?"

"Tin Blackaby owns no white horse," Heart replied.

"You're certain?" Simon demanded.

"Yes," Heart said clearly. "I like horses. I always stop and—"

"Good, then," Simon interrupted. "Lord Dunraven would not own or want this wreck of an animal—nor would any merchant. She's some Gypsy's runaway." He smiled. "Luck has smiled upon me."

Heart felt her belly tighten. "It has?"

Simon looked astonished. "Of course. I can sell this old mare to the knacker now. Or maybe later, after you feed her up a bit. I can make a bit of silver."

Heart felt the mare's breath on the back of her neck. "I want to keep her."

"Keep the horse?" Simon slowed, frowning. "We can't feed it. Nobles, rich merchants, and Gypsies have horses, not people like us."

Heart walked after Simon in silence. The mare struggled to keep the pace he set. They crossed the broad arch of the bluff, then started downward again, passing Dunraven's orchards. There were fallen apples just inside the fence.

Heart spotted one that had rolled into the road.

The mare ate it whole, without slowing, tickling Heart's palm when she took it.

"I'll get up early to cut grass," Heart said. "She'll get sound and strong."

Simon turned. "She might get fatter. The knacker wants them fat."

Heart risked a quick smile.

Simon hadn't said no. There was hope. And once the mare was well, Heart would try to find work for them both, hauling or plowing. If the

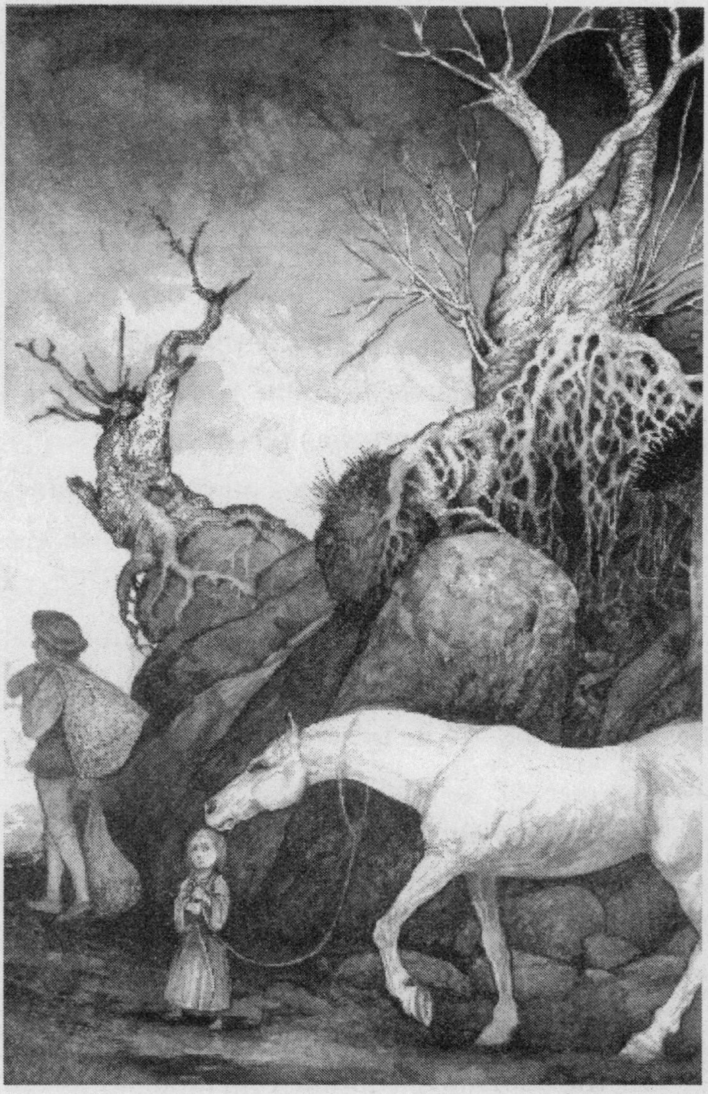

mare brought in money, Simon would keep her.

Heart touched the mare's scarred face. "Meadowsweet will help your leg, I think. Ruth Oakes will know what to do."

The mare lifted her head.

They went south along River Road, skirting along the edge of town. By the time they turned onto Crooked Lane, heading toward Simon's shack, the mare's limp was terrible.

There were only two places on Crooked Lane. Ruth Oakes's old stone house stood near the turnoff, neat and well kept.

Simon's shack was two miles off, at the lane's end where the land dropped down to the river.

Heart tried to keep it neat. Simon did not help.

Heart saw Ruth Oakes's lantern as they passed. "I should go see about the mare's leg," she said.

Simon looked back. "In the morning."

"But the mare—" Heart began.

"In the morning," Simon repeated. "And tell

that old woman I can't pay." Simon's voice was heavy as stone.

They walked on in silence.

Finally, Simon cleared his throat.

"You can put it in the old cow pen if you prop up the broken rails." He coughed, then spat. "I'm hungry. And I suppose that means fixing my own supper tonight."

Heart didn't answer. She let the mare set her own, halting pace.

Simon went ahead.

There was lantern light shining through the door planks when Heart finally passed the shack, leading the mare toward the old cow pen.

Simon was eating supper.

Heart's mouth watered at the smell of boiled barley. But she knew she had another hour's work before she could eat.

It would take at least that long to make the sagging fence fit to hold a horse. Even if the horse was starved and hurt and weary.

✦ CHAPTER THREE

Heart was used to getting up in the dark. She always struck a spark and made a little fire for Simon's barley water.

This morning she started the fire, then tiptoed outside.

The moon sailed silent overhead. The river's quiet voice came up the grassy hill.

Heart peered into the dusk toward the makeshift corral. The mare was lying down. Her white coat shone in the moonlight.

Heart's bare feet made almost no sound in the deep dust of Crooked Lane. She ran uphill, grateful to see the bright speck of Ruth Oakes's lantern shining through her window.

Ruth stayed up late.

She also rose early.

She was Ash Grove's only healer. There was always so much for her to do.

Heart hurried up the curving path, the scents of Ruth's herb gardens tickling at her nose.

Heart could see Ruth through the window and knocked quietly.

"Yes?" Ruth called. "Come in!"

Heart pushed on the door. The light from the lantern made her blink.

"Child!" Ruth said. "And why are you at my door so early?"

Heart explained about the mare.

Ruth tipped her head and listened.

"A scarred forehead?" she asked, when Heart was finished.

Heart sighed. "Yes, but that's all healed. It's the wound on her leg that worries me."

"Let's go see," Ruth said, slinging her worn leather herb bag over her shoulder. She picked up her lantern, then headed for the door.

"Simon won't pay anything."

Ruth looked back, smiling. "And when did he ever pay me?"

Heart shrugged, uneasy. "I'll do chores. I'll work and—"

"And when did you ever *not* pay me in some way?" Ruth asked, starting off, quickly settling into her long-striding walk.

Heart ran to catch up.

The mare was standing when Ruth ducked through the fence.

"Oh, my," she said quietly.

"Is it that bad?" Heart whispered.

Ruth didn't answer. She placed one hand on the mare's withers and spoke to her in a quiet, soothing, singsong voice.

"Hold the lantern," she said after a moment.

Heart held the light steady and high, wincing when she saw the wound on the mare's leg clearly. It was deeper than she had thought.

"Fresh water," Ruth said, straightening. "We'll wash the road dust out of it, then seal it with meadowsweet salve."

Heart ran for the well.

The bucket was heavy, but Ruth took it in one

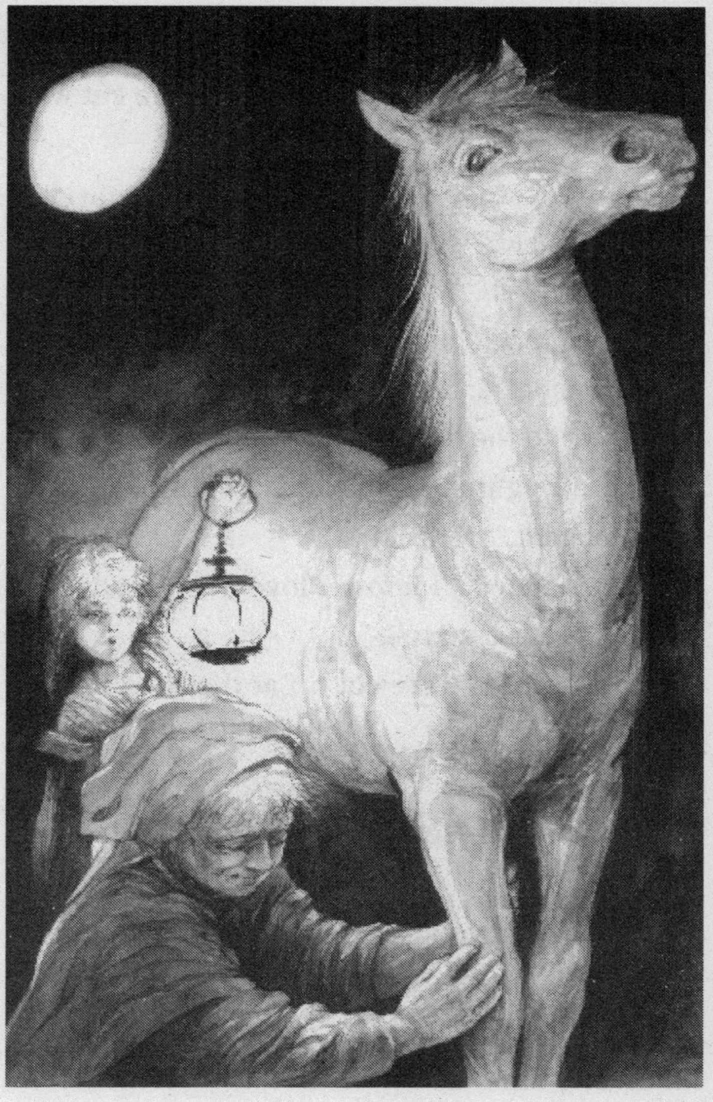

hand and tipped it to pour water slowly over the wound. Twice she stopped to dab at the cut with clean cloths from her bag.

The mare stood still, her head high.

"Will it heal?" Heart asked, biting at her lip.

Ruth nodded. "Yes. Another scar, but the lameness is just that it hurts her. The tendons aren't cut."

Heart exhaled. "I want to keep her. Simon wants to sell her to the knacker but—"

Ruth straightened and turned abruptly. "You can't let him."

Heart nodded. "I know. I love her already. She is the sweetest mare—"

Heart's words were cut off at the sound of the door banging open.

"Girl!"

"Her name is Heart Avamir," Ruth called out. "Not *Girl*."

"Did she tell you I won't pay a penny?" Simon groused.

Ruth laughed. "She did. The shock of it nearly killed me, Simon."

He growled something and went back inside.

"I'd better go cut grass for the mare," Heart said, looking at the horizon. "Sunup is coming and we have another field to glean today."

Ruth reached out suddenly and touched Heart's face. "You are a good-hearted child."

Heart smiled, wishing, as she had a thousand times, that Ruth had been the one to find her in the river grass instead of Simon.

Owing her life to Old Simon was a misery.

Owing Ruth Oakes would have been a joy.

Ruth stepped back. "Starting tomorrow, walk her just a little. Go a bit farther each day. It'll make her eat, and keep her leg from stiffening."

"I will," Heart promised.

Ruth handed her the pot of salve. "Twice a day, nice and thick."

Heart nodded, glancing at the door. "I had better go cut grass."

Ruth patted her arm. "Don't let that old man work you so hard."

✦ CHAPTER FOUR

No one in Ash Grove noticed the white mare.

Heart was careful.

She cut grass before dawn, hidden by the mists that rose from the Blue River.

She walked the mare only at dusk and always led her south, away from town.

To the south, the land was too dry and rocky to plow. No one farmed it. No one lived there.

People often came to Ruth Oakes's house, seeking her help. But no one walked two extra miles down to the end of Crooked Lane.

Adults had no business with Simon. He shouted and threw rocks at children who came too close—so they almost never did.

"Ready?" Heart said to the mare every evening.

And every evening, the mare tossed her mane and whickered quietly.

Ruth had given Heart a soft rope of woven flax.

Heart had made it into a knotted halter. The mare didn't like it, Heart could tell. But she allowed it.

Day by day the mare's limp faded. The cut closed and was healing well.

The heavy bundles of grass Heart brought were working magic. The mare gained weight. Her flesh smoothed over the bony ridges of her ribs. She stood with her head held high.

Heart found apples that had rolled beyond the fences around Lord Dunraven's orchards.

All the village children hunted these apples. Heart went before first light. Twice she had to run from boys who wanted to steal the ones she'd found. Both times, they had given up before the turnoff onto Crooked Lane. None of them wanted to be seen by Ruth Oakes—or to cross Old Simon's path.

"The horse is looking grand," Simon said one evening.

His voice startled Heart into whirling around. "I didn't hear you coming."

Simon nodded. "You were too busy talking to the mare." He shook his head, laughing, then ran one hand through his stubbly gray hair. "We can sell her soon. You've got her fat enough for any knacker."

"In another month or two, you could sell her as a saddle horse," Heart said quickly.

Simon stroked his chin with one hand. "Is she still limping?"

"A little," Heart fibbed. The mare hadn't limped for more than two weeks.

"You think she's strong enough to bear a rider?" Simon asked.

"Not yet," Heart said, pretending to consider the question. "But soon, I think."

"But that scar ruins her looks," Simon said, shaking his head. "What gentleman would want such an ugly saddle mare?"

Heart frowned at him. “She isn’t ugly!”

“Lower your voice,” Simon scolded.

Heart looked at her feet. Making Simon angry was foolish. “I’m sorry,” she said.

Simon puffed out his cheeks. “Well, then. Keep feeding it,” he said, jabbing one finger at the mare. “If no one else wants it, the knacker will.”

“I thought maybe . . .” Heart began, then stopped.

“Thought what?” Simon asked.

“Maybe I could find an old plow. We could find work.”

“We?” Simon repeated. “You mean you and the horse?”

Heart nodded.

Simon laughed. Then he spat. “Plowmen are *men*,” he scoffed.

Heart stood tall. “I could plow.”

Simon laughed. “You couldn’t. It takes weight and strength.”

Heart felt the mare tug her sleeve, nibbling at

the ragged cloth. Heart glanced at the sky. The sun was setting. "I need to take her out to walk."

"That where you go every evening after supper?"

Heart nodded. "Ruth Oakes said I should."

"That old faker," Simon said. "Her herbs aren't worth a half-penny." He headed back toward the house.

Heart waited until she heard the door slam.

Then she let out a long sigh.

"I will think of something," she told the mare, turning back. "Maybe we can get ahold of an old cart somehow. Would you pull a cart?"

The mare shook her mane.

Heart smiled; she loved it when the mare seemed to understand her. "We could carry messages. They say there's a man in Derrytown who carries letters for the merchants and nobles there."

The mare shook her mane again, snorting.

Heart frowned. "If we can earn a few pennies,

Simon will let me keep you." The mare lifted her head and flared her nostrils.

Heart pulled the halter down from its peg. The mare lowered her head as Heart slid it over her ears.

They passed Ruth Oakes's place and turned south as always. Out on River Road, the mare kept a good pace. As usual, she walked alongside Heart, not behind her.

The road was quiet. The air smelled of clean, fresh sage. The sounds and smells of town did not carry this far.

Heart glanced at the mare. She had never seen anyone but Dunraven's men or nobles like Tin Blackaby riding—and then only from a distance. She wanted to learn how.

Abruptly, the mare leapt sideways, wrenching hard at the halter.

Heart wasn't expecting it.

She lost her grip as the mare sprang into a canter.

Heart stood, stunned, as the mare galloped

away. Then she lunged after the horse, knowing it was useless. Aching inside, her eyes filling with tears, Heart ran on and on down the dusky road. The mare was a blurred speck of white in the dusk.

Finally, when Heart could run no more, she stumbled to a stop.

She bent over, gasping for breath.

In the distance, the muffled clatter of hooves had faded into silence.

The mare was gone.

Heart felt sick.

How could she have been so careless?

She trembled, still dragging in long breaths. Someone else would find the mare. Or wolves would.

Heart looked back toward Simon's shack. In the deepening dusk, it looked smaller and sadder than ever.

Heart stared at it.

Simon would be furious.

Ruth Oakes would be disappointed in her.

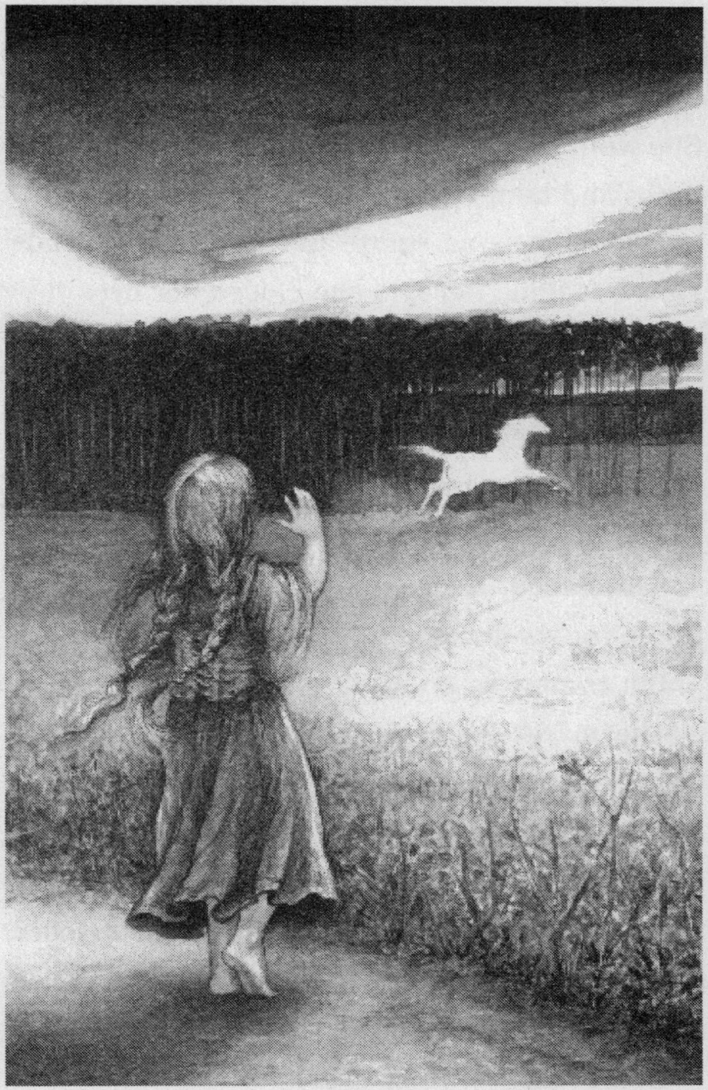

But that wasn't what hurt.

Now there'd be no reason to wake up excited. She would no longer have to get up early to cut grass and hunt extra apples—or hurry home.

A loneliness as sharp as thorns grew inside Heart. It filled her and she closed her eyes.

She was startled by a sudden cadence of distant hoofbeats. She caught her breath and opened her eyes, staring into the murky dusk.

Finally, she saw a blur of white.

The mare was galloping back toward her.

Astonished, Heart set her feet wide, ready to lunge for the halter.

But there was no need.

The mare dropped back to a canter, then a trot. She kept coming, her neck arched, breathing hard from the long gallop.

Heart felt joy rising inside her.

The mare looked grand indeed, trotting closer. She was stout now, her sides filled in, even swollen.

Heart narrowed her eyes.

There was something heavy in the mare's gait. Not the limp. That was gone. This was something different.

The mare stopped, standing so close that Heart simply lifted one hand to take hold of the halter.

The dusk around them had deepened. They stood in near darkness, so close Heart felt the warmth from the mare's run seeping into the chilly air. The mare pushed her muzzle into Heart's chest, blowing out deep breaths.

Keeping hold of the halter, Heart slid one hand over the mare's side. The tiniest flutter of movement beneath the white coat made Heart step back, blinking.

"You're in foal?" she breathed.

The mare shook her mane and stared off to the west. The sky was pink and orange now, the clouds colored like fire.

Heart pressed her palm against the white flank. The movement didn't return, but the fullness was unmistakable. Heart smiled.

The mare was going to have a baby.

Simon couldn't sell her now, not to the knacker or anyone else.

He *wouldn't*.

All he had to do was wait.

Two horses would be worth much more than one.

Heart put her arms around the mare's neck and began to cry.

✦ CHAPTER FIVE

Ruth Oakes knocked at the door early one morning. "I need to hire Heart," she told Simon. "I can't manage all my work."

"After she feeds the mare."

Heart stood up from her winnowing baskets and came to the door. "I cut grass before dawn, like always, Simon."

He turned away.

Halfway up Crooked Lane, Heart told Ruth the news. Ruth stopped, her hands on her hips. "Have you told Simon?"

Heart nodded.

"And his reaction?"

"He's whistling and humming over it." Heart scuffed her bare feet, making long marks in the dust.

They walked onward. "A foal," Ruth said softly. "Lovely. Any birth is like magic."

Heart smiled. "Her belly is getting bigger. She's eating as much as I can bring her."

"What have you named the mare?"

Heart glanced at Ruth. "I haven't. I don't know a name to give her."

"You could give her part of yours," Ruth said.

Heart liked the idea. Then the mare would be connected to her forever, like family. "Avamir?"

"It's a lovely name," Ruth agreed. "And an ancient one. That's why I chose it for you."

"Avamir, then," Heart agreed. She wanted to run back and tell the mare. But that was silly, of course. Horses didn't care about names.

Someone had left a box of fresh beets at Ruth's door.

Most of her patients paid her in trade.

She swung the box up and carried it inside. "Let's bundle the dried borage and hyssop, then we'll walk to market, if you're willing."

Heart smiled. "Of course."

Walking to town with Ruth meant no one would taunt her.

Every family in Ash Grove owed Ruth Oakes. Many of them loved her. No one wanted to offend her. Who could know when they would need the healer to come at midnight?

"These?" Heart asked, pointing at the drying racks.

Ruth nodded. "And the borage on the other side. I'll make packets of lobelia and verlane and . . ." She looked around the room. "Lemon-grass, I think."

Heart fetched the cloth bags from the bin in the sunny kitchen.

She laid them out, then set to work. She was careful not to let too many crisp leaves scatter onto the floor.

"You do that better than I do now," Ruth said.

Heart grinned.

She loved being in this house.

"We'll use the peachwood baskets," Ruth said.

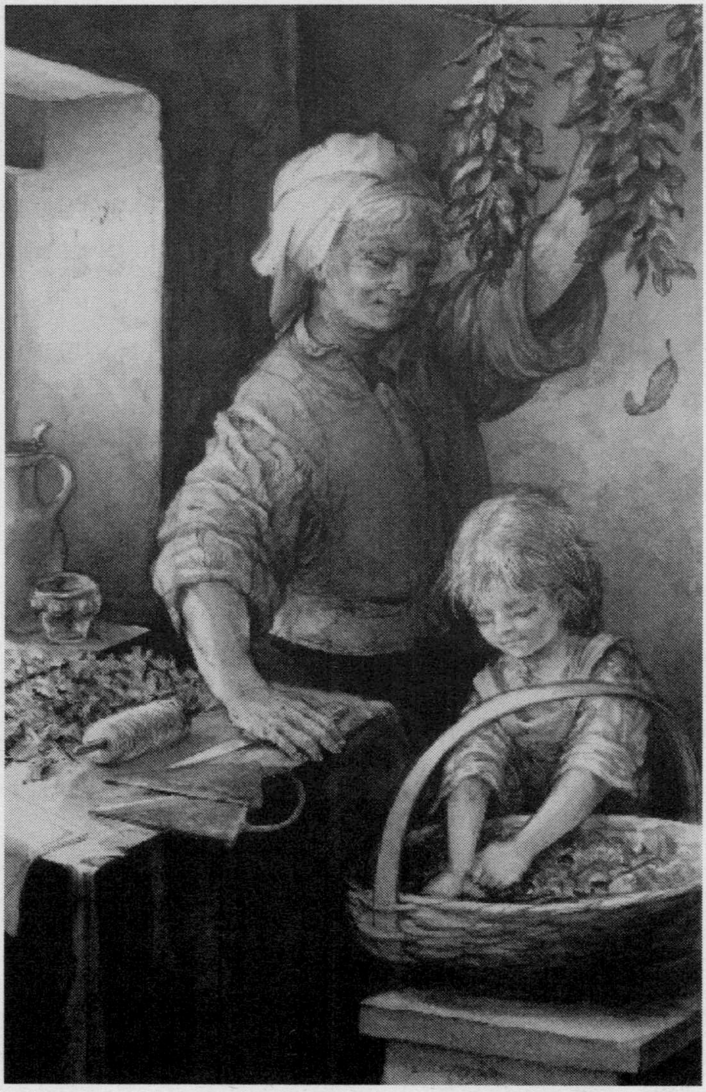

Heart ran to the storage room. The big peachwood baskets were reddish with arched handles.

"Perfect," Ruth said. "And a lovely day for the walk."

They followed River Road north, then turned on Crosswater Street.

The cobblestones were uneven.

Heart walked carefully—she didn't want to stub her bare toes.

After a few minutes, they crossed the creaking planks of the Tirin Creek Bridge and went on downhill.

"Look," Ruth said, pointing.

A mile ahead, coming across the long and narrow Blue River Bridge, carts and wagons turned toward Market Square. Derrytown merchants were arriving.

Ruth sighed. "A lot of them this morning. Maybe I should have brought more herbs."

"I would like to see Derrytown one day," Heart said aloud. "Maybe even Dunraven's castle."

Ruth patted her shoulder. "Then you shall."

It was not the answer Heart had expected. She laughed aloud.

"Good morning, Healer," someone called from across the street.

Heart saw Mrs. Renner; her husband ran the tallow works.

People moved away from Mrs. Renner as she walked. Tallow stink always clung to her clothes and hair. She had one son. Tibbs Renner was teased almost as much as Heart. She felt sorry for him, but she was afraid of him, too.

Ruth crossed the street to say hello to Mrs. Renner.

Heart waited, standing aside to let others go past.

"Psst. River foundling!"

Heart had been expecting this. Tibbs Renner was the biggest ten-year-old in Ash Grove. And the meanest.

Heart tensed as he walked up.

"I saw you with that horse," he said. "Where'd you steal it?"

Heart's breath caught. She had hoped no one had seen Avamir. "I found her. In the woods," she told him.

"Found her?" Tibbs sneered. "No one ever just *finds* a horse."

"I did," Heart said as evenly as she could.

"Liar," he said. "Why are you hiding the horse then?"

Heart blinked. "I'm not, really. I just thought people might—"

"Spread the word about it? Find the real owner?" Tibbs interrupted.

Looking past him, Heart saw Ruth saying good-bye to his mother.

"She was loose in the woods, no bridle or saddle and she was hurt terribly and—"

"Liar," Tibbs said. "That's one thing the healer can't cure—lying."

"Heart needs no such cure," Ruth said from behind him.

Tibbs jumped. "I was joking," he said quickly.

Ruth looked at him sternly. "I would hate to think you were insulting my friend."

Tibbs mumbled something and walked away. But he glanced back, flushed and scowling.

Ruth sighed. Then she led off, turning down Trader's Path when they came to it.

Trader's Path was the oldest—and the shortest and narrowest—street in Ash Grove. It veered toward the river, then back to run along the edge of Market Square. People on foot used it. The wagons went around to Market Street.

Heart loved the smells and colors of the Market Square.

She wished they could stay all day.

But they never did.

The booths were setting up.

Ruth walked fast, going up and down the aisles, saying hello to nearly everyone they passed. She stopped at a few booths.

The herbs sold quickly.

Ruth's medicines were known to be pure and strong.

Walking home, Heart saw Tibbs coming toward them. He gave a quick nod, and hurried past.

"That boy makes me worry," Ruth said.

Heart's stomach knotted up.

It didn't loosen until she ran the length of Crooked Lane and saw the mare standing safe in her fence.

Heart hugged her neck, clinging hard.

"Avamir?" she said when she stepped back. "Do you like that name?"

The mare shook her mane and rubbed her broad cheek against Heart's shoulder.

"Was there a boy out here today?" Heart asked.

Avamir shook her mane and stamped a fore hoof.

Then she went back to picking at scattered blades of grass in the apple crate that served as her hay rick.

✦ CHAPTER SIX

Heart worked for Ruth every chance she got.

At first, Simon complained about cleaning barley by himself.

Then, in October, he groused about digging potatoes without her.

He was upset having to make his own supper in December and January. By February, Heart finally reminded him loudly of all the pennies she was earning.

He frowned. And he kept complaining.

"Are you feeding that mare well enough?" he asked at least once a week.

"Of course," Heart said evenly, every time he asked.

Heart was happier than she had ever been.

Tibbs still stared at her. But he left her alone.

And every evening when she walked Avamir, she let go of the halter as soon as they were far from town.

Avamir loved to gallop, free as wind.

Heart loved to watch her.

The galloping had slowed somewhat, of course.

Avamir was very heavy now, her belly full with her growing foal.

Heart felt it moving nearly every time she pressed her palms on Avamir's flank.

Ruth said that meant the foal was close. She said she would come to help if Avamir needed her.

"When will she drop that foal?" Simon asked every single evening in March.

Heart just shrugged.

She didn't know. She couldn't know. When Ruth needed to go to the market, Heart was impatient to get back.

"Give me the pennies," Simon said every time she got home from Ruth's house.

Heart handed them to him.

Then he would ask his second question.

"Is that all?"

Heart had never hidden or kept back even one penny. The question insulted her.

"Would it be wrong to keep a few pennies?" Heart asked Ruth one fair morning in May.

The healer stopped her work and turned. "Doesn't he let you?"

Heart shook her head. "Never. Nary a one."

Ruth frowned. She looked out the window toward Simon's shack. "Keep half. But be honest. Tell him. Then hide them well."

"Half?" Heart breathed. "Is that fair?"

"Half." Ruth said it flatly. "More than fair," she added. "He's gotten dawn to dusk work out of you since he found you." She reached up and took down a wooden box. "Here. Bury it outside somewhere safe."

"I wish I had parents," Heart heard herself saying. Then she blushed.

"You do have parents, of course," Ruth said softly. "It's a matter of finding them."

Heart looked down at her hands.

Flecks of red mallow leaves were stuck to her nails.

"Do you think I ever will?" she asked.

Ruth exhaled. "I do. Now help me with the valerian roots, will you? I have them soaking in the copper tub."

A few days later, Heart told Simon she was keeping half her pennies.

He roared, then whined.

Then he went silent for a few hours.

The next morning he acted as though the argument had never happened.

That night, after he was asleep, Heart buried the box beside the corral.

One evening, going home, Heart saw someone dodge between two trees on River Road, running back toward town.

The sun was low and glaring, but it looked like Tibbs Renner.

Heart's skin prickled.

What was he doing?

Heart ran all the way from Ruth's house to Simon's shack, and headed straight for Avamir's corral.

The mare whickered as Heart ducked between the crooked rails.

"Are you all right?" Heart asked her. "Was Tibbs here? Did he scare you?"

The mare nudged Heart, pushing her back gently. She seemed fine.

Heart felt herself calming down. "I'm a little late," she apologized to the mare. "We better go or it'll be too dark."

Heart slid the rails aside. But, for the first time, Avamir wasn't eager to get out.

"Did he hurt you?" Heart searched the mare's silky white coat for wounds or lumps from rock bruises. Tibbs was a great aim with a rock. He liked to show off.

Avamir turned away, then paced a tight circle, switching her tail.

Then she lay down, dropping heavily to her knees. She groaned quietly.

Heart caught her breath, scared, but beginning to understand. "Avamir? Is your baby coming?" she asked softly. "Are you ready to foal?"

Avamir didn't respond to the sound of her name as she usually did. Heart could tell she was listening intently to something else.

Something inside herself.

Heart ran for clean rags and was glad when she saw Simon asleep on his cot.

She tiptoed in, then out, carrying her own cot blanket along with the rags.

Avamir was groaning.

It was a deep sound unlike anything Heart had ever heard.

The mare strained, then relaxed, gulping in long breaths.

Stars came out overhead one by one. The moon rose and climbed in the sky, full and round.

Avamir strained over and over, until her white coat was soaked with sweat.

Heart stayed close, draping the blanket over the mare's back so she wouldn't get chilled.

"Should I get Ruth?" Heart asked the sky. "Does Avamir need help?"

Avamir shook her mane, then lifted her head and nudged at Heart's shoulder.

"Do you want me to stay?" Heart pleaded.

She was afraid to leave the mare alone.

She was just as afraid to wait any longer to run for help.

What if Avamir was having trouble?

Suddenly, Avamir groaned, her whole body trembling with effort.

Heart saw two tiny hooves emerge.

The next push brought spindly front legs and a muzzle small enough to drink from a teacup.

Heart held her breath.

Avamir made an odd sound, somewhere between pain and joy. She strained again.

The foal slid into the world and lay still on the ground.

Then it curled like a fish without air.

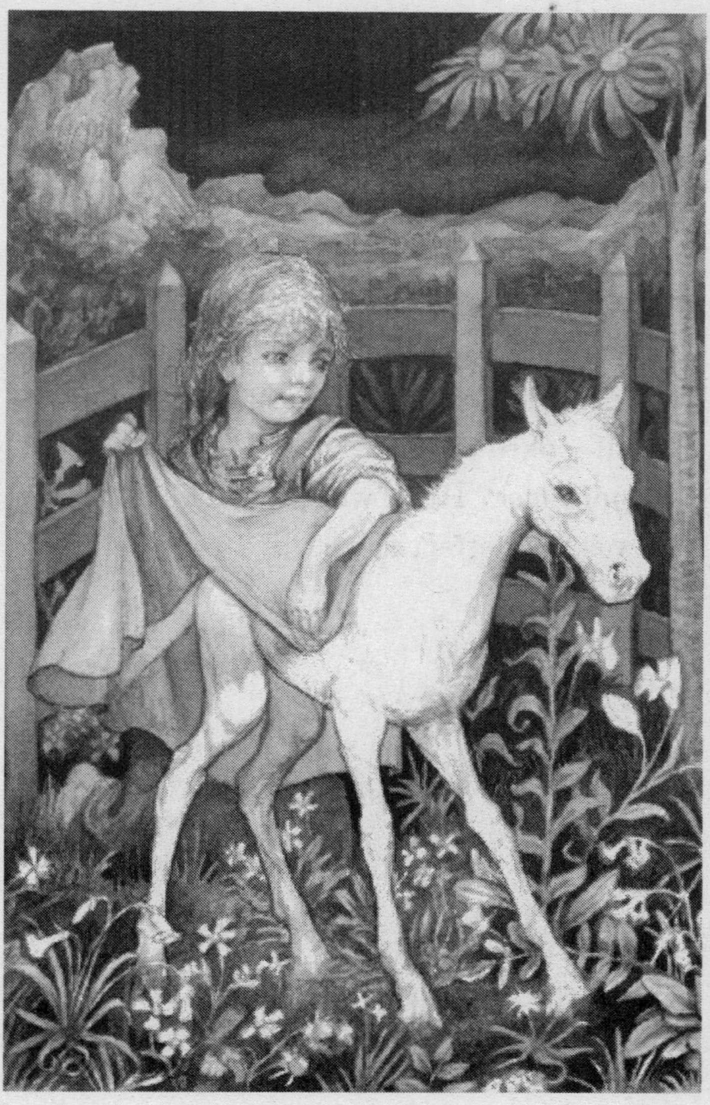

Heart frantically wiped away the birth water from its nostrils and eyes. She soaked one rag and picked up another.

The foal wriggled in her arms.

Avamir turned to lick at her baby.

Heart kept rubbing. Together they dried the foal and helped it stand on its own skinny legs. The foal's coat was purest white. In the moonlight, it looked silvery.

"Moonsilver," Heart whispered, and smiled.

It was the perfect name.

✦ CHAPTER SEVEN

The morning after the foal was born, Simon stood by the fence, frowning. "Look at it! It's ugly."

Heart stared at the baby horse that had slept in her arms. "He's only a little small. He'll grow and—"

"Small?" Simon exploded. "It's sickly like its mother!"

Heart shook her head, moving a step closer to Avamir. "She was half starved, Simon. And hurt. Not sickly."

He rubbed his chin. "What's wrong with its face?"

Heart bit her lip. The foal's head was oddly formed. It worried her. "Nothing," she said aloud.

"Its forehead is misshapen. It's swollen. Maybe it has brain fever?"

"No," Heart said.

"Tonight, you should walk them up the road for that old woman to take a look," Simon said.

Heart glanced at him. "I will."

"Tell her I won't pay her a penny."

Heart lifted her chin. "I will pay her."

Simon flashed her an angry look. "I suppose you can do what you like with *your* pennies."

"He isn't sickly," Heart said as Simon turned away.

But all day she was worried.

She did her work. She hoed their little garden and swept the house and cleaned the hearth.

She went to gather deadwood with Simon for their fire. Walking home with the heavy sacks, Heart walked as fast as Simon would go.

The worry knot in her stomach had been tightening all day. Passing Ruth's house, she peered inside. The old woman was there. Good.

Once the firewood was stacked, Simon sat in

his chair with a sigh. Heart ran for the horses. The dusk was thickening.

"Moonsilver isn't sick," Ruth told her. They stood outside her door, the lantern on the garden wall.

Heart let out a breath. "Are you sure?"

"I am," Ruth said, keeping her eye on Avamir.

The mare's ears were back. She kept circling to stand between Ruth and her foal.

"His forehead—"

"I see that," Ruth interrupted. "It is odd. But look at how quick he is. He seems very strong for a new foal."

Heart let out a long breath. Of course Ruth was right.

"Just feed Avamir every bit you can manage. The foal will grow strong and straight if her milk is rich."

"I will," Heart promised.

She kept her word.

Every day, she walked a mile down to the river and back to cut heavy bundles of tender grass.

She hunted by moonlight for fallen early plums along Lord Dunraven's fence.

She even saved boiled barley or wheat from her own suppers.

Avamir had plenty of milk.

Moonsilver nursed constantly.

But he stayed small and thin.

In the warm June evenings, Heart took the horses up to River Road. Avamir galloped as fast as ever. Moonsilver kept up with her. His legs were spindly, but he ran like lightning.

As summer nights warmed, Ruth's herbs needed setting. Then they needed weeding, and, finally, they had to be cut and dried. Heart learned that each plant was different.

Some loved damp soil, others rotted in it.

Some grew fast in bright sun, others died without shade.

Some days they gathered wild herbs.

Heart loved the long walks into the woods. Meadowsweet and velvety verbain, lobelia and prickly Colter's Wart . . . Heart learned where each herb hid in the forest.

And she was learning what they were used for.

On market days, Heart usually went to town with Ruth Oakes.

But it was different now.

Ruth started selling her herbs at one end of Market Square.

Heart began at the other.

They visited every customer's booth, selling everything they had brought and doing it twice as fast.

Heart often saw Tibbs Renner. He never spoke to her, but she caught him staring, sometimes. In a way, she was glad when she saw him. At least she knew he wasn't out poking around Simon's place, bothering Avamir.

Ruth always said hello to Tibbs—but then Ruth said hello to everyone.

"I saw Tibbs on River Road," Heart told Ruth on the way home after the first market day in July.

"Where?"

"Up by your place, headed back into town.

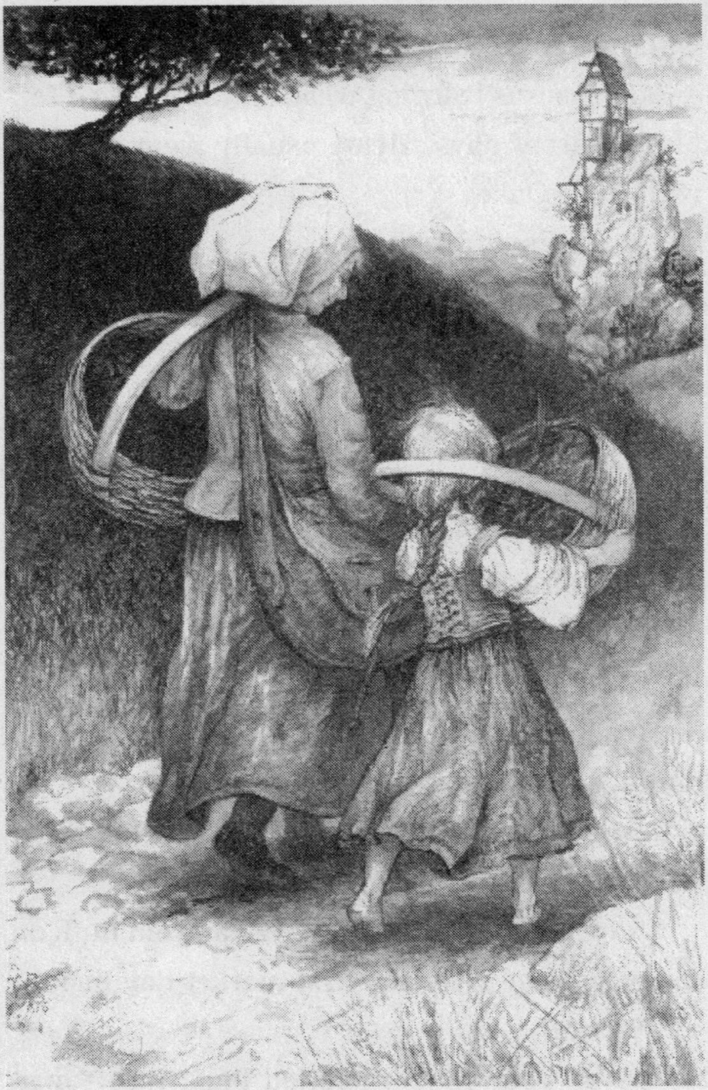

I was afraid he had done something to Avamir."

Ruth looked sad as they walked on. Her silence lasted a long time.

Finally, she straightened her apron, jingling the day's coins.

"Tibbs is mean because his father is mean to him. And the children taunt him."

"They taunt me, too," Heart said.

"Yes, but his father . . ." Ruth began, then fell silent again.

Heart wondered if her own father had been kind or cruel.

She tried, for the thousandth time, to follow her memories backward. They stopped where they always had. Before that day in the river grass, she had no memories at all.

"I do wish Simon hadn't sold the blanket," she said quietly.

Ruth sighed, understanding her. "It was lovely. Silver thread embroidery of unicorns."

"Unicorns," Heart echoed. Simon had not told her that.

Ruth smiled. "I saw it. Old fashioned, by a hundred years. No one believes any of those old stories now."

"My parents must be rich, then," Heart said. "If they owned a fine old blanket like that. So why would they just leave me?"

"I don't know." Ruth reached out to touch Heart's cheek. "But you will find out one day, I am sure."

Heart was unable to think of anything to say. She pulled in a deep breath. "Tibbs stares at me. He hates me, I think."

"We'll both watch for Tibbs," Ruth said, turned down Crooked Lane and headed for her house. "If he causes trouble, I'll help." She opened her front door and went inside. "Just leave Tin Blackaby out of it. The boy has enough trouble."

Heart followed Ruth into the kitchen, thinking.

If children stole or set fires, or did other terrible things, Tin Blackaby could arrest them. There were prisons in Dunraven's castle.

Heart could recall three boys being sent away.

None had ever come back.

"I won't tell Tin Blackaby anything," she promised.

"Thank you," Ruth said. "If Tibbs gets his chance, he'll turn out all right."

Ruth found her lantern and lit it, then spilled the day's money out onto her kitchen table. Heart added the coins she had collected.

Ruth made two stacks. One was a little smaller. She pushed it toward Heart.

"You've learned a great deal these past months," she said. "We can be partners now."

Heart was astonished. "I haven't learned nearly enough."

Ruth smiled. "I agree. But you will."

Heart stared at the money.

If Ruth made her partner, she might someday have enough to buy *shoes*. And she would save every penny after that so maybe she really could see Derrytown and Dunraven's castle one day.

Heart imagined herself riding Avamir into Derrytown. Moonsilver would run along loose behind them, strong and beautiful, his hooves dancing on the road.

She would wear a new red coat and soft leather boots.

People would wonder who she was.

"Take it," Ruth said. "You have earned it."

Heart stared at the coins, then swept them up and put them into her pockets.

"Thank you." The words seemed far too small so she said them again.

"Thank you."

Heart's partnership with Ruth meant she was gone all day every day.

She gave Simon some of her money, so he didn't scold her. As August passed and September came, he began gleaning the fields. The harvesters had been too quick again. They had been careless. The fields were full of missed grain.

Simon came home with a heavy sack every evening, smiling.

Then one evening, Simon met Heart at the

door. He was frowning, but said nothing until supper. "Tin Blackaby has called a meeting," he told her then. "One of his men pounded at the door today to tell me."

Heart looked up from her bowl of boiled wheat.

"No one knows what it's about," Simon said in a low voice. "Can't be anything good. His meetings never are."

Heart nodded, her stomach tightening. "When?"

"Tomorrow evening. You'll have to skip the mare's gallop."

Heart nodded and stood, her appetite gone.

Simon saw the barley in her dish and reached to pick it up. "That fool mare and colt," he muttered.

Heart didn't answer, but she knew what he was thinking.

He was afraid something they had done was the cause of the trouble.

Everyone in Ash Grove would be afraid of the same thing tonight.

✦ CHAPTER EIGHT

River Road was as full of people as Heart had ever seen it. Everyone was walking slowly, quietly. Simon was silent, frowning.

Where River Road met Crosswater Street, they turned toward Market Square with all the rest.

"There are hundreds coming," Simon muttered as they slowed with the thickening crowd. "Even the old ones and babies. Blackaby must have sent messengers to every door."

Heart looked around as they walked.

Simon was right.

There were people so old that their grandchildren had to help them walk.

She saw Tibbs just as they turned onto Trader's Path.

He was with his family.

Mr. Renner looked angry.

Heart saw Mr. Renner shove at Tibbs, saying something close to his ear. Tibbs looked scared.

"Stop staring at them," Simon said, tugging at Heart's sleeve. "I want no arguments with the knacker."

Tin Blackaby had had his men build a platform at one end of Market Square.

He stood upon it, his mouth a thin, angry line.

In front of the platform, a row of his men faced the crowd, their arms crossed.

The back of the square filled up first.

No one wanted to stand near Blackaby's men.

Heart and Simon ended up in the middle. People stood close together, but no one spoke.

Tin Blackaby stared at them until people began to clear their throats and glance around uneasily.

"The harvesters this year were careless," he shouted, finally, startling everyone. Heart felt her pulse quicken.

"No one bothered to tell me this," he accused them. "No one told me, so I could not tell Lord Dunraven."

Heart noticed a tall figure in a black cloak standing behind Tin Blackaby.

Had the man been there all along?

"I could not tell our lord that he had been cheated." Tin Blackaby's voice was rough and loud.

Heart noticed people drawing even closer together.

Everyone looked straight ahead.

"How many of you noticed that the fields had been harvested poorly these past two seasons?"

Heart waited.

No one put up a hand.

No one called out.

Tin Blackaby muttered something Heart couldn't hear, then he raised his voice again. "You have all shamed me before Lord Dunraven," he said. "I told him you were honest.

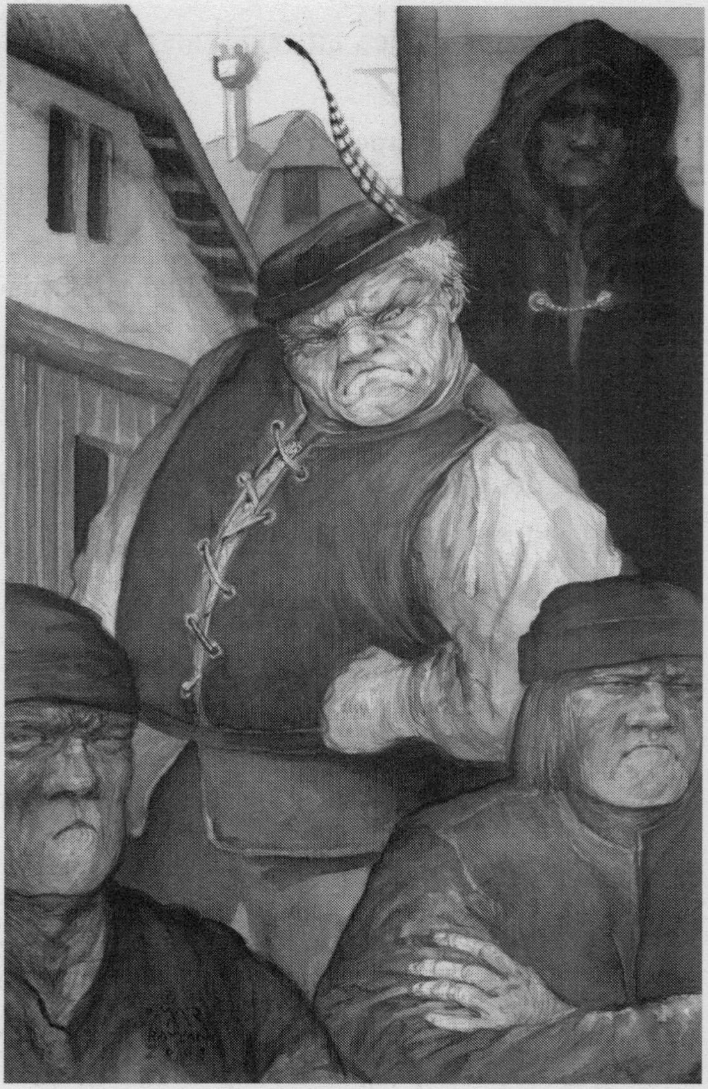

I said you would admit a mistake. But I see I was wrong."

The tall figure stepped forward suddenly and Tin Blackaby dropped to one knee. He bowed his head.

The man in the black cloak pushed back his hood.

Heart had never seen Lord Dunraven, but she knew that's who he was.

He had long silver hair. Even from where Heart stood she could tell that he had narrow, angry eyes. And when he spoke, his voice was like thunder.

"People of Ash Grove. Be grateful that I am honest and fair. Be glad I will not punish you."

The crowd stirred as people exchanged nervous glances. No one spoke.

"Tomorrow at dawn, men will come to your homes. They will collect my share of the wheat and barley you have gleaned from my fields: Half."

Lord Dunraven paused nearly a full minute

before he spoke again. "And if you ever cheat me again, I'll make you sorry."

He waited another full minute, then he gestured like a farmer shooing away pesky dogs. "Go home."

Heart followed Simon out of the square.

No one was talking.

Even the smallest children were quiet.

Heart scanned the crowd.

Where was Ruth Oakes? Maybe she was tending someone too sick to leave?

"It isn't fair," someone said clearly.

"Shhh!" an old man hissed.

"He's right though," someone else muttered.

No one responded.

They trudged back up the hill to River Road. The sun set and dusk darkened the sky. By the time they got to Crooked Lane, it was nearly dark. Only then did Simon speak.

"Get a halter on that mare."

Heart was startled. "Why?"

"As soon as it's pitch dark, you're taking

her to the knacker's. Her and the colt."

Heart shook her head. "Why? No one said anything about them."

"Maybe Blackaby's man didn't notice them. But Dunraven's man will." Simon made a chopping motion with one hand. "If they go to the knacker's tonight, I get paid. And there's no trouble with Dunraven's man come morning."

"No!" Heart breathed. "You can't ask me to do that."

"Why not?" Simon demanded. "I will do it if you won't. That colt isn't worth raising. I'll give you some of the money, of course," he added, softening his voice.

Heart wanted to scream at him.

She held it back.

She bit her lip.

And she nodded. "I'll take them, then."

"Good girl," Simon said. Then he went inside, slamming the door behind him.

✦ CHAPTER NINE

Heart put the halter on Avamir.

She told Simon she was cold and carried her ragged coat and her blanket outside.

She waited five minutes.

Then she went back in.

"I need some rags," she told Simon calmly. "I want to braid a halter for the colt, too. He might run off."

"That's my girl," Simon said proudly. "Thinking and planning." He was sitting by the fire.

He yawned. The long walk to town on top of the day's work had worn him out.

Heart hummed softly as she made a braided halter for the colt. She saw Simon yawn again.

Still humming, Heart took two of the four

apples on the sideboard. She filled a sack with cleaned barley. She took a striking flint and steel to make a fire. She packed the smallest cook pot. She took twine, bobbins, and a needle and everything else she could think of that Simon owned and could spare.

Then she went outside and dug up the little box that held her money. She left a stack of copper pennies on Simon's table to pay for what she was taking, then went outside again.

Shivering in the evening chill, Heart haltered Avamir. She put the braided halter on the colt, but let him run free behind as she started off, walking slowly.

She half-expected Simon to hear the hoof beats and come running out the door.

He didn't.

She thought Ruth might come out to ask where she was going.

But that didn't happen, either.

Ruth's windows were dark. She was probably at someone's house, nursing a sick person.

Heart blinked back tears.

Ruth's advice—a warm hug—Heart wanted both more than anything else in the world. But she was on her own and she knew it. She wasn't even going to get to say good-bye.

Heart tried to think clearly.

She and the horses would starve on the empty plains in winter. Open wheat and barley fields were useless to her.

The forests and mountains across the Blue River were her only hope of hiding.

Heart walked the mare toward town, trembling and afraid. Moonsilver came behind, staying close to his mother.

River Road was dark.

Crosswater Street was empty.

After she crossed the Tirin Creek Bridge, Heart could hear men's voices in Market Square. If they heard Avamir's hooves clopping they paid no attention.

She glanced eastward and saw a glow on the horizon.

The moon was rising.

Halfway across the bridge over the Blue River, the moon came up. Heart kept walking, clenching her teeth.

Then suddenly, shouts broke out behind her. Heart began to run, pulling at the halter.

Avamir balked, jerking Heart to a halt.

"Come on!" Heart whispered, dragging at the flaxen rope. The voices were getting louder. "I think they saw us," Heart pleaded, her pulse pounding in her temples. If they were caught now, with Tin Blackaby already so angry . . .

Avamir shook her mane.

Then she bent one knee and sank down on the bridge planks, kneeling like a trick horse.

For a long second, Heart thought the mare was hurt.

Then she understood.

Heart swung one leg awkwardly over Avamir's back.

The mare straightened.

Heart nearly fell, grasping at Avamir's mane

as the mare trotted, then cantered, her hoofbeats thunderous in the silent night. Moonsilver galloped after his mother, his own hoofbeats a rain-patter on the bridge planks.

Heart could not sit upright.

She had never ridden a horse in her life.

The quick rhythm of the mare's gait terrified her.

Heart closed her eyes and tangled her fingers in Avamir's mane, bouncing awkwardly on the mare's back as the voices faded behind them.

After a long time, Avamir slowed, breathing hard. Then she stopped and stood still.

Heart opened her eyes. Slowly, she released her grip on the mare's mane. Her hands were cramped.

Swinging down to the ground. Heart faced Avamir.

"You are the smartest horse I ever heard of," Heart said.

Avamir lifted her head and began to walk.

Moonsilver trotted after her.

Heart ran to catch up, grabbing at Avamir's halter. Side by side they walked deeper into the forest.

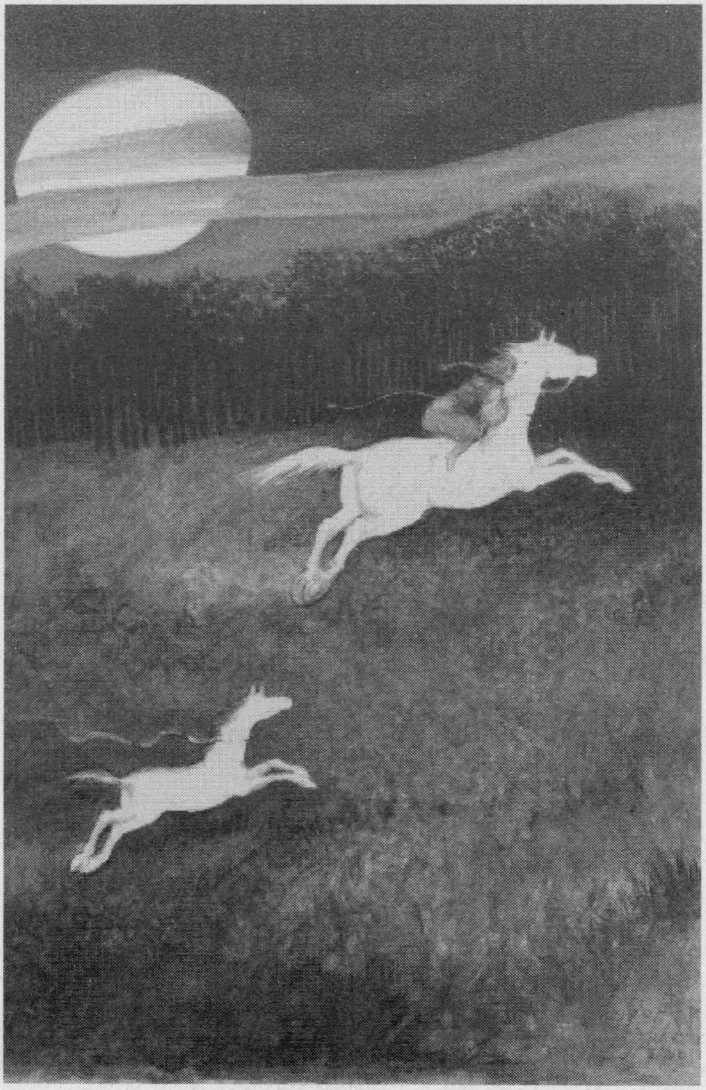

They walked until the moon was high overhead.

Then Heart stopped.

Her legs trembling from weariness and fear, Heart found a dense stand of trees—a safe place to build a tiny fire.

Too nervous to sleep, she sat still as Avamir and the colt settled onto beds of pine needles close by.

Heart ringed the fire with rocks and warmed a little barley in her cook pot.

She heard wolves howling far away and shivered.

Staring into the flames as the horses dozed, she tried to figure out what to do.

She could just keep going and try to live in the deep woods. Or she could try to find a village where she might manage to earn a living.

But Heart knew everyone she met would think she'd stolen the horses.

Girls dressed in raggedy clothes never owned horses, after all.

Heart looked at Avamir, her white coat shining in the firelight. Moonsilver slept beside her. An odd shadow darkened his odd, bulging forehead, making him even less pretty than usual.

Heart stood up, narrowing her eyes. Was the colt hurt?

Stepping around the fire, Heart knelt beside him. The shadow was a stain. Blood was seeping into his smooth white coat.

He must have cantered into a low branch, she decided, touching the wound. But it wasn't bad, no more than the skin broken.

Heart sighed in relief.

Then a strange glitter caught her attention.

She peered at Moonsilver's forehead.

There, peeking through the edges of the colt's broken skin, was a gleam of silver.

Holding her breath, Heart touched it carefully, knowing what it was, but not ready to believe it.

The hard, slick nub of a horn felt cold, like winter ice.

A unicorn's horn.

The awful scar on Avamir's face suddenly made sense.

So did her amazing intelligence.

"You're unicorns?" Heart whispered.

Avamir shook her mane and extended her muzzle. Heart felt the warm sweet breath on her cheek. Then Avamir lowered her head and closed her eyes to sleep.

Heart sat very still.

Unicorns?

Unicorns weren't real. They were legends, nothing more.

Heart tried to remember the tales she had heard. She was pretty sure people in the old stories were afraid of unicorns. She remembered something about people killing them for their magical horns.

Heart looked up at the sky.

Ruth had told her once that her blanket had had unicorns embroidered on it.

Heart shivered and moved closer to the fire.

Simon would sell her unicorns to Lord

Dunraven. So would Tibbs Renner if he got a chance. A lot of people would. And Dunraven might kill Moonsilver to cut off his horn.

Heart shuddered, feeling sick. This much was certain: Lord Dunraven would never let her see Avamir or Moonsilver again.

A breeze whispered through the treetops.

Heart stared into the flames of her campfire.

Maybe she could gather herbs and trade them for food at the Ash Grove Market, leaving Avamir and Moonsilver in the forest.

Ruth Oakes would help, if she could.

Heart took a deep breath and promised the starry sky that she would protect Avamir and Moonsilver.

She loved them both.

Whatever it cost—even her life—she would keep them safe.

THE UNICORN'S SECRET

The Silver Thread

✦ CHAPTER ONE

Heart shivered on a high ridge.

The sun was rising over Lord Dunraven's vast forest.

She couldn't see the village of Ash Grove or the Blue River.

But she knew where they were—a long day's walk, straight east on the Derrytown road.

Heart stretched, shaking off her dream.

Every night in the woods, she'd had the same one.

In it, she was always running; something was chasing her.

She woke every morning to the sound of forest birds singing.

Her pulse would slow and her fear would fade.

Heart sighed, looking down the slope. The trees spread out in every direction. Lord Dunraven's forests really were *endless.*

Heart wondered, as she did every morning, if Tin Blackaby's men were searching for her. They had seen her running away from Ash Grove.

But how important was a ragged girl with a scarred mare and a spindly colt?

Would they care where she went?

Heart had stayed away from the Derrytown road.

Both Avamir and Moonsilver were white, after all.

Any sharp-eyed traveler might spot them.

Heart glanced at them. From a distance, they *did* look like any mare and colt.

They weren't, of course.

As strange as it still seemed to Heart, they were unicorns.

Unicorns!

Heart smiled.

No one back in Ash Grove believed in unicorns

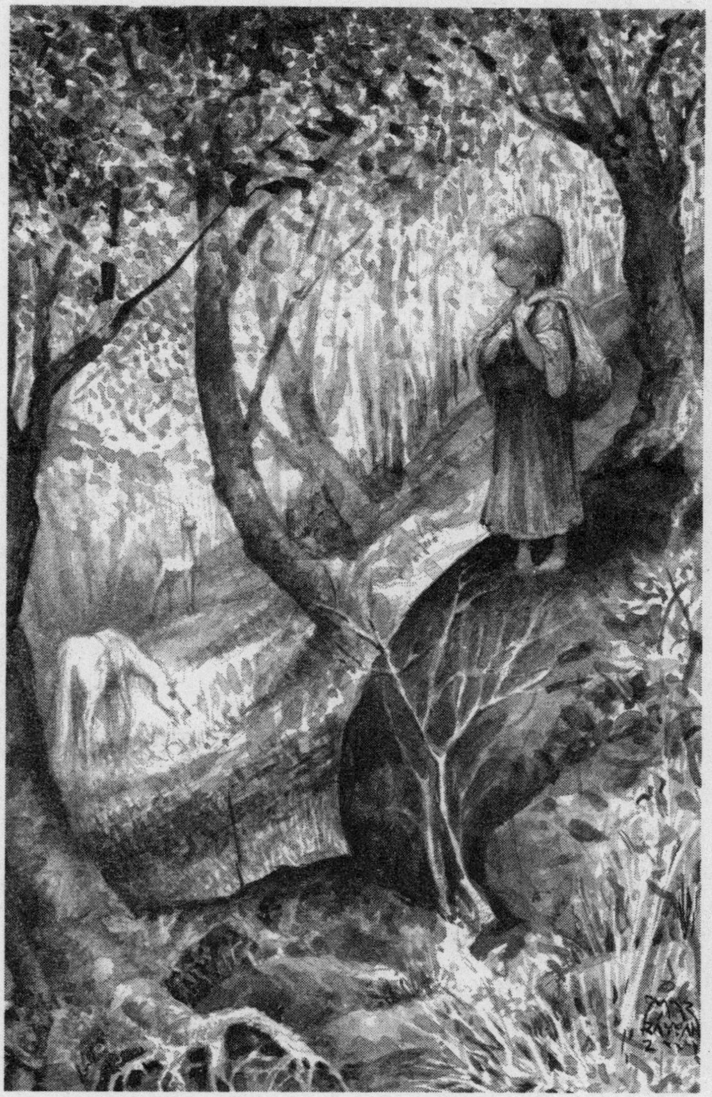

even though everyone knew the legend about the town's name.

It was an odd story. Storytellers said a unicorn had touched the Blue River with her horn. The water had exploded into steam so hot that the grove of ancient oaks on the bank had fallen in piles of ash.

Simon Pratt had thought the story was foolishness.

Ruth Oakes had said no one believed it anymore.

Heart had thought it sounded like someone's fancy.

Now, she wasn't so sure.

She glanced at the unicorns. Avamir had lost her horn somehow. Her face was scarred. Moonsilver was beautiful now, but he had been born small and skinny.

He'd had an odd-looking bulge on his forehead when they'd run away from Ash Grove.

Heart had been worried the first time she'd noticed the small, bloody split in Moonsilver's skin—until she realized it was his horn pushing through.

It was growing fast now. The colt rubbed his forehead on trees constantly, trying to ease the itching and stinging.

Heart blinked as the sun edged above the distant mountains.

She missed Ruth Oakes so much.

Ruth had started teaching her about herbs and healing. She had even paid Heart to help her with her work.

"Not that the coins do us any good here," Heart said aloud.

Heart missed Simon in an odd way too.

Her eyes filled with tears.

Simon had not loved her.

But maybe he had never loved anyone.

He had fed her and taught her, and for that she was grateful.

But he was cruel. If he had gotten his way, the unicorns would have been slaughtered for a few pennies.

If Simon had known Avamir and Moonsilver were unicorns, though, he'd have sold them to Tin Blackaby instead.

Heart shivered. If Blackaby learned the truth, he'd send a hundred men into the forest. He'd try to capture the unicorns so he could sell them to Lord Dunraven.

"And if Lord Dunraven ever finds out that you're unicorns, he'll have a thousand men searching," Heart said aloud.

The only way to stay safe was to stay hidden. She changed camps every night. She kept her cook fires small.

Avamir shook her mane and made a low, whickering sound. Moonsilver cantered to stand close beside his mother.

He was wilder every day, more independent. He had rubbed off the braided-rag halter and lost it on their first day in the woods. Now, he wouldn't let Heart touch him very often.

Heart's stomach growled and she sighed.

The barley she had brought from Simon's

house was more than half gone. She was trying to make it last.

She saw rabbits and squirrels, but had no way to hunt them.

And winter was coming.

Soon it would snow and the grass would be buried. And they had no shelter from the cold.

Heart kicked at a loose rock and listened to it rattle its way down the slope.

The mare looked up, then went on with her grazing.

"What should I do?" Heart asked the sky.

✦ CHAPTER TWO

The chilly nights came and went. Every day, Heart searched for shelter and food.

Then, one misty morning, she saw a shadow at the base of a cliff.

After a long moment, she began to walk up the mountainside.

Avamir lifted her head from grazing as Heart passed.

"Maybe it's a cave," Heart said aloud.

She was getting into the habit of talking to Avamir. She knew it was silly, but it made her feel less lonely.

Avamir whickered at Moonsilver, and they followed as they always did.

Heart waded across a clear little creek.

She slowed, coming up out of the little valley. She was afraid to hope.

Moonsilver galloped in wild circles.

He leaped from one boulder to another.

Heart smiled. No horse colt ever leaped like that. No horse colt ever *could.*

Moonsilver snorted, ducking his head to arch his neck. Avamir leaped sideways, startling him. He bolted into another boulder-jumping circle.

Heart smiled.

Avamir was such a good mother.

"I think it *is* a cave," Heart whispered.

She held her breath, pushing her way through a patch of deer brush. There *was* an opening in the rock!

Avamir slowed, her ears pricked forward.

Caves made good homes for bears, Heart knew. And wolves.

Avamir held her head high. Moonsilver stayed behind her. Heart was ready to run at the slightest sound.

But there was only the silence of the forest.

In front of the opening in the rock, Heart laid one hand on Avamir's withers.

They stood still for a long moment, listening. Then Heart picked up a handful of pebbles and tossed them into the darkness of the cave.

The pebbles hit and rolled to a standstill, then there was silence.

Heart set down her sack.

The silence continued.

She dug through the things she had brought from Simon Pratt's house. Near the bottom of the bag she found the two stubbed candles.

It took several tries to strike a spark into a little pile of dry pine needles.

Once they were burning, Heart lit a candle-wick.

Her pulse thudding, she protected the little flame with one hand. "You stay here," she said to Avamir.

The mare blew out a breath and twitched her tail.

Heart started forward, every muscle in her body tense and ready.

Just inside the cave, she stopped, blinking.

The candlelight flickered in a golden globe around her.

Beyond it, there was midnight darkness.

Heart took one more step. Then another.

The cave was *big*—much bigger than she had dared to hope. She had taken sixteen steps when her candle's light finally struck a wall of gray stone.

Heart lifted the candle, looking straight up.

The rock arched pretty high.

Avamir would be able to walk without lowering her head.

The floor was gritty with sand and pebbles. And it was dry as salt.

Heart allowed herself a hopeful smile.

She would gather firewood every day until they had enough.

She would cut grass and dry it as much as she could before the first snow settled in.

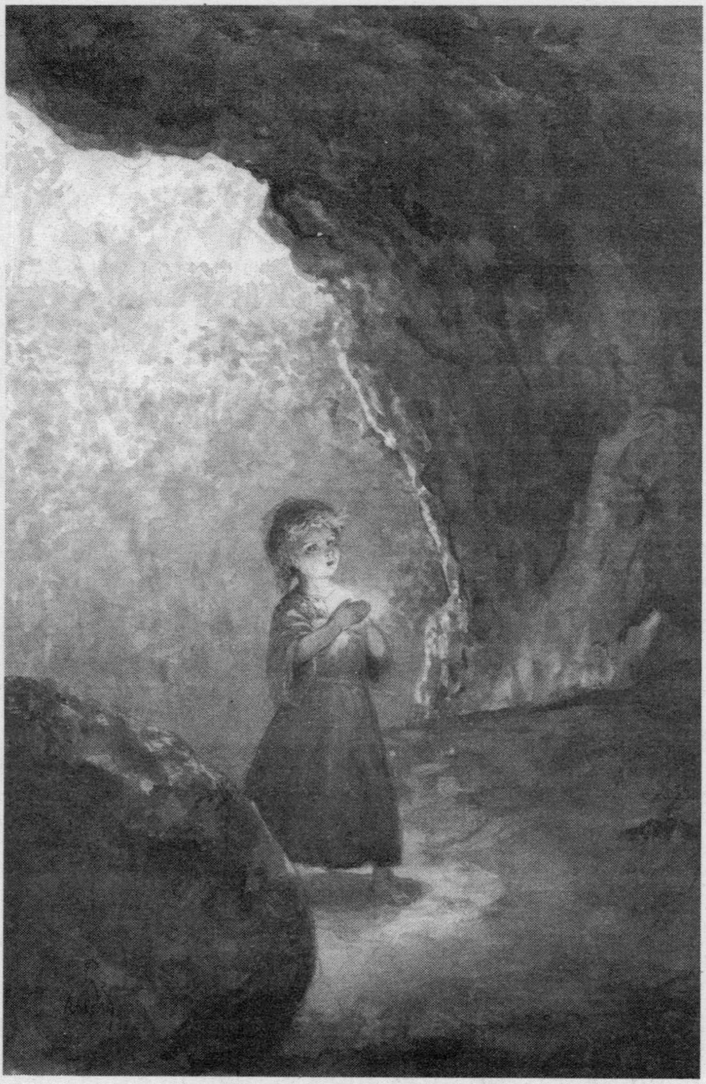

And she would manage, somehow, to build a gate across the entrance to the cave. "We will be safe here," she said aloud.

Her voice sounded hollow and strange.

She felt a sudden wrench of loneliness. But why should she be any lonelier now than she had been in Ash Grove?

Only three people there had ever really talked to her.

Simon had ordered her around. Tibbs Renner, the knacker's son, had found ways to be mean to her. Only Ruth Oakes had been her friend.

Heart turned back toward the entrance.

Avamir and Moonsilver were waiting for her. "It's wonderful," Heart said to Avamir. "Dry and warm and bigger than I thought."

The unicorn mare blew out a long breath and flicked her tail.

Then she came forward lightly.

Moonsilver was right behind her.

✦ CHAPTER THREE

Heart walked downhill with the unicorns every morning. Once they had found a meadow with good grass, she set about her own chores.

There was so much to do.

Heart swept a rock shelf in the cave and dried the grass and herbs upon it. She gathered grass and firewood. She found pine nuts and acorns and stored them. She gathered purslane and cress to eat. She built a fire ring of flat stones. She dragged in a wide log to sit upon.

And everywhere Heart walked, she looked for fallen branches.

She searched for long, straight ones.

At night, by firelight, Heart worked on her gate.

Using sharp sticks and a knife she had taken from Simon's house, she dug deep, narrow holes. When each hole was finished, she set a branch upright in it.

But before the gate was finished, she ran out of barley.

"I can eat pine nuts and purslane for a while," she told Avamir one afternoon.

The white mare shook her mane.

She switched her tail sharply.

"I've dried a lot of grass for you," Heart said. She reached out to lay her hand on the mare's neck.

Moonsilver was galloping in wide arcs as usual, playing.

"But I have to go back to Ash Grove to buy food before long," Heart whispered.

She knew Avamir couldn't really understand.

But she needed to say it, anyway.

"I'm afraid to go back," she admitted, "but I want to see Ruth Oakes. She'll worry."

Avamir ticked one forehoof on a pebble, and

it rolled ahead of them. Then she shook her mane and cantered away. Heart watched her gallop, then slow to a trot, then stop in a patch of tall, green grass.

A breeze rising from the valley below rustled the leaves.

Heart looked down the slope, toward the tree-hidden road.

Maybe she should follow it toward Derrytown, not back to Ash Grove.

Derrytown was twenty times the size of Ash Grove, people said. No one would know who she was. No one would notice one more poor girl.

"Look there!"

Heart stumbled to a stop.

It was a man's voice—not close, but not too far away.

Whirling around, Heart scanned the trees.

"Is that a white deer?" a second voice called. "Can you see it?"

Heart followed the shout with her eyes and

spotted a movement in the trees far downhill. A tiny bit of red flashed among the branches, then was gone. A hunter's cap?

"Moonsilver!" Heart whispered frantically, starting to run.

The colt had been cantering joyously.

Heart could tell he had heard the voices.

He was scared, turning sharply to start back toward his mother.

He galloped toward a fallen log, then rose to jump it. His forehooves tucked with a dancer's grace.

Avamir whickered anxiously. Then the air was torn by a terrible shriek.

For an instant, Heart was sure the scream was human.

As she ran, she imagined one of the men doubled over a sprained ankle.

Then she saw Moonsilver pitch to one side, the beautiful arc of his leap ending in a crashing fall.

Avamir lunged into a gallop, her hooves light and nearly soundless on the soft forest soil.

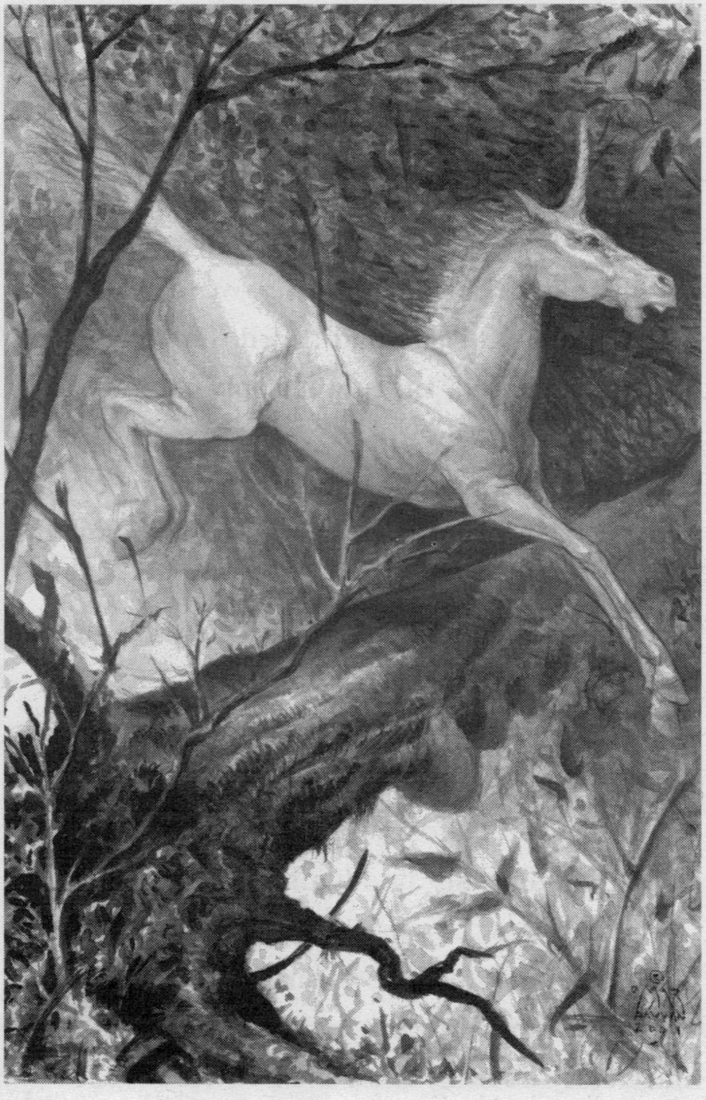

Heart dropped her gathering sack to run faster.

"Can you see it?"

The voice was closer, echoing among the trees. The hunters were coming through the thick forest, making their way up the rocky slope.

"No!" came the curt answer. "But I hit it. You heard it cry out."

Heart ran harder, holding her ragged skirts with one hand. If they got close enough to see Moonsilver clearly . . .

As Avamir plunged to a stop beside her colt, Heart veered to run almost straight across the slope. She sprinted, reckless and desperate.

She glanced back twice. Once she was sure that the unicorns were well behind her, she let out a high-pitched wail.

"There it is! Hear it?" came a shout.

"It's heading north," the second voice accused. "You only wounded it!"

The men's voices were still far down the mountainside—so far that Heart realized something as she ran.

To hit Moonsilver from that far, they had to be using crossbows.

Ordinary village men hunted with short bows. Lord Dunraven forbade any other weapon. Only his own men were armed with crossbows.

Heart put every ounce of her will into running.

She ignored the stab of sharp sticks and rocks bruising her bare feet.

She let out another trailing scream as she ran, then fell silent again.

Breathing hard, she heard the men shouting behind her. Good. They were following *her* now.

Heart ran desperately, pounding through the thickest stands of trees to keep the men from seeing her.

She screamed again over her shoulder.

After a long time, Heart veered to the east. She circled, leading the men farther and father from the unicorns.

Finally, she slowed, then stopped, dragging in gasping breaths.

Silent and careful, she found a tall tree to climb.

Breathing hard, she waited, high in the branches.

The afternoon light was fading.

The forest was thick with shadows.

The men passed close enough for her to hear what they were saying.

"I saw it clearly before I shot," one hunter insisted wearily. "It was a snow-white deer."

The other man laughed. "I'll bet it was an old gray pony some Gypsy let loose."

"An old pony wouldn't have made it this far," the first voice argued.

Heart waited until their voices had faded away.

Then she slid down the tree and doubled back.

The sun was setting.

How long had she been away from the unicorns?

Was Moonsilver still alive?

The thought that he might not be struck her with a pain so deep that for a moment, she could not draw in a breath.

CHAPTER FOUR

Heart made her way back through the forest. Fear weighed her feet and chilled her skin.

When she saw Moonsilver standing beside his mother, her spirits leaped upward.

But then she got close enough to see the blood streaming down his hind leg.

The arrow lay half buried in the dirt on the slope above Moonsilver. It had cut a long gash on his right back leg, just above the hock.

Moonsilver's wounded leg would not bear his weight. He stumbled against his mother, then stood trembling.

Heart found her gathering sack where she had dropped it.

She tore the soft cloth into wide strips.

Then she looked intently at Avamir. "Tell him he has to let me do this," she pleaded, wishing the mare really could understand her.

Avamir pawed the ground uneasily.

"I have to bind it," Heart said, trying not to cry, trying not to stare at the blood staining the pine needles.

She talked to Moonsilver in a low, murmuring voice.

Moonsilver looked at Heart. His eyes were distant, glassy. She could tell he was in terrible pain.

She risked a single step forward.

Moonsilver lifted his head sharply, but he didn't move. She took another step.

Avamir reached out to touch Moonsilver's back with her muzzle.

The colt twitched his skin, then held still.

One more step and Heart stood beside him. She reached out very slowly, placing her hand gently on his neck.

Heart paused again, giving Moonsilver time to calm down.

Then she slid her hand along, an inch at a time. The colt stood still.

Heart pressed the cloth against the wound.

Moonsilver had his muzzle almost on the ground. He swayed a little as she wrapped the strips around his leg.

Heart glanced up the mountainside. It was getting darker—and chillier.

Suddenly, Moonsilver fell forward onto his knees.

Heart rushed to put her arms around him, holding him upright. Avamir came close, whickering low.

Heart pulled Moonsilver back up.

He could barely walk.

Still, he managed to start uphill. He had to stop every few steps.

When they finally reached the entrance to their cave, he stumbled inside.

Heart staggered along, helping him, finally letting him sag to the sand near the fire ring.

She built up the fire and warmed creek water to wash the wound.

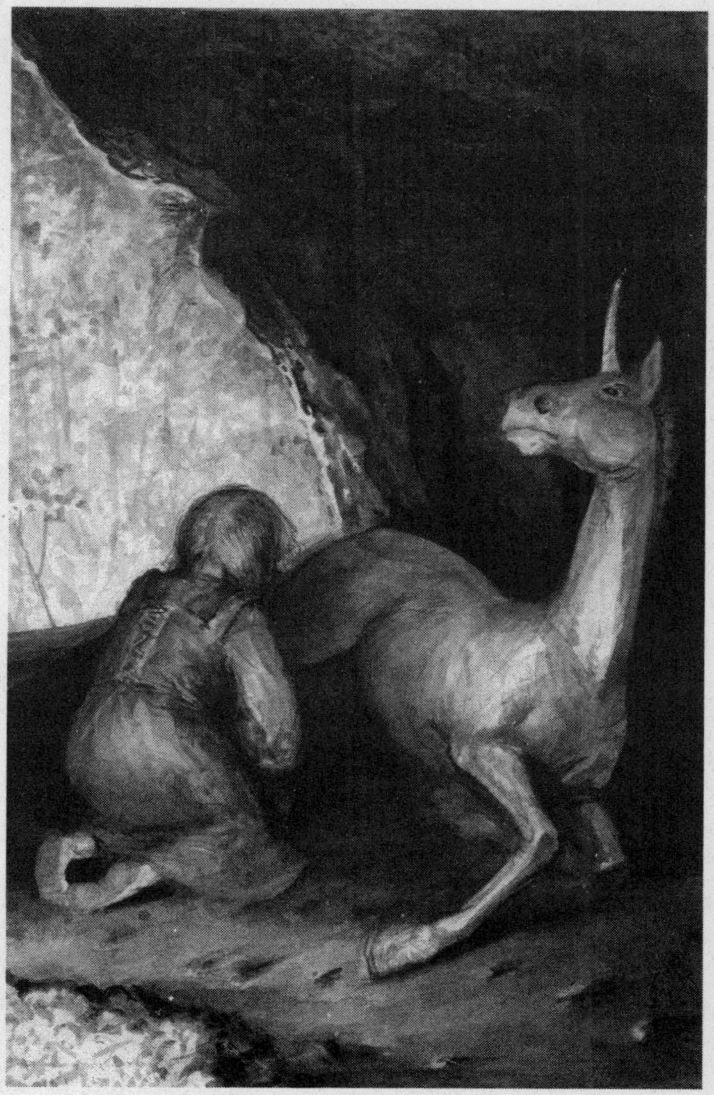

The bleeding had slowed, but it hadn't stopped.

The wound was deeper than she had thought.

Much deeper.

Once it was clean, Heart tightened the bandages a little.

"We need Ruth Oakes," she said to Avamir.

Moonsilver leaned against her.

He laid his head in her lap. Avamir nuzzled him.

"Maybe he'll be stronger in the morning," Heart said aloud.

Of course he would, she thought as she stared into the embers of the fire.

He *had* to be.

Heart lay awake worrying, listening to Moonsilver's breathing. Then sleep overcame her.

But she slept uneasily.

This time it was hunters who chased her across the rocky ground in her dreams.

✦ CHAPTER FIVE

In the morning, Heart woke up suddenly, breathing hard.

Then, her dreams faded away.

Except for her own pounding pulse, the cave was quiet.

Moonsilver was asleep beside her. Avamir was standing over him, her eyes closed and her head low.

Heart got to her feet.

She peeked out the cave entrance, listening.

Morning birds were singing. That meant there were no strangers in the forest.

Heart turned to kneel beside Moonsilver.

She touched him lightly. He did not awaken. His skin felt too warm beneath her hands. Fever?

Heart bit at her lip. He wasn't stronger. He

was weaker. And if the wound went bad—if it swelled and the flesh rotted—he could die. She tried to wake Moonsilver again. He opened his eyes, then closed them again.

A terrible thought came to her.

Every hunter carried one or two poisoned arrows for mountain lions or bears—dangerous animals that weren't easily killed.

Heart stood up, feeling almost dizzy with fear.

She went outside, trying to think.

The treetops below her rolled like a green ocean in the breeze.

Heart caught a distant glimpse of the Derrytown road through the swaying branches.

She took a long breath.

The hunters would come back.

They would search for the mysterious animal they had shot.

Now that it was light out, they'd find her barefoot prints and the unicorn's tracks—and the blood where Moonsilver had stood, trembling.

Heart told herself it would be all right—so long as the hunters didn't see Moonsilver.

The unicorn's hoofprints looked no different from any ordinary horse's. The hunters would think that they had shot a horse colt.

But then what would they do?

Would they keep looking? They might, if they had used poison and thought the animal had to be dead somewhere nearby.

Or maybe they would ride back to Dunraven's castle and never tell anyone, afraid they had killed an old pony by mistake.

Either way, it'd be safe to come back to the cave eventually, Heart thought.

For now, it was a very dangerous place.

Heart ducked back inside.

Avamir was wide awake now, still standing close to Moonsilver.

"Eat all you can," Heart whispered to the mare, piling dried grass beside her.

Heart buried her fire ring with clean, dry sand and hid her cook pot. She hid everything except her flint fire striker and one candle stub—and her coins. She knotted them up in a strip of cloth. Then she took down her unfinished gate.

Last, she used a leafy tree branch to smooth their tracks from the sandy floor.

Walking slowly, with Moonsilver between Heart and Avamir, they left the cave.

The sun was warm and it seemed to strengthen Moonsilver a little.

It was still hard going.

They walked close to the Derrytown road, but stayed out of sight.

Moonsilver would have fallen a dozen times if Heart and his mother hadn't been propping him up from both sides.

Heart's arms ached by noon. By dusk, her legs hurt too, strained from bracing Moonsilver upright.

Heart finally stopped, weary, in a stand of sycamore trees.

They were close.

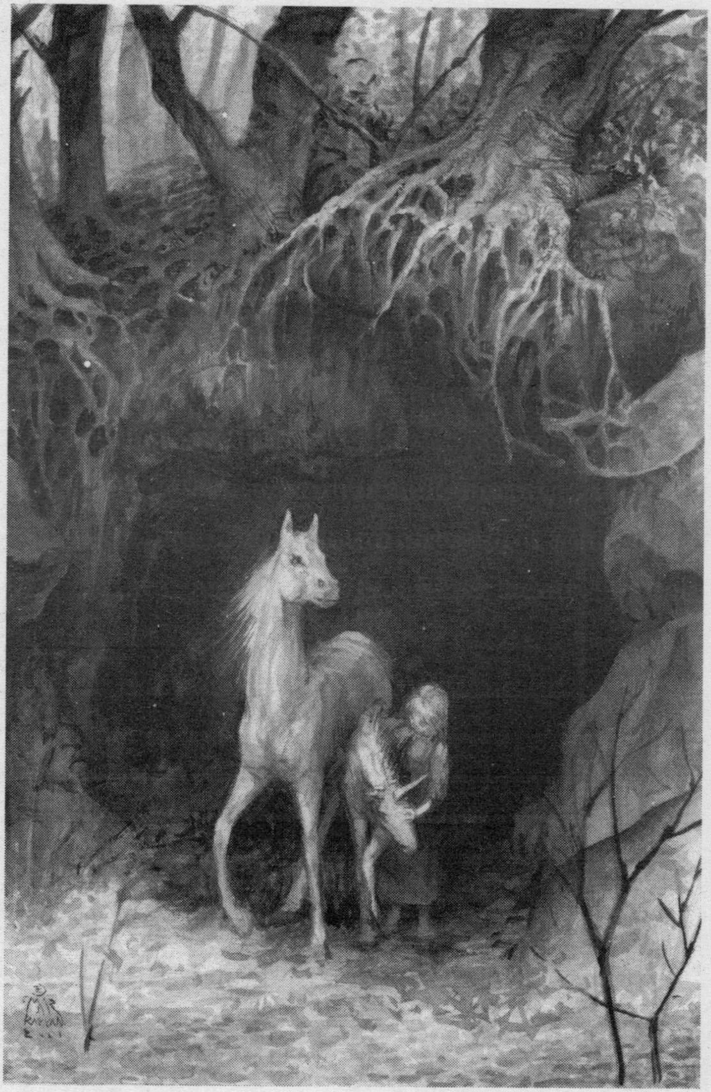

She could see the shine of the Blue River half a mile ahead.

"We can rest," Heart whispered to Avamir. "We'll wait until dark to cross the bridge."

Heart sighed. Moonsilver was too weak even to consider trying to swim the river. They had to go through the village.

Heart settled Moonsilver on a bed of leaves. He sank to the ground, his eyes closing. Avamir stood over him.

Heart curled up beside Moonsilver, worry numbing the pain of hunger in her stomach.

She lay silently, thinking.

They would have to go straight up Crosswater Street, right through town.

The shops would all be empty and closed, but there were some houses, too.

Suddenly, the clopping of hooves broke the silence of the night.

Heart caught her breath and opened her eyes.

✦ CHAPTER SIX

The moon had risen, full and bright.

Heart lay perfectly still, listening as the hoofbeats got closer.

"Stop following me!"

Heart flinched at the sound of the low, furious voice.

She got to her feet.

Through the trees she saw the shadowy shape of an old flat-bedded farmer's wagon.

The oak wheels were sun bleached, almost shining in the moonlight. The horse drawing it was swaybacked.

Heart glanced at Avamir.

The mare's head was high, her nostrils flared.

Moonsilver was still asleep. His breathing was deep and slow.

"Go back!" the man said over his shoulder.

Heart leaned close to Avamir. "Be still," she breathed. "Be quiet."

Heart heard the creaking of old wood as the wagon passed.

Then she listened hard.

The silence stretched out.

There was no sound of footsteps—nothing. Whoever the man had been arguing with must have followed him.

Heart closed her eyes again and tried to rest.

When she opened them, it was still dark, but Heart sensed it was time to go.

She sat up.

Avamir lowered her head, touching Moonsilver's back with her muzzle. The colt moved a little.

"We have to be careful," Heart whispered.

Moonsilver shivered the skin on his shoulders and back, as though there were summer flies biting him.

Then he opened his eyes.

Avamir nuzzled him again.

Moonsilver lurched up awkwardly, stumbling against his mother.

The stained bandage was tight over his wound.

But Heart could see dark streaks in his white coat. It was still bleeding.

"Wait here," Heart said, reaching out to pat Avamir's scarred forehead gently. "Do you understand? Stay hidden."

The unicorn mare looked into Heart's eyes.

Then Heart turned, making her way through the trees.

She looked both directions down the hard-packed dirt road.

It was empty.

It was hard to get Moonsilver moving again. His leg had stiffened. Avamir and Heart braced him up as well as they could.

Slowly, stopping every few minutes, they made their way eastward.

Heart glanced at the sky.

It wasn't getting light yet, and the moon was still high.

Maybe, with luck, they could make it through the town without being seen.

For a second, Heart imagined Ruth Oakes's warm kitchen, and her eyes flooded with tears.

A short, sharp bark startled her into an abrupt stop. Moonsilver nearly fell, and Heart struggled to steady him.

A patchy-colored puppy was standing stiff-legged in front of them, peering at them in the moonlight. Now Heart understood whom the wagoneer had been scolding.

She looked past the pup, squinting.

The road was empty, and there was no sound of hooves or footsteps.

"Come here," she whispered to the puppy, kneeling down.

The pup tilted its head.

"Come on," Heart said quietly. "I won't hurt you."

The puppy still didn't move.

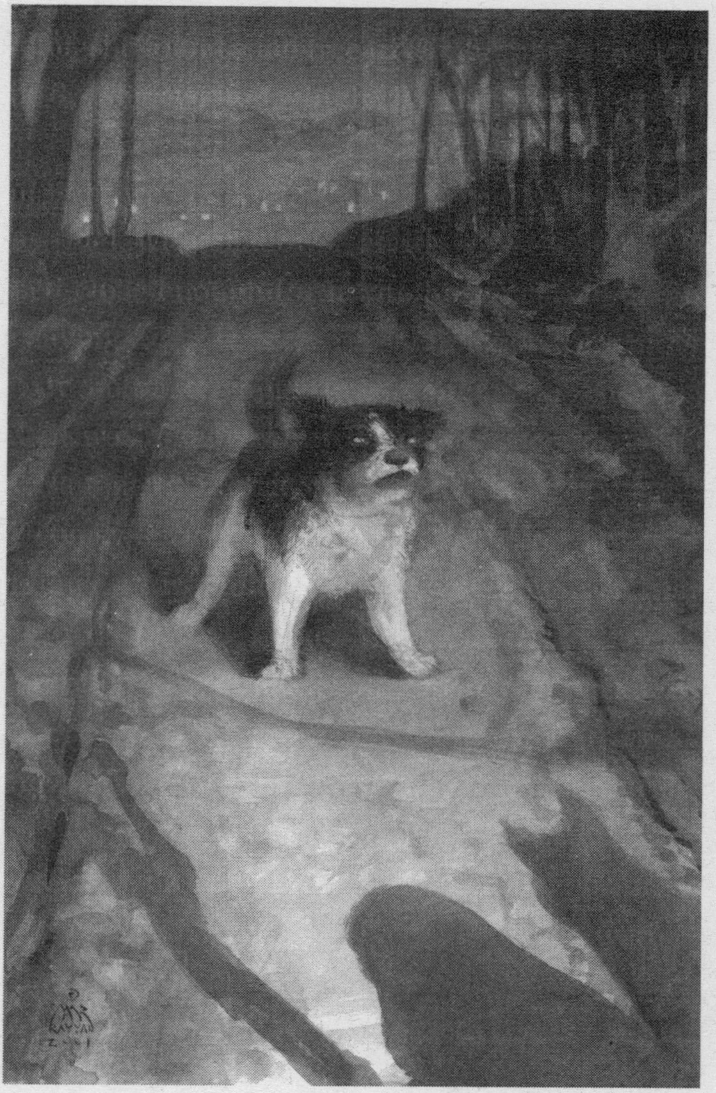

Heart heard Avamir blow out a soft, fluttery breath.

The puppy whined, a sad, reed-thin sound. Then he lifted his head, and the moonlight lit his face.

One of the puppy's eyes was deep brown.

The other was light blue.

Heart knelt and reached out to the puppy. He bolted into her arms. He was shaking, whimpering. He was almost too big to hold.

Avamir let out a longer, noisier breath.

Heart looked at her. "I know."

Avamir stamped a forehoof.

Heart stood up, gently sliding the pup back to the ground.

He let out another sharp bark.

"Kip?" Heart said, making the sound into a word. "I'm sorry, but you can't come with us, Kip."

Heart knew she had no choice.

If the pup barked going through town, he'd start every dog in Ash Grove howling. *Someone* would come look.

Moonsilver had lowered his head, his muzzle nearly touching the ground again.

Heart moved away slowly, making sure the colt was leaning against Avamir.

She clapped her hands suddenly, startling the puppy into leaping backward. "Shoo!"

The pup scrambled to get away from her.

Heart's eyes filled with tears.

She hated scaring him.

But what else could she do? It was too dangerous to let him follow them through Ash Grove. If she could have carried him—but she couldn't.

"Go on!" she said, clapping once more. "Go!" The puppy ran this time, disappearing into the darkness of the trees.

Heart took her place by Moonsilver, and they began to walk.

She glanced back.

The pup wasn't coming.

Her eyes stung and overflowed. She freed one hand long enough to swipe at the tears.

Then she went on.

✦ CHAPTER SEVEN

The sound of the unicorns' hooves on the bridge planks made Heart uneasy.

The night around them seemed too quiet.

At least there were no houses at this end of Crosswater Street.

As they came off the bridge onto the cobblestones, Heart pushed gently at Avamir's neck, guiding her to the side of the street.

In the gutter, mud and leaves muffled their hoofbeats.

They passed Market Square.

Heart barely breathed as they went.

There was no stirring of wind, no rain or distant thunder—nothing to cover the sound of their passing.

Moonsilver was unsteady.

They passed the last of the shops across from Market Square.

Avamir walked slower and slower—because Moonsilver did.

"Please, just keep going," Heart whispered to him as they passed the first of the houses.

The windows were all dark.

The second and third houses were dark as well.

So was the fourth.

The fifth and sixth houses were silent and lifeless.

But inside the seventh, a dog began to bark.

Heart tried to go a little faster.

It was impossible.

Moonsilver was tottering, barely able to walk.

The barking got louder.

The colt suddenly staggered and fell forward, crashing onto his knees. Heart stood over him, trying to drag him upright. He did his best, his hooves skidding on the cobblestones.

The dog kept barking, a quick, jarring rhythm.

Heart glanced at the house.

The front door opened.

The flicker of a candle-lantern shone dimly.

"Is someone there?" a voice from inside the house asked.

"I can't see anything." The answer came from the doorway.

A sudden sharp bark near Heart's feet made her spin around.

"Hush," she hissed at the pup. "Hush!" But the puppy yapped again.

"It's just some stray dog," the doorway-voice announced.

There were footsteps.

Then the amber glow of the candle-lantern disappeared. Heart heard the door close.

Kip stopped barking and stood close to her leg.

Heart touched his head gently.

Then she tried once more to help Moonsilver up.

This time, he made it.

Shaking with effort and fear, Heart steadied the colt as they went on.

She glanced back.

The puppy was trotting off to one side, stopping to sniff at the cobblestones.

His patchy colors made him look like a small cluster of moving shadows in the fading moonlight.

When Heart looked again, he was gone.

Tirin Bridge arched over its creek. On the far side, the cobblestones were older, rougher. Heart tried not to scrape her bare toes.

They made the turn at the end of Crosswater Street.

Heading south on the River Road was easier. The soft dust gave them firmer footing, and Moonsilver could go a little faster.

Heart looked up.

The moon was setting, and the sun would rise soon.

It didn't matter now.

They were getting close to Crooked Lane.

When Heart saw a lantern shining in Ruth Oakes's window, she felt tears rise in her eyes again.

Ruth was up very early, as usual.

The unicorns stood quietly on the garden walk, Moonsilver leaning on Avamir.

Heart inhaled the strong scent of rosemary and hyssop.

Then she stepped up to the door and knocked.

Ruth Oakes opened her door and looked out. Her eyes went wide. "I was so worried, child," she said, opening her arms to hug Heart.

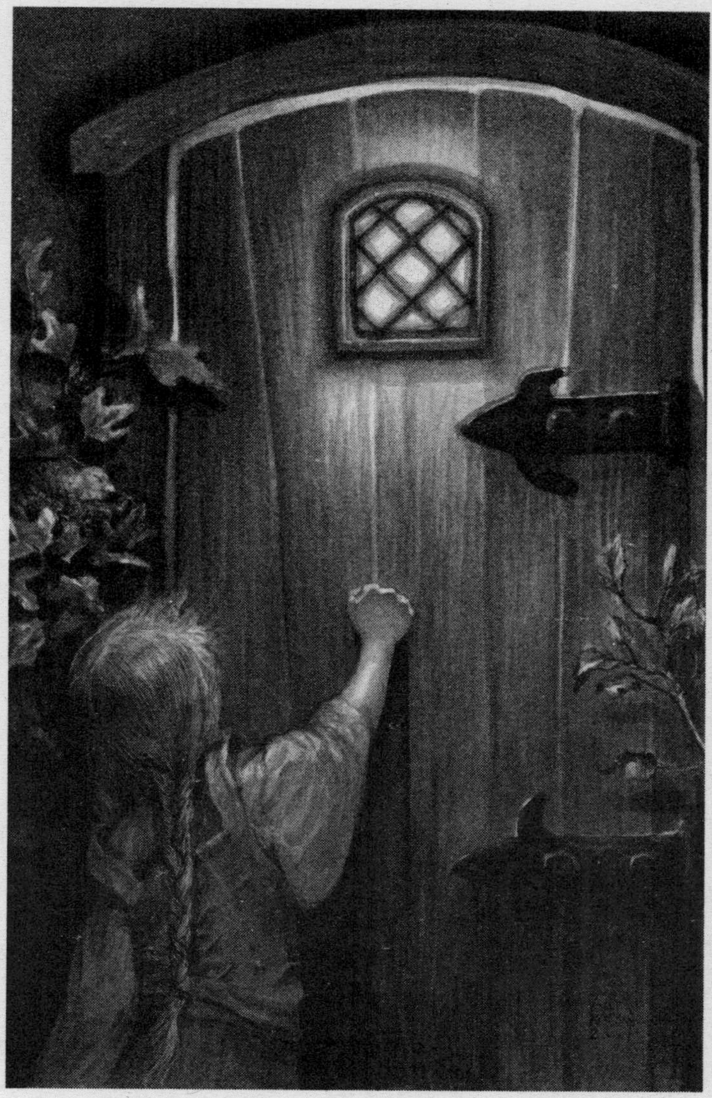

✦ CHAPTER EIGHT

"A hunter shot the colt . . . ," Heart began. The breathless story came rushing out.

Ruth listened, then raised one hand. "Let's put the mare in the old pasture and—"

"No," Heart interrupted. "No one can see them."

"Dunraven's men have long gone," Ruth said calmly. "There's no reason to—"

But before she could finish, Heart stood aside. The lantern light spilled out the door onto Moonsilver and Avamir.

Moonsilver's horn gleamed in the amber glow.

Ruth pulled in a sudden breath. "Oh, my." She covered her mouth with one hand. "Then the mare's scar . . . ? Oh, my!"

Heart stood still, waiting.

Ruth Oakes motioned. "Let's bring them both inside, then."

Heart nodded, grateful for Ruth Oakes's calmness, for her steadiness.

In half an hour, the healer had them all settled.

A storage room became an open stall for Avamir.

The mare stood looking at her colt as Heart told Ruth Oakes everything that had happened.

Moonsilver was lying in front of the hearth as they talked.

Ruth had put herbs and a clean bandage on his wound. He was sound asleep.

It was such a heavy, deep sleep that it scared Heart.

"Will he be all right?"

Ruth arched her brows. "Why don't you wash your face and sleep a few hours before you start to worry about—"

"Will he?" Heart interrupted.

Ruth sighed. "I don't know."

Heart felt her stomach tighten. "Is it poison?"

Ruth shrugged. "I used the spikenard in case."

"The hunter thought Moonsilver was a white deer. I heard him say it," Heart told her.

Ruth Oakes nodded. "Then he wouldn't care if the meat was spoiled. He just wanted to prove what he'd seen."

Heart winced. "I had the same thought."

Ruth nodded. She put another log on the fire.

Then she wiped her hands on her apron.

When she spoke again, her voice was soft. "The legends say unicorns can heal with their horns and—"

Avamir stamped a forehoof, and Ruth turned to face her.

Heart turned too.

Avamir had no horn now, only the wide, leathery scar.

Heart looked at Moonsilver again.

The colt lay so still.

His ribs rose and fell a little with his breathing.

Heart glanced at Avamir. The mare's eyes seemed full of sadness.

Ruth seemed to have the same thought. "It's hurting her not to be able to help."

"I love them," Heart said, without meaning to.

Ruth Oakes smiled. "Clearly. And they love you." She straightened her apron. "Unicorns!" her voice was full of wonder. "I always hoped the stories were true."

A sharp bark outside the door made Heart look up.

"Is this someone else you know?" Ruth asked, smiling.

Heart nodded slowly, explaining about the puppy.

Ruth rose and went to the door.

The puppy came in slowly, his head low, his tail tucked.

Then he saw Heart and bounded into her arms.

In the lantern light she could see his eyes more

clearly. The blue one was summer-sky blue.

"I thought Kip stopped following us," Heart told Ruth. She told her how the puppy had saved them by barking.

Ruth nodded. "Kip?"

The puppy looked up.

Ruth met Heart's eyes. "If you've named him, he's yours."

Heart shook her head. "I can't take care of him. I can't take care of anyone." She covered her mouth with one hand, fighting tears.

"You already have," Ruth said firmly.

Without another word she brought blankets and made a pallet beside Moonsilver.

Heart managed to wash her face and hands.

Then she lay down. Kip curled up against her back.

Heart closed her eyes, and sleep came almost instantly. For once, she didn't dream.

She woke by noon.

That first day was terrible.

Moonsilver barely stirred.

When he did, his eyes were clouded. He would not eat.

Kip whined and circled the room. Avamir stood uneasily in the storeroom doorway, staring at her colt.

Ruth cleaned the wound twice, sealing it with meadowsweet salve after each washing.

She steeped a pot of feverfew tea.

Then she added a dark powder Heart had never seen before.

"Cohosh and spikenard, in equal parts," Ruth said when she noticed Heart was watching.

Moonsilver drank a little of the mixture, then closed his eyes and sank back into sleep.

Heart watched, wishing she could stay forever in this sunny house.

The day went by very slowly.

Moonsilver slept most of the time.

When he woke for a few minutes, in the afternoon, he would not eat. He drank a little more of the tea.

Heart sat beside him.

Avamir stood close, all day, watching her colt.

Ruth Oakes gave Kip a bone to chew. He gnawed it and carried it around. Then he settled into a nap.

On the third morning, Heart woke early.

Ruth was sleeping—so were the unicorns.

Heart slipped outside. Kip wanted to follow, but she shut him in.

In the cover of the morning fog, she ran down to the river to cut grass. Going each way, she passed just within sight of Simon's house. It looked smaller and sadder than ever.

In the evening, once it was almost dark, Heart took Avamir out for a gallop.

Waiting for the mare to canter back to her, Heart was swept with sadness.

Everything felt so familiar.

It felt safe—even though she knew it wasn't.

She wanted to learn about herbs and healing from Ruth Oakes like she had before.

She wanted to stay in Ash Grove.

And she knew she couldn't.

On the fourth morning, Moonsilver untangled his long legs and stood up.

Heart ran outside to bring in a bundle of grass she'd cut by the river.

The colt ate eagerly.

Ruth Oakes smiled. "He's past it now."

Heart looked at her. "Was it poison?"

Ruth nodded. "The hunter chose an arrow to make sure he died, good shot or bad."

"I want to stay here," Heart said quietly.

"You could," Ruth Oakes said. "But they cannot." She gestured at Avamir and Moonsilver.

Heart nodded. "So as soon as Moonsilver is strong, we'll leave."

"Back to the cave you told me about?" Ruth Oakes asked.

Heart shrugged. "We'll be safe there."

Ruth Oakes leaned toward her and touched her cheek. "I will bring you whatever you need. We'll meet on the road."

Heart found herself grinning. "You would do that?"

Ruth laughed. "That and more."

"You will have to be very careful," Heart said quietly.

Ruth nodded. "Indeed, we both will." She stretched. "I'll be gone when you get up tomorrow. I'll be home around noontime."

"Is someone sick?" Heart asked.

Ruth nodded. "A sweet old woman. I should have gone yesterday."

Heart nodded.

"I want to give you something, before you go," Ruth said. She reached into her apron pocket and took out a tiny silk pouch. "My grandmother gave me this."

Heart opened the pouch. Inside was a silvery thread, coiled into a circle.

"My grandmother gave it to me when I was your age. She said it was magic, that it would protect me."

Heart touched the shining thread. It felt warm.

Ruth smiled. "Now it can protect you."

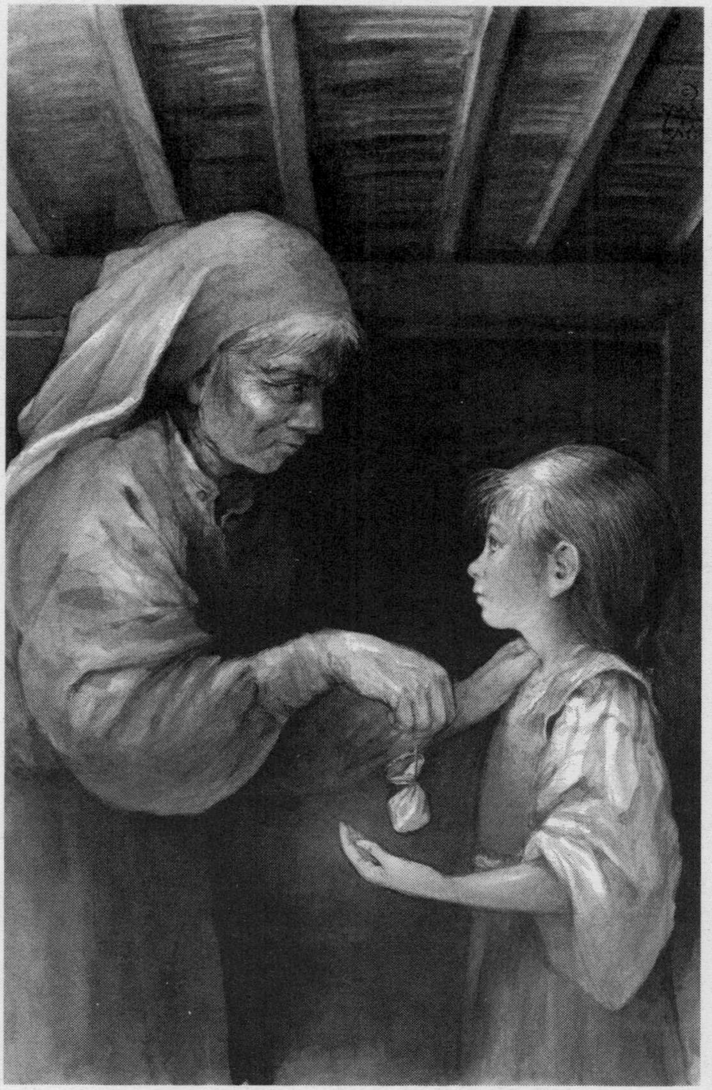

“Thank you,” Heart said, then hugged Ruth Oakes.

The old woman smiled again. “Now sleep, child.”

Heart nodded. She was tired. She straightened out her blankets and settled in for the night.

In her dreams she was running, as always, but she wasn’t as afraid this time. She ran faster—so fast that the rocky ground blurred beneath her feet.

✦ CHAPTER NINE

The next morning, Heart woke early, as always.

Ruth had already left.

The house felt empty without her in it. Heart got up and dressed, careful to be quiet.

Avamir was awake.

Moonsilver slept, but it was a normal sleep, a healing sleep now.

Kip sat up, watching her. When she went out, he slipped past her and scrambled through the door before she could close it.

Heart tried to catch him to put him back inside. He ran in circles, dodging her easily.

"I'm not playing, Kip," Heart whispered. "You have to go inside!"

Kip ignored her.

He leaped aside when she reached to grab him.

Heart clenched her fists. "I have to go get grass!" she scolded.

Kip reversed direction and ran close enough for her to lunge at him—and miss.

Heart frowned.

There was no real reason the pup couldn't come with her.

The fog was as thick as cotton.

They would be well hidden.

Almost no one ever came this far south of town—especially not this early in the morning.

There was nothing but sagebrush past Simon's house—sagebrush and the Blue River.

Heart started off.

Kip stayed close to her heels.

She followed Crooked Lane until she could see Simon's place through the fog.

Then she veered off through the sage.

Kip ran ahead, then came back.

The Blue River was beautiful, Heart thought as she walked down the long slope.

As always, she glanced toward the place Simon had found her, lying asleep in the grass.

As always, she tried to recall something from before that day.

Maybe I never will, she told herself.

The thought didn't upset her as much as usual.

She wasn't sure why, but she was grateful.

Heart set about her work.

The fog made her shiver, but she was glad it was so thick this morning. Kip splashed in the shallows. He chased a rabbit, then came back.

"Come, Kip," Heart called once she had the grass bundled.

The pup stopped playing and ran toward her.

They started back.

Heart stayed well away from Simon's house, angling northward toward Crooked Lane.

When she stepped out of the sagebrush onto the road, she sighed in relief. Her feet were sore from walking.

"Girl? Is that you?" Simon's rasping voice startled Heart so badly that she dropped the bundle of grass.

"Where have you been?"

Heart opened her mouth to say something, but no words came out.

"Where are the horses?" he demanded. "Did you put them back into the old pen?"

"They aren't here," Heart said.

Simon spat into the sagebrush. "Did you sell them?"

His face was even sharper than Heart had remembered.

She saw him step forward, but she could not move.

She saw him reaching out to grab her arm.

She still could not move.

Kip barked suddenly. Simon jerked backward as the pup jumped between them. Kip stood stiff-legged and solid, growling at him.

"And a pup now, too?" Simon demanded. "You can't come home with a pup."

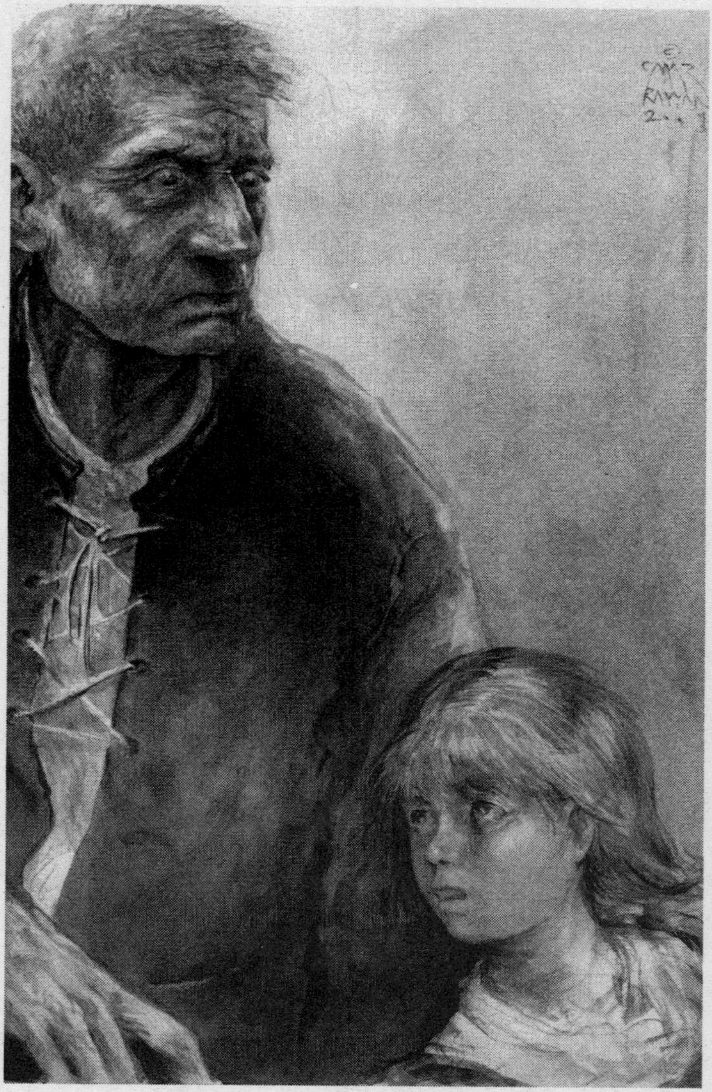

"I'm not," Heart said, cutting him off.

Simon looked like she had slapped him. "What?"

"I'm not coming back," Heart said. She scooped up the grass. "Avamir and Moonsilver are mine. I have taken care of her and fed her and I've taken care of the colt. And I left you money for everything else."

"You are ungrateful—" Simon began, but she interrupted him.

"I am not. But I am never coming back."

Heart strode away, Kip following at her heels.

Back at Ruth Oakes's house, she laid down the grass. Moonsilver ate eagerly. Avamir crossed the room to join him.

Simon would be angry, Heart knew. He would be watching.

Heart clenched her fists. She wanted so much to stay. But she couldn't. Not now.

Heart went into the kitchen.

She filled the gathering sack with leftover bread and some dry barley. She took a few carrots, and some herbs, too.

Then she unknotted the strip of cloth that held her coins.

She left half her money beside the kitchen basin.

Ruth would never ask her to pay, Heart knew. But she felt good doing it, anyway.

Heart took a length of flax rope from Ruth's storeroom.

She knotted it into a halter.

From a distance, at least, Avamir would have to look like an ordinary horse.

"We have to go now," she told the unicorns.

They were busy with the grass. "We have to go now," Heart repeated urgently, touching Avamir's neck. The unicorn mare allowed Heart to slide the halter on.

She lifted her head and looked into Heart's eyes. Then she turned and nuzzled Moonsilver.

Together they left Ruth Oakes's house.

Kip stayed close to Heart's heels.

Moonsilver limped, but he walked with his head high. Heart closed the door softly, silently, wondering if she would ever see Ruth again.

✦ CHAPTER TEN

Heart was afraid to go through town—but she was more afraid to try to swim the unicorns across the Blue River.

"Stay close, Kip," she said as they turned off the River Road and started down Crosswater Street.

The fog was thick.

It was as if the town had disappeared.

Heart could hear a cow mooing in someone's pens, ready to be milked.

The sound seemed muffled and far away.

Even the clopping of the unicorn's hooves on the cobblestones seemed softer in the fog.

Wagon wheels grinding on the stones warned Heart in time to push Moonsilver behind his mother. Then she walked close to Avamir's head, holding the rope, as though she was leading the mare.

The cart driver barely glanced at them.

Heart swallowed hard.

There were going to be more wagons. But what choice did she have? She had to leave before Simon managed to see Moonsilver's horn.

Avamir stayed close as they walked—just the right distance for a horse being led along. Moonsilver stayed behind her. Kip barked at vague shapes in the fog, but he was quiet when a wagon passed.

"Good, Kip," Heart praised him, glad that the pup knew better than to startle cart horses.

They were almost past Market Square and heading for the Blue River Bridge when Heart saw two familiar shapes in the fog ahead.

Tibbs Renner and his mother were on their way to market.

No one walked with them.

Heart knew why. They always smelled of the knacker's yard.

Mrs. Renner turned toward Market Square without seeing Heart, but Tibbs stared.

Heart felt her stomach tighten. She glanced over her shoulder. Moonsilver was staying close to Avamir's flank. Tibbs couldn't have seen him.

As Heart watched, he walked on with his mother.

He'd wait for a chance to say something mean to her at market, she was sure.

"But I won't be here," Heart whispered, watching the fog swallow him and his mother.

Heart gripped the rope and walked faster.

Her feet were cold and sore.

The cobblestones grated at her skin.

When they finally reached the Blue River Bridge, Heart pulled in a long breath.

They were going to make it.

And they were in luck.

The bridge was empty. If they hurried, they wouldn't have to pass too close to a wagon headed to market.

The fog had wet the planks as though it had rained.

Heart slipped once and steadied herself against Avamir.

Kip stayed close, trotting carefully.

Heart saw him looking downward through the cracks between the planks at the water below.

Stepping off the bridge, Heart listened.

There was no sound of hooves or wagon wheels.

"Halt!"

The man's voice seemed to come out of nowhere.

Heart spun around, trying to spot him.

"Stop where you are," the voice ordered.

Then the man stepped close enough for Heart to see him. She didn't know his face, but she knew who he was. Or what he was, anyway. He wore the gray shirt that all of Tin Blackaby's hired men wore.

"Where'd you get these horses?"

Heart glanced back at Avamir. She had

positioned herself between the man and Moonsilver. He could not see the colt.

"I found the mare in the forest," she said, telling the truth.

"We have someone here who says different," the man said.

It was only then that Heart saw Simon standing off to one side. The old man was sweating, breathing hard. He must have run all the way from his house, straight across the fields to Tin Blackaby's house.

Heart glanced around.

"The horses are mine, of course," Simon was saying. "I bought the mare from a Gypsy. I took this child in. Everyone knows that."

Tin Blackaby's man nodded.

"You are free to go, if you like," he said. "But the horses are Simon's property. He complained of the theft weeks ago."

The man stepped closer.

He reached out so quickly that Heart could not react. He caught her arm.

Heart stared at Simon.

He looked angry.

At what? She had been grateful to him for taking care of her, for teaching her how to cook, how to gather barley. She had worked so hard in his house.

"I'll buy the horses from you, Simon," she said aloud.

She stepped toward him, then glanced back.

Moonsilver was still hidden behind Avamir. Only his legs and hooves showed.

Tin Blackaby's man laughed again. "Buy? With what?"

Heart pulled her arm free and reached into her carry sack. She untied the cloth and took out some coins.

"Where'd you steal that?" the man asked.

Heart looked at Simon.

He knew very well she had worked for the coins.

He had taken a share of the money Ruth had paid her. She pressed her lips together.

She didn't want to give Tin Blackaby's man any reason to watch Ruth Oakes.

The sound of boot heels on the bridge behind her made Heart look up.

She saw two more of Tin Blackaby's men coming through the mist.

In seconds, they would be able to see Moonsilver.

"We've caught old Simon's horse thief," the man beside Heart called to them.

"Goat thief, too," the other man shouted back. "Hey, what *is* that? A colt?"

Heart whirled around and pulled the halter off Avamir so the rope wouldn't tangle and trip her. "Run! Get away!"

Heart jumped aside as the unicorn mare reared, lunging into a gallop.

Tin Blackaby's man was knocked sideways.

Moonsilver leaped over him to follow his mother.

In an instant, they were gone, their white coats blending with the fog.

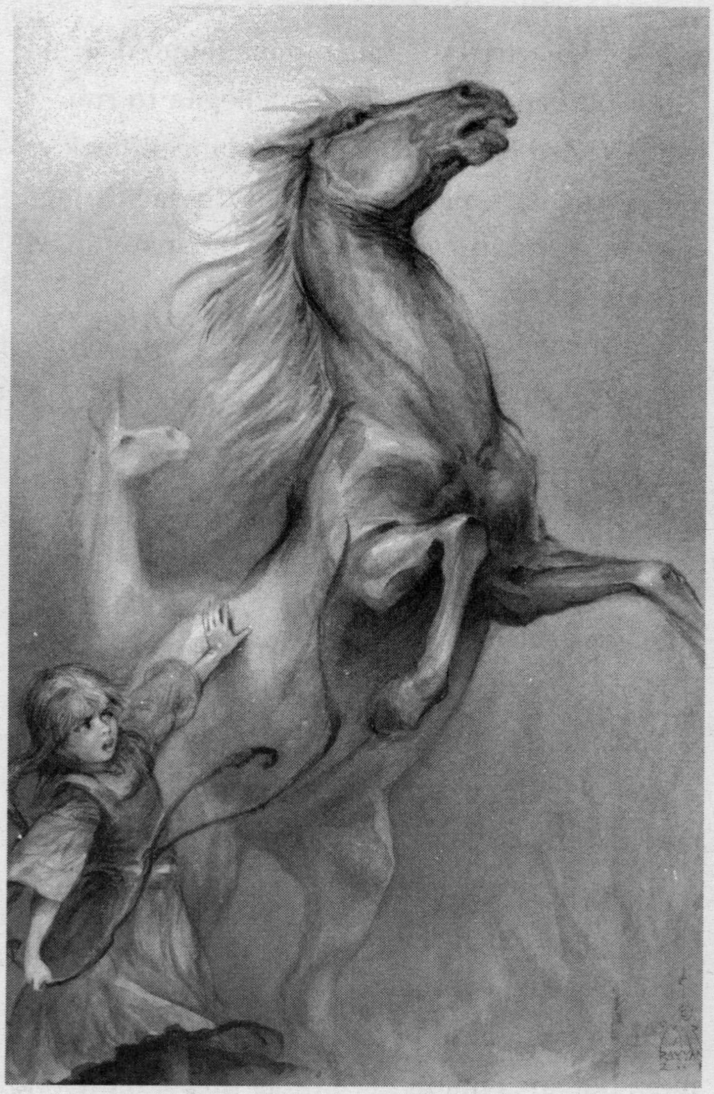

"Get that girl!" the fallen man shouted.

Kip barked sharply as Heart began to run.

She heard him snarling, and glanced back.

Kip was darting in and out of the men's legs, snapping and growling. One of them stumbled, cursing.

Kip sprang away and raced after her.

Heart headed for the trees, clutching her bag as she ran.

"Hurry!" a man's voice came through the fog. "She won't get far!"

Heart veered away, guided by the men's voices as they shouted to one another.

Her bare feet were silent in the dust.

Their boots thudded heavily.

She changed direction again when she reached the edge of the forest.

Heart heard Simon's voice, muffled in the fog, shouting her name.

She slowed enough to look back.

She could hear Simon and Tin Blackaby's men, but she couldn't see them through the fog.

That meant they couldn't see her.

Heart dodged around a huge oak tree, then ran on, heading into the deep woods.

Kip appeared out of the fog. He ran beside her.

Heart angled her direction again. Slowly, the shouts behind them faded.

Heart ran until her legs ached. She ran until her breath was painful.

Then, finally, she stopped—and listened.

She held perfectly still.

Kip stood leaning against her leg, panting.

Heart picked him up and held him close. "Be quiet," she whispered to him.

Kip wriggled in her arms, but he didn't bark. And all around them, there was only silence.

After a long time, Heart began making her way through the woods, staying well back from the road.

It was almost dark when she got back to the cave.

She walked slowly, coming up the slope carefully, listening.

It was silent.

There were no voices, no hoofbeats, nothing beyond the normal stirrings of mice in the pine needles.

Heart bit at her lower lip. If the unicorns weren't here . . . if they were lost, or hurt . . . Her eyes flooded with tears.

She wiped them away and started upward, Kip at her heels.

The pup yipped once as they topped the rise.

He bounded ahead of her, then ran straight into the cave.

Heart listened to be sure nothing had moved into the cave during her absence. Then she followed Kip inside.

If the unicorns weren't here tonight, she told herself, they would be in the morning.

"If nothing happened," Heart whispered, and her eyes filled with tears again.

Kip barked sharply.

"Hush!" Heart scolded, setting down her sack.

She felt her way along the cave wall for the place where she had hidden her supplies.

Fumbling through the little pile, she finally found a candle stub.

Then she patted the sandy floor until she had found a few wisps of dried grass.

She twisted them together.

The spark from her striker caught the grass on fire.

As the little flame came to life, Heart stood up straight.

Kip yipped again.

Heart turned to shush him.

Then she caught her breath and stared.

Avamir was standing near the back wall of the cave. Beside her, Moonsilver lay sleeping peacefully.

Heart ran to hug the mare's neck.

Avamir lowered her head, and Heart felt her warm breath on her cheek.

Heart felt an odd lightness inside herself. It took her a long moment to realize what it was.

She didn't know where she would get more food now that she couldn't go back to Ash Grove. Blackaby's men would be searching the woods, and she didn't want to endanger Ruth.

She wasn't sure where they could go or what they could do.

She knew only one thing.

For the first time in her life, she wasn't lonely.

Just before Heart fell asleep, she put her hand into her pocket.

She touched the little silk pouch that held Ruth Oakes's silvery thread.

Maybe it *could* protect her. Maybe it already had.

THE

UNICORN'S SECRET

The Silver Bracelet

✦ CHAPTER ONE

Heart stood behind the lightning-split pine tree, waiting.

It was cold.

She envied Moonsilver and Avamir, still warm and asleep back in the cave. Kip would be curled up between them, warmest of all.

"Please be careful, Ruth," she whispered.

Little clouds of her breath hung in the air.

Heart rubbed her mittened hands together.

Somewhere above her on the mountainside, she heard a quail waking, piping sleepily.

Heart was nervous even though they had been very careful. Sometimes Ruth came in the evening, sometimes in the morning.

Sometimes the visits were ten days apart.

Sometimes five or seven or twelve.

They never met in the same place twice.

Ruth always went to visit a patient first. She checked on a number of older people farther out on the Derrytown road. She met with Heart on her way back to Ash Grove.

So far, it had worked.

Tin Blackaby's men were used to Ruth coming and going to tend to the sick. There had always been baskets of apples and bags of wheat in her wagon. Her patients paid her with whatever they had.

Heart sighed and glanced out at the empty road.

They had worked out a signal. If Ruth wore her red hat, it meant she had seen someone on the road. Her blue hat meant everything was safe.

The red hat warned Heart to stay hidden, that Ruth wouldn't slow—or even glance at her—as she passed.

Ruth had worn her red hat only twice. The

first time, Tin Blackaby's men had been following her. The second time it had just been a farmer's wagon.

Heart rubbed her hands together harder, trying to keep them warm.

Finally she heard a faint clopping sound and held her breath as it got louder. She peeked out from behind the tree and grinned. Ruth was wearing her blue hat, pulled low over her ears.

As the wagon came closer, Heart stepped forward just far enough for Ruth to spot her.

"Whoa, Banjo," Ruth called to her bay gelding. She pulled him to a stop, then sat, looking straight ahead. "Hello, dear girl," she said without turning.

"Hello," Heart whispered back.

Ruth got down from the wagon and walked around to lift the bay's rear hoof.

She always did this when she and Heart met. In case someone came up the road it would look as if Ruth had stopped to see if her horse had picked up a stone.

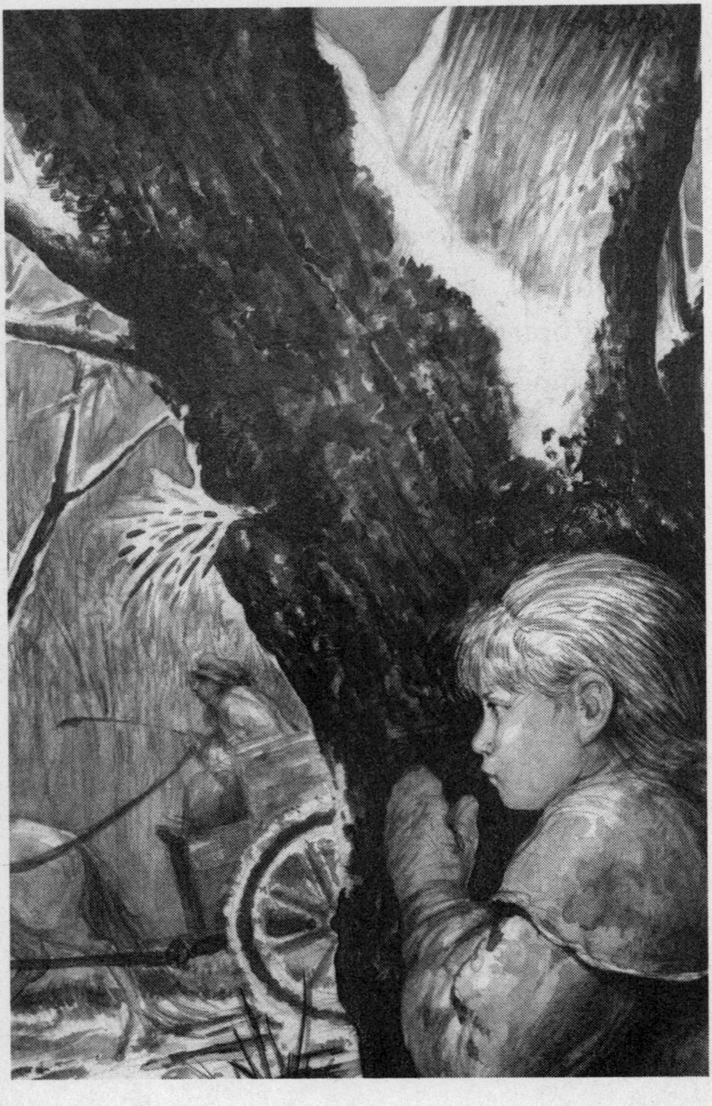

"You are well?" Ruth asked, using a stick to clean Banjo's hoof.

"I am," Heart assured her. "Kip is still catching rabbits almost every day. Avamir and Moonsilver are finding enough grass." Heart stepped forward. "How are you?"

Ruth let go of the bay's hoof. She fiddled with the harness, her back to Heart. "I can outwork any mule I ever met."

Heart smiled. "Have the rumors died down?"

Ruth shrugged. "The man who thought Moonsilver was a goat is still boasting about what fools the others are. Simon still claims you stole *his* horses."

"But have the unicorn rumors stopped?" Heart asked.

Ruth shrugged again. "No. Everyone loves the old stories too much. But people laugh. No one really *believes* there was a unicorn in Ash Grove."

Heart sighed. It was the best she could hope for. "Will you hide the wagon and come up to the cave with me?" Heart asked. She wanted Ruth to stay.

"Better not," Ruth said. "I am expected back to tend Tibbs Renner's twisted ankle."

Heart frowned. Tibbs had always been mean to her, but she pitied him and understood him. The children of Ash Grove made fun of them both.

"He's being apprenticed in Derrytown," Ruth said. "Wants to learn blacksmithing, his mother says. I suspect he just wants to get away from that cruel father of his."

Ruth walked around her horse, her fingers going through the motions of harness checking. "Simon has been ill."

Heart gasped. "He has?"

"Oh, he will soon recover," Ruth told her. "I made him pay me this time, though."

Heart covered her mouth with one hand. "He *paid* you?"

"Yes," Ruth said. She glanced up the road, then back toward Ash Grove. "With these." She pulled a little woven bag out of her coat pocket.

She tossed it to Heart, meeting her eyes for an instant. “Simon said they’re from the blanket you were wrapped in when he found you. They’re silver threads like the one my grandmother gave me. You still have it?”

Heart nodded. “Of course.”

“It hurt Simon to give these up,” Ruth said.

Heart pressed her lips together. She slipped the little bag into her pocket. “Poor Simon.”

Ruth nodded. “Poor indeed. He does not have a single friend.”

Heart wiped her eyes.

“Don’t pity him too much, Heart,” Ruth said. “If he had known for an instant that Moonsilver and Avamir were unicorns—”

“He’d have sold them to Tin Blackaby—or even Lord Dunraven,” Heart finished for her.

Ruth nodded. “Even knowing it would break your heart.” She looked up the road again, then down it.

Ruth shook her head. Then, swiftly, she

pulled three cloth sacks out of the back of the wagon. She tossed them neatly into the trees.

Heart saw a little tin of cheese roll out the top of one of the sacks and her mouth watered.

"Thank you so much, Ruth," she said quietly.

Ruth looked straight at her for just a moment. "It worries me to death, you being out here alone."

Heart blinked back tears. Ruth smiled at her and walked back around the wagon. She kicked at the narrow iron footrest to knock the snow and mud off her boots. Then she climbed up.

"I will repay you for all this," Heart said.

Ruth made a quiet sound of dismissal. "There is nothing to repay. I just wish I could make things right, that's all."

Heart sighed. "Be careful, please. Tin Blackaby might—"

"No, he won't hurt me," Ruth interrupted her. "I tend to him, same as everyone else."

Heart nodded, knowing that Ruth couldn't see her. She was looking straight ahead again.

"Let's meet in five days, by the white boulder on the straightaway before this one," Ruth said. "Come at noon."

Heart knew the flat-topped white rock that stood near the road. "I will be waiting," she said. "Thank you, Ruth."

Ruth glanced at her. Heart felt the look like a warm touch.

A single instant after that, Heart heard the thudding of hooves on the snow-packed road.

Someone was coming fast and riding hard.

✦ CHAPTER TWO

"Ruth!" Heart whispered. The hoofbeats were getting louder.

"Take care, little one," Ruth answered quietly. She shook the reins hard.

Banjo lurched into a gallop.

Heart ducked back into the trees.

Just then, Tin Blackaby's men burst around the bend, their horses galloping. They saw Ruth's wagon and reined in, surrounding her.

Heart watched through the tree branches, her breath uneven. She couldn't hear what they were saying.

Suddenly Ruth jumped down from the driver's bench. She came striding back, then faced the men, her hands on her hips. She looked furious.

"I dropped my coin purse when your horses startled mine," she accused. She walked toward Heart, staring down at the mud and ice in the road.

Heart crouched, hiding.

"I meant to see my patient again in five days," Ruth shouted angrily at the men. "Why do I have to wait two weeks?"

One of the men spurred his horse toward Ruth. "It's Blackaby's decree, Healer. "

"Why is he closing the road?" Ruth asked, pretending to grab something from the ground, then walking toward the rider.

"He hasn't told us anything," the man growled.

Heart watched Ruth get into her wagon. The riders trotted alongside as Banjo started off.

Heart stood still until they were out of sight.

Ruth had found a way to make sure Heart understood what had happened. Heart was grateful. But she was still worried.

She gathered the supplies Ruth had brought, then started uphill, tears in her eyes.

As she walked into the cave, Kip opened his blue eye, then his brown one. He wriggled his way out from between the unicorns.

Moonsilver lifted his head. Avamir scrambled upright.

"Something terrible happened," Heart said aloud, talking to the animals the way she always did. "Tin Blackaby's men came."

She set the food down, then reached into her pocket for the little woven bag Ruth had given her.

She opened it carefully.

There were two long silver threads inside. She passed them between her fingers. They were round and silken.

Heart pulled the tiny pouch Ruth had given her months before from her carry-sack. It held the single silver thread Ruth's grandmother had passed down to her. Heart placed it with the two new threads, then carefully closed the little woven bag.

Heart smiled. Ruth's grandmother had given

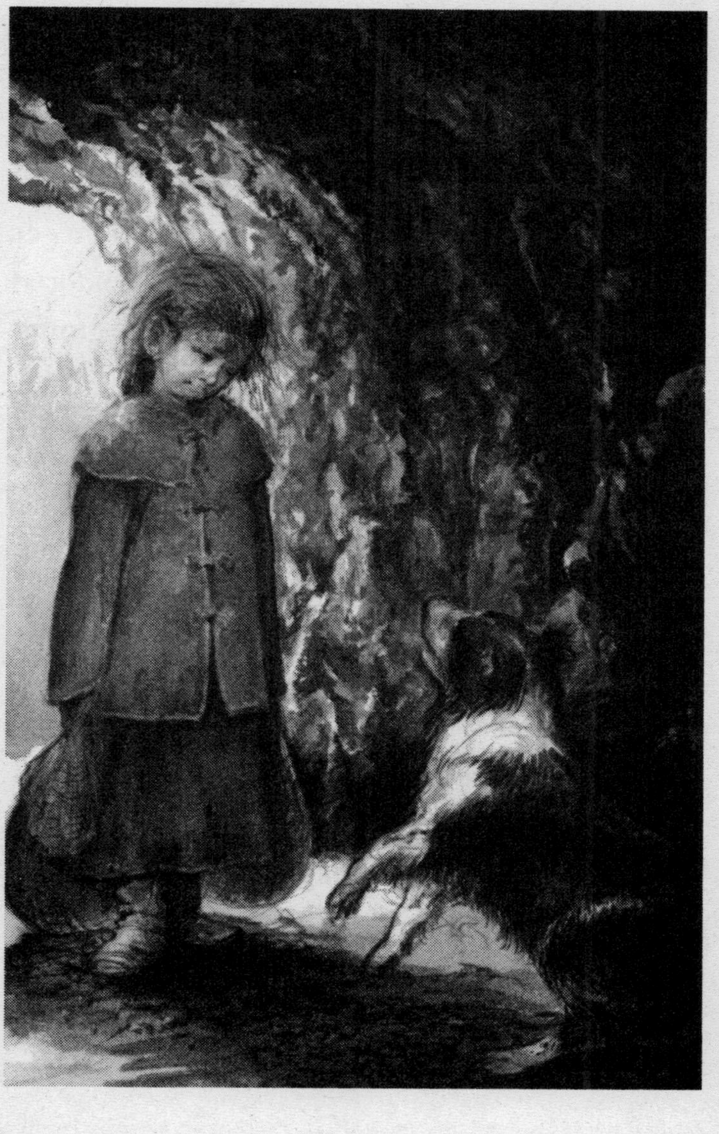

her the single silver thread as a luck-charm. Ruth had told Heart it would protect her, too.

Heart sighed.

It had . . . until now.

But how odd that her own mother—whoever she was—had owned a blanket embroidered with thread just like the thread Ruth's grandmother had handed down.

And where was the shop that held such wondrous things?

In Derrytown?

In the village at the foot of Dunraven's castle?

People said these places were full of wonders. Why not a shop that sold silver embroidery thread?

Kip barked softly. Heart turned. "You want your bone?" He barked again.

Heart began to go through the supplies.

As always, Ruth had packed a few surprises. The tinned cheese was for her. She gave Kip his bone. There was corn and oats for the unicorns.

Heart gave them a little of each, then tucked the rest away.

Heart swept the night's ashes aside, then laid kindling on the glowing coals.

Within minutes she had a cook fire to boil her barley.

She ate half as much as she usually would. If Ruth couldn't come for two weeks—or longer—she would need to stretch the food.

Heart cleaned up then walked outside. Kip followed, leaving his bone behind. The unicorns came out a moment later.

Heart looked up at the sky. The worst of the winter storms were over.

Kip leaped into his morning run. He had grown—his legs were getting long. He tore along, circling her.

Moonsilver danced into a canter to play with Kip.

Usually it made Heart smile to watch them. Today she just sighed and leaned against Avamir.

"This is awful," she said aloud. "I don't want to cause trouble for Ruth."

She knew she should leave.

But where could she possibly go?

✦ CHAPTER THREE

The next morning, Heart heard voices. Picking her way downhill, staying hidden, she saw Tin Blackaby's men pass on the road. The following afternoon, they passed by again.

Were they looking for *her*?

Would they look this hard for two horses and a ragged girl? It seemed impossible. Unless they suspected the truth about Moonsilver and Avamir

The idea they might know about the unicorns made Heart's throat ache.

"It doesn't matter," Heart told Kip the next day as they sat beside a snowy meadow.

Moonsilver and Avamir were grazing above them, pawing at the snow to uncover the frozen grass.

Kip tilted his head and stared at her.

"It doesn't matter why they are searching," Heart went on. "If they keep at it, we'll have to leave."

The next day, Heart watched the road.

She saw no one at all.

The morning after that, her spirits lifted a little. She found herself hoping.

Maybe Ruth would come to the white-rock meeting place after all. Maybe she would explain that Tin Blackaby had been upset about something else, that it had nothing to do with her or Heart or the unicorns.

Heart started up to the meadow.

As always, she led the unicorns and Kip across the rockiest ground she could find.

They left no tracks among the rocks.

It was safe. The unicorns *never* stumbled.

Kip was as surefooted as any dog.

Heart was the one who had to be careful on the rough ground.

The rising sun made the snow sparkle.

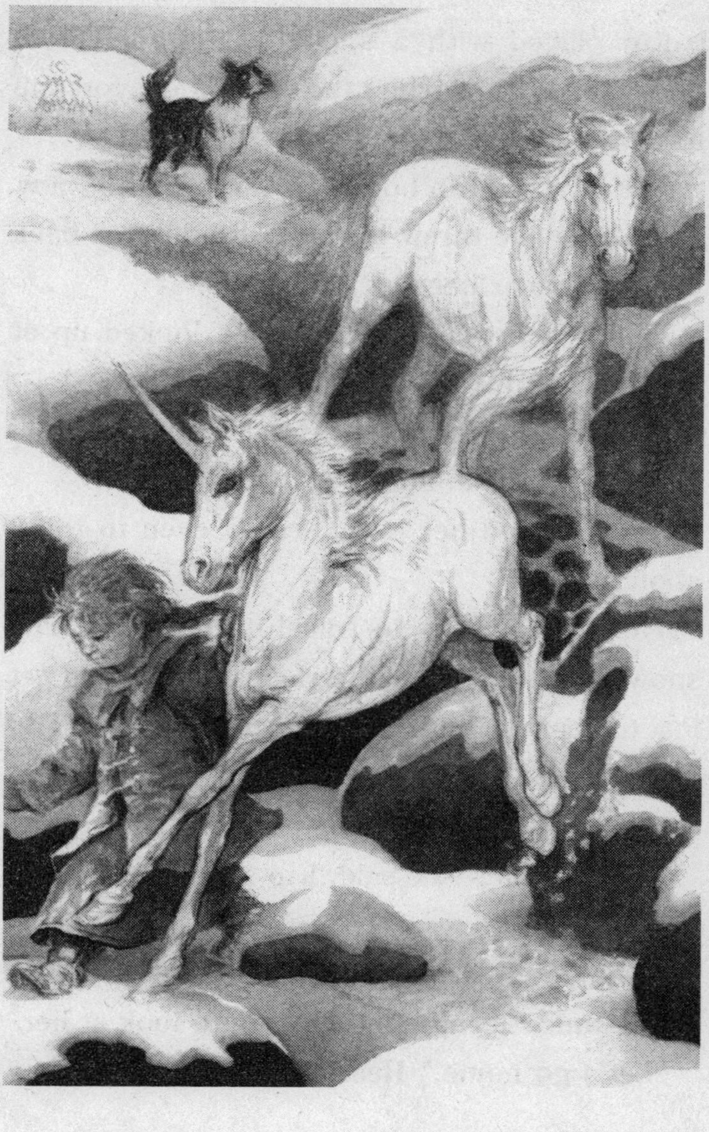

Kip played with a stick for a while. Then Heart made snowballs, throwing them for him to chase.

She watched Kip bounding through the snow. Each time she threw a snowball he raced back to drop it near her feet.

"Kip?" Heart said. He stopped looked up at her, his ears high. "We have to leave here."

Kip's ears went down. Heart knew he could hear the worry in her voice.

Heart closed her eyes, scared even to think about it.

They would have to travel on the road. The snow was too deep on the slopes; they could get lost too easily. But if they stayed in the cave and were found . . .

By early evening, Heart was tired of worrying.

"Suppertime," she said. Kip shook snow from his coat.

"Avamir?" Heart called. "Moonsilver?"

The unicorns stopped grazing to look at her.

"Let's go home," Heart called to them. They

turned and began to pick their way through the deep snow toward the rocks.

Once the fire had warmed the cave a little, Heart poured out a little barley to boil.

"You catch rabbits, Kip," she said. "The unicorns graze. I'm the only one who needs Ruth's help all the time."

Kip tilted his head. Then his ears jerked upward. He faced the cave entrance.

Heart scrambled to her feet. "What?"

Kip whimpered. He lifted one forepaw. Then he growled low in his throat.

Heart heard something faint, far away.

Voices?

✦ CHAPTER FOUR

"Kip!"

He looked up at her.

"Stay there!" Heart said.

She ran to the entrance. When she peeked out, she saw people coming out of the trees at the far end of the meadow.

They were dressed in bright colors. Some led ponies. And as they walked, they *jingled.*

Gypsies?

Heart ducked back inside.

She had heard about Gypsies all her life. But they rarely passed through Ash Grove. Why would they? Tin Blackaby wouldn't pay for their shows and the villagers had no money to spare.

Heart inched forward to peek outside again.

Some of the women wore long, swirling skirts. Some had wide, billowing trousers like the men's. The men's sleeves were gathered and full. All of them—even the toddling babies—wore wide sashes that dangled rainbows of silk tassels.

Heart watched them come up the slope in a ragged line. They were heading straight toward her. They were carrying bedrolls and blankets. Heart's stomach tightened as she realized that her cave was *their* cave. And they intended to shelter in it for the night.

Heart knew one thing.

She couldn't let them see Moonsilver.

"Stay inside, Avamir," Heart pleaded. The mare shook her mane and tossed her head. "Keep Moonsilver with you too," Heart added, then stared at the colt. He switched his long tail back and forth.

Heart took a deep breath.

If she waited any longer the Gypsies would be

too close. She stepped out of the cave into the late afternoon sunlight.

The Gypsies stopped, hands on hips, glancing at each other. Heart's pulse was a quick-time hammer.

Would they hurt her?

Heart stood still, her breath uneven. Suddenly, the Gypsies walked back downslope. They picked a place in the meadow to set up camp.

Heart stepped back into the cave entrance, then watched.

The Gypsy women made a fire—a big fire. They stood around, talking. Bursts of laughter came from the children.

The sun was setting.

It'd be dark soon.

Heart clenched her teeth.

She had been so careful with her cooking fires. And now these Gypsies had built a bonfire anyone could see.

"Wait here," she told to Avamir and Moonsilver.

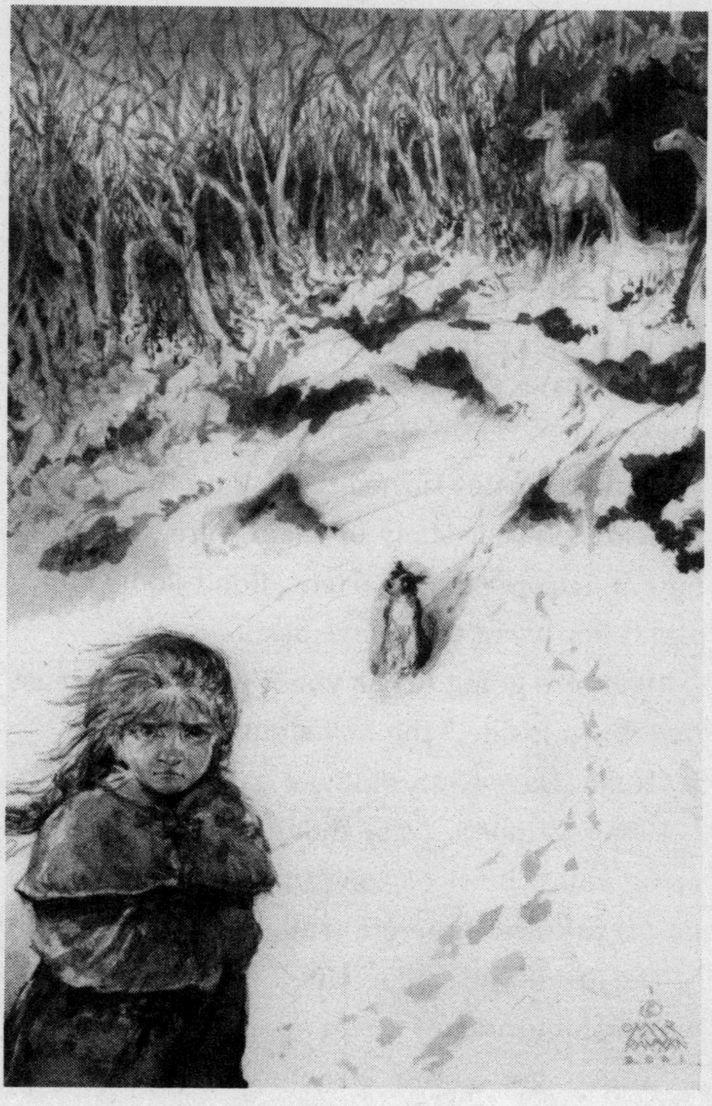

"You have to stay hidden." She looked at Kip. "Don't follow me."

Kip tilted his head and whined, which meant he had understood and didn't like it one bit.

Heart started down the slope, her feet heavy as lead.

One of the Gypsy children looked up. "She's come out!"

All the Gypsies turned to look up the slope.

Heart slowed. Many of them were smiling at her. It surprised her. They didn't look angry about her using their cave at all.

"We were going to ask you if we could at least bed down inside," the boy shouted.

"Hush, Davey," an old man said to him.

Davey grinned. "Zim thought it'd be best to bring you a bowl of stew to bargain with." He gestured toward the old man.

The instant he said it, Heart smelled the deep, wonderful aroma of a real supper cooking.

"We've got grand biscuits, too," a merry-faced girl called. Davey smiled. “That’s Fiona. She made the biscuits.”

Heart blinked as the Gypsies laughed. She had never, in her whole life, been around so many friendly people.

“Where are your folks?” Davey asked. “Where are you from?”

She looked at him. “Ash Grove. But I don’t have any folks.”

One of the older women made a clucking sound of dismay. “None? You can’t be out here by yourself, can you, dearie?”

Heart backed up a step, sorry she had spoken. She couldn’t explain herself to these people. And if they saw the unicorns . . .

“You could come with us, then,” Davey said.

There was a general sound of agreement. The old woman who had called her “dearie” was nodding. “Do you juggle? Can you dance?”

Heart shook her head, confused.

“I’ll teach her,” Davey said. “Look how little her feet are. She’d be a perfect doll up there.”

Heart stared at him. Up where? She had no idea what he was talking about.

"You'll need an act of some kind," the older woman said.

A man across the fire nodded. "A little thing like you can do most anything and people will applaud. But you'll grow. So it's best to learn something and—"

He stopped suddenly and stared past her. Heart turned to see Kip racing down the hill.

"Kip!" she shouted. "Stop right there!"

Kip slid to a stop and sat down, tilting his head.

A murmuring went around the fire.

"Has a touch with animals, don't she?" the man said, and laughed.

Heart sighed.

The fire was warm and they were all smiling at her.

She smiled back, wishing she belonged to them.

"Will you look at that!" one of the men said in a low voice.

He was pointing.

Heart turned back toward the cave.

Avamir was standing in the opening, peering out. And beside her was Moonsilver. His horn glistened in the dusk.

✦ CHAPTER FIVE

Everyone was staring, talking in excited voices.

"You clever child," the older woman said, coming around the bonfire to look into Heart's face. "We've heard the tales, of course. Some guard claims he saw a unicorn?"

Heart swallowed hard, confused and uncertain what to say.

"I'm Binney," the woman said, smiling. "That one named me." She pointed at Davey.

"She's my Granny Binnadell," he explained. "When I was little, I couldn't say it right."

"So he called me Binney and Binney I became," the woman added. She faced Heart. "Now, tell us how you did it."

"Please," Davey added.

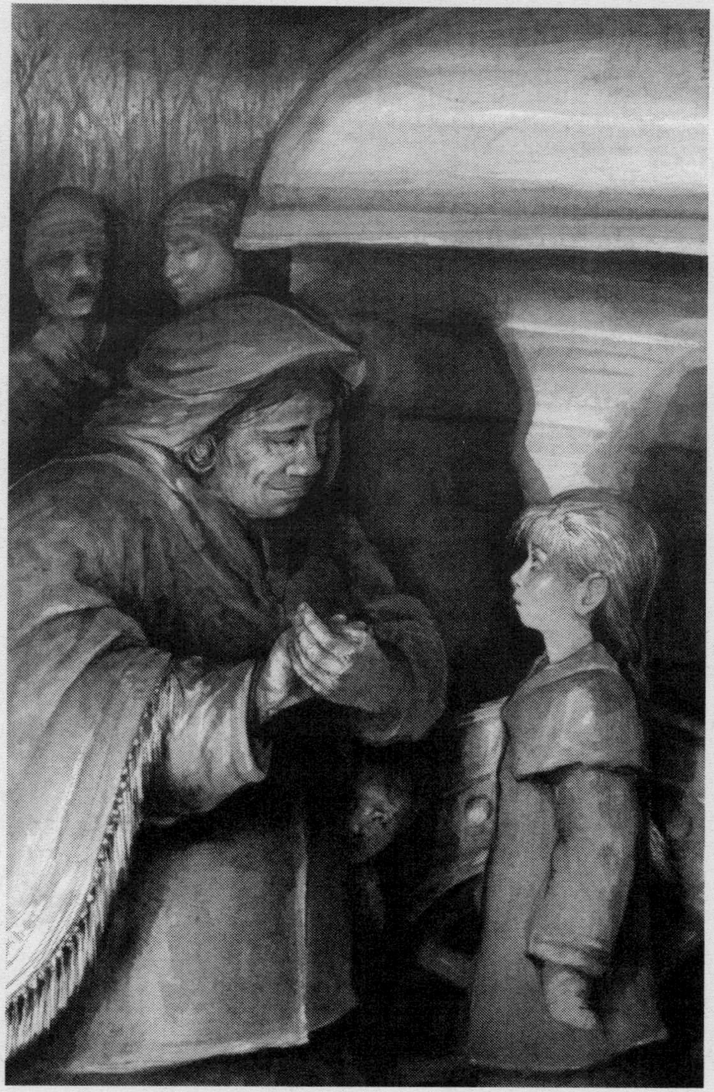

Heart glanced at him, her pulse speeding up.

"Pine gum to stick it on?" Davey asked. "What is it, a goat horn?"

"Whatever it is, we should have thought it up," Heart heard a man mutter. "Folks are going to line up to see this."

All at once, Heart understood.

The Gypsies thought Moonsilver was a colt with an old goat horn stuck on his forehead with sticky tree sap. They thought she had done it to make money.

Heart exhaled loudly. Then she cleared her throat. "Well, he's white, like all the legends say, and . . . so I . . ." Heart trailed off.

She was not used to lying.

Binney laughed, lifting her eyes to the dusky sky. "Rumors also say a little girl stole the horses. Did you?"

Heart straightened her spine. "I *paid* Simon. He lied. And I—"

"That's plenty." Binney waved one hand in the air. "I can hear the truth in your voice. The rest is your business." She gestured up at Moonsilver. "Jacob is right. People will line up. You are very clever."

Heart let out a slow, careful breath.

Binney looked at her, dark eyes steady. "Why you're alone is your business, so long as your troubles bring us no harm."

Heart told the truth. "Tin Blackaby's men might be searching for me."

Binney nodded slowly. "People look for us, too, sometimes." Everyone laughed. Binney hushed them. "Do you want to be found?"

Heart shook her head.

"Will they follow you to Derrytown and beyond?" Binney's eyes were sharp.

Heart thought about it.

Beyond Derrytown?

Tin Blackaby's men never even rode all the way *to* Derrytown. No one from Ash Grove went that far.

"No," she answered.

"What's your name?" Binney asked.

Heart told her.

"Then join us, Heart, do," Binney said. "We're off to Derrytown with many stops in between here and there. Then on to Yolen's Crossing and San Coville and—what?" she asked, peering into Heart's face.

"I've never heard of those places," Heart said quietly.

Binney laughed again. "Nor have the people there heard of your little thatched-roof Ash Grove. If you go far enough, you will find people who haven't heard of your Lord Dunraven."

Heart caught her breath. "Is that true?"

Binney nodded, her eyes twinkling.

Heart smiled. Then her eyes flooded with tears. Maybe she'd never see Ruth again.

Zim pointed to Kip. "How well is he trained?"

Heart realized Kip was wagging his tail, staring at her.

"He's smart," Heart said. "I've never taught him tricks."

"Call him," Zim said quietly.

"Kip?" Heart said. "Will you come down here?" She heard the Gypsy children giggling.

Kip lunged into a headlong run. Sliding on the snowy patches, he charged down the slope. He skidded to a stop beside Heart.

"There's a dog that knows good biscuits when he smells them," Fiona said.

Everyone laughed again.

Heart let the sound wash over her. Ruth would love these people, she was sure.

Heart glanced back at the cave entrance. The dusk was deepening. Moonsilver and Avamir had gone back inside.

Zim ladled stew into a bowl. Then he scooped in clean snow to cool it.

"Tell him not to eat it," he said to Heart.

"Why?" She frowned, puzzled.

"To see if he really listens to you."

"Kip," Heart said somberly as Zim set the bowl in front of him. "Don't touch it, please." Kip looked sad, but he didn't move.

The Gypsies stared, then applauded.

"You have the gift," Zim said approvingly. He caught Heart's eye. "Tell him it's his."

"You can eat it, Kip," she said quietly.

Kip buried his muzzle in the bowl, lapping noisily.

"Are the horses trained like this?" Zim asked her.

Heart shrugged. "The . . . horses are smart too. Moonsilver is shy—"

"The colt?" Zim interrupted.

Heart nodded.

"I'm surprised he stands for the spirit gum and the goat horn."

Heart hoped he couldn't see her blushing in the soft dusk. "I mean, he's shy with everyone but me," she explained.

"Would it be all right with him if we slept inside the cave, do you think?" Davey asked. He shivered and grinned.

Heart glanced around at the eager faces. It was getting chilly. Binney was ladling stew and Heart knew it was for her.

"Of course," she said slowly.

Zim pulled a silver flute from beneath his coat. He began to play. The melody was like rainwater, quick and clear.

Heart stared at his fingers. The firelight polished the silver flute into gold.

"Do you play?" Zim asked, when he finished the tune.

Heart shook her head.

"I will teach you if you like."

Heart nodded, smiling. She ate fast.

The Gypsies were standing, stretching. They were gathering their blankets and carry-sacks.

It was nearly dark as they trudged up the hill behind Heart.

She was grateful.

The unicorns came to the entrance when they heard the voices. Avamir led Moonsilver to stand in the meadow while the Gypsies settled in for the night.

Heart moved her things to the front of the cave.

It was strange to hear so many voices inside it.

One by one they quieted, calling good night to her.

Only when it was silent did the unicorns come back to the cave.

She waited until they had lain down just inside the entrance. Kip curled up between them.

Then, being as quiet as she could, Heart went through went her carry-sack. She finally found the empty cheese tin.

She placed it beside her blankets and lay down to wait.

She bit at her lip to keep from falling asleep.

She had to wait for the moon to rise.

And she had to be careful.

If even one of the Gypsies heard her leave the cave, it would ruin everything.

✦ CHAPTER SIX

When the moon finally came up, Heart tiptoed out so quietly that even Kip did not waken.

She used clean snow to scrub out the little cheese tin. Then she made her way, shivering, to the edge of the woods.

Working in the pale light, she found a thick gob of pinesap oozing from a limb low enough to reach.

She scraped it into the tin.

Back in the cave, she held the closed tin against her belly to warm it.

When the pine gum was softened, she gently wakened Moonsilver.

"Hold still," she begged him. "Hush."

She smeared a circle of the sticky pine gum

around the base of his horn.

Then she lightly kissed his muzzle and put the tin away.

She managed to doze a little, but she dreamed that she was running uphill. She woke up breathing hard, as though the steep rocky hillside of her dream had been real.

She lay still, until the Gypsies rose at daybreak. Then she got up.

The unicorns moved away to the meadow, pawing up grass to eat.

Heart thought the tree gum looked perfect. No one else seemed to notice.

The Gypsies sang as they broke camp. The bells on their sashes jingled. The children chased each other, laughing.

Heart packed her carry-sack. It did not take long. All of her possessions fit inside.

Kip stood close to her as the Gypsies left the cave.

The children stared wide-eyed at Moonsilver, giggling.

Binney and Zim smiled broadly.

"Do you need help?" Fiona asked on her way past Heart. Davey was right behind her. Heart shook her head, and they went on.

"Moonsilver was a baby when we found this place," Heart whispered to Avamir once they were alone. "Now he's nearly as tall as you are."

Avamir's breath smelled like sweet grass.

"I'm afraid," Heart said softly.

Avamir nudged her shoulder, then whinnied softly at Moonsilver.

Heart watched the colt canter up, then slide to a halt. She laughed. "You two aren't scared, are you?" She took Ruth's little woven bag from her pocket and opened it to touch the silver threads.

Heart caught her breath.

Simon's threads had knotted themselves into a circle with Ruth's. *How?*

"Heart!"

Davey's shout made her whirl around. She pushed the silvery circle back inside the woven bag.

She started down the mountain, Kip at her heels.

Avamir followed. Moonsilver cantered in a wide arc, then caught up. Heart wondered what the Gypsies would think. The unicorns never had on a rope or a halter.

She wouldn't be able to make them act like horses.

Maybe the Gypsies would think she had trained them.

Heart could hear Gypsies singing and talking. They had hidden their wagons in the trees. They were moving them back onto the road now.

Heart took a deep breath and stepped out of the forest.

The unicorns were right behind her.

Sighs and murmurs rose from the Gypsies.

Moonsilver *was* beautiful, even with the sticky ring of pinesap on his snowy white forehead. Avamir was stately, like a queen in a story. Both were more graceful than any horse ever born.

Heart was uneasy standing out in the open. She was used to *hiding*. What if Tin Blackaby's men came galloping up? Glancing around, she recognized a flat-topped white boulder.

Heart sighed. This was where she was supposed to meet Ruth next time.

Avamir and Moonsilver drifted back into the trees. They began to paw at the snow.

Kip ran to meet a small, black dog tagging after Fiona.

"Sadie won't fight," Fiona called. "We'll all watch out for Kip."

"Heart?"

She turned. Davey was pointing at the unicorns. "Binney wondered—don't they just wander off?"

Heart shook her head. "Never."

Davey's smiled. "That horn looks amazing from a distance. Maybe you won't need to learn to wire walk." He waved and went back to help the men who were rolling wagons back onto the road.

The sun was coming up.

It made the wagons shine. Each was painted differently, with bright patterns sweeping along its sides. Binney's was meadow-flower blue.

Heart watched the laughing Gypsies, her own spirits sinking lower and lower. Ruth would look for her. Then she would worry.

Heart watched a girl her age standing on a box to fasten harness buckles.

Some of the children were gathering pinecones.

Older ones brought buckets of icy creek water to fill the oaken barrels on the wagons.

Heart saw a glimmer of silver in the frozen mud.

It was a tiny Gypsy bell, fallen from someone's sash.

She scooped it up, smiling. Maybe there *was* a way to let Ruth know she was with the Gypsies.

Heart took the circle of silver thread out of its woven bag and put it on her wrist, like a bracelet.

Then she put the bell in Ruth's little woven bag.

She found a stone the size of a supper plate and pried it loose from the frozen ground.

Glancing around, she made sure no one was watching her.

Then she placed the little bag on the white boulder and hid it with the smaller rock.

Heart glanced around again.

No one had seen her.

She walked back toward the wagons.

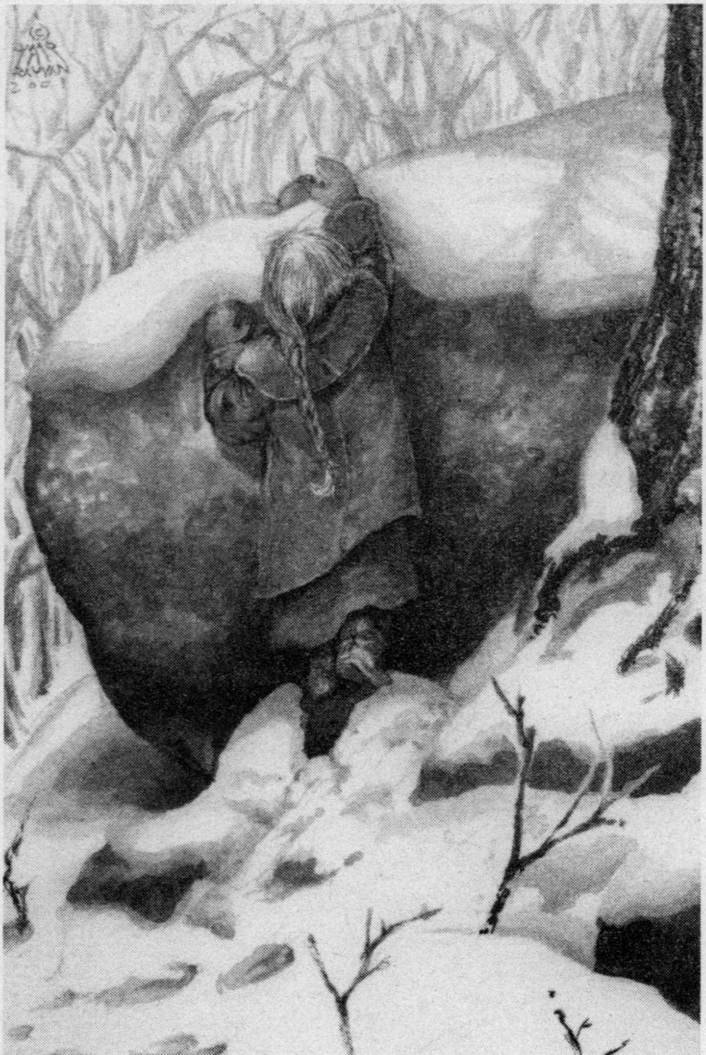

✦ CHAPTER SEVEN

The next day, Zim walked beside Heart. He played his silvery flute.

The melodies were like waterfalls, like quick-winged birds flying through a forest.

That evening Zim taught Heart a simple scale. He lent her a flute so she could practice. She had to slide the circle of silver thread higher on her arm or it would get in her way. She didn't take it off. She never wanted to lose it.

Once she had learned the first scale, Zim taught her another. The silvery flute felt cool and smooth beneath Heart's fingers.

Every night, Heart slept in Binney's warm, clean wagon. It smelled like herbs and apples, and she felt safe inside it. Binney gave her a soft blanket and a pillow. Binney's heart was clear as creek water. She was like Ruth.

Every morning, Binney's blue wagon led the way. The other drivers followed in a long line.

As they wound their way down out of the mountains, the weather warmed. Soon there was no snow on the ground at all.

Dozens of roads crossed the Derrytown road. The Gypsies knew which ones to take.

Heart was happy—and *busy*. There were enough hands for every chore—and enough work to keep all hands moving.

Every morning, the Gypsies folded their blankets, shook out their pillows, and made breakfast. They tended their babies, washed their children's faces, and fed their dogs.

They left nothing behind but boot prints.

Every evening, away from the wagons where no one could see, Heart redrew the sticky pinegum circle on Moonsilver's forehead.

He did not seem to mind.

The unicorns slept near Binney's wagon. The

Gypsies admired them, but no one tried to touch them.

Heart was grateful. Moonsilver's secret had to be kept.

At first Heart walked with Kip, Avamir, and Moonsilver. Then things began to change.

Kip often visited Sadie, Fiona's dog.

Sometimes Heart joined Binney or Fiona and her friends.

She showed them how to pick and dry meadowsweet and how to make the healing salve Ruth had used on Moonsilver's wound back in Ash Grove.

Zim walked beside Heart to teach her the scales. She carried the flute and practiced each day.

Davey sometimes walked where he could watch the unicorns. Avamir was friendly with the children, but Moonsilver remained shy. Heart was glad. She didn't want anyone to realize his horn was real.

In the camps at night Heart learned what

Davey had meant by wirewalking and juggling.

The Gypsies tied wires between two trees. One was low so the children could practice. The higher one was for the adults.

It looked impossible.

How could anyone balance?

Heart was afraid to try it.

"Have you planned your act yet?" Binney asked gently, almost every day.

"No," Heart answered every time.

Binney would smile. "It will come to you."

"Everyone is so good," Heart said to Davey one evening as they watched the wirewalkers.

He glanced at her. "Of course. We practice hard."

Heart thought about it as she snuggled into her soft blanket inside Binney's wagon that night.

The next day she started playing the flute every moment she could.

"You are ready," Zim said a few days later. He showed her a song. It was harder than the scales.

Heart practiced. Once she could play the song, she found herself adding notes to make it prettier.

Then she made up a song of her own.

Kip loved it.

He came running whenever she played it.

Zim grinned. He told her to give Kip a bit of bread every time he came to hear the tune.

Heart did. Soon Kip leaped into a mad dash the instant he heard the first few notes. Moonsilver noticed. He began to follow Kip.

It became a race between them.

They would slide to a stop in front of Heart.

Then Moonsilver would go back to graze with Avamir.

Kip would wander through the wagons.

He played with all the dogs, but Sadie adored him. He followed Binney asking for leftover stew.

They came to a village named Fallbrook. It was small, its hills covered with fruit trees and farms.

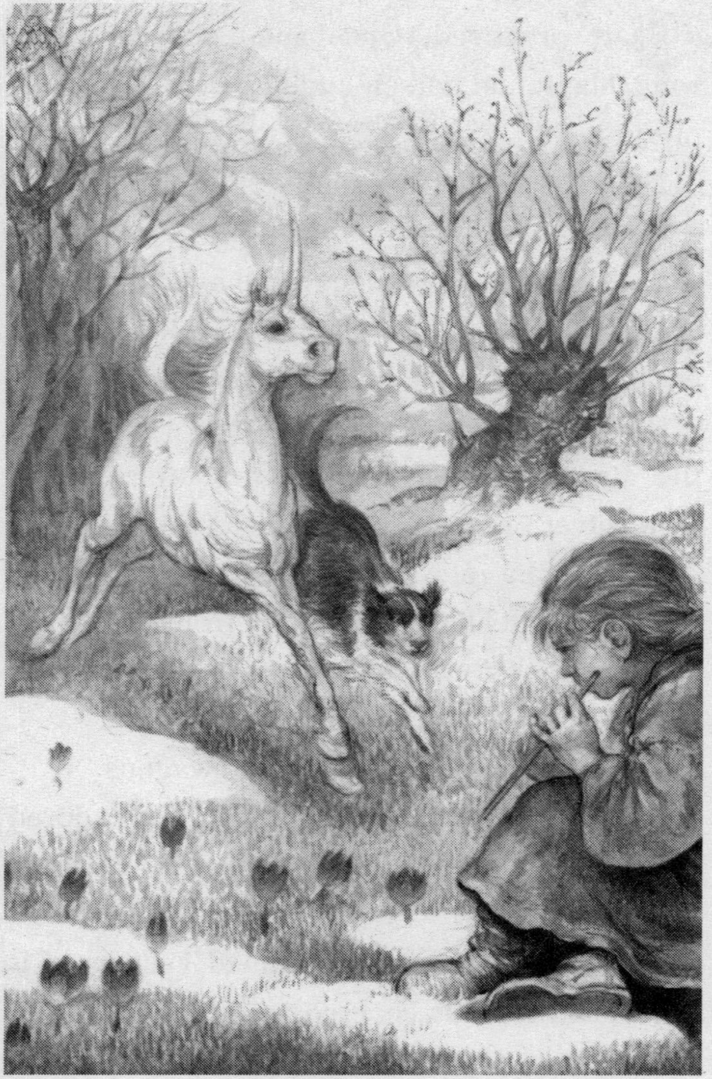

It's prettier than Ash Grove, Heart thought. The people had better houses.

Heart walked close to the unicorns. They seemed calm—much calmer than she was.

"We'd like to show Moonsilver tonight," Binney said. "Have you planned an act?"

Heart shook her head, blushing.

Binney patted Heart's cheek. "Let us do it, then. You can change it later to suit yourself." She touched Heart's arm. "Look."

Heart glanced around.

People had stopped. They were staring at Moonsilver.

✦ CHAPTER EIGHT

Binney raised her hand and signaled.

The Gypsies pulled in their ponies.

Zim jumped down to play his flute. He gestured for Heart to join in. She pushed the silver thread-bracelet higher on her arm and lifted the flute. She played as well as she could.

The Gypsy children appeared in a long, laughing line.

They turned flips and danced.

They shouted to the people they passed, inviting them to a show in a few hours.

"Tell your neighbors!" Binney shouted. "Come to see Dunraven's Rumor—a real unicorn!"

People waved and called back, laughing.

Binney gestured, and the wagons creaked back into motion.

Heart felt breathless. The Gypsy wagons followed a cobbled road to a meadow at the edge of the town.

Avamir and Moonsilver walked a little ways off to graze on the fresh spring grass. Kip stayed close to them.

Heart fidgeted when Lord Dunraven's steward came to talk to Binney. But he was a jolly-faced man—nothing like Tin Blackaby.

He joked with Binney.

His eyes went wide when he noticed Moonsilver.

Heart's breath stopped in her throat.

"Now that's clever," the man remarked.

Binney was counting coins into his hand. She smiled. "You've heard the tales?"

He shrugged. "Some wheat-gleaner in a thatch-roofed village claiming he saw a herd of unicorns in Dunraven's forest?" He chuckled. "Who hasn't? But people will get a smile out of this."

Binney half bowed. “That is our trade. We sell smiles.”

The man laughed. “I’ll bring my family to the show.”

Binney made him a curtsy as he left. “He takes a big share, but they all do,” she said wearily. “At least he’s more pleasant than most. That’s why his town does well.”

Heart was trembling. Maybe this was foolish. What if someone guessed Moonsilver really was a unicorn?

“You’re shaking like a leaf in high wind,” Binney said gently. She nudged Heart’s shoulder. “Go. Get ready.”

The Gypsies’ everyday clothes were colorful. Their costumes were embroidered, trimmed, mirrored, and beaded.

Heart was dazzled.

Fiona loaned her a loose-sleeved raspberry blouse and an embroidered pinafore of columbine blue.

Talia’s aunt gave her a copper-colored scarf

with a lacey edge. Josepha smiled and clapped. Heart felt beautiful.

When people began to arrive at dusk, Binney told her to hide Moonsilver behind the wagons. "And put this in your pocket." She handed Heart bits of bread.

Heart helped set out the circle of Gypsy lanterns.

The meadow became a magical place.

The jugglers began the show.

Davey was amazing. He juggled heavy clubs, then balls, then sticks that had been set on fire! Two grown men juggled with him. They threw balls between them, their hands flashing.

Then came the wirewalkers.

The wire was strung high, between two elm trees.

The girls did graceful tricks. One of them did a slow somersault, gripping the wire in her hands, then coming back up onto her feet.

The crowd clapped and shouted.

Heart clapped with them, staring.

Then Davey walked the wire. Heart blinked. She had never even seen him practice! He pretended to fall, but caught the wire and swung around it, then stood up again.

The crowd gasped, then clapped.

While they were still clapping, Binney danced forward on the grass. She wore a sparkling gold skirt. She put a flaming torch into her mouth, then breathed out a long plume of fire.

The audience fell silent.

Binney breathed out fire like a dragon in a bedtime tale.

Then, from somewhere in the dark, Zim began to play. After a moment, he stepped into the lantern circle. The light sparkled off his flute.

He played a melody that made Heart's skin prickle.

The people clapped and whistled.

Then Binney walked out again. "We have something very special tonight," she said. "A girl who plays a magic flute."

The people applauded.

Heart stood still, trembling.

She felt Davey pressing her flute into her hand. "Go on," he whispered in her ear. "You'll be wonderful."

Heart managed to walk forward and bow.

"She plays many melodies," Binney was saying. "But there is one tune that sometimes calls up magical beasts!"

Binney bowed to the audience, then backed out of the light.

Heart touched her pocket. The bread was there. She took a deep breath.

Heart began to play. Her breathing was a little uneven, but the tune sounded all right.

The second song was better. She danced a little. People clapped. For the third song, she played Kip's melody.

As he had dozens of times before, Kip came running the instant he heard the first notes.

Moonsilver was right behind him. They raced in a long circle, Moonsilver leaping and tossing his head.

Heart stood with her head high, her back straight.

She kept playing as Kip and Moonsilver plunged to a stop in front of her.

The melody whirled and spun across the soft evening air.

The people stared at Moonsilver. They stared at Kip. Only then did Heart notice a ruff of false hair around Kip's neck. Someone had gummed a tuft on the end of his tail, too.

He looked like a tiny, patchy-coated lion.

She saw Davey grinning from beyond the lanterns.

Moonsilver pawed the ground. Kip ran in a tight circle around him. The audience roared its approval.

The noise startled Moonsilver into another headlong gallop.

He circled the whole meadow, tossing his head. His snow-white coat gleamed in the lantern light.

Coming back, Kip crossed in front of

Moonsilver. The colt leaped over him, landing as lightly as a cat.

The audience stood and cheered.

Moonsilver reared, pawing at the summer night.

"They just think you are beautiful," Heart said to him, lowering the flute. "Don't be afraid."

Moonsilver calmed down. He stood on all four hooves and tossed his head. Then he bent to rub his muzzle on one foreleg.

It looked like he was bowing.

The audience clapped and cheered again. They applauded for a long time.

The show was over, and Binney told them good night.

It took a long time for them to leave. Heart stood beside Moonsilver, waving good-bye, smiling and smiling.

"You were wonderful," Binney told her the next morning. "You made them happy."

Davey was standing nearby. He turned and nodded. "They'll talk about that for months."

Moonsilver tossed his head.

"You were wonderful too," Davey assured him.

The colt pricked his ears and listened.

"He likes you," Heart said.

Davey grinned.

✦ CHAPTER NINE

The next show was in a smaller town called Bonsall.

The one after that was in Finley, a town built around a water-wheeled flourmill.

Then came Cusick's Farm, Mayes, Harlan Bend, and Werlinburg.

Heart began to dance more while she played the flute. Fiona taught her steps. She practiced playing. She learned to make each note shine like a star.

Moonsilver seemed to like making people clap and whistle.

Heart taught him signals. If she raised one finger, he would bow. Two fingers made him gallop in a circle. She taught him to rear when she lifted her head and crossed her eyes.

Kip learned fast, too.

Every show got better.

The Gypsies were delighted.

Heart taught Kip to bare his teeth like a lion. It made people laugh aloud.

Fiona helped sometimes. She began to think up new tricks to teach Sadie, too. Fiona—and her friends Talia and Josepha—began to sit next to Heart at the campfire.

Talia and Josepha had a balancing act. They could spin plates on their fingers. They could dance with swords balanced across their foreheads. They practiced nearly every evening.

"Heart! Watch!" Davey called one night in camp.

She turned to see him climbing the ladder to the low wire.

Holding his juggling clubs, he stepped onto the slender line.

Heart stared as he set his feet.

Then he began to juggle. The whole camp went quiet. Heart realized she was holding her breath.

How could he do it? Juggling looked hard enough standing on firm ground.

Davey took a step forward, then another, then a third.

He caught all the clubs, then dropped them so he could raise his hands high and bow.

Everyone cheered and clapped.

Davey leaped down from the low wire, grinning. Heart shook her head as he came toward her. "When have you been practicing that?" she demanded.

Davey shrugged. "After everyone goes to sleep."

Heart frowned. "Why keep it a secret?"

He lowered his head. "In case I couldn't do it. I'll try the high wire next."

Heart shook her head. "But then, if you lose your balance, you'll—"

Davey waved one hand in the air to stop her. "But I won't!"

"No one juggles up there," Heart argued. But Davey's eyes were shining and he only smiled at her.

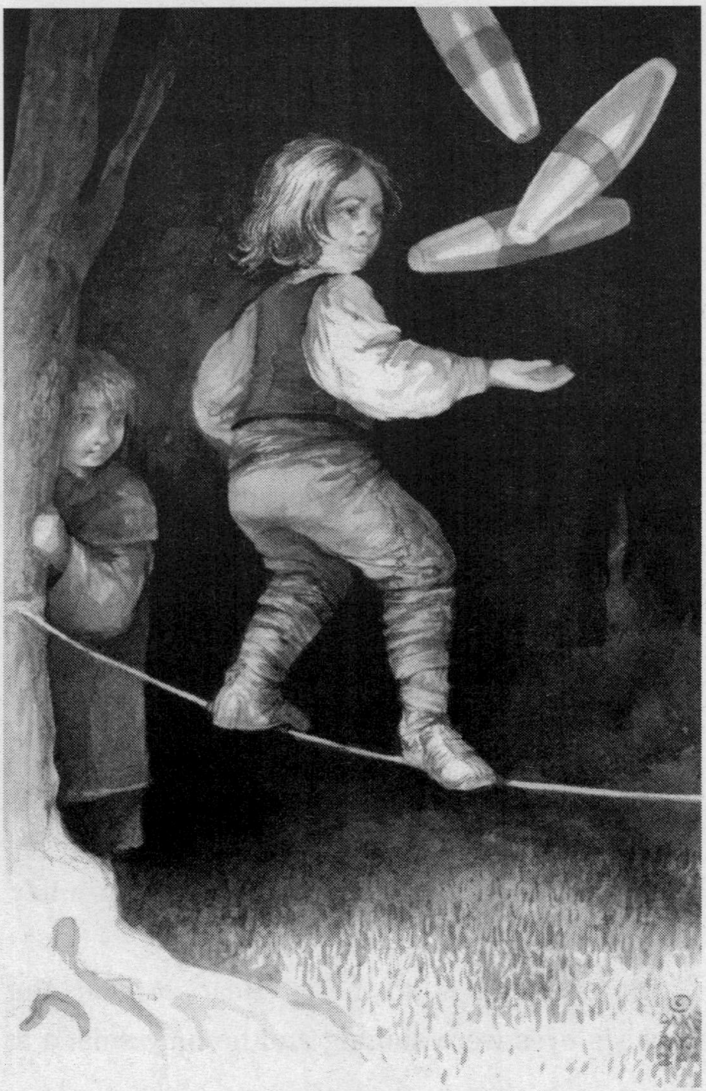

Seven days later, they came to Derrytown, late at night.

Binney had insisted they travel past dark.

She didn't want the whole town to see Moonsilver before the show.

Derrytown amazed Heart. There were tall posts with lanterns hanging from them on street corners.

The shops were all closed, but there were so many of them!

Everything was sold here.

Maybe she would find a shop that sold silver thread.

"I dreamed of coming here when I first found you in the forest," she whispered to Avamir as they walked.

Then she smiled. She had long ago imagined *riding* into Derrytown on Avamir, wearing fancy boots and a nice coat.

"This is better," she whispered to Avamir. "I am walking next to a dear friend." She turned the silver circle on her wrist, thinking about Ruth.

Kip barked at a cat.

The unicorn mare shook her mane, startled. Heart heard a faint jingling. Heart smiled. One of the Gypsy girls had braided a few tiny bells into Avamir's mane.

The unicorn mare was making new friends, too.

Heart hoped they could stay with the Gypsies forever.

The hanging lanterns made perfect globes of yellow light.

"Have you ever seen a real town?" Davey asked, falling into step beside her.

"No." Heart tilted her head to see the tops of the buildings. Many of them were as tall as a tree. "Do birds nest on the roofs?" she asked Davey.

He narrowed his eyes. "Probably."

"What kind of stone is that?" Heart asked him, touching the rough red surface of the building.

"It's not stone, it's brick," Davey explained. "Made from baked river clay."

Heart touched it again. It *felt* like rock.

They made camp on the level, green meadow in the center of the town square. The steward came to see them, of course. He left with so many coins that Binney spent a few minutes muttering to herself in anger.

Then she cleared her throat and started shouting instructions.

Heart led the unicorns and Kip out of the way.

Binney had the wagoners back into place. The finished circle looked like a spoked wheel.

"There," Binney said wearily, coming to stand by Heart. "We can hide the unicorn inside the circle."

The unicorn.

It made Heart's skin prickle to hear her say it. She settled Moonsilver and Avamir near Binney's wagon for the night. Kip lay down with them.

"How long will we be here?" she asked as she climbed into bed.

"A day or two, no more," Binney told Heart as

they settled down. "Then we'll go on."

"I still can't believe there is anyplace beyond Derrytown," Heart told her.

Binney chuckled. "Oh, there is. You'll see. Remember what I said about people not knowing your Lord Dunraven?"

"Yes," Heart said softly.

"To the west they worry about Lord Irmaedith. East it's Lord Kaybale, to the south it's Lord Levin. But northward . . ."

Binney stopped midsentence.

Heart propped herself on one elbow, staring into the dark. "What's to the north, Binney?" she asked.

The Gypsy sighed. "Dunraven's Manor, of course, but past that, no one knows. There was a road once, people say. But if there was, Lord Dunraven has let the forest take it back."

Heart lay back down. "Will we go that way?"

Binney sighed. "No, child. No one does. Not for as long as I have lived, anyway."

✦ CHAPTER TEN

They spent the whole day getting ready. Heart kept glancing at the town girls who walked past.

Their skirts were perfect.

They wore little leather shoes without scuffs or mud on them.

Josepha caught Heart's eye. "They're jealous of us, you know," she whispered. "They get bored keeping clean." Beside Heart, Talia giggled.

Heart smiled at them both.

Men were shouting as the high wire was strung between two huge oak trees.

It was higher than Heart had ever seen it.

"Derrytown audiences see lots of Gypsies," Binney said. "It's harder to amaze them."

Heart walked around playing her flute, staying inside the circle of wagons.

Everyone was busy.

Davey was practicing his juggling.

Moonsilver and Avamir let her lean against them for a while. Then they moved away, restless.

When dusk finally came, Heart helped set up the lanterns in a circle. The townspeople started coming.

Whole families strolled down the streets. They paid their admission and found places to sit on the grass.

Heart had never *seen* so many people.

The show began with the Gypsy children singing, then doing flips across the grass.

When the people applauded, it sounded like thunder. Heart had goose bumps watching the performers.

Fiona and Sadie made the audience laugh out loud.

Josepha and Talia did their balancing act perfectly.

Heart was nervous. She glanced at Kip, sitting beside the unicorns.

Kip would do his part perfectly, she was sure. So would Moonsilver.

If she played her flute well . . .

Heart looked down at the silver flute. She fingered the keys, arching her hands the way Zim had taught her.

There was a round of applause and shouting.

Then another, even louder.

Heart looked up.

There, way up on the high wire, was Davey.

And he was *juggling*.

The heavy pins danced in a blurred circle between his hands.

The crowd gasped.

Davey took a step forward, walking the wire as he flipped the heavy clubs in a twirling circle.

Heart heard the audience draw in a breath. She held hers.

Davey was smiling. He walked in an even,

slow rhythm. He began to toss the heavy clubs higher and higher.

And then, suddenly, he lost his balance.

Heart stared. It was just a tiny loss of rhythm at first. Then he lurched to one side, bending sharply to recover.

But it was too late.

The audience went still as Davey plunged to the ground.

Binney screamed and ran toward him.

Heart found herself running too, her flute forgotten in her hand. The Gypsies formed a worried ring around Davey.

He wasn't moving.

"Davey? Davey!" Binney pleaded.

But he didn't move.

Heart could hear the audience murmuring.

She glanced at them. People were standing up, trying to see better.

The thudding clatter of hooves didn't make sense to Heart at first.

Then she heard the audience's murmuring

rise to a roar and she knew what had happened.

She turned to see Moonsilver galloping toward her.

Binney saw him too, and she stood.

The audience was pouring toward them.

"Stand back," Binney shouted. "Get out of the unicorn's way!"

Heart could only watch as Moonsilver came forward, his neck arched, his horn lowered.

He touched Davey gently, the tip of his horn crossing Davey's lips.

A wind, a song, the sound of the moon sighing rose into the air.

Then it was gone and Heart wasn't sure she had heard it at all.

She could hear the audience talking, though, their voices a tangle of pitches and rhythms.

And she could hear Binney weeping.

Then Moonsilver stepped back.

Davey opened his eyes and sat up.

Heart covered her mouth with one hand.

She heard a soft, astonished murmur and

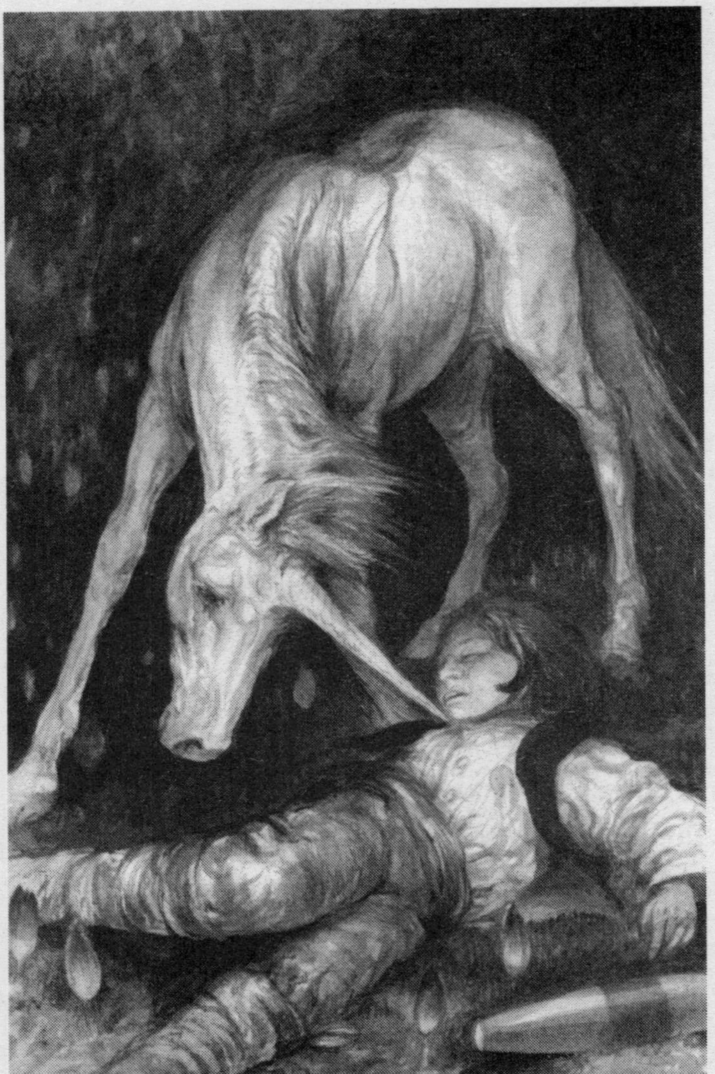

turned to see hundreds of people standing in a loose circle. The audience had mixed with the Gypsies, and they stood, shoulder to shoulder, staring.

Davey didn't seem to notice them.

He put his arms around Moonsilver's neck.

It was Zim who stepped forward and bowed, sweeping his hand out toward Davey and Moonsilver.

"Ladies and gentlemen," he said loudly. "Please be seated."

The crowd moved back across the grass. They found their places and sat down.

✦ CHAPTER ELEVEN

A tense hush fell, and Heart helf her breath.

"We are delighted that you have enjoyed our play, *The Unicorn's Secret*," Zim said loudly.

Before the audience could applaud, he raised his flute to his lips.

His eyes caught Heart's, and she realized she was holding her flute as well.

She raised it and walked to stand beside him. Zim led off, playing the melody that Heart had used to train Kip.

Kip dashed up from out of nowhere.

He and Moonsilver fell into their usual act. Leaping and galloping, the unicorn circled the ring of lanterns. Then he pranced to a stop. And he bowed.

The audience applauded wildly, shouting and whistling.

"Good night!" Zim called, and all the Gypsies bowed.

Heart played one of her own melodies, a lively tune, to make people walk faster as they left.

Only once the green was empty of townspeople did she stop playing.

"Let's build our fire," Binney said. "And then we had better have a talk."

The Gypsies all nodded and set about changing their clothes and setting up camp for the night.

Heart found Davey. "Why did you do that? You scared your grandmother half to death. And me," she added.

Davey frowned. "I just thought I could," he said quietly. "Moonsilver saved my life. He's . . . real, isn't he?"

Heart nodded.

Binney was calling for everyone to sit down.

Heart and Davey walked toward the fire to join the circle.

The grass was damp with night dew.

"Thank you, Heart," Binney said softly. "And Moonsilver. Without you my Davey might not be alive."

The Gypsies nodded and smiled at Heart. Fiona winked.

Moonsilver was standing at the edge of the circle with Avamir. The mare shook her mane. The tiny bells tinkled in the soft night air.

Binney cleared her throat. "I want to give Heart a gift."

Heart shook her head, but Binney walked toward her, one hand out.

"These belonged to my mother. She was told that they were strands of hair from a unicorn's mane." Binney paused. "The Queen of the Unicorns."

The Gypsies leaned and stretched, trying to see.

Heart looked into Binney's eyes.

They hugged, hard. Then Binney released her and put three threads into her hand.

Heart stared at them.

They were silver, thick and round.

They were exactly like the thread Ruth had given her.

They were the same as the strands of thread from the blanket Simon had sold. Her blanket.

Heart felt the silver threads around her wrist begin to turn, and tighten.

She looked down and caught her breath. The new threads were weaving themselves into the circle!

In an instant there were no loose ends. The bracelet of uneven knots had become a finely woven silver lace.

Heart saw Binney's eyes widen, but she said nothing aloud. No one else was close enough to have seen. Heart lowered her hand and let her sleeve cover the silver bracelet.

"We all need supper," Zim called out.

A round of laughter rose into the warm night.

Heart ate, but she kept touching the bracelet.

It was magical.

It had to be.

Finally everyone started for bed.

As Heart rose to go to Binney's wagon, she saw flickering shadows along the edge of the green.

She heard a soft, rough voice, talking low.

" . . . a real unicorn. Didn't you see?" it demanded. "We have to tell someone!" There were murmurs of agreement.

Heart's stomach wrenched. She knew that voice! And Ruth had said Tibbs Renner was coming to Derrytown.

Heart's eyes stung with tears.

Tibbs had always tried to cause her trouble.

He would make sure the rumors flew.

And the whispers from Derrytown would reach important ears, no matter where the Gypsies went. Heart bit at her lip. Which of the lords would not want a unicorn?

Moonsilver would soon be hunted *everywhere*. And if the Gypsies tried to help her, they would be in danger, too.

Heart blinked and wiped at her eyes.

She loved Binney and Zim and Davey. Fiona and Josepha and Talia were so nice she was starting to love them, too.

Heart crawled into her blankets and told Binney good night. Then she lay awake long enough for the stars to trace their way across half the sky.

Where could she go?

How could she save Moonsilver and Avamir from Dunraven and the other powerful lords?

Finally she slid into a tense sleep.

Her dreams were fierce.

She was running for her life in stark, treeless mountains. The massive boulders were white and gray, the colors of a full moon. She saw a mountaintop far ahead and knew it was safe—if she could reach it.

Heart woke breathing hard.

Was the dream real? It *felt* real.

Heart touched the silver bracelet on her wrist,

then sat up. She slipped out of the wagon into the darkness, taking her carry-sack with her.

If she left now, the Gypsies would be safe.

They wouldn't know where she had gone.

Moonsilver and Avamir woke silently. Kip stretched.

Heart knew she had to find the moon-colored mountains.

Every lord in every forest would soon be hunting for Moonsilver.

Avamir shook her mane and the Gypsy bells jingled.

Heart smiled.

Ruth would know why she left. And Binney would know she loved them all too much to put them in danger.

The moon rose as Heart led the way into the forest.

Avamir and Kip walked side by side.

Moonsilver stayed close.

Heart could feel his warm breath on her shoulder.

THE

UNICORN'S SECRET

The Mountains of the Moon

✦CHAPTER ONE

Heart led the way through the midnight forest.

Moon shadows striped the ground.

Kip trotted close beside Avamir, his ears high, his tail raised like a flag.

Behind Heart, Moonsilver blew out a long, soft breath. He touched her shoulder lightly with his muzzle.

As they started walking downhill Heart sighed, thinking about the silver bracelet on her wrist.

How had the silver threads woven themselves together?

Was it magic?

What else could it be?

A whisper of breeze touched the treetops.

Heart looked up at the full moon, then back at the rocky hillside. They had to hide.

But *where?*

Heart shifted the carry-sack on her back. Where were the moon-colored mountains she had dreamed about? Were they real? She shook her head. Chasing dreams would hardly help.

Heart tried to remember what Binney had told her.

"To the west is Lord Irmaedith," Heart whispered to herself.

She knew nothing about Lord Irmaedith.

Was he cruel?

Worse than Lord Dunraven?

"And to the East, it's Lord Kaybale," Heart said aloud, repeating Binney's words.

Lord Kaybale.

She had never heard of him, either.

No one in Ash Grove had known anything about the world beyond the village. No one ever talked about it. Not even Ruth Oakes.

In the moonlit dusk ahead a boulder took

shape, rising out of the ground as big as a farmer's house.

Heart led the unicorns around it.

The dry pine needles crumbled beneath her feet and the unicorns' hooves, scenting the still night air.

Heart could hear Kip's quick, panting breath. At least he was excited about this journey. No one else could be.

Ruth would be so worried.

Heart's Gypsy friends would be sad when they discovered she was gone.

But Binney and Zim would understand, Heart knew. They would know that she didn't want to bring them trouble.

"I am afraid," Heart breathed, glancing down at the silver bracelet on her wrist.

The six silver threads were now a lacy circle.

"They tell the story of my life," Heart whispered to herself. "Or as much of it as I can remember."

It was true. Two had come from the blanket

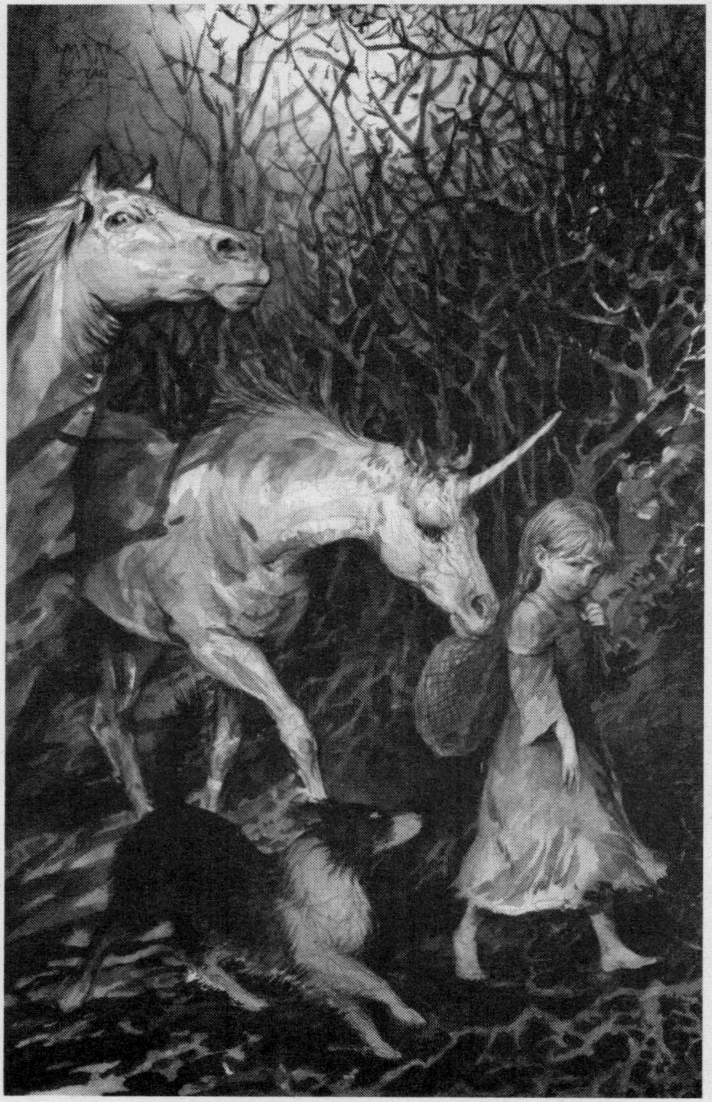

she'd been wrapped in when Simon found her by the Blue River.

One was a gift from dear Ruth Oakes.

Three were from Binney in thanks for Moonsilver saving Davey's life.

Heart stared at the intricate woven pattern in the bracelet.

Binney had said her threads were from the Queen of the Unicorns' mane.

Heart glanced at Avamir.

The white mare was beautiful, and her mane was long and silky. But it was white, not silver.

So maybe that part wasn't true?

Avamir tossed her head.

The tiny Gypsy bells in her mane jingled against the vast silence of the forest, then stilled.

Heart felt Moonsilver's muzzle against her shoulder, another quick, warm touch. She wished desperately that she knew what to do, where to go. Derrytown was on the edge of Lord Dunraven's lands—his castle lay somewhere to the north. He would be the first to hear the rumors about Moonsilver healing Davey.

"Lord Kaybale," she said aloud, trying to break the panic-circle of her thoughts. "Lord Kaybale is to the East."

Heart liked the rounded, strong sound of the name Kaybale.

It was plain and sturdy.

It sounded like an everyday word—like *rainwater* or *hearthstone.* But Lord Kaybale's lands lay to the East of Lord Dunraven's—beyond Ash Grove.

Heart was afraid to go back that way.

Lord Dunraven's men would search there first. He would send his men to watch the Derrytown Road and the village—and Ruth Oakes's house.

Heart took a deep breath.

Everyone in Ash Grove had heard the old stories about the unicorn and the Blue River.

But no one had thought unicorns were *real.*

Now the rumors would spread. They would wonder. They would watch.

"Where can we go?" Heart asked the sky.

Northward was Lord Dunraven's manor. Southward lay Lord Levin's lands, according to Binney.

North, south, east, west.

There was no reason to think any direction led to safety.

Heart felt a familiar ache rising inside her.

Her family might help her—if she could find them.

But she had no idea where they were—or even *who* they were.

A rustling sound up the slope made Heart turn.

She caught her breath.

A vague shape was slipping in and out of the moon shadows.

Someone—or something—was at the top of the slope, following her.

✦CHAPTER TWO

Ahead in the moonlight Heart saw another huge boulder. She hurried the unicorns toward it.

Kip trotted beside her.

"Shhh," she whispered to him.

Kip's eyes were bright. He lifted his muzzle. He did not bark.

The unicorns moved almost silently. Heart walked carefully, leading Moonsilver and Avamir around to the far side of the huge stone.

She set down her carry-sack.

Kip and the unicorns stood close together in the deep shadows cast by the enormous boulder.

After a few moments Heart heard footsteps coming closer.

She could hear a voice, too.

It was so familiar her stomach turned over.

Simon? What was *Simon Pratt* doing here?

Avamir breathed out, lifting her head.

"He might offer me silver on the spot," Simon was saying to himself as he came closer.

Heart pressed herself against the rock. The stone was rough and hard beneath her hands. What was *he* doing this far from Ash Grove?

"Or he might be angry," Simon was muttering. "But at Ruth Oakes, not at me. . . ."

Heart strained to hear more, but the sound of Simon's voice and footfalls dimmed, then disappeared. He hadn't seen her.

"Who will be angry?" Heart breathed.

Moonsilver tossed his head.

Kip was looking up at Heart.

Shivering with dread, she waited until Simon was well ahead of them, then she followed. Kip stayed at her heels. The unicorns were graceful and quiet as always.

Simon never looked back.

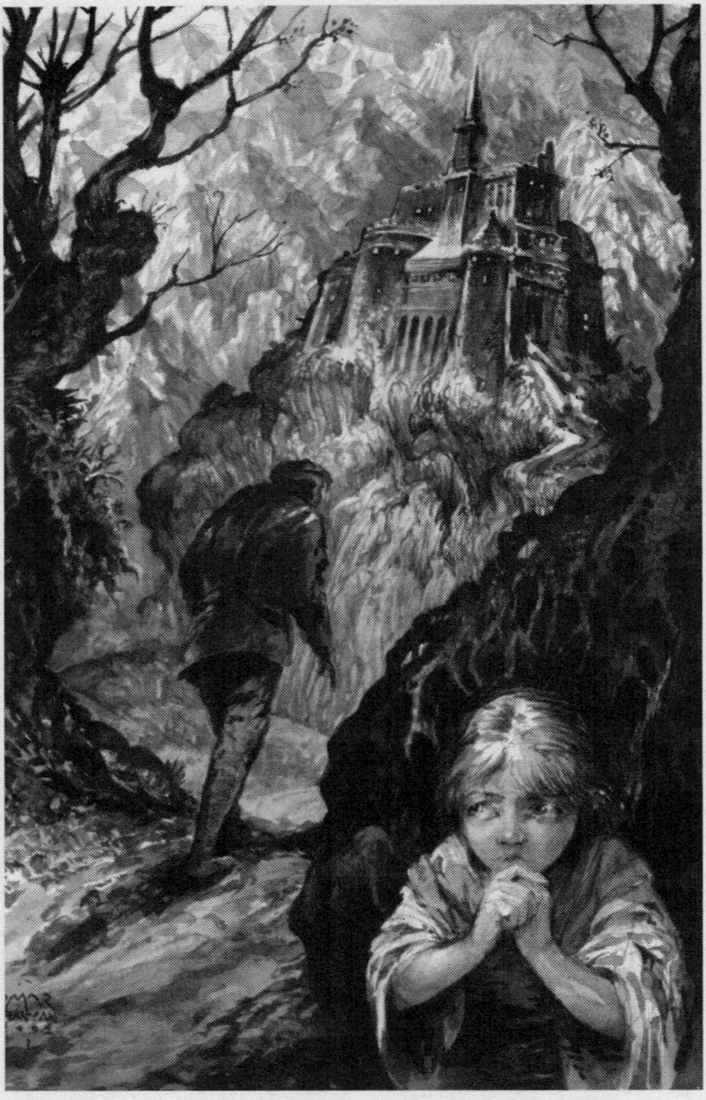

He kept muttering to himself.

Heart was afraid to get close enough to understand what he was saying. She glanced at the moon.

It was shining low through the trees on her left.

She caught her breath.

The moon *set* in the west.

That meant the road had curved northward—the direction of Lord Dunraven's castle.

Was that where Simon was headed?

Heart felt numb. Simon was afraid of Lord Dunraven. Everyone was. Why would Simon be walking toward the castle in the middle of the night like this?

She could think of only one reason.

He had heard the rumors.

He had figured out the truth.

Now he was going to tell Lord Dunraven all he knew about her, about Ruth Oakes . . . and about the unicorns.

"You will have to hide and wait for me," Heart whispered to Avamir.

The unicorn mare lifted her head. Her eyes were calm.

Heart veered off the road and found a rocky point.

In the distance she could just see the high walled castle. Beyond it rose steep mountains that disappeared into the night sky.

"Stay hidden," Heart pleaded with Kip. "Stay here with Moonsilver and Avamir."

She set down her carry-sack on the rocky ground.

There was a tiny clinking sound.

Her flute!

"Dear Zim," Heart breathed. What a gift he had given her, teaching her to play. Maybe one day she would find a way to repay the Gypsies for all their kindness.

Kip whined softly.

Avamir blew out a disapproving breath and Kip sat down and hushed. Moonsilver moved uneasily. Heart put her hand on his neck for an instant.

"I'll be back as quickly as I can," she promised them all.

Avamir shook her mane.

The silvery jingle of the Gypsy bells made Heart sigh.

Heart hugged Avamir's silky neck and patted Kip's head.

Then she set off.

Once she was back down on the road, Heart couldn't see the castle.

There was a village along the road.

Heart had heard stories about it. She had always wanted to see what might be sold in such fancy shops for lords and ladies.

Now she was only glad no lanterns were lit.

All was dark. She couldn't see into the shops.

But no one could see her either—and she was grateful.

CHAPTER THREE

Heart trailed behind Simon, keeping him in sight and trying to think of a way to talk him out of betraying her.

She could promise him money, but Lord Dunraven might reward him a thousand times more than she could ever earn.

She could plead with him—but she was pretty sure he would not listen. He might even force her to go with him to Lord Dunraven's castle.

Heart followed silently, unsure what she could do.

But she had to try *something.*

Simon was still muttering to himself.

Heart tried to get a little closer.

She heard Ruth's name once more, then her

own. He was rehearsing what he was going to say!

As they came around a bend in the road, Heart raised her head to call out to Simon.

Then she looked past him and caught her breath. Ahead in the dark, arched windows glowed with warm lantern light.

Dunraven's castle!

Shouts startled Heart.

She whirled and ran into the trees.

When she peeked out she could hear Simon's voice.

There were two men in dark shirts.

Lord Dunraven had guards on his road.

She crept closer.

"I just came to talk to Lord Dunraven," Simon was saying. He sounded scared.

Heart bit her lip.

"About what?" one guard demanded.

"I will tell *him* that," Simon insisted in a shaky voice.

"And what could a ragged field-gleaner

possibly know that our master does not?" the second guard scoffed.

Heart couldn't hear Simon's answer.

When the guards led him away, she followed.

She hid behind one tree, then another. She ducked under a wagon in a stable yard, waiting until the men were a little ahead of her.

The guards walked heavily, one on each side of Simon.

Heart stared at the castle as they got closer.

The bright moonlight traced its walls and towers with a silvery outline.

It was huge! It made the buildings in Derrytown seem as small as toys.

Dunraven's guards walked faster. They pushed Simon along.

Beyond the castle she could see mountains rising into the sky. Was that where the old road ran?

Binney had said it was ruined, that it had been closed for years and years.

Heart tried to keep close enough to hear what

Simon was saying, then realized he had fallen silent.

There was no sound except the guards' heavy boots on the gritty soil.

Around the castle there were no trees at all—nothing Heart could hide behind.

She stopped and watched as Dunraven's men led Simon along.

They headed straight for the castle wall.

Heart blinked. Where were they going?

One of the guards stepped forward and reached out. Heart couldn't see the round-topped door until it opened.

The guards marched Simon through the door.

Then it closed and it was impossible to see again. Heart was startled by the complete silence. There were no night birds here, no crickets. Even the sound of the guards' boots was gone.

The stone walls and towers stretched upward, taller than any tree.

Heart was afraid to move, but she made herself do it anyway.

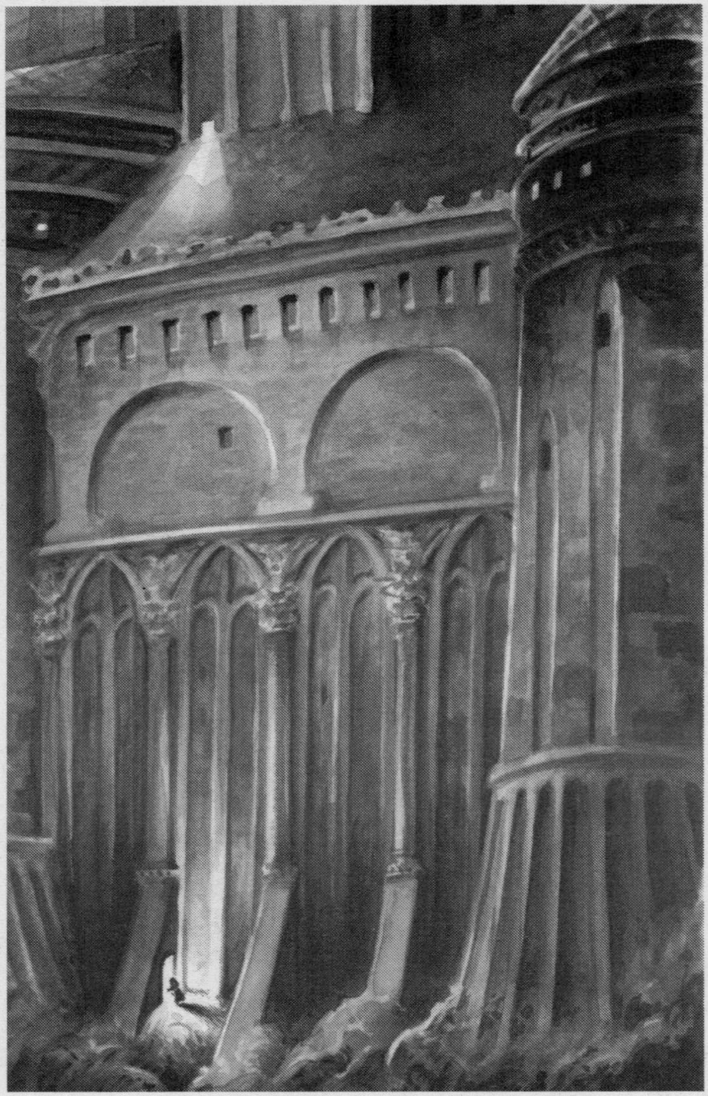

She ran her hands along the stone wall, searching for the hidden door. She finally saw a tiny mark in the stone. When she touched it the door opened.

Heart squeezed inside and stood in a long corridor. Candlelight flickered dimly within.

Heart could see faint outlines of the wide arches leading into rooms on each side of a long hallway.

She could hear Simon's voice.

She took a step forward.

CHAPTER FOUR

"It is the truth," Simon was saying.

Heart slid along the cold stone wall, inching closer. The shadows piled along the walls, thick and ink-black.

"I found her by the river," Simon added in a trembling voice. "Raised her myself. Fed her from my hearth."

Heart's hands tightened. Simon was talking about *her.*

"There was a fancy blanket, but I . . . ," Simon began. He cleared his throat. "I sold it."

Heart peeked into the arched doorway.

There was a single candle on the table.

She was careful to stay in the darkness beyond the flickering light.

Simon was facing a tall man with long, silvery hair.

Heart knew him from that long-ago day in market square. It was Lord Dunraven. She held her breath.

Lord Dunraven gestured. One of the guards lit another candle. Lord Dunraven opened a massive wooden trunk.

He pulled out a child's blanket of fine woolen cloth.

Candlelight caught the silver embroidery.

The design was beautiful. There were two unicorns, rearing. Between them was a setting sun.

"That's it," Simon muttered. "But I sold it to a—"

"Bring him along," Dunraven said. His voice rumbled like summer thunder.

Heart felt her knees go weak. It was her blanket?

She twisted the bracelet on her wrist.

She wanted to leap out of the shadows and

take the blanket from Dunraven. She knew she couldn't.

Simon was cowering.

The guards held his arms.

Heart cringed backward into the dark shadows just as they turned.

She longed to see the blanket. *Her* blanket. She wanted to touch it.

Lord Dunraven led the way.

He carried a candle high.

Heart watched Simon and the guards follow him down the hallway.

She pressed her back against the stone wall, holding her breath. The amber candlelight was too weak to push the deep shadows aside. No one looked back. No one saw her crouching by the wall.

As the footsteps dimmed, Heart let out her breath.

She glanced down the corridor, back toward the round-topped door.

Then she risked a single step forward and

peeked in to the room where Dunraven and Simon had been.

It was filled with mysterious objects.

Heart glanced up the hall. She strained to listen.

The voices were distant now. There was no other sound.

She tiptoed into the room.

Candle shadows twitched and shivered; every breath of air moved the flames.

Heart struggled to open the trunk lid.

There were many things inside it, strange things for which she had no names. But her blanket was not there.

Lord Dunraven must have taken it with him.

Heart blinked back tears.

She looked around the room. There was a dark wooden table with legs carved in the shape of unicorns.

There was a set of shelves with bits of colored glass set into the wood.

Each shelf was full of peculiar, slender boxes.

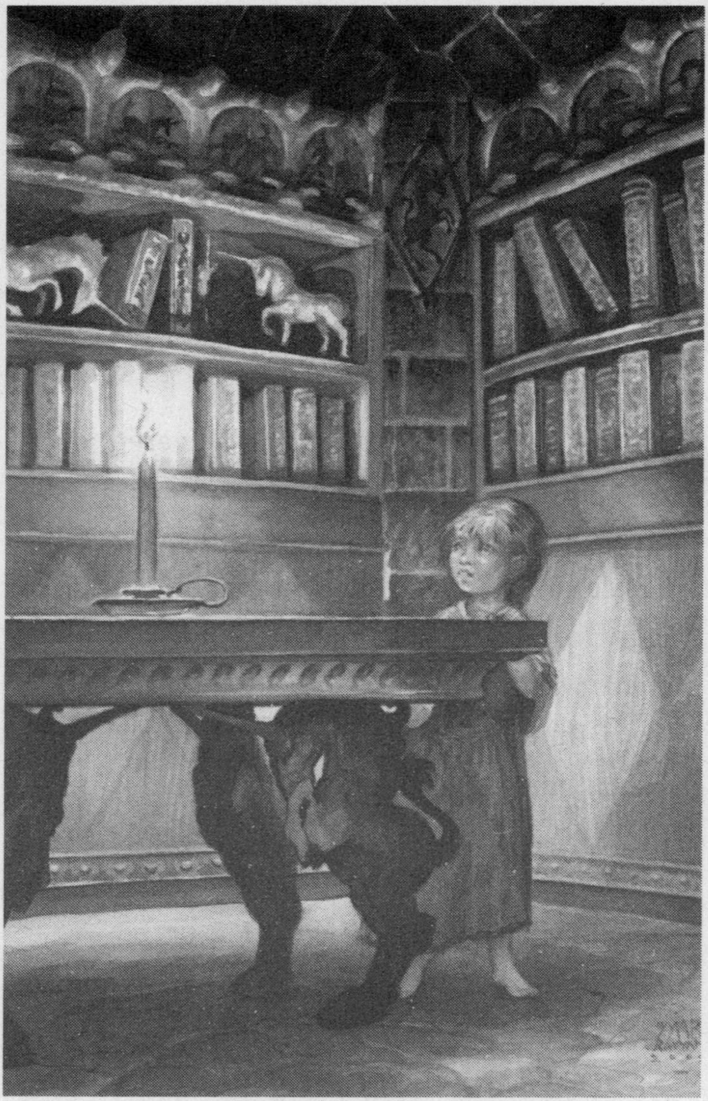

Heart touched them.

They weren't boxes.

She pulled one out.

Two squares of dark leather enclosed a neat stack of paper.

Heart had seen Derrytown merchants figure sums on rough brown paper.

This was different. It was smooth and the color of cow's milk. It had rows of odd-shaped marks all over it—dark, perfect, tiny shapes.

Heart tugged at the top sheet.

The paper was fastened along one edge so it could not fall loose.

Heart turned over more leaves of the paper. The shapes were endless, like rows of ants marching after a rain.

Why would someone draw so many of the tiny designs?

They weren't even very pretty.

She turned two more leaves of the paper, then shook her head and flipped through the rest.

Something caught her eye, and she pressed the paper flat.

Heart exhaled slowly.

There was a drawing on the paper.

It showed two rearing unicorns with a sunset between them—exactly like the embroidery on her blanket.

Had this belonged to her family too?

Heart looked around the room again.

High on one wall there was a drawing of two unicorns, one white, one black.

Heart turned in a slow circle.

There was a cabinet with glass doors over the shelves. There were small carved statues of unicorns lined up inside. A carving of a long, slender unicorn horn lay in front of them. It looked like old oak. The tip was broken.

Heart shivered. She reached up to touch the glass. Her sleeve caught on the silver bracelet. It pinched her wrist. She dropped her arm to loosen her sleeve.

Then she bent down, staring through the glass.

The lowest shelf held a halter braided of thick golden cord.

"A reward?" The voice was sudden and deep. The words were followed by a harsh, deep laugh.

Lord Dunraven!

Heart heard heavy footsteps in the hallway.

She spun around and ran out of the room.

She fled down the corridor, staying bent over, keeping close to the wall, and hoping the shadows would hide her.

The round-topped door swung open easily.

The night air rushed in, cool and clean. Heart hesitated just long enough to glance back up the passage.

She could still hear muffled voices and the sound of heavy boots. Had they seen her?

She slipped outside and closed the door.

Then there was only the silence of the night.

Heart ran again, her pulse pounding in her throat. Every second she expected to hear angry shouts.

She ran until her lungs ached. The road

slanted uphill past the village, but she didn't slow down.

She was back to the trees before she realized she still had the strange paper box in her hand.

She stumbled to a halt and stared at it in the moonlight.

She *had* not meant to take it.

She wasn't a thief!

Would Lord Dunraven notice it was gone? Would he send his guards to find her?

Heart kicked at the ground, furious at herself.

If only she had put it back on the shelf! Lord Dunraven would never have known she'd been there.

But would he notice it was missing? The shelves had been full of paper boxes, and all of them had looked pretty much the same.

"I can only hope that he doesn't," Heart whispered to herself.

Around her the forest was deep and silent except for a silk-rustle breeze in the highest branches.

Heart was glad to be away from candles and dusty stone—back in the pure light of the moon.

She stood still, catching her breath.

Whatever Simon had told Lord Dunraven—and no matter how much of it Lord Dunraven had believed—men would soon be searching for her. Would they let Simon go home? Would Lord Dunraven give him a reward?

She would lead Kip and the unicorns westward tonight.

That was the quickest way out of Dunraven's lands.

She tightened her fists.

She would have taken the blanket if she'd been able to find it.

That blanket was *hers*.

Her mother and father had wrapped her in it and . . .

Heart's thoughts came to a stop, and she blinked back tears.

Simon Pratt had nearly stepped on her the

morning he had found her by the river. He had told her that much. The tall grass had nearly hidden her.

But why had she been left there? Heart wiped her eyes. It was so hard not knowing who her parents were.

She took a deep breath. The rearing unicorns were on her blanket and on the paper. For the first time, she had a clue that might lead to her family.

Heart squared her shoulders.

She would find them someday.

Her family would help her keep the unicorns safe.

But she would have to avoid Dunraven's men when they began to search.

Heart began to run again, light-footed with both hope and fear.

✦CHAPTER FIVE

Ten days later, Heart was a long way from Dunraven's castle.

She had been very careful.

No one had spotted the unicorns.

Moonsilver and Avamir grazed beside forest streams. Heart had found berries and wild plums to eat. A farmer's wife had given her a mincemeat pie. Kip had caught mice and squirrels.

At first they had traveled by moonlight.

But the moon had waned now.

Traveling in the daytime, Heart stayed off the road. She led the unicorns and Kip through the forest alongside it.

She wanted to find a town.

She needed to earn a little money to buy food.

She wanted to show the drawing of the unicorns to people too. Maybe someone would recognize it.

"We have to find my family," she said out loud.

Avamir shook her mane. She reached out to touch her velvet muzzle to Heart's cheek. Her breath smelled of sweet grass.

Heart often caught glimpses of people passing on the road.

She saw a ladies' carriage, with matched bay horses snapping their hooves upward, necks arched.

There was a boy in rich clothing leading a horse.

Heart stared.

The horse's back and sides were covered with gray-silver metal.

Even its head was fitted with smooth silver.

A silver spike stuck out like a unicorn's horn. It had white plumes on it.

Heart had never seen a horse like this one. It was huge. Its hooves were broad as pie pans.

The next morning Heart heard something.

She listened, tipping her head to one side.

It was a rooster crowing. Later she heard a donkey bray.

There were farms up ahead.

That meant they were probably within a day's walk of a town.

Heart spent the morning heading uphill. They found a high valley with a thick stand of trees. There was a noisy stream and deep grass.

Avamir and Moonsilver would have to wait for her again. She hated to leave them, but if anyone saw them trouble would begin.

Heart kissed Avamir on the muzzle, then turned to Moonsilver. "You will stay hidden?"

Moonsilver's dark eyes were calm. Avamir switched her tail and arched her neck.

"Will you wait for me right here?" Heart asked her.

The mare lifted her head and looked at Heart. Heart knew they both understood. They would stay out of sight.

But Kip ran in circles around her legs.

Heart laughed softly. “You can come, but you have to be good.”

Kip barked once, a high, happy sound. He sat down, thumping his tail.

Heart lifted her carry-sack. Kip watched her, his eyes bright. When she began to walk he leaped after her. Together they made their way back down the steep hillside.

The road was wide and level. There were thousands of wheel ruts. There was a jumble of cloven tracks, hoof prints, and boot marks.

Far ahead Heart saw a farmer’s wagon. But no one was close enough to see her step out of the forest.

The sun was warm.

Billowing clouds drifted across the sky.

Heart smiled as she walked. It was a fine, wide road.

Coming around bend, Heart noticed something lying in the dirt.

She picked it up.

"A goat's horn?" she wondered aloud.

Kip sniffed at it. He tried to take it from her.

"No," Heart said firmly.

She shuddered, pitying the goat, thinking about the scar on Avamir's face.

Kip whined, wagging his tail.

Heart knew he would chew it like he would a bone.

She ran her fingers over the long, smooth horn.

She didn't want Kip to ruin it. She put it in her carry-sack.

Then she set off again and walked faster, taking deep breaths of the warm air.

After a time, she stopped and took her flute out.

She wasn't hiding now.

It would be all right to play as she walked.

She hadn't practiced in a long time. It would be good to warm up a little before she got to the town.

She tied the corners of her carry-sack together and slipped it over her shoulder.

Then she raised the flute to her lips.

Heart blew softly. Her hands were a little stiff at first. She kept playing. Soon her fingers flew over the silver metal. A tune as light as dandelion down floated into the air.

Kip ran ahead, then came back. He saw a squirrel and chased it. Heart could hear him crashing through the vines.

He came back panting, his tail high.

Heart lowered the flute to smile at him.

The first farm was around the next bend.

Heart waited until she was on the edge of the town to start playing again.

Then she walked straight to the market square.

People turned when they heard the flute.

Heart kept walking.

Some of the people followed her.

It was a pretty town.

The streets were clean.

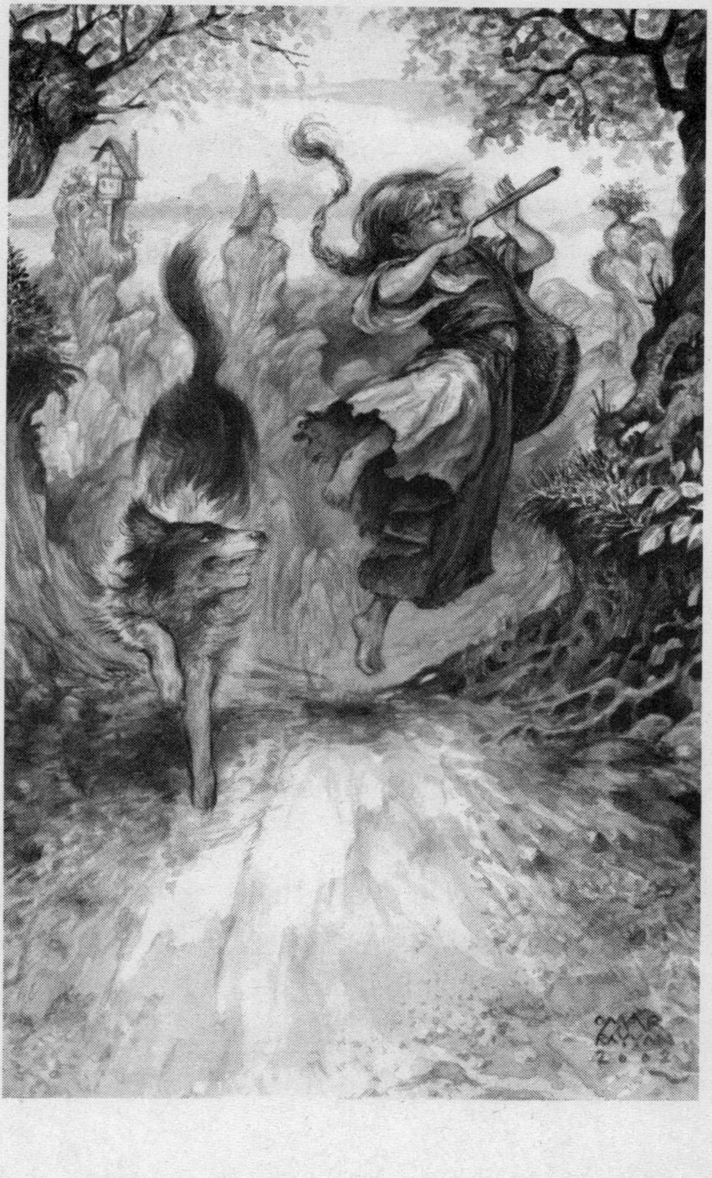

Many people were dressed in velvet with shiny silver buttons.

No one wore rags—and they all smiled at her.

Heart found a place on a street corner by the square. She pulled the winter hat Ruth had given her from her carry-sack. She turned it upside-down and set it front of her.

Then she played.

She chose quick, lively tunes.

The notes rushed out, fast as creek water.

Heart danced. Kip sat up to beg. He rolled over and over. He walked on his hind legs. He did all the tricks he had learned from the Gypsies.

People laughed at Kip. They tapped their feet to the melodies. They applauded. They put pennies in the hat.

When she had enough, Heart stopped playing. She put the flute away and looked around.

There were a hundred market stalls. Most were selling wonderful food. Her mouth watered.

Heart bought cheese, fragrant, dark bread,

and a little box of butter. She bought a pair of new socks and some rosy apples. The butcher sold her a bone for Kip.

Heart put everything in her carry-sack.

Then she walked slowly out of the market place. Kip stayed close.

She turned down a long, narrow street.

It was shady.

Big trees arched over the houses. Heart saw a small cottage with a yard full of roses.

A tall, thin woman came out of the front door.

She waved. "What a lovely dog!"

Kip trotted toward her. Heart stared. Tucked beneath the woman's arm was a paper-box like the one from Lord Dunraven's castle.

"What is that?" Heart asked politely, pointing.

The woman smiled. "A book. Haven't you ever seen a book?"

✦CHAPTER SIX

The woman's name was Toni Doohan. Her dark hair was a cloud around her face.

She held the book out, turning the leaves of paper. There were no pictures.

"This one was my great grandmother's," she told Heart. Heart smiled. Toni Doohan seemed very nice.

"It's about Yolen's Crossing," she added.

"Where is that?" Heart asked, puzzled.

Toni laughed and leaned down to pat Kip's head. "Here. This town is Yolen's Crossing. See?"

She turned the book toward Heart.

She ran her finger beneath some of the tiny patterns.

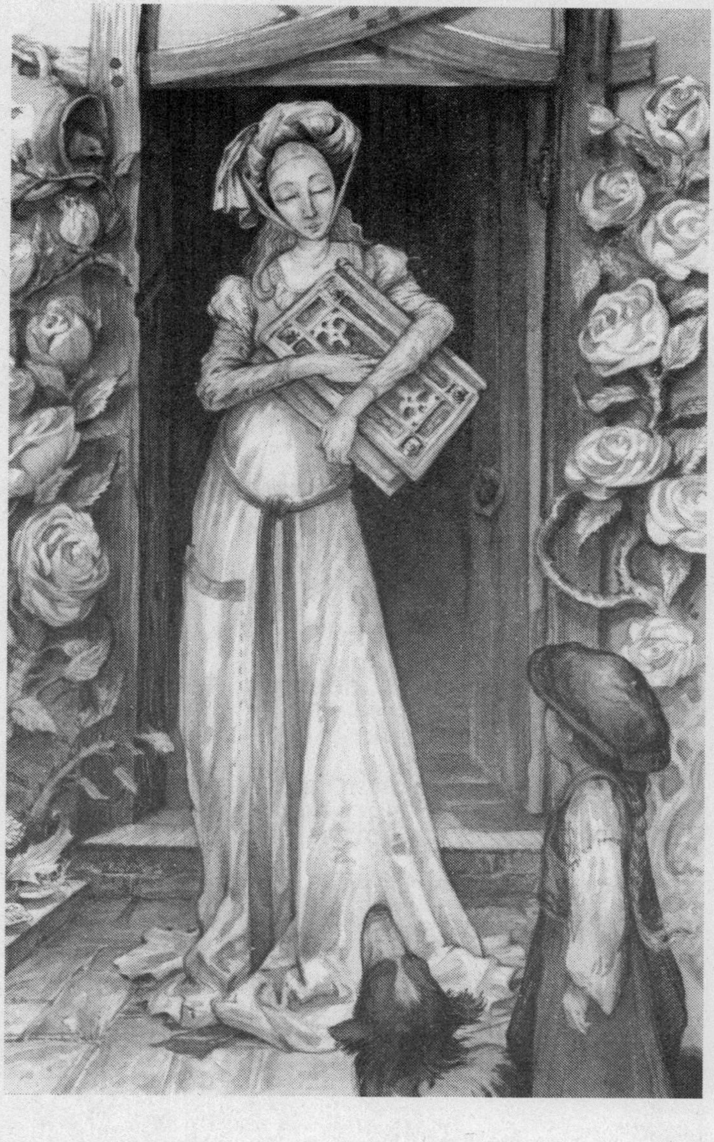

Heart met her eyes. “I don’t understand.”

Toni sighed. “Where are you from?”

Heart hesitated. If Lord Dunraven’s men came looking they would ask people questions.

“A little village a long way from here,” she said, finally.

Toni looked sad. “So many people never learn to read.”

Heart blinked. “Read?”

Toni nodded. “Read. It’s rare enough. But at least Lord Irmaedith doesn’t forbid books the way most the others do.”

Heart saw the anger in Toni’s eyes.

“Listen,” Toni said suddenly.

She opened the book.

She looked down at it and began speaking. “The two largest towns are now Yolen’s Crossing and San Coville, farther west,” she said. She kept talking.

She traced a zig-zag line with her finger as she spoke, sliding line by line down the paper.

It took Heart a long time to figure it out.

When she did, she got the shivers.

This was amazing! The little patterns were words somehow.

Toni could look at them and say them aloud!

Heart listened intently.

She watched Toni's eyes go back and forth.

The story began with the people who had come to this place long ago. A family named Yolen had been the first.

They had made a fine farm in the valley.

They had built the first little store and a flour mill on the river. Other farmers had come to settle. The book told their names and where they had lived.

"And then Talman Irmaedith was named lord of the land," Toni read.

Heart nodded to let Toni to know she was listening.

"He claimed the fields and mountains. He took a share of every harvest. He hunted the unicorns in the forests."

Heart made a little sound.

Toni glanced up.

Heart got a second set of shivers. Ash Grove's story had a unicorn in it, too, but no one had believed it.

"Please go on," she said quietly.

"You could learn to read it yourself," Toni said.

Heart swallowed. "Is it hard?"

Toni smiled. "A little. But it's worth it. I could teach you."

"Could you teach me right now?" Heart asked. She didn't want to leave the unicorns alone any longer than she had to.

Toni smiled. "It would take a few weeks to get you started."

Heart thought about the book in her carry-sack.

She longed to find out what it said about the rearing unicorns.

But she was afraid to show it to Toni.

She wanted to learn how to read too—but she couldn't stay for weeks.

She shouldn't stay even another hour.

"I have to go," she said sadly. "But thank you very much."

Toni closed the book and straightened. "You could come back tomorrow."

Heart looked at the ground.

"Are you staying on a farm near town? Would your family mind?" Toni asked.

Heart let out a careful breath. She couldn't tell this kind woman about the rearing unicorns—or where she was from, or anything else. She shouldn't even be talking to her.

"I can't," she said carefully. "But thank you very much."

Toni sighed, then nodded, then tapped the book with one graceful finger. "This book was written by a woman who died two hundred years ago."

Heart was amazed. She started to ask who the woman had been and how she'd made all the little marks so neatly.

Then the sound of hoofbeats made her turn.

Two men had turned their horses down the lane. They were riding at a clattering trot.

They wore dark shirts.

Both had crossbows and swords.

Toni slid the book into a pocket in her skirt. She nodded at the riders.

Heart glanced at the men as they passed.

"Lord Irmaedith is sending his men all the way past San Coville," Toni said once they were gone. "No one seems to know why." She twirled the clover between two fingers. "Have you heard anything about it?"

Heart didn't answer for a moment. Then she stepped back. "I have to go," she repeated.

Toni nodded. "Come back any time. I will teach you to read."

Heart smiled and thanked her again.

She called Kip, and they headed back toward the main road.

She would walk out of town the way she had come in.

If she saw Lord Irmaedith's men again they

would think she was a farm girl, just as Toni had.

Heart could feel the corner of the book pressing against her back.

She had to learn to read somehow.

She had to find out what it said about the rearing unicorns. Maybe the book would tell her where her family lived.

But first she had to get as far away from Lord Dunraven and the rumors about Moonsilver as she could.

Maybe in San Coville she could find someone to help.

Heart walked faster.

CHAPTER SEVEN

Heart kept going. She tried to travel fast.

It was hard to keep the unicorns hidden, but they seemed to understand that they had to stay where the forest was thickest.

Heart played her flute in two tiny mountain villages.

The people were poor. They gave her food instead of pennies. They tossed Kip bits of meat from their own dinners.

Then the roads began to lead downhill and the land leveled out. The river Heart followed was wide and lazy.

Every day more people and wagons passed on the road.

Heart could see them in glimpses through the trees.

There were farmers' wagons.

People in fancy carriages went by too.

The women wore long dresses and hats with flowers and feathers.

There were people leading cows and goats too. Their clothes were clean and plain.

"San Coville must be a big town," Heart said to Avamir. "All kinds of people are going there."

The unicorn mare tossed her head.

The Gypsy bells jingled.

Then they jingled again.

Heart stared. Avamir hadn't tossed her head a second time. The bells sounded again, distant and silvery. Heart turned to peer through the branches.

There was no one on the road.

"You're imagining it," she told herself.

Moonsilver reached out to nudge her shoulder with his muzzle. An instant later the sound of tiny Gypsy bells came again.

Heart peeked out of the trees. Moonsilver and Avamir followed. They stood close behind her.

Kip wagged his tail, his ears raised forward.

"That's Binney's wagon!" Heart breathed.

The whole caravan of bright-colored wagons was coming around a bend in the road. Heart ached to run toward her friends, but she knew she couldn't.

"Stay back," she said to the unicorns. "We'll just wait until they pass."

Kip barked.

"Hush," Heart scolded him. He barked again.

Heart reached down to hold him back, but it was already too late. Kip bounded out of the trees.

Heart covered her mouth with one hand. She could only watch as Kip streaked toward the road.

She heard the shouts when Binney spotted Kip. He raced in circles around Sadie, Fiona's dog.

The Gypsies reined in their ponies. They lined up along the edge of the road, shading their eyes, looking out over the meadow.

Heart ducked back into the trees. "We would only bring them harm," she began, but Avamir pawed at the ground with a forehoof. Moonsilver reared, striking at the air. Then they

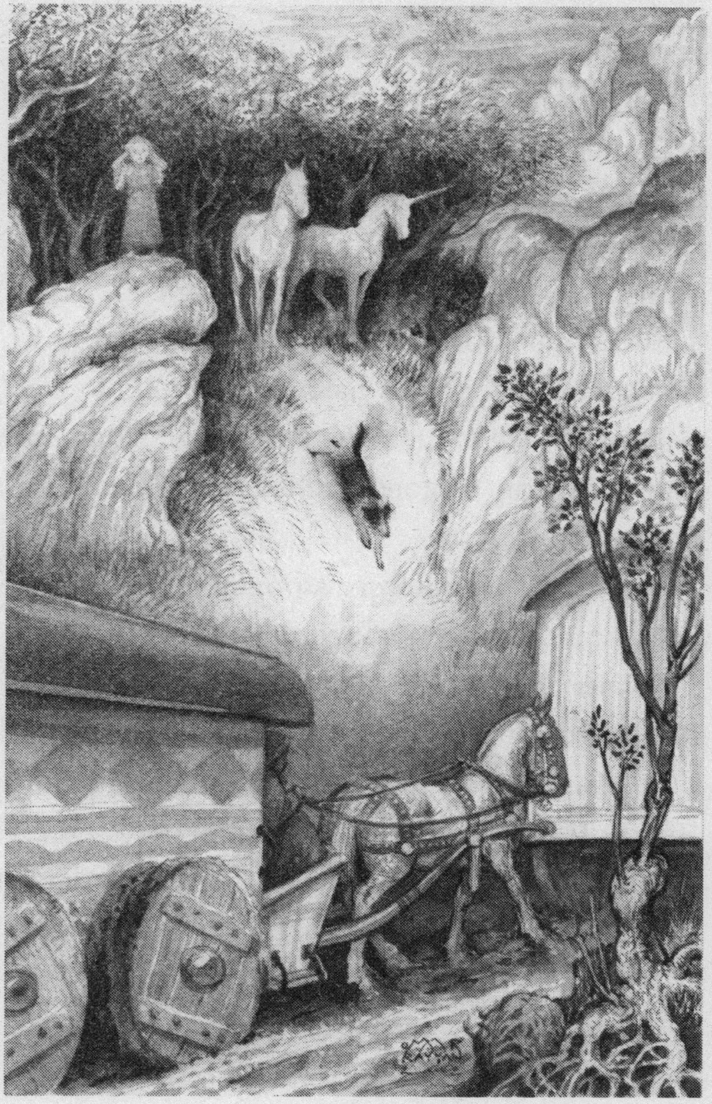

walked past Heart into the open meadow.

On the road the Gypsies saw them and cheered.

Binney waved joyously. Josepha and Talia shouted Heart's name, their hands cupped around their mouths.

Heart felt her eyes flood with tears.

She stepped out of the trees and waved.

Whistles and cheers made her grin.

The Gypsies found a gentle enough slope and one by one the wagons lurched down it and into the meadow.

Once the wagons were stopped in their usual neat circle, Binney jumped down.

"Binney!" Heart cried out. She ran toward the Gypsy woman.

"Oh, we missed you," Binney said. She swung Heart off her feet and turned in a circle.

When Binney set her down Heart saw Davey smiling at her. Behind him Zim was grinning.

"They are beautiful," Binney said, looking at the unicorns. "I love watching them. And I will always be grateful to Moonsilver for saving Davey."

Heart smiled at her. "I missed all of you so much."

"The rumors have run this way," Binney told her.

"I know," Heart said.

Binney glanced up at the sky. "We have an hour before sunset." She raised her chin and her voice. "A celebration tonight! Our dear Heart has come back to us."

Heart smiled at her, then glanced at Avamir and Moonsilver. They were moving back into the trees. It would be all right if they stayed with the Gypsies for a night or two, she thought.

She was so glad to be with them.

It felt wonderful to be with people who cared about her, people who loved Kip and Moonsilver and Avamir.

That night it was chilly. Kip curled up between the unicorns behind a copse of trees.

Heart slept soundly in Binney's wagon.

Her dreams were shadowy and dark.

The mountains she ran in were steep and bleak.

When she cried out, Binney reached out to soothe her.

✦CHAPTER EIGHT

For two days the Gypsies traveled the road. Heart and the unicorns walked along a wooded creek that ran below it.

Kip ran back and forth between them.

Heart told the Gypsies everything that had happened to her—except for the part about accidentally stealing the book.

She wanted to show it to them.

She decided not to.

It would only put them in more danger.

She didn't want Lord Dunraven to be able to blame the Gypsies for *anything.*

The next morning they came to a village.

Heart and the unicorns went around it.

They all met on the other side.

When they stopped for noon dinner Davey brought Heart a bowl of sweet, spicy beans. They were steaming hot and delicious.

"A woman in that last town said Lord Irmaedith's men rode through yesterday."

Heart set down the bowl.

Davey's eyes were deep and sad.

Avamir stopped grazing and lifted her head.

Heart sighed. "We should leave today. We should get as far away from you as we can."

Davey shrugged unhappily. "I almost wish Moonsilver wasn't a real unicorn."

Heart felt an idea bloom inside her. "Davey," she began carefully, "if they found a fake unicorn, they'd stop looking for a real one."

Trembling with hope, she pulled the goat horn from her carry sack.

Davey turned it over in his hands.

He looked up, puzzled.

"We can teach the act to Avamir," Heart said. "At the next show, you can pretend to fall and she can touch you and—"

"That's it!" Davey shouted. "I'll tell Binney."

Heart watched him splash across the little creek as he headed back toward the wagons.

Avamir sidled closer. She lowered her head to sniff at the goat horn.

"Will you stand for sticky pine gum on your forehead?" Heart asked her.

Avamir wrinkled her upper lip.

Heart laughed.

Moonsilver came close, reaching over Heart's head to nuzzle his mother's shoulder.

Heart stepped back and watched them.

Moonsilver was tall now, nearly as tall as Avamir.

Avamir was still a good mother, kind and gentle.

Moonsilver wasn't timid anymore, though.

"Performing with the Gypsies cured your shyness," Heart told him. Then she laughed again. "And mine, I think."

The next day, walking, Heart made up a tune for Avamir's act.

By midmorning the unicorn mare understood perfectly.

Heart saved bits of bread from her noontime meal.

Every time she played the tune she tossed a piece to Kip. By evening he had learned to come when he heard the new melody.

The next morning, Avamir and Kip both came running when Heart played the tune. Avamir raced with Kip, just as Moonsilver had.

Moonsilver watched them practice for a while. Then he wandered off to graze

Heart liked the new melody. It was a slower, more serious melody than the one Kip had liked.

It fit Avamir better.

As they walked, Heart kept glancing up the slope to the road.

It felt wonderful to be with the Gypsies again.

Playing the flute made her feel happy.

Heart kissed Moonsilver on the muzzle as he

and Avamir settled in to sleep that evening. Kip lay between them as usual.

Heart walked up to the Gypsy camp.

By the bright campfire, she explained her idea to Binney.

"Avamir is nearly trained," Heart finished.

"In two days?" Binney asked.

Heart smiled.

Binney nodded thoughtfully. "It'll work, I think. We'll be in San Coville in four days. Will you be ready by then?"

"Of course she will," Zim said from behind Binney.

Heart nodded, grinning.

The firelight flickered, lighting the Gypsies' faces.

"Heart, watch!" Talia called.

Talia and Joseph had learned how to balance full pitchers of water on their heads.

Heart played them a slow, graceful melody.

Talia and Josepha danced in gliding circles.

Their arms rose and fell.

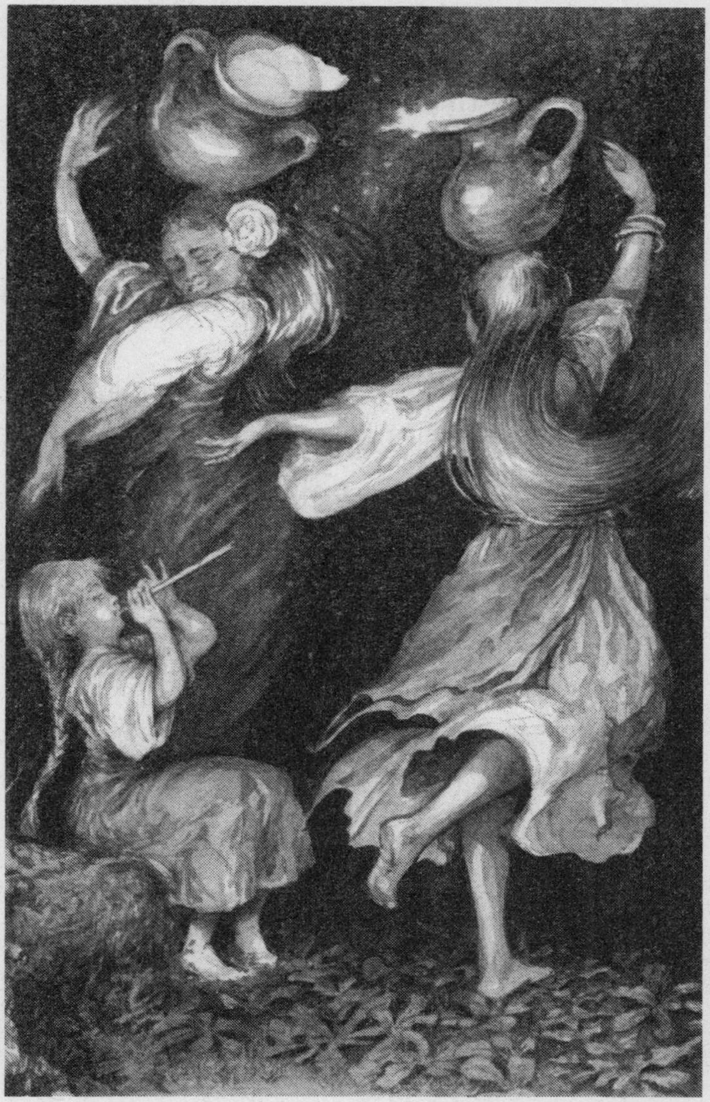

Their fingers and hands seemed to dance.

The water in the pitchers swayed gently.

"Will you play for us in San Coville?" Talia asked.

Heart nodded.

"We made the most beautiful shawls to wear," Josepha told her.

"I have more cloth," an older woman said from the fireside. "I'll stitch one for Heart."

Heart recognized her. It was Talia's aunt—the one who had loaned her a costume in Derrytown.

It seemed so long ago.

Heart raised the flute and began to play.

Her sleeve slid up over her wrist.

The silver sparkle of the bracelet was burnished into sunset colors by the firelight.

CHAPTER NINE

All the way to San Coville, Heart rehearsed the act.

At first the horn wouldn't stay on Avamir's forehead at all.

Heart borrowed Davey's knife.

She hollowed out the horn until it was a light, thin shell that weighed almost nothing.

Then the pine tar worked.

Avamir could toss her head.

She could shake her mane.

The horn stayed in place.

When Kip chased Avamir around in a circle, she reared and looked magnificent.

Davey was practicing the fall.

He would use the low wire this time—and

of course he wouldn't really get hurt.

Avamir understood her part of the act the first time they practiced it.

"Well," Binney said. "All the old stories talk about unicorns healing people. She knows all about how to do that part."

In the evenings Heart played a dance melody for Talia and Josepha to practice. They decided it should start slowly, then speed up.

"You have gotten very good," Zim told her.

Heart smiled. Zim played so well. His praise made her blush.

"Do you think Moonsilver would get into a wagon and hide there while we put on our show?" Binney asked.

Heart's smile faded.

She had been so busy rehearsing that she hadn't given Moonsilver a single thought. "Maybe," she said slowly. "But maybe not."

"We could send someone to stay with him in the woods," Binney said. "But I'd rather have him close."

Heart nodded. "I'm just not sure he will understand."

"We had better see," Binney said. "We emptied Zim's second wagon is empty just now."

Heart nodded.

She walked back to the trees. Moonsilver was standing up, not yet asleep.

He followed her quietly to the wagons.

Avamir came with them. Her forehead was smudged with pine gum.

Heart watched Zim make sure there was nothing in the wagon.

Then she walked up the little ramp. "Moonsilver?" she asked quietly. "Would you mind coming inside here?"

The unicorn touched his muzzle to the ramp. He stretched out his neck, sniffing at the wagon gate.

Then he lowered his head and stepped up into the wagon.

There wasn't much room.

Heart scrambled out of his way.

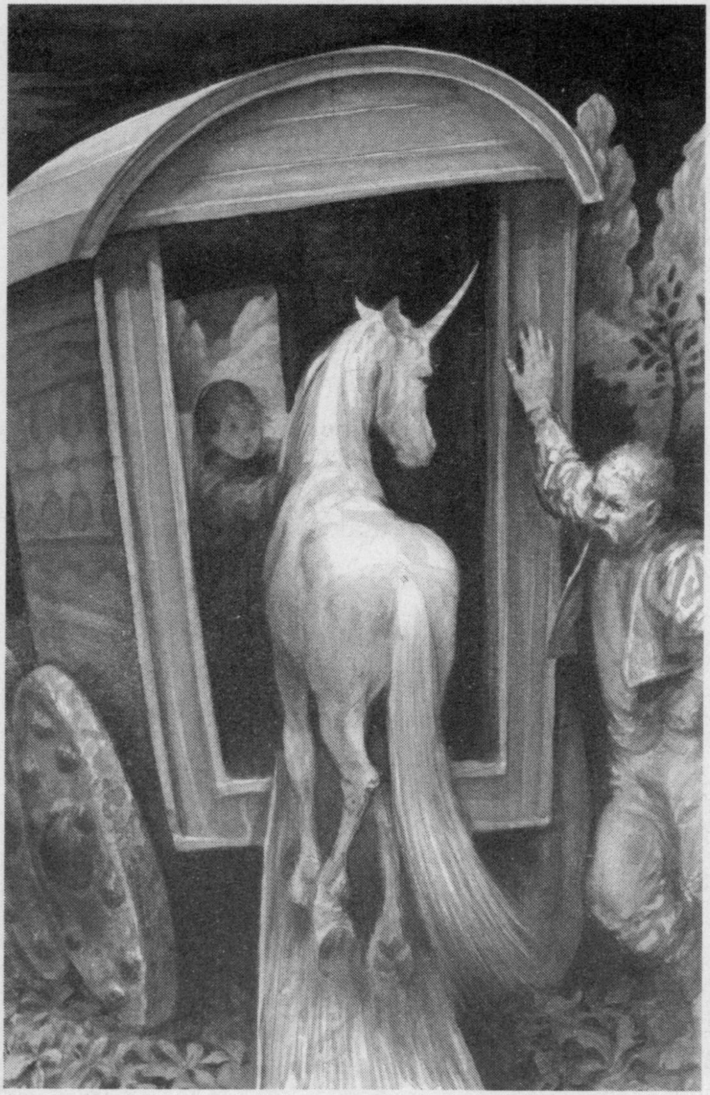

Moonsilver stood calmly while Zim closed up the back of the wagon.

"We'll fill it with sweet straw and fresh grass when we get to San Coville," Binney said.

Moonsilver nickered.

Everyone laughed.

Zim opened the wagon gate and Moonsilver backed out. He nuzzled Heart's cheek, then went off to sleep beside his mother and Kip. Heart yawned.

"Bed for you, too," Binney said. "We'll make sure we get to San Coville at dusk to be safe."

✦CHAPTER TEN

San Coville's green was wide and sloped. The people sat uphill from the circle of lanterns.

Moonsilver had ridden into town inside the wagon.

He stood quietly, eating the grass Heart had gathered.

When the show started Heart watched the other acts.

It was amazing how many new tricks the Gypsies had added.

Talia and Josepha danced to her flute music.

The audience clapped and clapped.

Heart swirled her shawl as they all three bowed.

The other acts went on.

Binney made jokes. Everyone laughed.

Then came the last act.

Heart held her breath, standing next to Avamir in the dark. Inside the ring of lanterns Davey and the other jugglers began.

They threw their clubs high in the air.

Their hands blurred in the lantern light.

Then Davey walked out on the low wire. He threw the clubs high, walking forward.

Then he pretended to lose his balance.

He dropped the clubs, then fell sideways, catching the wire and swinging himself back up.

The audience gasped in relief.

But then Davey dropped to the ground. He landed for just an instant on his feet, then sprawled on the ground, his eyes closed.

It looked very real.

The audience gasped, then groaned.

They thought he was really hurt.

"Go ahead," Heart said to Avamir. She nudged the mare's side.

Avamir galloped forward, and the audience

made a low sighing sound when they saw her.

She bent to touch her goat horn to Davey's lips. He slowly opened his eyes and stood up.

Heart walked forward then, playing her flute.

Avamir galloped in graceful circles as they had practiced. Kip ran alongside her.

Then Heart changed melodies, and they both came to her.

Avamir had even learned to bow like Moonsilver had.

The audience stood up, whooping and clapping.

"Psssst!"

Heart looked around to see Binney gesturing to the side of the field.

There, standing in the shadows, were five or six men in dark clothes. The lantern light glinted from their sword scabbards. They were laughing, shaking their heads.

Heart grinned. Perfect. Lord Irmaedith's men had seen the whole thing.

She walked to their side of the field and

played the melody again. Avamir and Kip ran to her.

She patted Avamir's neck and reached up to the goat horn.

The pine gum was working perfectly, but she pretended to press the horn in place.

She could hear the men laughing behind her.

Across the field, she saw Binney grin.

She led Avamir and Kip out to bow again.

Then she and Zim played a lively tune as people left.

Heart couldn't stop smiling.

"They'll tell everyone that the unicorn is a fake," Davey said happily. "You can stay with us."

"Let's camp outside town," Binney shouted. "I know a good meadow close to the road."

All the Gypsies went about their work.

Heart was grateful. They were tired, but they knew Moonsilver would hate being cooped up all night. And the truth was they all liked the open country better than any town.

The wagons rolled onto the road.

Binney knew exactly where the field was.

The fire was made quickly.

Supper was warm bread and apples.

Moonsilver and Avamir grazed quietly in the dark behind the wagons.

After supper everyone else went to bed, but Heart stayed by the fire playing quietly.

She was too relieved and too happy to go to sleep.

Zim came to stand beside her.

He played a melody that danced with hers.

Heart closed her eyes and lost herself in the music.

"I wonder if anyone in my family plays," she said after they let the song drift into silence.

"Where are they?" he asked.

Heart shrugged. "All I can remember is Simon Pratt finding me."

Zim stared into the fire. "He's the one you followed to Dunraven's castle?"

Heart nodded. "I want to find my family."

"You should learn to read," Zim said.

Heart blinked, startled. “Read?”

He nodded. “My mother could. There are books that tell about different towns, about the families who settled them.”

“Can you read?” Heart asked, trying to keep her voice even.

Zim shrugged. “Not really. A little, maybe.”

Heart pressed her lips together. “Will you keep a secret?”

Zim nodded somberly. “All Gypsies know how to keep secrets.”

Heart ran to get the book. She took it out of her carry-sack without waking Binney.

Coming back, she glanced around the camp.

No one else was awake.

“I didn’t mean to take it,” Heart began. She opened the book to the drawing and held it out to Zim. “It’s the same design as the embroidering on my blanket.”

Zim arched his eyebrows. “It is?”

Heart nodded. “Exactly. But you can’t tell Binney or anyone else about the book, Zim.”

He frowned. "None of us would tell an outsider."

"But if Dunraven's men ever question them, they don't have to lie if they don't know anything," Heart insisted.

Zim nodded slowly. "I won't tell anyone else."

He looked at the rearing unicorns. Then he placed his finger beneath the tiny patterns. He squinted and stared, then made sounds that seemed not to be words at first.

"Th . . . th . . . the," he said. "The."

Heart watched his eyes. They didn't go back and forth like Toni's had. They were glued to a single word as he tried to puzzle it out.

"The M . . . m . . . The Mooo, Moun . . . Mount . . . t . . . t . . . t . . . tain . . . tains?" Zim said. He looked up at her, then back at the book. "Then it says o . . . o . . . of . . . Of. Th . . . the . . . M . . . M . . . Moun . . . Moun . . . tains of th . . . the . . . mmmm . . ." He stopped and looked at the sky, then took a big breath and started over on the last word. "Mo . . . No. Moun . . . No, it is mooo . . . then . . . nnnn.

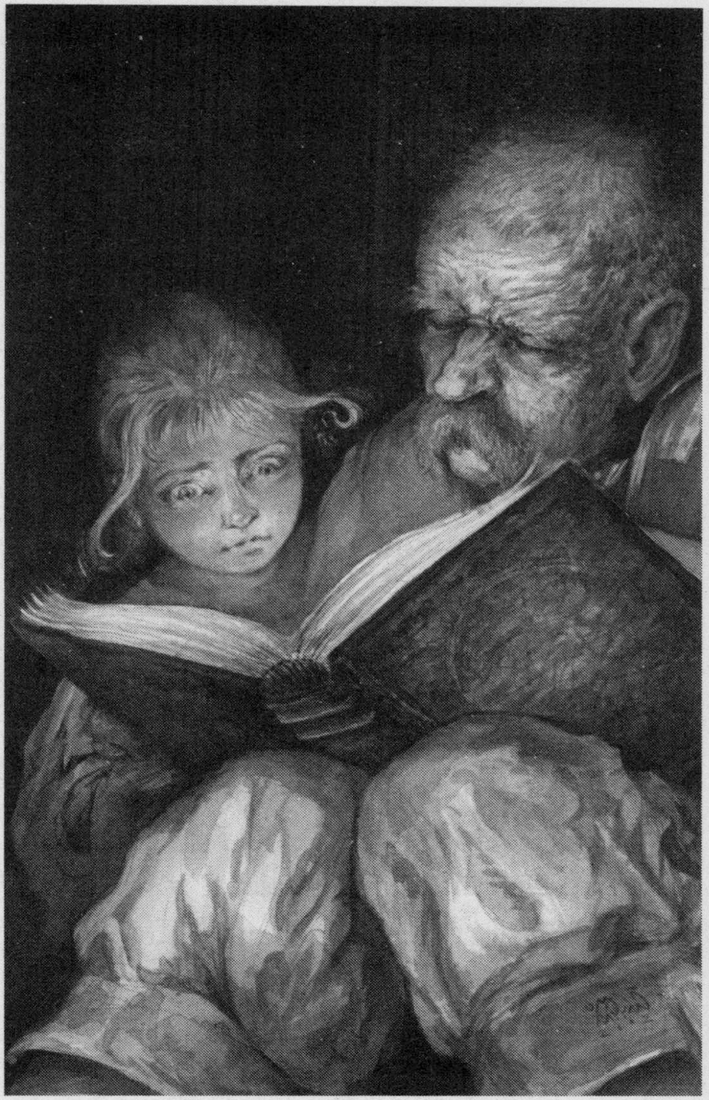

Moon." He looked up, smiling.

Heart waited, holding her breath.

"The Mountains of the Moon," he said slowly. Then he frowned. "That must be wrong, Heart. It makes no sense at all."

Heart stood completely still.

In her dreams the mountains were the color of the full moon. Did the book say something about her dreams?

"Have you ever heard of The Mountains of the Moon?" Heart asked.

Zim shrugged. "No. But, Heart, you need someone who can truly read. Gypsies don't. My mother was a town woman. She taught me a little, but I've forgotten most of it."

"Try again," Heart pleaded.

Zim tried.

He wrinkled his face and stared at the book.

He pushed his finger back and forth over the same place a dozen times.

"Th . . . the . . . A . . . A . . . A . . . A . . . An . . . An . . . ," he began. Then he looked up. "It's a long word. I can't remember enough of the letters." He stared at it again.

"Letters?" Heart echoed.

"That's what the little designs are called. Letters." He handed the book back to her. "I'm sorry, Heart."

Heart hugged him. "I love you all so much," she said, not knowing that she was going to say it.

"Everyone missed you," Zim said. Then he smiled. "Avamir and Moonsilver are lucky that you found them. And Kip."

He rose and stretched.

As he walked toward his wagon Heart glanced up at the sky.

Zim had done his best.

She would have to learn to read—somehow.

She smiled up at the sky. At least she could travel with the Gypsies now.

That meant she might be able to find someone who knew something about the drawing of the rearing unicorns.

It might lead her to her family. To her real home.

"Home."

Heart whispered the word as Zim started off to bed.

It was a magic word for her.

Heart turned toward Binney's wagon.

Past it, on the horizon, the moon was rising. It was almost full again. Heart watched it. The bracelet on her wrist felt snug and warm against her skin.

She breathed in the chilly night air.

The unicorns were asleep and so was Kip. They were all safe for now. And her family would help her. All she had to do was find them.

KATHLEEN DUEY has written more than forty books for children. She grew up thinking about fanciful things. The Unicorn's Secret series is based on a dream she had in the third grade. She lives in southern California, is in love, happy, and gets up smiling every single day.

She loves to get letters at www.kathleenduey.com and answers every single one.